Rheumatology: A Clinical Appro

Rheumatology: A Clinical Approach

Editor: Travis Reagan

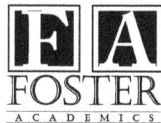

FA FOSTER
ACADEMICS

www.fosteracademics.com

www.fosteracademics.com

FA
FOSTER
ACADEMICS

Cataloging-in-Publication Data

Rheumatology : a clinical approach / edited by Travis Reagan.
    p. cm.
Includes bibliographical references and index.
ISBN 978-1-63242-806-6
1. Rheumatology. 2. Rheumatism. 3. Rheumatism--Diagnosis.
4. Rheumatism--Treatment. I. Reagan, Travis.
RC927 .R44 2019
616.723--dc23

Foster Academics,
118-35 Queens Blvd., Suite 400,
Forest Hills, NY 11375, USA

ISBN 978-1-63242-806-6 (Hardback)

Contents

Preface

This book has been a concerted effort by a group of academicians, researchers and scientists, who have contributed their research works for the realization of the book. This book has materialized in the wake of emerging advancements and innovations in this field. Therefore, the need of the hour was to compile all the required researches and disseminate the knowledge to a broad spectrum of people comprising of students, researchers and specialists of the field.

Rheumatology is a branch of medicine, which is concerned with the diagnosis, and treatment of rheumatic diseases. There are more than 200 different types of rheumatic diseases, such as osteoporosis, arthritis, back pain, gout, lupus, etc. A significant focus of this field lies in the treatment of immune-mediated disorders of the musculoskeletal system, autoimmune diseases, vasculitides and soft tissue. Rheumatology may also be assumed to be the study of medical immunology. Physical examination and specialized tests including X-rays, ultrasounds, rheumatoid factor test, erythrocyte sedimentation rate, cytopathology, etc. are performed for the diagnosis of rheumatic diseases. After diagnosis, their treatment strategy comprises of a prescription of analgesics, steroids, non-steroid anti-inflammatory drugs, monoclonal antibodies or disease-modifying anti-rheumatic drugs. Corrective interventions such as arthrodesis, removal of cartilage fragments or loose bone, joint replacements, etc. can also be performed for improving function, soothing pain and limiting disease activity. This book provides comprehensive insights into the field of rheumatology. There has been rapid progress in the understanding of rheumatic diseases, their diagnoses and treatments, which have been included in this extensive book. It is an essential guide for both academicians and those who wish to pursue this discipline further.

At the end of the preface, I would like to thank the authors for their brilliant chapters and the publisher for guiding us all-through the making of the book till its final stage. Also, I would like to thank my family for providing the support and encouragement throughout my academic career and research projects.

Editor

Fears and beliefs of people living with rheumatoid arthritis

Penélope Esther Palominos[1,2]*, Andrese Aline Gasparin[1], Nicole Pamplona Bueno de Andrade[1], Ricardo Machado Xavier[1,2], Rafael Mendonça da Silva Chakr[1,2], Fernanda Igansi[1] and Laure Gossec[3]

Abstract

Objective: To assess the main fears and beliefs of people with rheumatoid arthritis (RA) and their effect on treatment outcomes;

Methods: A systematic literature review was conducted in Pubmed/Medline; original articles published up to May 2017, reporting fears and/or beliefs of adult patients with RA were analyzed. Fears and beliefs were collected by two independent researchers and grouped into categories.

Results: Among 474 references identified, 84 were analyzed, corresponding to 24,336 RA patients. Fears were reported in 38.4% of the articles ($N = 32/84$): most studies described fears related to pharmacological therapy (50.0%, $N = 16/32$) and fear of disability (28.1%, $N = 9/32$). Beliefs were reported in 88.0% of articles ($N = 74/84$) and were found to moderate the patient-perceived impact of RA in 44.6% ($N = 33/74$), mainly the emotional impact (18.9%, $N = 14/74$); measures of function, quality of life, fatigue and pain were also found to be affected by patients' beliefs in 8.1% ($N = 6/74$), 6.8% ($N = 5/74$), 2.7% ($N = 2/74$) and 2.7% ($N = 2/74$) of the articles, respectively. Beliefs about therapy were linked to adherence in 17.6% of articles ($N = 13/74$) and beliefs about cause of RA predicted coping patterns in 12.2% of publications ($N = 9/74$). Only 9.5% ($N = 8/84$) of articles reported fears and/or beliefs of patients living outside Europe and North America: there was only one work which recruited patients in Latin America and no article included patients from Africa.

Conclusion: In RA, patients' beliefs are linked to impact of disease and non-adherence. Further research is needed on fears/ beliefs of patients living outside Europe and North America.

Keywords: Fears, Beliefs, Rheumatoid arthritis

Background

Despite the growing interest of rheumatologists into the patients' perspective in the last decade and the wide use of patient-reported outcomes in the assessment of Rheumatoid Arthritis (RA), the main fears and beliefs of this group of patients and their consequences on treatment outcomes are unclear [1, 2]. This theme has been explored through qualitative and quantitative methodology in different populations with a large amount of

fears and beliefs being reported and even conflicting data being published about the consequences of patients' perceptions [3–5]. While some authors, for example, found an association between higher concern scores about drugs with non-adherence, other found no association between patients' beliefs and maintenance of disease-modifying antirheumatic drugs (DMARDs) [3–5].

The subjectivity of fear and beliefs, the small patient samples in some studies and the limited knowledge about the consequences of patients' fears and beliefs on treatment outcomes may lead some rheumatologists to be unconvinced about the importance of the theme.

A systematic literature review would help to obtain an overview. Furthermore, cultural background may play a role in fears and beliefs [6, 7].

* Correspondence: penelopepalominos@gmail.com
[1]Universidade Federal do Rio Grande do Sul (UFRGS), Programa de Pós Graduação em Ciências Médicas (PPGCM), Rua Ramiro Barcelos 2400, segundo andar, Porto Alegre 90035-903, Brazil
[2]Department of Rheumatology, Hospital de Clinicas de Porto Alegre, Rua Ramiro Barcelos 2350, sexto andar, Porto Alegre 90035-903, Brazil
Full list of author information is available at the end of the article

This systematic literature review aimed to obtain an overview on fears and beliefs of patients living with RA reported in the medical literature, as well as assess the consequences of fears and beliefs on impact of disease and treatment outcomes. It also investigated if published studies reporting fears and beliefs are representative of all continents.

Methods

A systematic literature review was conducted in PubMed Medline up to 25 May 2017, using the Preferred Reporting Items for Systematic Reviews and Meta-Analyses statement as a guideline in the development of the study protocol and reporting of the results [8].

Search and selection process

Publications were identified through the following research strategy:

("interviews as topic"[MeSH Terms] OR "narration"[MeSH Terms] OR "surveys and questionnaires"[MeSH Terms] OR "qualitative research"[MeSH Terms]) AND ("arthritis/psychology"[MeSH Terms] OR "arthritis, rheumatoid"[MeSH Terms]) AND ("fears"[All Fields] OR "beliefs"[All Fields] OR "attitude to health/psychology"[MeSH Terms] OR "behavior and behavior mechanisms/psychology"[MeSH Terms] OR "affective symptoms/psychology"[MeSH Terms])

Inclusion criteria

All original articles reporting fears and/or beliefs of adult patients diagnosed with RA were included in the analysis; fears and beliefs were defined according to the Cambridge English Dictionary respectively as "a strong emotion caused by great worry about something dangerous, painful or unknown that is happening or might happen" and "the feeling of being certain that something exist or is true". These concepts were useful for making the distinction between articles reporting fears/beliefs and articles reporting coping patterns and psychological status. Articles written in English, Spanish, French, Italian and Portuguese and published up to 25 May 2017 were considered.

Both qualitative studies (data obtained through individual interview and/or focus groups), quantitative studies (information obtained through questionnaires) and mixed designs (articles including qualitative and quantitative methods) were included.

When RA and other clinical conditions (i.e. systemic lupus erythematosus, osteoarthritis, chronic pain etc) were included in the same study, the article was included in the analysis only if fears and/or beliefs of patients with RA were described separately from the other clinical condition.

Exclusion criteria

articles not reporting fears and/or beliefs, articles reporting fears and/or beliefs of patients with other rheumatic and non-rheumatic diseases, articles assessing children's fears and/or beliefs, studies assessing fears and/or beliefs of patients' spouses, partners and caregivers as well as reviews, letters and editorials were excluded.

Data collection

The selection process was performed by two authors (PEP and AAG) based on the titles and abstracts of the articles, and then on full texts. The articles included were then reviewed by two authors (PEP and NPD) and disagreements were solved by consensus.

General data extraction

Data were obtained on year of publication, study design (qualitative, quantitative or mixed design), number of patients, sampling method (convenience, consecutive, purposeful, systematic random sample), number of centers recruiting patients, the method used for data collection (individual interview, focus groups, questionnaire or mixed methods). When qualitative methodology was employed, the method used for qualitative analysis and for sample size definition was obtained. Demographic data of participants such as gender, mean age, mean disease duration was recorded for each report.

Collection of fear and beliefs

Fears were grouped in categories by PEP and LG (e.g. fears related to pharmacological therapy, fear of falling, fear of exercise relating injury, etc.). Beliefs were grouped in categories according to their consequences (e.g. beliefs about cause of disease predicting coping patterns, beliefs about pharmacological therapy affecting adherence, beliefs affecting impact of disease etc.).

Statistical analysis

Analysis was mainly descriptive; characteristic of articles and patients included were expressed as mean and standard deviation as estimates of central tendency and dispersion, respectively.

Categories of fears and beliefs were presented as number of articles which were included in that category and percentage of articles reporting that specific category among the total number of publication assessing fears or beliefs, respectively. The recruitment of patients worldwide was described as percentage, with the number of articles recruiting patients in each region as numerator and total number of studies reporting that category of fears/beliefs in the denominator.

Results

Description of publications and participants

Of the 474 publications identified by the literature search, 84 were included in the analysis. The list of all articles included in the analysis is provided as Additional file 1.

The main reasons for exclusion were articles assessing fears and/or beliefs from patients with other clinical conditions (52.3%, $N = 204$) and articles not assessing fears and/or beliefs (45.6%, $N = 178$) (Fig. 1).

The 84 articles considered in the analysis included 24,336 subjects with RA; mean age of participants was 54.9 ± 5.0 years old, mean disease duration was 10.7 ± 6.0 years and 74.0% ($N = 18,032$) were females (Table 1).

The sample was recruited by convenience in the majority of analyzed articles (57.1%, $N = 48$), followed by the recruitment of consecutive patients ($N = 14$; 16.7%). Systematic random sampling was described in only 4.8% of articles (N = 4).

The majority of trials employed exclusively quantitative methodology (69.0% of the 84 articles analyzed, $N = 58$) with the cross sectional design being the most commonly found (77.6% of the publications reporting only quantitative methods, $N = 45$). Thirty-one percent ($N = 26$) of the 84 articles employed some method of qualitative analysis (both solely or associated with quantitative methods). Among these 26 articles, the majority described the methodology used for analysis of qualitative data (55.5%, $N = 15$) and the inductive thematic analysis/grounded theory was the most cited ($N = 12$, 80.0% of those articles describing the methodology used for qualitative analysis) (Table 1). Six articles (23.0% of the 26 articles employing qualitative methodology) described that the saturation method was used to define the sample size [9].

Fears and/or beliefs were assessed through questionnaires, individual interviews and focus groups in 75.0% ($N = 63$), 20.2% ($N = 17$) and 6.0% ($N = 5$) of articles, respectively (Table 1).

All articles employing quantitative methodology ($N = 58$) assessed beliefs trough questionnaires and more than 50 different tools assessing fears and/or beliefs were described; the most frequently used were the original, and brief versions of the "Illness Perception Questionnaire" (IPQ) [10, 11] (22.4%, $N = 13$) and the "Beliefs about Medicines Questionnaire" (BMQ) (18.9%, $N = 11$) [12].

Disagreements between the two authors collecting the characteristics of publications, demographic data

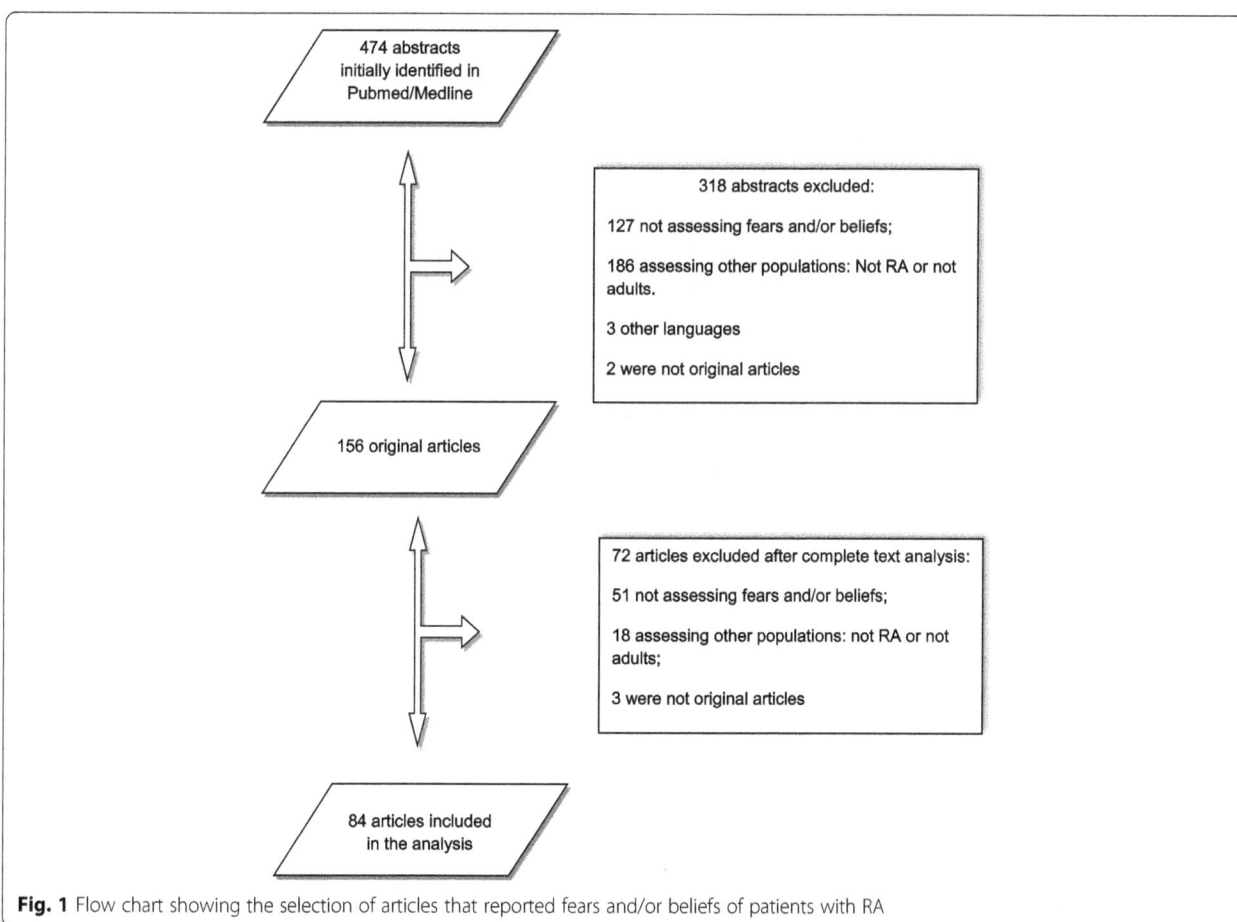

Fig. 1 Flow chart showing the selection of articles that reported fears and/or beliefs of patients with RA

Table 1 Characteristics of the publications and patients included in the analysis

	All articles (N = 84)	Studies employing only qualitative methodology N = 18	Studies employing only quantitative methodology N = 58	Studies with mixed (qualitative and quantitative) methodology N = 8
Total number of patients	24,336	334	23,539	463
Female sex N [a]	18,032	201	17,577	254
Age of participants (mean ± SD)[a]	54.9 ± 5.0	56.4 ± 7.2	54.5 ± 4.8	56.3 ± 2.1
Disease duration in years (mean ± SD) [a]	10.7 ± 6.0	13.9 ± 7.2	10.1 ± 5.9	11.2 ± 4.2
Method used for assessment of fears and/or beliefs N (%) of articles using the method [b]				
Individual interviews	17 (20.2)	13 (72.2)	NA	4 (50.0)
Focus groups	5 (6.0)	4 (22.2)	NA	1 (12.5)
Individual interviews and focus groups	1 (1.2)	1 (5.6)	NA	0 (0.0)
Questionnaire	63 (75.0)	NA	58 (100.0)	5(62.5)

SD standard deviation, *N* number, *NA* non applicable
[a]Numbers calculated on available data
[b]The final result can be greater than 100% since some articles employed more than one method to assess fear and/or beliefs

of participants and fears/beliefs occurred in 7.1% of articles when describing study design and in 5.7% of publication when demographic data of patients were analyzed. All disagreements were solved by consensus. There were no disagreements about fears and beliefs presented in the publications.

Fears

Thirty two articles (38.0% of the 84 analyzed publications) reported fears experienced by AR patients (Table 2). Articles reporting patient's concerns about pharmacological therapy and/or reporting factors that influenced these fears about drugs were the most

Table 2 Fears of people living with RA reported in the analyzed articles

Fears	Articles N (% of the 32 articles reporting fears) [a]	Total number of patients	N (%) of studies recruiting participants in Europe in each category/ Number of patients recruited in Europe	N (%) of studies recruiting participants in North America / Number of patients recruited in North America	N (%) of studies recruiting participants outside Europe and North America / Number of patients recruited outside Europe and North America
Fears related to pharmacological therapy	16 (50.0)	1085	13 (81.3) / 867 (760 in UK, 101 in Netherlands, 6 in Sweden)	2 (12.5) /78 (60 in Canada, 18 USA)	1(6.2)/140 (140 in Egypt)
Fear of consequences of disease in the future and disability	9 (28.1)	1049	6 (66.7) / 707 (460 in UK, 199 in Greece, 48 in Sweden)	1 (11.1)/ 30 (30 in USA)	2 (22.2) /312 (101 in United Arab Emirates, 211 in Australia)
Fears related to pregnancy and parenting role	3 (9.4)	211	3 (100.0) / 211 (102 in UK, 25 in France, 84 in Netherlands)	–	–
Fear of falling	3 (9.4)	5172	1(33.3)/48 (48 in Sweden)	1 (33.3) / 128 (128 in USA)	1 (33.3) / 4996 (4996 in Japan)
Fear of exercise related injury/ fear of exercise increasing RA symptoms	3 (9.4)	4289	3 (100.0) / 4289 (4283 in Sweden, 6 in UK)	–	–
Fear to disturb other people	2 (6.3)	38	1 (50.0)/ 8 (8 in UK)	1 (50.0) / 30 (30 in USA)	–
Fear of infections	2 (6.3)	54	2(100.0)/ 54 (48 in Sweden, 6 in UK)	–	–
Fear of negative evaluation from other people due to appearance	1 (3.1)	89	1 (100.0)/89 (89 in UK)	–	–

[a]Some articles reported more than one category of fears
N number; *UK* United Kingdom, *USA* United States of America

reported (50.0% of the 32 articles reporting fears, $N = 16$). Fears about pharmacological therapy were related to both synthetic and biological DMARDs (Table 3). Beliefs about drugs seemed to change with the course of disease and personal experiences with the drug [4, 13–15]; according to Ostlund et al., for example, initial beliefs and expectations about methotrexate were challenged as patients initiated treatment and began experiencing varying degrees of effectiveness and side effects [13]. Demographic factors, such as age and educational level were also found to influence fear about drugs, with older patients and subjects with lower educational level experiencing higher concern about DMARDs [5, 6, 14]. People with RA and different ethnicities may have different views about DMARDS even when they are living in the same country: Kumar et al. described higher concern about drugs among RA patients with an Asiatic origin living in United Kingdom when compared with White British patients who lived in the same country [6, 16].

Fear of disease progression and disability was the second most described category ($N = 9/32$ articles reporting fears, 28.1%) (Table 2);

Fears related to pregnancy and parenting roles were reported in three articles (9.4% of the 32 articles

Table 3 Fears related to synthetic and biological DMARDs

Fears	Author and year of publication
Fear of treatment failure	Sanderson 2009 [60]
Fear of being taken of a drug	Sanderson 2009 [60]
Fear of side effects of treatment (mainly long- term side effects)	Goodacre 2004 [4] Popa-Lisseanu 2005 [61] Wong 2007 [5] Sanderson 2009 [60] Fitzcharles 2009 [62] Kumar 2011 [43] Van den Bent 2011 [63] Hayden 2015 [14] Gadallah 2015 [42] Pasma 2015 [15] Nota 2015 [64]
Fear of "too many pills/too many drugs", fear of over-prescription	Popa-Lisseanu 2005 [61] Wong 2007 [5] Fitzcharles 2009 [62]
Fear of drug interaction	Fitzcharles 2009 [62]
Fear of addiction	Goodacre 2004 [4] Wong 2007 [5] Sanderson 2009 [60] Fitzcharles 2009 [62] Kumar 2011 [43] Van den Bent 2011 [63] Nota 2015 [64]
Fear of masking disease	Fitzcharles 2009 [62]
Fear of drugs causing reduced life expectancy	Goodacre 2004 [4]
Fear of being disappointed with a new treatment	Nyman 1999 [46]
Fear of too many changes in therapy	Kumar 2011 [43]

reporting fears) (Table 2). Patients who participated in these articles were recruited in Europe and reported the fear of drugs causing birth defects, fear of genetic transfer, fear of being unable to fulfill parenting roles, fear of not being able to prevent accidents and fear of dropping a small baby or toddler [17–19].

Other reported concerns were: the fear of falling ($N = 3/32$ articles, 9.4%), the fear of exercise related injury/ fear of having symptoms increased by exercise ($N = 3/32$ articles, 9.4%) and fear of negative evaluation from other people due to appearance ($N = 1/32$ articles, 3.1%).

Some examples of the fear to disturb other people ($N = 2/32$ articles, 6.3%) included: the fear to disturb family members and partners at home due to night pain, fear to disturb other patients and nurses in the hospital due to night pain, the fear of taking the spouses' time and giving them too much responsibilities [20, 21].

Patients with RA also reported fear of infections such as catching colds; these fears were reported in 6.3% ($N = 2$) of those articles reporting fears. Some patients were afraid of taking exercise in public places such as swimming pools because they thought that having RA made them more susceptible to infections [22, 23].

Only four articles (12.5% of those reporting fears) included patients living outside Europe and North America. No articles reported fears of patients from Latin America or Africa.

Beliefs
Seventy-four articles, corresponding to 88.0% of the total 84 analyzed articles, reported at least one belief. Main categories of beliefs and their consequences were described in Table 4.

Patient's beliefs about RA influenced impact of disease and assessment of health domains
Patients' beliefs were reported to influence the impact of RA ($N = 33$, 44.6% of the 74 articles assessing beliefs), mediated by their consequences in 8 health domains (Table 4).

Beliefs affecting the emotional domain were reported in 14/74 articles (18.9%). Perceptions of greater symptomatology and greater stress, beliefs on serious consequences of RA, beliefs on lower ability to handle or cope with disease and beliefs on its owns responsibility in the development of RA were reported to amplify the negative emotional impact of disease and contribute to depressive mood and anxiety [24–29].

Patients' beliefs affecting measures of function were reported in 6 publications (8.1% of articles reporting beliefs). Among RA patients, helplessness (patients' beliefs that they were not able to control pain and the course of disease) has a lower but statistically significant correlation with disability [30]. People who attributed more symptoms to RA, believe in a long illness duration, and held stronger beliefs that it would have negative consequences also presented greater disability on disease-specific measures of functioning; on the other side, stronger beliefs of personal control were associated with lower levels of disability, as were stronger beliefs in the ability of treatment to control RA [6, 26, 31–33].

Health-related quality of life (HRQOL) was found to be influenced by patients' beliefs in 5 articles (6.8% of the 72 publications assessing beliefs). Fears about the consequences of the RA were independently correlated to physical HRQOL, i.e., patients who believe in worse consequences of RA had worse scores in the physical component of quality of life measures; patient global assessment of disease activity was also a significant predictor of poor mental and physical HRQOL [6, 33–36].

Other health domains affected by patients' beliefs were: fatigue (2.7% of the publications assessing beliefs, $N = 2$ articles), pain (2.7%, N = 2), well-being (2.7%, N = 2), disease activity (1.4%, $N = 1$) and sexual life (1.4%, N = 1).

Among the 33 articles reporting consequences of patients' beliefs on health domains, only one manuscript recruited RA patients living outside Europe and North America.

Beliefs about pharmacological and non-pharmacological therapy affected patients' adherence

Beliefs about pharmacological and non-pharmacological therapy, including exercise and devices, were sometimes found to affect adherence to therapy (17.6% of articles reporting beliefs, $N = 13$). Among the 13 articles in this category, four publication (30.8%) studied the influence of patients' beliefs on adherence to physical activity. These references concluded that patient's beliefs about the usefulness of exercise for managing disease and their perceptions of positive social support for participation in exercise were highly correlated with physical activity participation [37–40]. Other eight articles in the same category (61.5%) analyzed the consequences of patients' beliefs about drugs on adherence. Although most patients with RA believed their synthetic and biological DMARDS were necessary to preserve joint structures, reduce pain and increase quality of life, levels of concern about side effects were high and related to non-adherence [3, 5, 15, 16, 41–44].

Table 4 Beliefs of people living with rheumatoid arthritis reported in the analyzed articles

Beliefs and their consequences	Articles N (% of the 74 articles reporting beliefs)[a]	Total number of patients	Studies recruiting participants in Europe N (%) / Number of patients recruited in Europe	Studies recruiting participants in North America N (%) / Number of patients recruited in North America	Studies recruiting participants outside Europe and North America N (%) / Number of patients recruited outside Europe and North America
Beliefs about the RA affecting impact of disease	33 (44.6)	9146			
Emotional impact	14 (18.9)	6404	6 (42.9) / 901	7 (50.0) / 945	1 (7.1)/ 4558
Function	6 (8.1)	715	4 (66.7)/ 370	2 (33.3) / 345	–
Quality of life	5 (6.8)	1034	4 (80.0) / 623	1 (20.0) / 411	–
Fatigue	2 (2.7)	186	1 (50.0) / 64	1 (50.0) / 122	–
Pain	2 (2.7)	299	–	2 (100.0) / 299	–
Well being	2 (2.7)	123	–	2 (100.0) / 123	–
Disease activity	1 (1.4)	322	1 (100.0) / 322	–	–
Sexual life	1 (1.4)	63	1 (100.0) / 63	–	–
Beliefs about pharmacological and non-pharmacological therapy affecting adherence	13 (17.6)	2464	10 (77.0) / 1999	2 (15.4) / 325	1 (7.6) / 140
Beliefs about cause of disease affecting coping strategies and adherence	9 (12.1)	961	8 (88.9) / 750	–	1 (11.1)/ 211
Beliefs affecting decision on therapy	1 (1.4)	142	–	1 (100.0) / 142	–
Beliefs affecting detection, tolerance and reporting of side effects	1 (1.4)	29	1 (100.0) / 29	–	–

N number; RA rheumatoid arthritis, [a]Some articles reported more than one category of beliefs

Beliefs about cause of disease predicted copping patterns and adherence

Beliefs about cause of disease expressed by RA patients in 9 studies (12.1% of articles reporting beliefs) included: hereditarity, stress, unexpressed grief, diet, occupational factors/overwork, lack of exercise, God's will, weather conditions, biological reasons/immune system failure/autoimmunity, accident/chance and karmic explanation (disease caused by past "bad" actions) [18, 36, 43, 45–50]. Beliefs about cause of disease predicted copping patterns: Salminem et al., for example, observed that 40.0% of RA patients believe diet contributed to their disease, more so if longer disease duration and higher education and 51% changed their diet after diagnosis, usually reducing consumption of animal fat and red meat [45].

Nyman et al. also showed that psychological factors, such as stress, overwork, anxiety or a distressing life event, for example bereavement or divorce were cited by 59.7% of AR patients as triggers factors leading to disease [46]. Other authors also demonstrated that most part of RA patients believe the cause of their disease was psychological in nature and that RA patients more readily admitted that psychological factors contributed to their illness compared to osteoarthritis patients [36, 50]. The psychological attribution as cause of RA seemed to have negative consequences: it was positively correlated with patient-related delay between beginning of symptoms and the first visit with general practitioner as well as with the tendency to use dysfunctional coping strategies [47, 49].

The analyzed work also described that patients who believed that the cause of RA was a biological one, viewed medicines less negatively than those who held the view that stress, God or fate were important causative factors [43].

Patients' beliefs influenced decision making during clinical visits

One article (1.4% of the 74 articles reporting beliefs) concluded that patient's beliefs about consequences of RA and high level of concern about disease were more likely to have their treatment escalated, independently of disease activity [51]. In this work, high disease activity was not associated with future escalation of treatment in patients reporting low levels of perceived consequences, concern, and emotional impact; the combination of disease activity and illness beliefs better predicted future escalation of treatment in RA patients than either factor in isolation [51].

Beliefs about DMARDs affected detection, tolerance and reporting of side effects

One qualitative study (1.4% of the 74 articles reporting beliefs) reported a relation between patients' beliefs about DMARDs and the reporting of side effects, with people more prepared to tolerate and do not report side effects when medication was perceived as beneficial or the number of alternatives perceived as limited. When DMARDs were not perceived as beneficial, concerns about side effects were voiced more frequently and the rationale for continued use was questioned [4].

Among the 74 articles reporting beliefs, only three (4.0%) described perceptions of patients with RA living outside Europe and North America (Table 4).

When all the 84 articles were analyzed, only 9.5% (N = 8) of them reported fears and/or beliefs of patients living outside Europe and North America: there was only one work which recruited patients in Latin America and no article included patients from Africa.

Discussion

This systematic literature review demonstrated that patients with RA have several beliefs about disease and its treatment and these beliefs influenced global impact of disease, adherence to therapy and copping patterns. Fears regarding the use of DMARDs and the fear of functional disability due to disease progression were the most reported in literature. It also highlighted areas where further original research is required: studies assessing patients' fears and beliefs were conducted mainly in Europe and North America and there is limited knowledge on fears and beliefs of patients living with RA in Asia, Africa, Latin America and Oceania.

Beliefs were shown to influence the patient-perceived impact of RA and, specially, the emotional / psychological impact of disease. This fact seems to be relevant since the prevalence of depression and anxiety is significant among people with RA [52]. Health professionals responsible for the management of RA patients should try to identify unjustified fears and erroneous beliefs that could amplify the psychological impact of disease. To minimize the patients' feeling of culpability by clarifying wrong beliefs about cause of disease, as well as to reinforce patients' ability to cope with consequences of RA are some strategies that can be adopted by health professionals. Since patients who attribute more symptoms to the rheumatic disease have higher psychological impact, it seems appropriate to help patients to recognize symptoms that are really attributed to RA and to differentiate them from those caused by comorbidities such as depression, anxiety and fibromyalgia [24, 28].

Although the emotional domain was the most cited, outcome measures evaluating other health domains as function, quality of life, pain and fatigue were also influenced by patients' perceptions. Since beliefs in more severe consequences of rheumatic disease and feelings of helplessness were associated with worse outcome measures of functioning it is convenient to consider beliefs when facing to patients with poor function not otherwise explained by disease activity [26, 30, 32, 33].

Moreover, this systematic literature review provides rheumatologists new evidence to consider patient's fears and beliefs when facing people with RA who are non-adherent to therapy. Recent work, which used pharmacy dispensing data to calculate medication possession ratios (MPR) and determine patients' adherence (MPR $\geq$ 0.80), demonstrated that patients with RA have low adherence to conventional and biological DMARDs [53, 54]. Mena-Vazquez et al. found that 88.8% of RA patients showed good adherence to biological drugs but only 61.2% also correctly took concomitant conventional synthetic DMARDs [54]. Another work from Calip et al. found lower rates of adherence to biological therapy: only 37.0% of RA patients were adherent, and the lower rates of adherence (17.0%) were found among young patients in their third year of treatment [53]. Fears related to pharmacological therapy were the most reported in our literature review and almost 20.0% of articles reported that patients' beliefs about therapy were found to affect adherence to treatment, reinforcing the idea that fears and beliefs may have an important role in explaining non-adherence. Since the fear of functional disability was the second most described patients' concern, it could be a strategy to increase adherence to DMARDS to instruct the patients about the ability of these drugs to avoid future structural damage and loss of function.

Although it seems plausible that to offer better knowledge on RA treatment could be a good strategy to improve non-adherence, some authors found that motivational-interviewing-guided group sessions about DMARDs use were not effective to change patients' beliefs about necessity of these drugs and concerns about therapy; this intervention did not improved rates of non-adherence [55]. Van den Bent et al. tested another intervention aiming to change patients' beliefs about medicines and improve non-adherence: a written report informing the physician about the medicine use and the adherence rate was sent to the rheumatologist by the researcher [56]. Adherence did not change after the intervention, compared to adherence assessment prior to the intervention and beliefs about medication were not significantly altered [56]. Further research is necessary to ensure effective strategies aiming to reduce erroneous fears and beliefs that could negatively affect the adherence to therapy in RA patients.

This work brings to light the paucity of published articles reporting fears and/or beliefs of RA patients living in Latin America, Africa, Oceania and Asia. Since nationality was found to influence, among RA patients, the perceptions about trust in physicians and the choice of the RA priority domains, it is convenient to rheumatologists working outside Europe and North America to gain more insight on fear and beliefs of their patients [7, 57].

In addition to differences among nationalities, the diversity of opinions among distinct ethnical groups living in the same country also exists; in United Kingdom, for example, Kumar et al. demonstrated that non-English-speaking RA patients (patients of South Asian origin) usually believe that RA is caused by a God's will and that they do not have an active role in therapy, while English-speaking patients usually believe that the cause of disease is a biological one and view DMARDs less negatively [43]. Salminem et al. also interviewed Punjabi women living in United Kingdom and remarked that this group made sense of the development of RA as a consequence of past "bad" actions. This "karmic explanation" to the development of disease lead patients to hide symptoms from others in order to avoid a moral judgement and stigmatization [48]. Further research comparing fear and beliefs among people of different ethnic and cultural backgrounds would be interesting.

Other gap in publications was remarked: most articles included only patients with long disease duration, and the perception of patients with early RA was rarely described [58]. Further studies allowing comparison of fear and beliefs of patients in different stages of RA is necessary since it has been shown that beliefs about the consequences of disease and expectations of patients varied according to the stage of RA and familiarity with other people with the same clinical condition [13, 18].

This study has some weaknesses. It is not exhaustive since the one database assessed was PubMed/Medline; however this is the most important database of biomedical research articles covering more than 5600 journals published in more than 80 countries; articles in five languages were included in the analysis and there was no limit of date for the search.

This work included all studies reporting fear and/or beliefs of patients with RA found with our search strategy regardless of their quality level to optimize the number of reported fear and beliefs. The appraisal of qualitative research, for example, is still a challenge since there is no consensus on a tool for quality evaluation in this type of studies. According to Dixon-Woods et al., there are over 100 tolls described to evaluate quality in qualitative research, some adopting non-reconcilable positions on a number of issues [59].

It is possible that among the studies employing some method of qualitative analysis, some work were probably not exhaustive since less than a quarter of those articles reported that the principle of saturation was used to define the sample size [9].

Despite its limitations, this work highlights several fears and beliefs of patients with RA, allowing rheumatologists and other health professionals to create strategies to minimize fears and beliefs that could affect negatively the management of disease.

Conclusion
In RA, patients' beliefs influenced global impact of disease, adherence to therapy and copping patterns. The most common fears of RA patients were related to the consequences of RA and the use of DMARDs. Further research is needed on fears and beliefs of patients living outside Europe and North America.

Abbreviations
BMQ: Beliefs about medicines questionnaire; DMARDs: Disease- modifying antirheumatic drugs; HRQOL: Health-related quality of life; IPQ: Illness perception questionnaire; MPR: Medication possession ratios; RA: Rheumatoid arthritis

Funding
The first author P Palominos conducted this project with own resources. Professor Ricardo Machado Xavier has received a grant for research from CNPq -National Council for Scientific and Technological Development.

Authors' contributions
All authors meet the authorship criteria, giving substantial contribution to the conception of the work, data acquisition and analysis, drafting or reviewing the work for intellectual content and giving final approval of the version to be published. The authors agree to be accountable for all aspects of the work in ensuring that questions related to the accuracy or integrity of any part of the work are appropriately investigated and resolved.

Competing interests
The authors declare that they have no competing interests.

Author details
[1]Universidade Federal do Rio Grande do Sul (UFRGS), Programa de Pós Graduação em Ciências Médicas (PPGCM), Rua Ramiro Barcelos 2400, segundo andar, Porto Alegre 90035-903, Brazil. [2]Department of Rheumatology, Hospital de Clinicas de Porto Alegre, Rua Ramiro Barcelos 2350, sexto andar, Porto Alegre 90035-903, Brazil. [3]Sorbonne Universités, UPMC Univ Paris 06, Institut Pierre Louis d'Epidémiologie et de Santé Publique, GRC-UPMC 08 (EEMOIS); Department of Rheumatology, Pitié Salpêtrière Hospital, AP-HP, 47-83 Boulevard de l'Hôpital, 75013 Paris, France.

References
1. Gossec L, Dougados M, Dixon W. Patient-reported outcomes as end points in clinical trials in rheumatoid arthritis. RMD Open. 2015;1(1):e000019.
2. Kalyoncu U, Dougados M, Daurès J-P, Gossec L. Reporting of patient-reported outcomes in recent trials in rheumatoid arthritis: a systematic literature review. Ann Rheum Dis. 2009;68(2):183–90.
3. Neame R, Hammond A. Beliefs about medications: a questionnaire survey of people with rheumatoid arthritis. Rheumatology. 2005;44(6):762–7.
4. Goodacre LJ, Goodacre JA. Factors influencing the beliefs of patients with rheumatoid arthritis regarding disease-modifying medication. Rheumatology. 2004;43(5):583–6.
5. Wong M, Mulherin D. The influence of medication beliefs and other psychosocial factors on early discontinuation of disease-modifying anti-rheumatic drugs. Musculoskeletal Care. 2007;5(3):148–59.
6. Kumar K, Gordon C, Toescu V, Buckley CD, Horne R, Nightingale PG, et al. Beliefs about medicines in patients with rheumatoid arthritis and systemic lupus erythematosus: a comparison between patients of south Asian and white British origin. Rheumatology. 2008;47(5):690–7.
7. Berrios-Rivera J, Street R Jr, Popa-Lisseanu M, Kallen M, Richardson M, Janssen N. Trust in physicians and elements of the medical interaction in patients with rheumatoid arthritis and systemic lupus erythematosus. Arthritis Rheum. 2006;55(3):385–93.
8. PRISMA: transparent report of systematic reviews and metanalysis. Acessed 1 May 2017.
9. Depoy E, Gitlin L. Introduction to research: understanding and applying multiple strategies. Fourth Edi. St. Louis: Elsevier, Mosby; 1998.
10. Weinman J, Petrie K, Moss-Morris R, Horne R. The illness perception questionnaire: a new method for assessing illness perceptions. Psychology and Health Psychol Heal. 1996;11:431–46.
11. Broadbent E, Petrie KJ, Main J, Weinman J. The brief illness perception questionnaire. J Psychosom Res. 2006;60(6):631–7.
12. Horne R, Weinman J, Hankins M. The beliefs about medicines questionnaire: the development and evaluation of a new method for assessing the cognitive representation of medication. Psychol Health. 1999;14(1):1–24.
13. Östlund G, Björk M, Valtersson E, Sverker A. Lived experiences of sex life difficulties in men and women with early RA – the Swedish TIRA project. Musculoskeletal Care. 2015;13(4):248–57.
14. Hayden C, Neame R, Tarrant C. Patients' adherence-related beliefs about methotrexate: a qualitative study of the role of written patient information. BMJ Open. 2015;5(5):e006918.
15. Pasma A, Van't Spijker A, Luime JJ, Walter MJM, Busschbach JJV, Hazes JMW. Facilitators and barriers to adherence in the initiation phase of disease-modifying antirheumatic drug (DMARD) use in patients with arthritis who recently started their first DMARD treatment. J Rheumatol. 2015;42(3):379–85.
16. Kumar K, Raza K, Nightingale P, Horne R, Chapman S, Greenfield S, et al. Determinants of adherence to disease modifying anti-rheumatic drugs in white British and south Asian patients with rheumatoid arthritis: a cross sectional study. BMC Musculoskelet Disord. 2015;16(1):396.
17. Barlow JH, Cullen LA, Rowe IF. Comparison of knowledge and psychological well-being between patients with a short disease duration (≤1 year) and patients with more established rheumatoid arthritis (≥10 years duration). Patient Educ Couns. 1999;38(3):195–203.
18. Berenbaum F, Chauvin P, Hudry C, Mathoret-Philibert F, Poussiere M, De Chalus T, et al. Fears and beliefs in rheumatoid arthritis and spondyloarthritis: a qualitative study. PLoS One. 2014;9(12):e114350.
19. Clowse MEB, Chakravarty E, Costenbader KH, Chambers C, Michaud K. Effects of infertility, pregnancy loss, and patient concerns on family size of women with rheumatoid arthritis and systemic lupus erythematosus. Arthritis Care Res (Hoboken). 2012;64(5):668–74.
20. Coady DA, Armitage C, Wright D. Rheumatoid arthritis patients' experiences of night pain. J Clin Rheumatol. 2007;13(2):66–9.
21. Foxall MJ, Kollasch C, McDermott S. Family stress and coping in rheumatoid arthritis. Arthritis Care Res (Hoboken). 1989;2(4):114–21.
22. Wang M, Donovan-Hall M, Hayward H, Adams J. People's perceptions and beliefs about their ability to exercise with rheumatoid arthritis: a qualitative study. Musculoskeletal Care. 2015;13(2):112–5.
23. Östlund G, Björk M, Thyberg I, Thyberg M, Valtersson E, Stenström B, et al. Emotions related to participation restrictions as experienced by patients with early rheumatoid arthritis: a qualitative interview study (the Swedish TIRA project). Clin Rheumatol. 2014;33(10):1403–13.
24. Van Os S, Norton S, Hughes LD, Chilcot J. Illness perceptions account for variation in positive outlook as well as psychological distress in rheumatoid arthritis. Psychol Health Med. 2012;17(4):427–39.
25. Strahl C, Kleinknecht RA, Dinnel DL. The role of pain anxiety, coping, and pain self-efficacy in rheumatoid arthritis patient functioning. Behav Res Ther. 2000;38(9):863–73.
26. Smith C. A, Wallston K a. Adaptation in patients with chronic rheumatoid arthritis: application of a general model. Health Psychol. 1992;11(3):151–62.
27. Lowe R, Cockshott Z, Greenwood R, Kirwan JR, Almeida C, Richards P, et al. Self-efficacy as an appraisal that moderates the coping-emotion relationship: associations among people with rheumatoid arthritis. Psychol Health. 2008;23(2):155–74.
28. Devins GM, Gupta A, Cameron J, Woodend K, Mah K, Gladman D. Cultural syndromes and age moderate the emotional impact of illness intrusiveness in rheumatoid arthritis. Rehabil Psychol. 2009;54:33–44. 12p
29. Nakajima A, Kamitsuji S, Saito A, Tanaka E, Nishimura K, Horikawa N, et al. Disability and patient's appraisal of general health contribute to depressed

mood in rheumatoid arthritis in a large clinical study in Japan. Mod Rheumatol. 2006;16(3):151–7.

30. Nicassio PM, Kay MA, Custodio MK, Irwin MR, Olmstead R, Weisman MH. An evaluation of a biopsychosocial framework for health-related quality of life and disability in rheumatoid arthritis. J Psychosom Res. 2011;71(2):79–85.

31. Scharloo M, Kaptein AA, Weinman J, Hazes JM, Willems LNA, Bergman W, et al. Illness perceptions, coping and functioning in patients with rheumatoid arthritis, chronic obstructive pulmonary disease and psoriasis. J Psychosom Res. 1998;44(5):573–85.

32. Serbo B, Jajic I. Relationship of the functional status, duration of the disease and pain intensity and some psychological variables in patients with rheumatoid arthritis. Clin Rheumatol. 1991;10(4):419–22.

33. Graves H, Scott DL, Lempp H, Weinman J. Illness beliefs predict disability in rheumatoid arthritis. J Psychosom Res. 2009;67(5):417–23.

34. Kotsis K, Voulgari PV, Tsifetaki N, Machado MO, Carvalho AF, Creed F, et al. Anxiety and depressive symptoms and illness perceptions in psoriatic arthritis and associations with physical health-related quality of life. Arthritis Care Res (Hoboken). 2012;64(10):1593–601.

35. Alishiri GH, Bayat N, Fathi Ashtiani A, Tavallaii SA, Assari S, Moharamzad Y. Logistic regression models for predicting physical and mental health-related quality of life in rheumatoid arthritis patients. Mod Rheumatol. 2008;18(6):601–8.

36. Kotsis K, Voulgari PV, Tsifetaki N, Drosos AA, Carvalho AF, Hyphantis T. Illness perceptions and psychological distress associated with physical health-related quality of life in primary Sjögren's syndrome compared to systemic lupus erythematosus and rheumatoid arthritis. Rheumatol Int. 2014;34(12):1671–81.

37. Ehrlich-Jones L, Lee J, Semanik P, Cox C, Dunlop D, Chang RW. Relationship between beliefs, motivation, and worries about physical activity and physical activity participation in persons with rheumatoid arthritis. Arthritis Care Res. 2011;63(12):1700–5.

38. Swardh E, Biguet G, Opava CH. Views on exercise maintenance: variations among patients with rheumatoid arthritis. Phys Ther. 2008;88(9):1049–60.

39. Sperber NR, Allen KD, DeVellis BM, DeVellis RF, Lewis MA, Callahan LF. Differences in effectiveness of the active living every day program for older adults with arthritis. J Aging Phys Act. 2013;21(4):387–401.

40. Iversen MD, Fossel AH, Daltroy LH. Rheumatologist-patient communication about exercise and physical therapy in the management of rheumatoid arthritis. Arthritis Care Res. 1999;12(3):180–92.

41. Morgan C, McBeth J, Cordingley L, Watson K, Hyrich KL, Symmons DPM, et al. The influence of behavioural and psychological factors on medication adherence over time in rheumatoid arthritis patients: a study in the biologics era. Rheumatol (United Kingdom). 2015;54(10):1780–91.

42. Gadallah MA, Boulos DNK, Gebrel A, Dewedar S, Morisky DE. Assessment of rheumatoid arthritis patients' adherence to treatment. Am J Med Sci. 2015;349(2):151–6.

43. Kumar K, Gordon C, Barry R, Shaw K, Horne R, Raza K. "It's like taking poison to kill poison but I have to get better": a qualitative study of beliefs about medicines in rheumatoid arthritis and systemic lupus erythematosus patients of south Asian origin. Lupus. 2011;20(8):837–44.

44. Lendrem D, Mitchell S, McMeekin P, Bowman S, Price E, Pease CT, et al. Health-related utility values of patients with primary Sjögren's syndrome and its predictors. Ann Rheum Dis. 2014;73(7):1362–8.

45. Salminen E, Heikkilä S, Poussa T, Lagström H, Saario R, Salminen S. Female patients tend to alter their diet following the diagnosis of rheumatoid arthritis and breast cancer. Prev Med (Baltim). 2002;34(5):529–35.

46. Nyman CS, Lutzen K. Caring needs of patients with rheumatoid arthritis. Nurs Sci Q. 1999;12(2):164–9.

47. Van Der Elst K, De Cock D, Vecoven E, Arat S, Meyfroidt S, Joly J, et al. Are illness perception and coping style associated with the delay between symptom onset and the first general practitioner consultation in early rheumatoid arthritis management? An exploratory study within the CareRA trial. Scand J Rheumatol. 2016;45(3):171–8.

48. Sanderson T, Calnan M, Kumar K. The moral experience of illness and its impact on normalisation: examples from narratives with Punjabi women living with rheumatoid arthritis in the UK. Sociol Health Illn. 2015;37(8):1218–35.

49. Ziarko M, Mojs E, Piasecki B, Samborski W. The mediating role of dysfunctional coping in the relationship between beliefs about the disease and the level of depression in patients with rheumatoid arthritis. Sci World J. 2014;2014:585063.

50. Ahern MJ, McFarlane AC, Leslie A, Eden J, Roberts-Thomson PJ. Illness behaviour in patients with arthritis. Ann Rheum Dis. 1995;54:245–50.

51. Fraenkel L, Cunningham M. High disease activity may not be sufficient to escalate care. Arthritis Care Res. 2014;66(2):197–203.

52. Isik A, Koca SS, Ozturk A, Mermi O. Anxiety and depression in patients with rheumatoid arthritis. Clin Rheumatol. 2007;26(6):872–8.

53. Calip GS, Adimadhyam S, Xing S, Rincon JC, Lee WJ, Anguiano RH. Medication adherence and persistence over time with self-administered TNF-alpha inhibitors among young adult, middle-aged, and older patients with rheumatologic conditions. Semin Arthritis Rheum. 2017 Oct;47(2):157–64.

54. Mena-Vazquez N, Manrique-Arija S, Yunquera-Romero L, Ureña-Garnica I, Rojas-Gimenez M, Domic C, et al. Adherence of rheumatoid arthritis patients to biologic disease-modifying antirheumatic drugs: a cross-sectional study. Rheumatol Int. 2017 Oct;37(10):1709–18.

55. Zwikker HE, Van den Ende CH, Van Lankveld WG, Den Broeder AA, Van den Hoogen FH, Van de Mosselaar B, et al. Effectiveness of a group-based intervention to change medication beliefs and improve medication adherence in patients with rheumatoid arthritis: a randomized controlled trial. Patient Educ Couns. 2014;94(3):356–61.

56. Van den Bemt BJF, den Broeder AA, van den Hoogen FHJ, Benraad B, Hekster YA, van Riel PLCM, et al. Making the rheumatologist aware of patients' non-adherence does not improve medication adherence in patients with rheumatoid arthritis. Scand J Rheumatol. 2011;40(3):192–6.

57. Wen H, Ralph Schumacher H, Li X, Gu J, Ma L, Wei H, et al. Comparison of expectations of physicians and patients with rheumatoid arthritis for rheumatology clinic visits: a pilot, multicenter, international study. Int J Rheum Dis. 2012;15(4):380–9.

58. Townsend A, Adam P, Cox SM, Li LC. Everyday ethics and help-seeking in early rheumatoid arthritis. Chronic Illn. 2010;6(3):171–82.

59. Dixon-Woods M, Sutton A, Shaw R, Miller T, Smith J, Young B, et al. Appraising qualitative research for inclusion in systematic reviews: a quantitative and qualitative comparison of three methods. J Health Serv Res Policy. 2007;12(1):42–7.

60. Sanderson T, Calnan M, Morris M, Richards P, Hewlett S. The impact of patient-perceived restricted access to anti-TNF therapy for rheumatoid arthritis: a qualitative study. Musculoskeletal Care. 2009;7(3):194–209.

61. Popa-Lisseanu MGG, Greisinger A, Richardson M, O'Malley KJ, Janssen NM, Marcus DM, et al. Determinants of treatment adherence in ethnically diverse, economically disadvantaged patients with rheumatic disease. J Rheumatol. 2005;32(5):913–9.

62. Fitzcharles MA, DaCosta D, Ware MA, Shir Y. Patient barriers to pain management may contribute to poor pain control in rheumatoid arthritis. J Pain. 2009;10(3):300–5.

63. Van Den Bemt BJF, Den Broeder AA, Van Den Hoogen FHJ, Benraad B, Hekster YA, Van Riel PLCM, et al. Making the rheumatologist aware of patients' non-adherence does not improve medication adherence in patients with rheumatoid arthritis. Scand J Rheumatol. 2011;40(3):192–6.

64. Nota I, Drossaert CHC, Taal E, Van De Laar MAFJ. Patients' considerations in the decision-making process of initiating disease-modifying antirheumatic drugs. Arthritis Care Res. 2015;67(7):956–64.

2

Work disability in fibromyalgia and other soft tissue disorders: analysis of preventive benefits in Brazil from 2006 to 2015

Ana Paula Monteiro Gomides[1][*] ⓘ, Josierton Cruz Bezerra[2], Eduardo José do Rosário e Souza[3], Licia Maria Henrique da Mota[1] and Leopoldo Luiz Santos-Neto[1]

Abstract

Background: Fibromyalgia is a common chronic disease characterized by persistent diffuse pain, fatigue, sleep disorders and functional symptoms.

The disease can have negative consequences in personal and social life, in addition to significant public health expenses caused by treatment and work leave.

The purpose of this article is to evaluate the number of social security benefits granted due to incapacity for work in Brazil in patients with ICD M79 and variants in the period 2006–2015.

There has been no previous study with data referring to work withdrawals caused by fibromyalgia in Brazil.

Methods: Data for this study were obtained through an official Social Security platform. The disability and retirement benefits were analyzed.

Results: A total of 95,882 social security disability benefits were granted to ICD M79 and variants in the period from 2006 to 2015.

Regarding gender, 69,420 benefits (72.3%) were granted to women and 26,562 (27.7%) to men. Regarding the types of benefits, we found 93,556 (97.5%) temporary withdrawals from work and 2426 (2.5%) permanent withdrawals. When comparing the initial and final years, we observed a significant reduction in the number of awards: 15,562 in 2006 to 6163 in 2015.

Conclusion: Fibromyalgia was an important cause of withdrawal due to incapacity for work in Brazil, with consequent public health expenditure.

These data may serve as a basis for new studies and can alert professionals of the need for adequate management of fibromyalgia to reduce work withdrawal and its consequences.

Keywords: Fibromyalgia, Incapacity for work, Social security benefits

Background

Fibromyalgia is a chronic disease characterized by persistent diffuse pain, fatigue, sleep disorders and, in most cases, other associated functional symptoms [1]. This disease has a common framework, with an estimated global prevalence of between 5 and 15% of the general population [2–4]. In recent years, several mechanisms have been studied, but their etiopathogenesis remains unknown [1, 5].

Patients with fibromyalgia often report worsening of quality of life, changes in social life and reduced productivity at work, especially when there are associated depressive symptoms. These facts can generate negative effects on personal and social life, along with significant public health expenditures caused by treatment and work withdrawals [6–11].

Although the complaints of productivity reduction in patients with fibromyalgia are frequent, there are few studies in the literature that can measure this probable consequence of the disease.

The objective of this article is to evaluate the number of work withdrawals in patients with fibromyalgia and

* Correspondence: anapmgomides@gmail.com
[1]Programa de Pós-Graduação em Ciências Médicas, Faculdade de Medicina, Universidade de Brasília, UnB, CEP, Brasília, DF 70910-900, Brazil
Full list of author information is available at the end of the article

Table 1 List of ICD-10 disease codes from group M79 and its variants

ICD-10 Disease code	Description
ICD M79	Other and unspecified soft tissue disorders, not elsewhere classified
ICD M79.0	Rheumatism, unspecified
ICD M79.1	Myalgia
ICD M79.6	Pain in limb, hand, foot, fingers and toes
ICD M79.7	Fibromyalgia
ICD M79.8	Other specified soft tissue disorders
ICD M79.9	Soft tissue disorder, unspecified

other soft tissue disorders (ICD M79 and variants) by analyzing the disability benefits granted by Social Security in Brazil over a period of 10 years.

Methods

A retrospective study was conducted in which the disability benefits (DBs) granted by Social Security in Brazil were analyzed as a function of fibromyalgia and other soft tissue disorders classified as ICD M79 and its ICD-10 variants, which are specified in Table 1.

The assessment consisted of two types of benefits: disease assistance (temporary work withdrawal) and disability retirement (permanent work withdrawal) during the period from 2006 to 2015.

The data for this study were obtained through the E-SIC portal and the official Social Security platform in which spreadsheets and graphs were composed of numerical and descriptive variables [12, 13]. A qualitative and quantitative analysis of the data was performed.

Results

A total of 24,815,916 disability benefits were provided by Brazilian Social Security in the period from 2006 to 2015. Among these benefits (provided for all diseases), 95,882 of the benefits (0.39%) were attributed to ICD M79 and variants.

When the DBs were analyzed according to the ICD M79 group, 69,420 benefits (72.3%) were granted to women and 26,562 (27.7%) to men. The age and salary distributions were also calculated and can be seen in Tables 2 and 3. In relation to the types of benefits, we found 93,556 (97.5%) benefits from temporary work withdrawal (disease benefit) and 2426 (2.5%) permanent retirements (disability retirement).

The distribution of concessions per year was analyzed, and more benefits were found in the years 2006 to 2008. The number of benefits per year and the total benefits in the period from 2006 to 2015 can be seen in Table 4.

Discussion

Fibromyalgia has the potential to cause functional impairment in patients when compared with the normal population, especially when there is exacerbation of painful symptoms or associated psychiatric conditions [14–17]. Limitations in work capacity caused by pain, fatigue, cognitive alterations, reduction of muscular strength and physical resistance have been described in the literature [18–20].

The evaluation of the number of work withdrawals for a given disease is important for measuring the disease's impact. In this article, we evaluated the number of work withdrawals by analyzing benefits granted by Social Security in Brazil between 2006 and 2015. We did not find similar articles in the literature for comparison.

In our study, we noted the granting of 95,982 benefits for this group of diseases (ICD M79 and variants) in the analyzed period. The occurrence of 72.3% of the benefits for the female sex can be easily explained by the very incidence of fibromyalgia and other diseases in this group.

In relation to the age group, the age with the greatest number of benefits was 40 to 49 years (30.3% of the total), with the greatest number of work withdrawals being between 30 and 59 years old: 88,867 (92.6%). It is important to emphasize that these withdrawals are predominant during the time of full professional capacity. Within this context, some authors have warned about the need for early evaluation and diagnosis and better management of fibromyalgia to minimize the personal consequences and expenses of withdrawals. The maintenance of the functional and working capacity of the individual, besides the improvement in the quality of life, has also been advocated [20].

Regarding the annual distribution of benefits, there were greater numbers in the years 2006, 2007 and 2008. The rest of the period remained similar. When comparing the initial and final years of the analyzed period, we observed a significant reduction in the number of concessions: 15,562 in 2006 to 6163 in 2015. It is believed that during the analyzed years, there was progressively greater knowledge on the part of the physician regarding fibromyalgia and the current recommendation that removal from work in general should be avoided [20]. Increased rigor when granting benefits by Social Security may be another explanation for the decrease in the number of benefits granted.

The amount paid for disability benefits was mostly up to two minimum wages (89%), which likely represents the income of most of those insured by the National Institute of Social Security / Social Security. No data were provided on the duration of each benefit.

Table 2 Number of disability benefits granted by ICD M79 (and variants) distributed by age group

Up to 19 years	20–29 years	30–39 years	35–39 years	40–49 years	50–59 years	55–59 years	60–69 years	70 years and over	Total
808	15.415	24.661	12.944	29.070	22.192	8.578	3.700	136	95.982

Table 3 Distribution of disability benefits for M79 (and variants) by salary range in minimum wages (MW) from 2006 to 2015

Distribution year	< 1 MW	1–2 MW	2–3 MW	3–4 MW	4–5 MW	5–6 MW	6–7 MW	Total
2006	7.833	5.355	1.308	527	397	127	2	15.562
2007	5.815	3.758	868	364	317	19	0	11.154
2008	5.319	3.009	743	284	246	9	0	9.615
2009	4.814	2.410	515	262	163	0	0	8.169
2010	5.449	2.500	463	268	120	1	0	8.811
2011	5.337	2.721	478	241	126	0	0	8.916
2012	6.015	2.455	433	268	45	0	0	9.224
2013	6.061	2.446	447	243	31	0	0	9.240
2014	5.934	2.511	411	241	20	0	0	9.128
2015	4.032	1.668	279	158	20	0	0	6.163
Total	56.609	28.833	5.945	2.856	1.485	156	2	95.982

Although the vast majority of the benefits granted (97.5%) were due to temporary withdrawals from work (disease assistance), the large number of such benefits represents an important measure of the financial impact of the disease. In addition, we observed 2426 cases of disability retirement, a fact that deserves extreme attention due to the great personal and social repercussions resulting from the early and permanent departure from the labor market.

Conclusions

In the present study, we analyzed the group of diseases defined in ICD-10 as M79 and its variants, which encompasses several soft tissue disorders. Future research with specific evaluation for fibromyalgia in patients diagnosed by a rheumatologist should be encouraged.

This paper presents some limitations, such as its retrospective character and the lack of data regarding the occupation of individuals and the duration of benefits. However, it is the first article that analyzes the social security benefits granted by ICD M79 in Brazil through an official and reliable database. The analysis covered an extended period, which provides us with relevant information on departures from the last decade. These data may serve as a basis for further studies and should alert professionals and specialist societies to the need for adequate management of fibromyalgia to reduce work withdrawal and its consequences.

Author's contribuitions
APMG performed the data collection, data analysis and writing of the manuscript. JCB performed data collection and data analysis. EJ do R e S, LMH da M and LLS-N revision and writing of the manuscript.

Competing interests
The authors have no competing interests to this article to disclose.

Author details
[1]Programa de Pós-Graduação em Ciências Médicas, Faculdade de Medicina, Universidade de Brasília, UnB, CEP, Brasília, DF 70910-900, Brazil. [2]National Social Security Institute, Brasília, Brazil. [3]Santa Casa de Misericórdia Hospital of Belo Horizonte, Belo Horizonte, Minas Gerais, Brazil.

Table 4 Disability benefits granted by social security for ICD M 79 and variants in the period from 2006 to 2015

Distribution year	Disease assistance	Disability retirement	Total
2006	15.158	404	15.562
2007	10.970	184	11.154
2008	9.289	326	9.615
2009	7.924	244	8.169
2010	8.579	232	8.811
2011	8.726	190	8.916
2012	8.991	233	9.224
2013	8.998	242	9.240
2014	8.912	216	9.128
2015	6.008	155	6.163
Total	93.555	2.426	95.982

References
1. Bazzichi L, Giacomelli C, Consensi A, Atzeni F, Batticciotto A, Di Franco M, et al. One year in review 2016: fibromyalgia. Clin Exp Rheumatol. 2016;34(2 Suppl 96):S145–9.
2. Walitt B, Nahin RL, Katz RS, Bergman MJ, Wolfe F. The Prevalence and Characteristics of Fibromyalgia in the 2012 National Health Interview Survey. PLoS One. 2015 Sep 17;10(9):e0138024.
3. Queiroz LP. Worldwide epidemiology of fibromyalgia. Curr Pain Headache Rep. 2013 Aug;17(8):356.
4. Neumann L, Buskila D. Epidemiology of fibromyalgia. Curr Pain Headache Rep. 2003 Oct;7(5):362–8.
5. Jiao J, Vincent A, Cha SS, Luedtke CA, Kim CH, Oh TH. Physical Trauma and Infection as Precipitating Factors in Patients with Fibromyalgia. Am J Phys Med Rehabil. 2015 Dec;94(12):1075–82.
6. Skaer TL. Fibromyalgia: disease synopsis, medication cost effectiveness and economic burden. PharmacoEconomics. 2014 May;32(5):457–66.
7. Tutoglu A, Boyaci A, Koca I, Celen E, Korkmaz N. Quality of life, depression, and sexual dysfunction in spouses of female patients with fibromyalgia. Rheumatol Int. 2014 Aug;34(8):1079–84.
8. Alok R, Das SK, Agarwal GG, Tiwari SC, Salwahan L, Srivastava R. Problem-focused coping and self-efficacy as correlates of quality of life and severity of fibromyalgia in primary fibromyalgia patients. J Clin Rheumatol. 2014; 20(6):314–6.

9. Lavergne MR, Cole DC, Kerr K, Marshall LM. Functional impairment in chronic fatigue syndrome, fibromyalgia, and multiple chemical sensitivity. Can Fam Physician. 2010;56(2):e57–65.

10. Vervoort VM, Vriezekolk JE, Olde Hartman TC, Cats HA, van Helmond T, van der Laan WH, et al. Cost of illness and illness perceptions in patients with fibromyalgia. Clin Exp Rheumatol. 2016;34(2 Suppl 96):S74–82.

11. Robinson RL, Kroenke K, Mease P, Williams DA, Chen Y, D'Souza D, Wohlreich M, et al. Burden of illness and treatment patterns for patients with fibromyalgia. Pain Med. 2012 Oct;13(10):1366–76.

12. Ministério da Previdência Social. Disponível em: http://www.previdencia.gov.br/

13. E-SIC - Sistema Eletrônico do Serviço de Informação ao Cidadão [Internet]. Disponível em: http://www.acessoainformacao.gov.br/sistema/site/index

14. Schaefer C, Mann R, Masters ET, Cappelleri JC, Daniel SR, Zlateva G, McElroy HJ, Chandran AB, et al. The Comparative Burden of Chronic Widespread Pain and Fibromyalgia in the United States. Pain Pract. 2016;16(5):565–79.

15. Soriano-Maldonado A, Amris K, Ortega FB, Segura-Jiménez V, Estévez-López F, Álvarez-Gallardo IC, et al. Association of different levels of depressive symptoms with symptomatology, overall disease severity, and quality of life in women with fibromyalgia. Qual Life Res. 2015 Dec;24(12):2951–7.

16. Bateman L, Sarzi-Puttini P, Burbridge CL, Landen JW, Masters ET, Bhadra Brown P, et al. Burden of illness in fibromyalgia patients with comorbid depression. Clin Exp Rheumatol. 2016;34(2 Suppl 96):S106–13.

17. Ghavidel-Parsa B, Bidari A, Amir Maafi A, Ghalebaghi B. The Iceberg Nature of Fibromyalgia Burden: The Clinical and Economic Aspects. Korean J Pain. 2015 Jul;28(3):169–76.

18. Tesio V, Torta DM, Colonna F, Leombruni P, Ghiggia A, Fusaro E, et al. Are fibromyalgia patients cognitively impaired? Objective and subjective neuropsychological evidence. Arthritis Care Res (Hoboken). 2015 Jan;67(1):143–50.

19. Kravitz HM, Katz RS. Fibrofog and fibromyalgia: a narrative review and implications for clinical practice. Rheumatol Int. 2015 Jul;35(7):1115–25.

20. Henriksson CM, Liedberg GM, Gerdle B. Women with fibromyalgia: work and rehabilitation. Disabil Rehabil. 2005 Jun 17;27(12):685–94.

3

Validation of the Brazilian version of the Hip Outcome Score (HOS) questionnaire

Rafaela Maria de Paula Costa[1,5*], Themis Moura Cardinot[2], Letícia Nunes Carreras Del Castillo Mathias[1,5], Gustavo Leporace[3] and Liszt Palmeira de Oliveira[4,5]

Abstract

Background: The Hip Outcome Score (HOS) was developed to evaluate physically active patients with hip disease but without severe degenerative change. A translation and cultural adaptation into Brazilian Portuguese was previously conducted. The aim of this study was to validate the Brazilian version of the HOS (HOS-Brazil) among a group of physically active patients with a diagnosis of femoroacetabular impingement (FAI) or greater trochanteric pain syndrome (GTPS).

Methods: The following questionnaires were applied: the HOS-Brazil; the validated Brazilian versions of the Nonarthritic Hip Score (NAHS) and the 12-Item Short-Form Health Survey (SF-12). The psychometric properties analyzed with regard to the validation process were reliability and validity. Internal consistency and intra-rater test-retest reliabilities were analyzed using Cronbach's alpha and the intraclass correlation coefficient (ICC) statistical tests based on test-retest agreement. Construct and content validities were examined using Pearson's correlation coefficient. Content validity was also analyzed based on evidence of floor, ceiling, or both types of effects from the questionnaires.

Results: A total of 70 male and female patients were selected, aged between 19 and 70 years old. The internal consistency and intra-rater test-retest reliability values were high (Cronbach's $\alpha > 0.9$; ICC > 0.9). The questionnaire showed acceptable convergent ($r > 0.7$) and divergent ($r < 0.4$) validities. No floor or ceiling effects were observed.

Conclusion: The HOS-Brazil was validated. Additional studies are underway to evaluate its responsiveness.

Keywords: Questionnaires, Hip, Hip outcome score, Validity, Reliability

Background

The Hip Outcome Score (HOS) is an instrument used to assess patients with hip disorders who are young, physically active, or both but who do not have severe degenerative abnormalities. Other hip assessment instruments do not address this population with the same degree of specificity [1–5].

Martin developed the HOS in the United States of America (USA) in 2005 to assess patients with acetabular labral tears who were physically active, young, or both [1]. The instrument was validated using two groups: individuals receiving hip arthroscopy and those with acetabular labral tears [6, 7].

Most quality of life instruments and orthopedic assessments were originally developed in English [1, 2, 8, 9]. For these instruments to be used across cultures and languages, several steps of translation and cross-cultural adaptation should be accomplished. These steps should be followed by validation to determine whether the new instrument conserves the psychometric characteristics of the original [10–12].

The standardized set of instructions for the translation and cultural adaptation of quality of life assessments includes five steps: translation, back-translation, review by a committee pretesting and final translation. Guillemin et al. [10] first described these criteria, which were later revised by Beaton et al. [11]. Following translation and cultural

* Correspondence: rafaelacosta87@gmail.com
[1]Medical Sciences, State University of Rio de Janeiro, Rio de Janeiro, Brazil
[5]Orthopedics Service, Pedro Ernesto University Hospital, State University of Rio de Janeiro, Rio de Janeiro, RJ, Brazil
Full list of author information is available at the end of the article

adaptation, the measurement (i.e., psychometric) properties of instruments should be tested (i.e., validated) [12–14].

The psychometric properties usually analyzed for the purpose of validation are reliability, validity, and responsiveness [12, 13]. These properties were standardized by researchers who developed consensus-based guidelines for the selection of measurement properties for the validation of health instruments (i.e., the *Consensus-based Standards for the Selection of Health Measurement Instruments*; COSMIN) to assess the methodological quality of studies that use these measurement properties [13–15].

The present study sought to validate the Brazilian version of HOS (HOS-Brazil) using a group of physically active patients diagnosed with femoroacetabular impingement (FAI) or greater trochanteric pain syndrome (GTPS). This validated questionnaire will provide doctors and other healthcare providers in Brazil with a more specific instrument to assess this population of patients. Importantly, the hip research group at Pedro Ernesto University Hospital, State University of Rio de Janeiro (Hospital Universitário Pedro Ernesto, Universidade do Estado do Rio de Janeiro; HUPE/UERJ) previously translated and culturally adapted the HOS [16].

Methods

The HUPE/UERJ research ethics committee approved the present study (CEP/HUPE no. 2674). The participants were informed of the study aims and methods before signing an informed consent document.

Patient selection

A total of 70 male and female patients who were literate and physically active who reported hip pain and were diagnosed with either FAI or GTPS (as confirmed by radiograph, tomography, or magnetic resonance imaging) were selected. The participants were recruited from the Orthopedic Institute of Tijuca, a private hip outpatient clinic in Rio de Janeiro. Data were collected between December 2015 and June 2016.

Patients were excluded if they showed visual or cognitive disorders that impaired the reading and interpretation of the questions; hip arthrosis, characterized by a minimum joint space of < 1.5 mm and a severe limitation in hip range of motion [17]; or incomplete responses to the questionnaires on day 1 and 48 h after the first application.

Study protocol

The study protocol included completing the identification form, which was composed of the clinical characteristics of the patients and the application of three quality of life assessments: the HOS-Brazil as well as the Brazilian-validated versions of 12-Item Short-

Form Health Survey (SF-12) and the Nonarthritic Hip Score (NAHS) [16, 18, 19]. The participants were instructed to complete all three questionnaires (1st application or test). Approximately 48 h later, they completed only the HOS-Brazil via e-mail (2nd application or retest).

HOS-Brazil

The HOS is a self-report questionnaire composed of 28 questions divided into two subscales: Activities of Daily Living (ADLs; 19 items) and Sports (nine items) [1, 16]. The total score of each subscale ranges from 0 to 100, where higher scores denote better hip function. The scores for each subscale were calculated separately [6].

The response options are the same for all 28 items and given specific scores that are added to the end of the assessment. Responses to the 19 items of the ADL subscale are scored from 0 to 4, where 4 is "No difficulty at all" and 0 is "Unable to perform." The scores of the individual items are added to obtain the total score, which is then multiplied by 4 to generate the highest potential score. Assuming the patients respond to all 19 items, the highest possible score is 76. The total score obtained is divided by 76. The resulting value is multiplied by 100 to express the score as a percentage. The nine items of the Sports scale are calculated in the same way, and the highest possible score is 36. A higher final score represents a better level of physical functioning with regard to both the ADL and Sports subscales [6].

In addition, the HOS includes two questions regarding how respondents rate their current level of functioning during ADLs and sports from 0 to 100 as well as one qualitative question asking them to rate their current level of functioning (normal, nearly normal, abnormal, or severely abnormal). The responses to these three questions are not considered in the HOS final score [20].

Psychometric properties

To validate the psychometric properties of the HOS-Brazil, its reliability and validity were assessed according to the COSMIN checklist [13–15].

Reliability is a psychometric property that measures the degree to which a questionnaire is free from measurement error; furthermore, this process establishes whether the scores remain similar after repeated application to the same sample on a different occasion and without the influence of treatment. The reliability of the HOS-Brazil was assessed based on the following properties: internal consistency, intra-rater test-retest reliability, measurement error, and concordance [12, 14, 21].

Internal consistency assesses the ability of a set of questions to measure a similar concept. Test-retest reliability is a measurement property that assesses the ability of a questionnaire to yield similar results when the same respondents are assessed on a different occasion without undergoing any change in health. Concordance is related to systematic and random errors in the respondents' scores that are not attributed to true changes in the construct to be measured [12, 14].

The reliability of the HOS-Brazil was investigated using a sample of 70 patients who responded to the questionnaire twice with a 48-h interval. In between applications, no new medications, therapies, or procedures were introduced that were likely to induce rapid changes to the patients' clinical conditions. The interval between the test and retest was selected based on two criteria: The period of time was held long enough for the respondents not to remember their previous responses but was simultaneously brief enough for no changes to occur to the patients' clinical conditions [12, 14].

The psychometric property of validity concerns the degree of instrument precision (i.e., whether it conserves the precision of the concept that it intends to measure). Validity assesses whether a new instrument retains the characteristics of the original version and is composed of three measurement properties: construct validity, content validity, and criterion validity [12, 14].

Construct validity corresponds to the degree to which an instrument's scores are consistent with the hypotheses based on the assumption that the instrument measures the intended construct. Content validity estimates the degree to which the content of a measurement instrument is considered as an adequate reflection of the construct to be measured. Criterion validity determines the degree to which an instrument's score adequately reflects the instrument considered as a "gold standard." Criterion validity was not assessed in the present study because, according to the COSMIN formulators, no health assessment instrument is considered as a "gold standard" [12, 14, 21]. Therefore, the validity of the HOS-Brazil was assessed based on only construct and content validity.

Statistical analyses

The intraclass correlation coefficient (ICC) and Pearson's correlation coefficient were used to analyze test-retest reliability [22, 23]. Internal consistency was assessed using Cronbach's alpha [24, 25]. This statistical technique is based on the number of items and their homogeneity within a scale. A paired-sample Student's t-test was used to compare the scores obtained for the first and second applications of the HOS-Brazil [23].

Measurement error was calculated based on the standard error of measurement (SEM) and minimal clinically important difference (MCID). SEM was calculated by multiplying the square root of 1 minus ICC times the standard deviation of the scores obtained for the first application of the HOS-Brazil. The MCID was calculated by multiplying the SEM times 1.96, which is equivalent to the z-score of the 95% confidence interval and the square root of 2 [12, 26].

Concordance was assessed based on the graphical representation of the measurement error between test and retest via Bland-Altman and concordance-survival plots [27–29]. The former quantifies concordance using limits of concordance based on the means of the test and retest as well as the difference between both assessments. These statistical limits are calculated using the mean and standard deviation of the differences. A linear regression curve of the Bland-Altman plot was modeled to assess the presence of proportional bias [27, 28]. The independent variable (x-axis) used for the linear regression was the mean of both assessments, and the dependent variable (y-axis) was the difference between both assessments. The null hypothesis stated that the slope of the regression line would not differ from zero. Proportional bias alludes to a situation in which the difference between the two measurements is not constant across the full range of possible scores as indicated by the p-value obtained for regression analysis ($p < 0.05$). If the difference between the scores obtained at two measurements is constant and independent of the scores' magnitude, then it is described as a fixed bias [27, 28].

Construct validity, both convergent and divergent, was assessed using Pearson's correlation coefficient. The HOS-Brazil was compared with the NAHS and SF 12, which have already been validated for Brazilian Portuguese. The aim of the construct validity assessment was to investigate the convergence and divergence of the HOS-Brazil relative to the NAHS and SF-12 [23]. Content validity was assessed based on the presence of completed questionnaires scored as zero or 100 (maximum score), i.e., floor or ceiling effects, respectively [30].

A descriptive statistical analysis was performed to characterize the study sample. The psychometric properties of reliability and validity were analyzed using Graph-Pad Prism software, version 7.00 for Windows (GraphPad Software, La Jolla, California, USA). The significance level was set at 0.05.

Results

Patient characteristics

Of the 70 selected patients, 46 (65.7%) were female, and 24 (34.3%) were male. The average age was 42.9 ± 12.9 years old (range: 19 to 70 years old). A total of 44 (62.9%) patients were diagnosed with GTPS, and 26 (37.1%) were diagnosed with FAI.

Questionnaire results

The scores on the three applied questionnaires ranged from 2 to 99; higher scores denoted better quality of life (SF-12) and hip function (NAHS and HOS-Brazil). Table 1 describes the means, standard deviations, minimums, and maximums associated with the applied questionnaires.

Psychometric properties

A. Reliability

1. Internal consistency

For the first application of the HOS-Brazil, Cronbach's alphas were 0.95 and 0.92 for the ADL and Sports subscales, respectively (Table 2). The elimination of any isolated question did not significantly change the Cronbach's alpha value for any subscale; therefore, no questions were eliminated from the HOS-Brazil.

2. Intra-rater test-retest reliability

The value obtained was 0.99 for both subscales, with 95% confidence intervals (95% CIs) of 0.986–0.995 and 0.990–0.996 for the ADL and Sports subscales, respectively (Table 2).

3. Measurement error and concordance

Paired-samples Student's t-tests did not show significant differences in the average test-retest scores for either the ADL ($p = 0.84$) or Sports ($p = 0.82$) subscales. The correlation between the test and retest scores was 0.992 (95% CIs = 0.986–0.996, $P < 0.0001$) for the ADL subscale and 0.994 (95% CIs = 0.990–0.996, $P < 0.0001$) for the Sports subscale.

Concordance limits and CIs were analyzed. The Bland-Altman plot showed a mean error of the difference between the test and retest scores of – 0.1 for both

Table 2 Psychometric property: Reliability

Internal consistency according to Cronbach's alpha			
Questionnaire	Subscale	Cronbach's alpha	
HOS-Brazil 1st application	ADL	0.95	
	Sports	0.92	
Intra-rater test-retest reliability			
HOS-Brazil test-retest	Subscale	ICC	Lower 95% CI	Upper 95% CI
	ADL	0.992	0.986	0.995
	Sports	0.994	0.990	0.996

HOS-Brazil Brazilian version of Hip Outcome Score, *ADL* activity of daily living, *ICC* intraclass correlation coefficient, *CI* confidence interval

subscales (95% concordance limits = – 4.5 to 4.5 for the ADL subscale and – 5.3 to 5.2 for the Sports subscale). The two dotted lines represent the upper and lower concordance limits. The P-value of the regression analysis showed that the curve slope did not deviate from zero ($P = 0.26$ for the ADL subscale, $P = 0.14$ for the Sports subscale; Fig. 1a and b).

The concordance and survival plots revealed two findings: a difference of 7 in the ADL subscale scores (Fig. 1c) and of 6 in the Sports subscale scores (Fig. 1d), representing 95% agreement between the test and retest scores.

The SEMs were 1.7 and 1.9 for the ADL and Sports subscale scores, respectively. The calculated MCID was 4.6 for the ADL subscale score and 5.5 for the Sports subscale score.

B. Validity

1. Construct validity

Convergent construct validity was estimated based on the correlation between the HOS-Brazil ADL and Sports subscale scores (1st application) and the NAHS total score and SF-12 Physical subscale score. The values of all Pearson's correlation coefficients were over 0.7,

Table 1 The questionnaire scores of 70 patients

Questionnaire	Mean	SD	Minimum score	Maximum score
NAHS 1st application – Total score	62.0	21.8	12.5	96.2
SF-12 1st application, Mental subscale	52.2	9.5	15.8	65.1
SF-12 1st application, Physical subscale	42.9	12.5	20.8	60.9
HOS-Brazil 1st application, ADL subscale	71.1	18.1	25.0	97.4
HOS-Brazil 1st application, Sports subscale	55.1	23.7	2.8	97.2
HOS-Brazil 2nd application, ADL subscale	71.0	17.8	26.3	98.6
HOS-Brazil 2nd application, Sports subscale	55.0	23.3	5.5	97.2

SD standard deviation, *NAHS* Nonarthritic Hip Score, *SF-12* 12-Item Short-Form Health Survey, *HOS-Brazil* Brazilian version of Hip Outcome Score, *ADL* activity of daily living

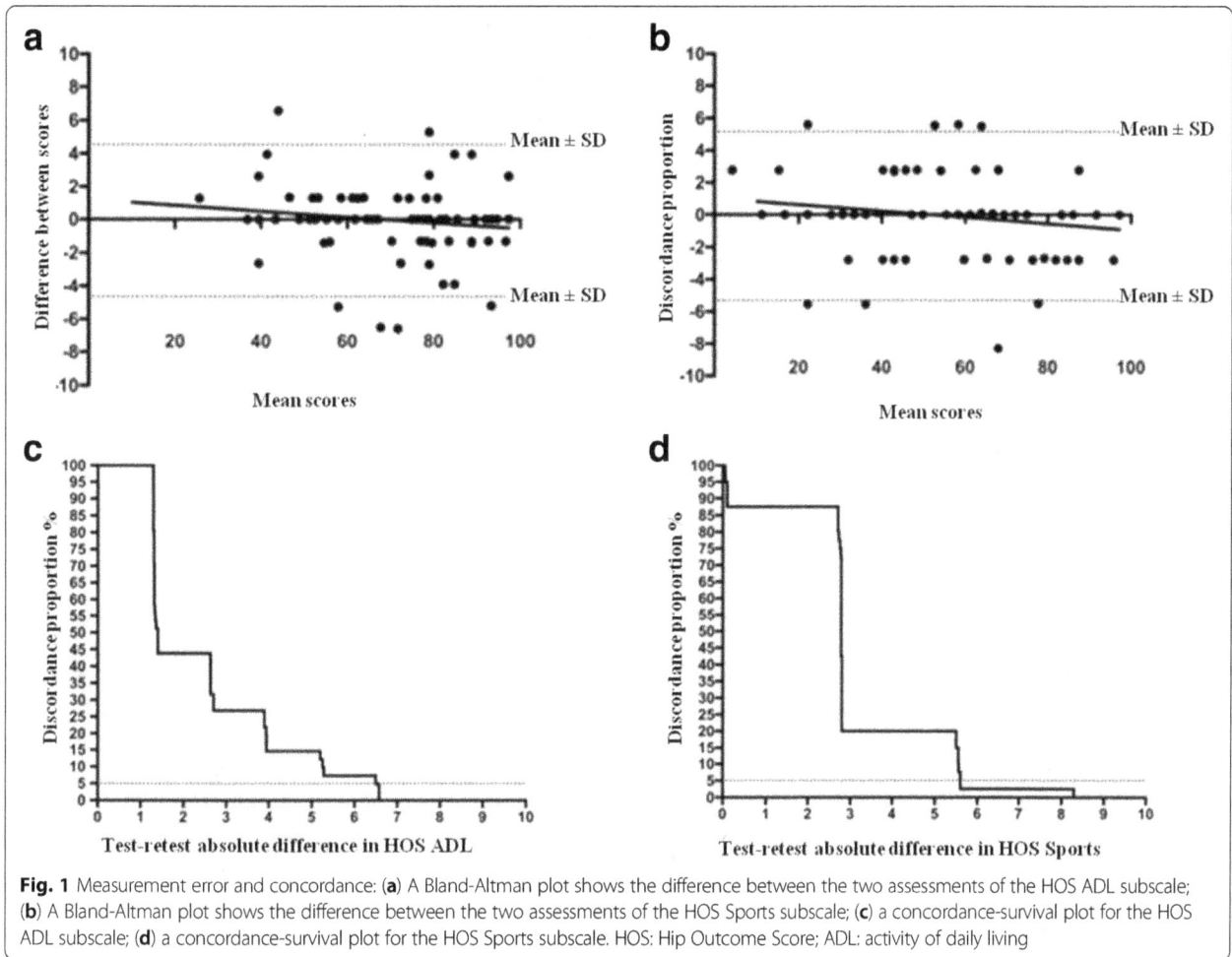

Fig. 1 Measurement error and concordance: (**a**) A Bland-Altman plot shows the difference between the two assessments of the HOS ADL subscale; (**b**) A Bland-Altman plot shows the difference between the two assessments of the HOS Sports subscale; (**c**) a concordance-survival plot for the HOS ADL subscale; (**d**) a concordance-survival plot for the HOS Sports subscale. HOS: Hip Outcome Score; ADL: activity of daily living

except for the correlation between the HOS-Brazil Sports subscale and the SF-12 Physical subscale, which was 0.685 (Table 3).

Next, the divergent construct validity between the HOS-Brazil and SF-12 was analyzed. Pearson's correlation coefficient was calculated to investigate the presence of a correlation between the HOS-Brazil ADL and

Table 3 Psychometric property: Validity

Questionnaires (subscale)	Pearson's r
Pearson's correlation coefficient for convergent validity	
HOS-Brazil (ADL subscale) vs. NAHS (total)	0.874***
HOS-Brazil (ADL subscale) vs. SF-12 (Physical subscale)	0.744***
HOS-Brazil (Sports subscale) vs. NAHS (total)	0.789***
HOS-Brazil (Sports subscale) vs. SF-12 (Physical subscale)	0.685***
Pearson's correlation coefficient for divergent validity	
HOS-Brazil (ADL subscale) vs. SF-12 (Mental subscale)	0.346**
HOS-Brazil (Sports subscale) vs. SF-12 (Mental subscale)	0.344**

HOS-Brazil Brazilian version of Hip Outcome Score, *ADL* activity of daily living, *NAHS* Nonarthritic Hip Score, *SF-12* 12-Item Short-Form Health Survey, *r* Pearson's correlation coefficient *** $p < 0.0001$; **$p = 0.003$

Sports subscale scores and the SF-12 Mental subscale score. The results obtained were less than 0.4, indicating a low correlation and, consequently, a lack of convergence (Table 3).

2. Content validity

The obtained content validity was satisfactory; no questionnaire exhibited scores of zero or 100 (maximum score); i.e., floor or ceiling effects were not found with regard to the HOS-Brazil (Fig. 2).

Discussion

The HOS is a quality of life assessment instrument specific to people with hip disease without severe degenerative abnormalities that was originally developed in English [1]. The HOS was translated and cross-culturally adapted into German, Korean, Spanish, and Brazilian Portuguese [16, 20, 31, 32]. The German, Korean, and Spanish versions are already validated for use in their corresponding countries [20, 31, 32]. A group of physically active individuals diagnosed with FAI or GTPS was

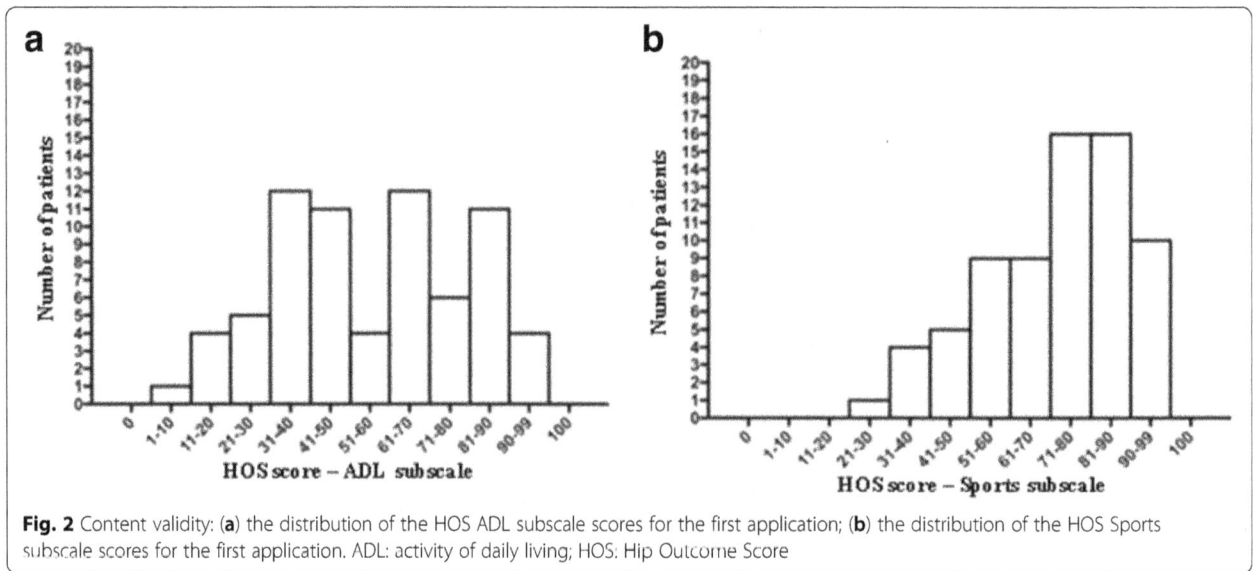

Fig. 2 Content validity: (**a**) the distribution of the HOS ADL subscale scores for the first application; (**b**) the distribution of the HOS Sports subscale scores for the first application. ADL: activity of daily living; HOS: Hip Outcome Score

selected for the present validation study of the HOS-Brazil.

A total of 70 patients with an average age of 42. 9 years were assessed for the present validation of the HOS-Brazil. In the validation studies of the German, Korean, and Spanish versions, the numbers of patients varied from 60 to 100, and their average age varied from 33 and 45 years [20, 31, 32]. Therefore, the average age of the patients included in the HOS-Brazil validation study was similar to that of the German, Korean, and Spanish studies. Females were more prevalent in the population included for the HOS-Brazil study, which matches the sample recruited to validate the original HOS as well as assess its reliability and responsiveness [6, 33].

The values for internal consistency were high (> 0.9) for both scales (0.95 and 0.92 for ADL and Sports, respectively). According to Hair et al. [25] the minimum recommended value is 0.7; 0.8 to 0.9 is rated as moderate to high; and > 0.9 is high. Therefore, the questions included in both subscales likely provide a clear reflection of the subject they investigate, which is indicative of sufficient homogeneity among all the items [24, 25]. These internal consistency findings are similar to those obtained in the validation of the original version (and other versions) of the HOS [6, 20, 31, 32].

The HOS-Brazil exhibited excellent intra-rater test-retest reliability, with an ICC of 0.992 for the ADL subscale and 0.994 for the Sports subscale. An ICC ranging from 0.4 to 0.75 is considered satisfactory, whereas values ≥0.75 are considered excellent [32]. The analysis showed that all of the ICC values resulting from the comparison of the first and second application were over 0.9 for both subscales. This finding indicates high intra-rater test-retest reliability and shows that the HOS-Brazil

is reliable. The time interval between the test and retest was 48 h.

In the validation studies of the German, Korean, and Spanish versions of the HOS, the median time between assessments was 10 to 21 days [20, 31, 32]. Perhaps these intervals were not brief enough to ensure that no changes occurred to the clinical conditions of patients. In addition, it is difficult to assert that the patients did not receive any therapeutic support during that time. Nevertheless, the results regarding the HOS-Brazil were similar to those obtained after assessing the reliability of the original HOS and the aforementioned translated versions, the overly long interval between test and retest notwithstanding [20, 31–33].

The SEMs for the HOS-Brazil ADL and Sports subscale scores were 1.7 and 1.9, respectively, and the MCIDs were 4.6 and 5.3 for these scores, respectively [12, 33]. In the reliability study of the original HOS, the MCID values were ± 4 and ± 8 for the ADL and Sports subscales scores, respectively [33]. For the German version, the SEMs were ± 4 and ± 8 for these scores, respectively, whereas the MCIDs were ± 11 and ± 22, respectively [31]. For the Spanish version, the SEMs were ± 5.1 and ± 8.5 for the ADL and Sports subscales scores, respectively, whereas the MCIDs were 13.7 and 22.8, respectively [20]. The discrepancies in the results of the HOS-Brazil compared with the German, Korean, and Spanish versions might be because of the overly long intervals between the test and retest of the latter. Knowledge of the amount of measurement error contributes to the assessment of the outcomes of surgery or other treatments received by patients as well as indicates whether clinical changes relevant to patients occurred [12, 14].

A linear regression curve was created for the Bland-Altman plot to investigate the presence of proportional deviation. The independent variable (x-axis) used in the linear regression analysis was the mean between the two assessments of the HOS-Brazil, and the dependent variable (y-axis) the difference between both assessments. The null hypothesis stated that the slope of the regression line would not differ from zero. Importantly, proportional bias alludes to a situation in which the difference between two measurements is not constant across the full range of possible scores, which demonstrates that the curve slope does not deviate from zero. When the difference in the scores between two assessments is constant, independent from the score's magnitude, it is described as fixed polarization. When the regression line is parallel to the x-axis, it provides a demonstration of a fixed bias. The differences between the values obtained in the two applications of the HOS-Brazil remained constant. This analysis quantifies concordance by constructing concordance limits [27, 28].

An analysis of the convergent validity between the HOS-Brazil ADL subscale and the NAHS showed a strong correlation (0.874). The same was true of the correlation between the HOS-Brazil Sports subscale and the SF-12 Physical subscale (0.744). In addition, the correlation between the HOS-Brazil Sports subscale and the NAHS was strong (0.789). The correlation between the HOS-Brazil Sports subscale and the SF-12 Physical subscale was only moderate (0.685). These significant (strong and moderate, respectively) correlations between the HOS-Brazil ADL and Sports subscales and the NAHS and the SF-12 Physical scale allows us to infer that the HOS-Brazil subscales are convergent with the scores of the other two instruments. The highest values correspond to the correlation between the HOS-Brazil and the NAHS, which shows that both instruments exhibit similar characteristics. This finding might be explained by the fact that the NAHS is also an instrument specific to hip disease, and its questions investigate pain, mechanical symptoms, function, and activity, whereas the SF-12 is a generic quality of life questionnaire.

An analysis of the divergent validity between the HOS-Brazil ADL and Sports subscales and the SF-12 Mental scale yielded values of 0.346 and 0.344, respectively. These are weak, non-significant correlations; on these grounds, the analyzed subscales do not converge. In this case, one might infer that a divergence exists between the scores on the HOS-Brazil ADL and Sports subscales and the SF-12 Mental subscale. As a result, one might conclude that the HOS-Brazil adequately converged and diverged relative to the target construct.

The HOS-Brazil exhibited satisfactory content validity because no questionnaire exhibited floor or ceiling effects. This result is similar to that of the validation study of the Korean version [32], but differs from the German and Spanish validation studies, which detected floor or ceiling effects [20, 31].

The validation studies of the Spanish and Korean versions of the HOS assessed the responsiveness of patients receiving surgery 6 months after treatment [20, 30]. The present validation study did not assess responsiveness because we did not apply the questionnaire to patients after a long period of time. However, the absence of this analysis does not hinder the validation of the HOS-Brazil. Additional studies assessing its responsiveness are currently in progress.

This aspect was one limitation of the present study, which was due to the lack of the prospective reassessment of patients to evaluate their sensitivity to changes in their quality of life following treatment. This limitation derived from a lack of treatment adherence. Another limitation arises from the fact that all participants were recruited from a single center that was part of a private health network in Rio de Janeiro. Therefore, the results might not reflect the experience of the entire Brazilian population.

Conclusions

The HOS-Brazil was validated using a group of physically active patients diagnosed with FAI or GTPS. The psychometric properties of reliability and validity demonstrated excellent internal consistency, intra-rater test-retest reliability, content validity and construct validity.

The present validation study of the HOS-Brazil shows that this instrument is a valid and reliable quality of life assessments in Brazilian Portuguese. Thus, it will provide doctors, physiotherapists and other healthcare providers in Brazil with the ability to assess physically active patients with hip disorders but without severe degenerative abnormalities.

Authors' contributions
RMdePC Elaboration of the article and critical review; Data collection; Data analysis and interpretation; Approval of the final version to be published. TMC Elaboration of the article and critical revision; Approval of the final version to be published. LNCDCM Critical review; Approval of the final version to be published. GL Data analysis and interpretation; Critical review; Approval of the final version to be published. LPdeO Design and study design; Data collection; Data analysis and interpretation; Critical review; Approval of the final version to be published.

Competing interests
The authors declare that they have no competing interests.

Author details
[1]Medical Sciences, State University of Rio de Janeiro, Rio de Janeiro, Brazil. [2]Medical Sciences, Rural Federal University of Rio de Janeiro, Seropédica, RJ, Brazil. [3]Biomedical Engineering, Federal University of Rio de Janeiro, Rio de Janeiro, RJ, Brazil. [4]State University of Rio de Janeiro, Rio de Janeiro, RJ, Brazil. [5]Orthopedics Service, Pedro Ernesto University Hospital, State University of Rio de Janeiro, Rio de Janeiro, RJ, Brazil.

References

1. Martin RL. Hip arthroscopy and outcome assessment. Oper Tech Orthop. 2005;15(3):290–6.
2. Christensen CP, Althausen PL, Mittleman MA, Lee JA, Mccarthy JC. The nonarthritic hip score: reliable and validated. Clin Orthop Relat Res. 2003;406:75–83.
3. Klässbo M, Larsson E, Mannevik E. Hip disability and osteoarthritis outcome score. An extension of the western Ontario and McMaster universities osteoarthritis index. Scand J Rheumatol. 2003;32(1):46–51.
4. Mohtadi NG, Griffin DR, Pedersen ME, Chan D, Safran MR. The development and validation of a self-administered quality-of-life outcome measure for young, active patients with symptomatic hip disease: the international hip outcome tool (iHOT-33). Arthroscopy. 2012;28(5):595–605.
5. Naal FD, Miozzari HH, Kelly BT, Magennis EM, Leunig M, Noetzli HP. The hip sports activity scale (HSAS) for patients with femoroacetabular impingement. Hip Int. 2013;23(2):204–11.
6. Martin RL, Kelly BT, Philippon MJ. Evidence of validity for the hip outcome score. Arthroscopy. 2006;22(12):1304–11.
7. Martin RL, Philippon MJ. Evidence of validity for the hip outcome score in hip arthroscopy. Arthroscopy. 2007;23(8):822–6.
8. Harris WH. Traumatic arthritis of the hip after dislocation and acetabular fractures: treatment by mold arthroplasty. J Bone Joint Surg Am. 1969; 51:737–55.
9. Marx FC, Oliveira LM, Bellini CG, Ribeiro MCC. Tradução e validação cultural do questionário algofuncional de Lequesne para osteoartrite de joelhos e quadris para a língua portuguesa. Rev Bras Reumatol. 2006;46(4):253–60.
10. Guillemin F, Bombardier C, Beaton D. Cross-cultural adaptation of health-related quality of life measures: literature review and proposed guidelines. J Clin Epidemiol. 1993;46(12):1417–32.
11. Beaton DE, Bombardie C, Guillemin F, Ferraz MB. Guidelines for the process of cross-cultural adaptation of self-report measures. Spine. 2000; 25(24):3186–91.
12. Scholtes VA, Terwee CB, Poolman RW. What makes a measurement instrument valid and reliable? Injury. Int J Care Injured. 2011;42:236–40.
13. Mokkink LB, Terwee CB, Knol DL, Stratford PW, Alonso J, Patrick DL, et al. Protocol of the COSMIN study: COnsensus-based standards for the selection of health measurement instruments. BMC Med Res Methodol. 2006;6:2.
14. Mokkink LB, Prinsen CAC, Bouter LM, De Vet HCW, Terwee CB. The COnsensus-based standards for the selection of health measurement instruments (COSMIN) and how to select an outcome measurement instrument. Braz J Phys Ther. 2016;20(2):105–13.
15. Mokkink LB, Terwee CB, Knol DL, Stratford PW, Alonso J, Patrick DL, et al. The COSMIN checklist for evaluating the methodological quality of studies on measurement properties: a clarification of its content. BMC Med Res Methodol. 2010;10:22.
16. Oliveira LP, Cardinot TM, Del Castillo LNC, Queiroz MC, Polesello GC. Translation and cultural adaptation of the hip outcome score to the Portuguese language. Rev Bras Ortop. 2014;49(3):297–304.
17. Croft P, Coope RC, Wickham C, Coggon D. Defining osteoarthritis of the hip for epidemiologic studies. Am J Epidemiol. 1990;132(3):514–22.
18. Silveira MF, Almeida JC, Freire RS, Haikal DS, Martins AEBL. Propriedades psicométricas do instrumento de avaliação da qualidade de vida: 12-item health survey (SF-12). Ciênc saúde coletiva. 2013;18(7):1923–31.
19. Del Castillo LN, Leporace G, Cardinot TM, Levy RA, Oliveira LP. Translation, cross-cultural adaptation and validation of the Brazilian version of the nonarthritic hip score. São Paulo Med J. 2013;131(4):244–51.
20. Seijas R, Sallent A, Ruiz-Ibán MA, Ares O, Marín-Peña O, Cuéllar R, et al. Validation of the Spanish version of the hip outcome score: a multicenter study. Health Qual Life Outcomes. 2014;12:70.
21. Mokkink LB, Terwee CB, Patrick DL, Alonso J, Stratford PW, Knol DL, et al. The COSMIN study reached international consensus on taxonomy, terminology, and definitions of measurement properties for health-related patient-reported outcomes. J Clin Epidemiol. 2010;63:737–45.
22. Bartko JJ. The Intraclass correlation coefficient as a measure of reliability. Psychol Rep. 1966;19:3–11.
23. Vieira S. Bioestatística: tópicos avançados. 3ed ed. Rio de Janeiro: Elsevier; 2010.
24. Cronbach LJ. Coefficient alpha and internal structure of tests. Psicometrika. 1951;16:297–334.
25. Hair Jr JF, Anderson RE, Tatham RL, Black WC. Análise multivariada de dados. In: Porto Alegre: Book. 6ed ed; 2009.
26. Bartlett JW, Frost C. Reliability, repeatability and reproducibility: analysis of measurement errors in continuous variables. Ultrasound Obstet Gynecol. 2008;31:466–75.
27. Altman DG, Bland JM. Measurement in medicine: the analysis of method comparison studies. Underst Stat. 1983;32:207–17.
28. Bland JM, Altman DG. Statistical methods of assessing agreement between two methods of clinical measurement. Lancet. 1986;1:307–10.
29. Luiz RR, Costa AJL, Kale PL, Werneck GL. Assessment of agreement of a quantitative variable: a new graphical approach. J Clin Epidimiol. 2003; 56(10):593–7.
30. Everitt BS, Skrondal A. The Cambridge dictionary of statistics. 4th ed. New York: Cambridge University Press; 2010.
31. Naal FD, Impellizzeri FM, Miozzari HH, Mannion AF, Leunig M. The German hip outcome score: validation in patients undergoing surgical treatment for femoroacetabular impingement. Arthroscopy. 2011;27(3):339–45.
32. Lee YK, Ha YC, Martin RL, Hwang DS, Koo KH. Transcultural adaptation of the Korean version of the hip outcome score. Knee Surg Sports Traumatol Arthrosc: Official Journal of the ESSKA. 2014;23(11):3426-31. https://doi.org/10.1007/s00167-014-2946-0.
33. Martin RL, Philippon MJ. Evidence of reliability and responsiveness for the hip outcome score. Arthroscopy. 2008;24(6):676–82.

4

Granulomatosis with polyangiitis in Northeastern Brazil: study of 25 cases

Francisco Vileimar Andrade de Azevedo[1*], Fabrício Oliveira Lima[1], Jozélio Freire de Carvalho[2], Andrea Rocha de Saboia Mont'Alverne[3] and Carlos Ewerton Maia Rodrigues[1]

Abstract

Background: Little has been published about the epidemiology of Granulomatosis with polyangiitis (GPA) in South America, especially in the intertropical zone, and no epidemiological data from Brazil are available. The purpose of the present study was to draw a clinical and demographic profile of GPA patients living in Northeastern Brazil based on laboratory, histological and imaging findings, and evaluate the frequency of organic involvement.

Methods: Clinical, epidemiological and treatment data of GPA patients were collected retrospectively and compared with the literature.

Results: The cohort included 25 GPA patients (84% female) aged 45.8 ± 16.1 years. Renal and ear-nose-throat (ENT) manifestations were the most common (both 64%). One third (32%) of the patients had 24-h proteinuria > 1 g, 50% had creatinine clearance < 50 mL/min at the time of diagnosis, and 33% had recurrent kidney damage during disease progress. The affected organs included lungs (60%), joints (44%), skin (32%), peripheral nervous system (28%), eyes (28%) and heart (16%). ENT involvement ($n = 16/64\%$) was less frequent in our region than in São Paulo ($n = 115/85.8\%$). Renal ($n = 16/64\%$) and pulmonary ($n = 15/60\%$) involvement was less frequent in our region than in the U.K. (renal $n = 30/90\%$; pulmonary $n = 28/84.8\%$).

Conclusion: Most of our patients were female, presented the generalized form and were diagnosed late. The frequency of the main clinical manifestations (ENT, renal and pulmonary) was lower than that observed at higher latitudes, suggesting the existence of a Northeast Brazilian clinical and epidemiological profile and adding to our knowledge of this rare condition.

Background

Granulomatosis with polyangiitis (GPA) is a rare systemic disease of the pauci-immune vasculitis spectrum associated with antineutrophil cytoplasmic antibodies (ANCA) [1] and affecting mainly the upper respiratory tract, lungs and kidneys [2]. Approximately 85% of GPA patients are ANCA-positive, with proteinase 3 (PR3) as the most commonly observed antigen (~ 75%) [3, 4].

GPA affects mostly adults, especially Caucasians, with no gender predominance [1]. The mean age at diagnosis is 50 years [5]. GPA is usually treated with a combination of glucocorticoids and cyclophosphamide, inducing remission in most patients [6]. The recent introduction of rituximab has further increased the rates of remission maintenance [7, 8].

The etiology of GPA is unknown, but the frequent early involvement of the upper respiratory tract suggests an environmental cause. Epidemiological studies from the northern hemisphere also support the notion of environmental risk, as reflected in regional differences in prevalence and incidence and the existence of a North-South negative gradient (the incidence of GPA is higher in Northern Europe than in Southern Europe) [5, 9, 10]. Genetic and geographical factors may explain these differences [10–12].

Little has been published about the epidemiology of GPA in South America, especially in the intertropical zone, and no epidemiological data from Brazil are

* Correspondence: vileimar@yahoo.com.br
[1]Post-Graduate Program in Medical Sciences, University of Fortaleza (UNIFOR), Fonseca Lobo 560 apto. 1202, Aldeota, Fortaleza, Ceará CEP 60175020, Brazil
Full list of author information is available at the end of the article

available [13–17]. The only two Brazilian studies investigating the clinical and laboratory profile of GPA patients reported a spectrum of clinical manifestations similar to that found in the international literature [13, 14]. However, these Brazilian studies on GPA were conducted outside the intertropical zone [13, 14].

The purpose of the present study was to draw a clinical and demographic profile of GPA patients living in Northeastern Brazil based on laboratory, histological and imaging findings, and evaluate the frequency of organic involvement in relation to data from the international literature.

Methods
Study design and patient selection
This descriptive, retrospective and cross-sectional multicenter study was based on medical records covering a period of 10 years (January 2006 to January 2016). The study area was the metropolitan region of Fortaleza, a state capital in Northeastern Brazil located in the intertropical zone (03° 43′S), with an estimated population just over 4 million [18].

Medical records of patients diagnosed as having "Wegener's granulomatosis", "granulomatosis with polyangiitis", "vasculitis" or International Classification of Diseases (ICD-10) code M31.3 were obtained from three public rheumatology referral centers and from private clinics located in the metropolitan region of Fortaleza to which GPA patients are referred for evaluation. The medical records were reviewed by a single investigator (FVAA). Ambiguous cases were discussed by two rheumatologists (CEMR and FVAA) until reaching a consensus. Two patients did not meet the clinical diagnostic criteria for GPA and were excluded.

To be eligible, patients had to be living in the metropolitan region of Fortaleza and meet the criteria of the classification algorithm of the European Medicines Agency (EMA) [19].

Data collection
The information retrieved from medical records included demographic data, comorbidities, disease extension (localized / early systemic / generalized / severe / refractory) [20], clinical manifestations (including signs and symptoms at diagnosis and during the course of the disease), treatment and histopathological, radiologic and laboratory findings. The clinical parameters and definitions of organ involvement were based on the Birmingham Vasculitis Activity Score (BVAS; version 3) and were actively searched for in the medical records [21].

The following clinical parameters were actively searched for:

- *Upper respiratory tract*: rhinorrhea, crusting, nosebleed, oral and nasopharyngeal ulceration, chronic sinusitis, otitis media, saddle nose deformity, mastoiditis, hearing loss and subglottic stenosis.

- *Lungs*: hemoptysis, alveolar hemorrhage, respiratory failure and pulmonary infiltrates (in the absence of concurrent infection), nodules or cavitations.
- *Kidneys*: fall in creatinine clearance > 25%, proteinuria > 500 mg/day, hematuria or red blood cell casts in urinary sediment.
- *Joints*: arthritis, polyarthralgias or morning stiffness for > 1 h.
- *Skin*: petechiae or purpura, nodules, skin vasculitis and skin ulcers.
- *Eyes*: conjunctivitis, episcleritis, scleritis, pseudotumor, amaurosis.
- *Nervous system*: peripheral neuritis, cranial neuropathy, pachymeningitis or CNS vasculitis.
- *Heart:* valvular lesions, pericarditis, myocarditis, conduction system abnormalities.
- *Gastrointestinal tract*: mesenteric vasculitis, bloody diarrhea, colitis.

The laboratory data included complete blood count, serum creatinine, urine analysis, 24-h urine protein output and immunological markers (ANCA and PR3/MPO). ANCA was detected by indirect immunofluorescence with ethanol-fixed neutrophils and specificity for PR3-ANCA and MPO-ANCA was determined by ELISA. The tests were carried out at two core laboratories. Creatinine clearance was estimated using the equation developed by the Chronic Kidney Disease Epidemiology Collaboration (CKD-EPI) [22]. Peripheral nervous system involvement was diagnosed based on electroneuromyographic changes. The histopathological examination was considered positive when findings were compatible with vasculitis with granulomatous changes, or necrotizing vasculitis, or pauci-immune necrotizing glomerulonephritis.

Limited GPA was diagnosed in cases with symptoms limited to a single organ and without kidney involvement. The extension of organ injury secondary to GPA was quantified with the Vasculitis Damage Index (VDI) based on the most recent medical appointment [23]. Disease activity at the time of diagnosis was quantified with the Birmingham Vasculitis Activity Score (BVAS, v.3) [21].

The evaluation of comorbidities included information on systemic arterial hypertension, thyroid pathologies, diabetes mellitus and obesity.

Refractoriness to treatment was defined as progressive decline in kidney function with active urine sedimentation and persistence of (or the appearance of new) extrarenal manifestations. Relapse was defined as post-remission recurrence of signs and symptoms of active vasculitis in any organ [24].

Statistical analysis
The prevalence was calculated by dividing the number of GPA patients on 31 January 2016 by the population of the metropolitan region of Fortaleza in 2016, as estimated

by the Brazilian Institute of Geography and Statistics. Demographic and clinical parameters were expressed as mean values ± standard deviation (continuous variables) and frequencies and percentages (categorical variables). Non-normally distributed continuous variables were expressed as median values (maximum and minimum). The clinical, epidemiological and laboratory data were collected and managed with a standardized instrument, creating a database with individual patient entries. Microsoft Excel© spreadsheets were used for descriptive statistics.

The study protocol was approved by the Research Ethics Committee of the University of Fortaleza (Unifor) and by the IRBs of the three participating referral centers.

Results

Patient characteristics and demographic profile

The demographic and clinical characterisitics of the 25 GPA patients included in the study are shown in Table 1. Caucasians accounted for 28%. The disease extension was predominantly generalized (52%). Twelve percent of the patients were classified as "severe extension" and 20% as "localized disease". Time between the onset of clinical manifestations and diagnosis varied greatly, and diagnosis took over 6 months to be established in 46%. The 2016 prevalence of GPA the metropolitan region of Fortaleza was estimated at 5.0/1,000,000 pop.

As for comorbidities at the time of diagnosis, 40% were receiving treatment for systemic arterial hypertension, one patient had Hashimoto's thyroiditis and one had type-2 diabetes mellitus. A summary of the demographic, clinical and laboratory data is presented in Table 1.

Clinical manifestations

Renal and ENT involvement were the most common manifestations in our cohort ($n = 16/64\%$). The type and frequency of the clinical manifestations at presentation and/or during the course of the disease are shown in Table 2.

Nephritic syndrome was the most frequent manifestation (52%) among patients with renal impairment. The lungs were affected in 15 patients (60%). One patient had a chest CT displaying bibasilar pulmonary infiltrate with tree-in-bud sign suggestive of pulmonary fibrosis with honeycombing.

Laboratory and anatomopathological findings

Most patients (88%) were ANCA-positive (c-ANCA 91%; p-ANCA 9%). Anti-PR3 ELISA was only performed on 4 patients, yielding 100% positivity. At diagnosis, the median ANCA titer on immunofluorescence was 1:320 (range: 20–640), the median 24-h urine protein output was 858 mg (range: 56–26,350) and the mean hemoglobin level was 11.3 ± 2.5 g/dL.

Biopsies were taken from 15 patients: four skin biopsies revealing leukocytoclastic vasculitis ($n = 3$) and Churg Strauss granuloma ($n = 1$), four kidney biopsies revealing pauci-immune crescentic glomerulonephritis ($n = 1$), focal segmental glomerulosclerosis ($n = 1$), diffuse proliferative glomerulonephritis ($n = 1$) and acute tubular necrosis ($n = 1$), two bronchial biopsies revealing granulomatous vasculitis, two pulmonary nodule biopsies revealing granulomatous vasculitis with organizing pneumonia, two nasal mucosa biopsies revealing granulomatous vasculitis, and one sural nerve biopsy revealing granulomatous vasculitis.

Frequency of clinical manifestations: Northeastern Brazil vs. other regions

Tables 3 and 4 show the frequency of clinical manifestations observed in the present study (Northeastern Brazil) and in studies from the northern and southern hemispheres.

- ENT involvement was less frequent in Northeastern Brazil ($n = 16$; 64%) than in São Paulo ($n = 115$; 85.8%) and New Zealand ($n = 63$; 86%) [11, 13].

Table 1 Demographic, clinical and laboratory data of a cohort of 25 patients from Northeastern Brazil diagnosed with granulomatosis with polyangiitis (GPA) between 2005 and 2016

Demographic, clinical and laboratory variables	$n = 25$
Female gender (%)	84
Months from diagnosis to present age, median (range)	45 (1–120)
ANCA positivity (%)	88
Months from onset of manifestations to diagnosis, median (range)	6 (1–192)
Biopsy performed (%)	60
Rate of biopsies positive for granuloma (%)	47
BVAS score at diagnosis, median (range)	6 (2–16)
VDI score, median (range)	4 (0–12)

ANCA antineutrophil cytoplasmic antibodies, BVAS Birmingham vasculitis activity score, VDI vasculitis damage index. Results expressed as mean values ± standard deviation, percentages or median values (maximum and minimum)

Table 2 Frequency of clinical manifestations in 25 patients from Northeastern Brazil diagnosed with granulomatosis with polyangiitis (GPA) between 2005 and 2016

Organ/system (n = 25)	n (%)	Clinical manifestation	n (%)
Kidney	16 (64)	Nephritic syndrome	13/16 (81)
		Creatinine clearance < 50 mL/min at diagnosis	12/16 (75)
		Microscopic hematuria at presentation	12/16 (75)
		Proteinuria > 1 g/day (mg/24 h)	8/16 (50)
		Proteinuria > 1 g/day (mg/24 h) at presentation	6/16 (38)
		Nephrotic-range proteinuria	5/16 (31)
		Chronic kidney disease requiring dialysis	4/16 (25)
Nose, ear, throat	16 (64)	Sinusitis	15/16 (93)
		Sensorineural deafness	3/16 (18)
		Mastoiditis	2/16 (13)
Lung	15 (60)	Pulmonary nodule	7/15 (47)
		Alveolar hemorrhage	4/15 (27)
		Bronchial stenosis	2/15 (13)
Constitutional manifestations	12 (48)	Fever	9/12 (75)
		Asthenia	2/12 (17)
Joints	11 (44)	Oligo/polyarthritis	11/11 (100)
Skin	8 (32)	Purpura of lower limbs	8/8 (100)
		Churg-Strauss nodule	1/8 (13)
Peripheral nervous system	7 (28)	Axonal polyneuropathy	4/7 (57)
		Multiple mononeuritis	2/7 (28)
		Facial nerve paralysis	1/7 (14)
Eyes	7 (28)	Orbital pseudotumor	3/7 (42)
		Scleritis	3/7 (42)
		Conjunctivitis	2/7 (28)
		Uveitis	1/7 (14)
Heart	4 (16)	Mitral insufficiency	2/4 (50)
		Congestive heart failure	1/4 (25)
		Third-degree atrioventricular block	1/4 (25)
Central nervous system	1 (4)	Transverse myelitis	1/1 (100)
Gastrointestinal tract	1 (4)	Bloody diarrhea	1/1 (100)

- Pulmonary involvement was less frequent in Northeastern Brazil (n = 15; 60%) than in the U.K. (n = 28; 84.8%) [25].
- Renal involvement was less frequent in Northeastern Brazil (n = 16; 64%) than in the U.K. (n = 30; 90%) [25].

Treatment

All 25 patients received corticosteroids as first-line therapy. Treatment for GPA consisted of a combination of corticosteroids and cyclophosphamide in 56% of the patients. All patients received intravenous cyclophosphamide

Table 3 Frequency of clinical manifestations in patients with granulomatosis with polyangiitis (GPA) from Northeastern Brazil (present study) and other countries in the southern hemisphere

Organ/system involved n (%)	Northeastern Brazil (present study)	Southeastern Brazil (Souza et al., [13])	Chile (Cisternas et al., [15])	New Zealand (Gibson et al., [11])
Number of patients	25	134	58	73
ENT symptoms	16 (64%)	115 (85.8%)	33 (57%)	63 (86%)
Lung involvement	15 (60%)	104 (77.6%)	36 (62%)	38 (52%)
Renal involvement	16 (64%)	101 (75.4%)	45 (78%)	57 (78%)

Table 4 Comparison of frequency of clinical manifestations in patients with granulomatosis with polyangiitis (GPA) from Northeastern Brazil (present study) and from three countries in the northern hemisphere

Organ/system involved n (%)	Northeastern Brazil (present study)	U.K. (Fujimoto et al., [25])	Japan (Fujimoto et al., [25])	Italy (Catanoso et al., [10])
Number of patients	25	33	8	18
ENT symptoms	16 (64%)	28 (85%)	8 (100%)	10 (55.6%)
Lung involvement	15 (60%)	28 (85%)	3 (38%)	10 (55.6%)
Renal involvement	16 (64%)	30 (90%)	3 (38%)	10 (55.6%)

in monthly pulses. Azathioprine was the drug most frequently used for maintenance (36%). Due to pulmonary-renal syndrome, 1 (4%) patient had plasmapheresis and 1 (4%) required immunoglobulin therapy. Nine (36%) were treated with rituximab: 4 due to glomerulonephritis refractory to cyclophosphamide, 1 due to recurrence of renal activity after one year of maintenance with azathioprine, 2 due to alveolar hemorrhage, 1 due to orbital pseudotumor and 1 due to sensory axonal polyneuropathy. The last four patients were refractory to cyclophosphamide therapy or presented recurrent infection during immunosuppression (Table 5).

Adverse events and mortality

Infections requiring hospitalization included 2 cases of recurrent pneumonia, 1 case of recurrent pyelonephritis and 1 case of lung abscess. No patient presented *Pneumocystis jirovecii* pneumonia or active tuberculosis, but 2 had a history of tuberculosis treated more than five years before GPA diagnosis.

Seven (28%) of the 25 patients presented new onset or worsening of systemic arterial hypertension and one patient developed diabetes mellitus after GPA diagnosis. Two developed osteoporosis, one of whom with pathological fracture.

Within the study period, 4 deaths were confirmed. Two occurred within one year after diagnosis due to severe pulmonary hemorrhage and rapidly progressing glomerulonephritis (pulmonary-renal syndrome), and 2 occurred years after diagnosis, due to diffuse alveolar hemorrhage in dialytic patients. The 5-year and 10-year mortality rate was 10 and 22%, respectively. The ability of BVAS scores at diagnosis to predict mortality was evaluated, however no association was observed between BVAS score and fatal outcome. BVAS > 6: (dead: $n = 1$; alive: $n = 9$); BVAS ≤6: (dead: $n = 3$; alive: $n = 12$) ($p = 0.627$).

Discussion

This is the largest retrospective multicenter study to draw a clinical and epidemiological profile of patients with GPA from Northeastern Brazil and the first to systematically use BVAS and VDI scores. Compared to the international literature, the upper respiratory tract and

the lungs were less frequently affected in our patients from Northeastern Brazil [11, 13, 25]. The most frequent disease extension was generalized, and time to diagnosis was relatively long (in one case, 18 years from the onset of symptoms).

Our sample was predominantly female (84%; M/F ratio: 0.2). Gender distribution is known to be influenced by geographical variables [10]. For example, the female gender was predominant in a study from Southern Europe while the male gender was predominant in a study from Northern Europe [5, 10]. Within the southern hemisphere, the male gender is predominant in New Zealand (43°S) (M/F ratio: 1.2) and Argentina (31°S) (M/F ratio: 1.2), while the female gender is predominant in Chile (33°S) (M/F ratio: 0.8) and São Paulo (23°S) (M/F ratio: 0.9) [11, 13, 15, 16]. In short, available data suggest a tendency for female predominance among GPA patients at low latitudes in both hemispheres [10].

The average age at diagnosis in the present study (42 years) was similar to that observed in studies from São Paulo (43.4 years) and the U.S. (41 years) [1, 13], but GPA patients from Chile (50.8 years), Australia (55 years), New Zealand (66 years) and Italy (58.8 years) were significantly older [10, 11, 15, 26], possibly due to differences in geographical variables and/or in methodology. In fact, populational studies suggest GPA is more frequent in older individuals whereas case studies conducted at hospitals show a lower age at diagnosis [5, 27, 28].

Matching the literature, ENT was the most frequently involved organ system, followed by the lung [1, 5, 10]. The most frequent pulmonary manifestation was pulmonary nodules, as observed in other studies conducted in the southern hemisphere [11, 13]. Sinus disorder was the main manifestation of ENT involvement observed, but the frequency was still significantly lower in our study than in studies from Southeastern Brazil and New Zealand [11, 13]. The observed prevalence of skin involvement (32%, all of which included purpura) was comparable to that reported in another Brazilian study and in studies conducted in the northern hemisphere. With a frequency of less than 30%, PNS involvement (predominantly axonal polyneuropathy) was within the range reported worldwide [1, 13, 29]. Ocular involvement was less frequent in Northeastern Brazil ($n = 1$; 4%) than in New Zealand ($n = 15$; 20%) [11].

Table 5 Clinical, histopathological, therapeutic, evolutional, therapeutic and laboratory data of 25 patients from Northeastern Brazil diagnosed with granulomatosis with polyangiitis (GPA) between 2005 and 2016

Patient	Sex	1stM → D (months)	Clinical manifestations	Current 24-h UPO	ANCA	Biopsy	Therapy
1	F	6	nephritic syndrome, hemoptysis, CKD	1461	c-Anca + Tu	n/a	CS, CFM
2	F	1	Hemoptysis, nephritic syndrome, AKI, purpura, sinusitis, mastoiditis, acral necrosis	816	c-Anca + 1:80	n/a	CS, CFM
3	F	3.5	sinusitis, scleritis, multiple mononeuritis, pulmonary nodule, polyneuropathy, CHF, nephritic syndrome; AKI	3760	c-Anca + Tu	Pulmonary nodule: granulomatous vasculitis with OP	CS, CFM, RTX
4	M	6	laryngitis, sinusitis, pulmonary nodule, hemoptysis, upper respiratory tract stenosis	150	c-Anca + 1:320	n/a	CS, CFM, RTX
5	F	66	sinusitis, polyarthritis, purpura laryngitis, bronchial stenosis	130	c-Anca -	Skin: LCV	CS, CFM
6	F	0.5	sinusitis, CKD, alveolar hemorrhage, death	n/a	c-Anca + 1:640	n/a	CS, CFM
7	F	84	sinusitis, polyarthritis, saddle nose deformity, pulmonary nodule	74	c-Anca -	Nasal mucosa: granulomatous vasculitis	CS
8	F	36	multiple mononeuritis, transverse myelitis, neurosensory deafness, sinusitis, uveitis, polyarthritis,, polyneuropathy, laryngitis, pulmonary nodule	150	c-Anca -	n/a	CS, CFM, RTX
9	F	216	sinusitis, saddle nose deformity nephritic syndrome, polyarthritis, dialytic AKI	n/a	c-Anca + 1:40	n/a	CS
10	F	12	neurosensory deafness, polyarthritis, nephrotic syndrome, nephritic syndrome, epistaxis, dialytic CKD, alveolar hemorrhage, death	385	c-Anca + 1:160	n/a	CS, AZA, RTX
11	M	120	polyarthritis, purpura; sinusitis, orbital pseudotumor, otitis media, pericardial effusion	64	c-Anca + Tu	n/a	CS, AZA, RTX
12	F	0.5	polyarthritis, nephritic syndrome; epistaxis, mastoiditis, scleritis, pulmonary nodule, facial nerve paralysis, CKD, mitral insufficiency	1680	c-Anca + 1:160	Bronchial lesion: granulomatous vasculitis	CS, AZA
13	M	5	neurosensory deafness, polyneuropathy, polyarthritis, purpura, acral necrosis, nephritic syndrome; pulmonary nodule	150	c-Anca + 1:640	Sural nerve: granulomatous vasculitis	CS, AZA
14	F	5	neurosensory deafness, sinusitis, nephritic syndrome, pulmonary nodule	1078	c-Anca + 1:40	Kidney: diffuse proliferative GN	CS, CFM
15	F	192	scleritis, polyarthritis, epistaxis, orbital pseudotumor, sinusitis, hemoptysis, AKI, amaurosis	511	p-Anca + 1:640	Kidney: acute tubular necrosis	CS, CFM
16	F	42	nodular scleritis, neurosensory deafness, polyarthritis, pulmonary nodule, third-degree AVB, cutaneous nodule	200	c-Anca + 1:640	Skin: Churg-Strauss granuloma; pulmonary nodule: granulomatous vasculitis with OP	CS, CFM
17	F	120	Purpura, hemoptysis, cutaneous nodule, polyarthritis, CKD, orbital pseudotumor,	900	c-Anca + 1:320	Nasal mucosa: granulomatous vasculitis	CS, CFM, AZA, RTX
18	F	0.5	purpura, pulmonary-renal syndrome, death	n/a	c-Anca + 1:320	Skin: LCV	CS, IMGN
19	M	1	polyarthritis, nephrotic syndrome, pulmonary-renal syndrome, death	26,350	c-Anca + 1:80	Bronchial: granulomatous vasculitis	CS, CFM, PLASMF
20	F	1	sinusitis, purpura, polyarthritis, nephritic syndrome	775	c-Anca + 1:640	Kidney: FSGS	CS, CFM, RTX
21	F	120	hemoptysis, otitis media, sinusitis	140	c-Anca + 1:640	n/a	CS, AZA, RTX
22	F	32	Raynaud phenomen, vertigo, polyneuropathy, purpura, sinusitis	150	c-Anca + 1:20	Skin: LCV	CS, AZA

Table 5 Clinical, histopathological, therapeutic, evolutional, therapeutic and laboratory data of 25 patients from Northeastern Brazil diagnosed with granulomatosis with polyangiitis (GPA) between 2005 and 2016 *(Continued)*

Patient	Sex	1stM → D (months)	Clinical manifestations	Current 24-h UPO	ANCA	Biopsy	Therapy
23	F	3	polyarthritis, hemoptysis, nephritic syndrome, AKI, nephrotic syndrome	4300	c-Anca + 1:160	Kidney: pauci-immune crescentic GN	CS, RTX
24	F	n/a	sinusitis, anosmia, pulmonary fibrosis	n/a	p-Anca + 1:640	n/a	CS, CFM
25	F	3	Scleritis, purpura, polyarthritis, sinusitis, Cushing's syndrome	n/a	c-Anca + 1:80	Skin: LCV	CS, MTX

M male, *F* female, *1stM → D* time in months from first manifestation of GPA to diagnosis, *ANCA* antineutrophil cytoplasmic antibodies, *UPO* urine protein output, *CFM* cyclophosphamide, *RTX* rituximab, *AZA* azathioprine, *CS* corticosteroids, *AKI* acute kidney injury, *IMGN* immunoglobulin, *PLASM* plasmapheresis, *GN* glomerulonephritis, *CKD* chronic kidney disease, *AVB* atrioventricular block, *CHF* congestive heart failure, *OP* organizing pneumonia, *LCV* leukocytoclastic vasculitis, *Tu* titer unavailable, *FSGS* focal segmental glomerulosclerosis

The observed frequency of cardiac involvement (16%) matched the findings of other epidemiological studies but was lower than the frequency reported in case studies (25–46%) [30]. CNS and gastrointestinal tract involvement was rare, as in most other studies [13, 29].

Two thirds (4/6) of our patients with 24-h proteinuria > 1 g at the time of diagnosis developed CKD after one year, with three patients requiring permanent dialysis. According to Neumann and coworkers, high levels of proteinuria at diagnosis in patients with ANCA-related glomerulonephritis may be predictive of poor renal prognosis [31]. The present study was limited by the unavailability of follow-up data to determine the frequency of development of CKD in patients with normal urine protein output (or < 1 g) at the time of diagnosis. An expressive number of patients in our sample presented proteinuria in the nephrotic range (31%). The degree of proteinuria in patients with GPA is most often subnephrotic [1]. High levels of proteinuria (> 3 g/day) seem to be most common in patients who present later in the course of the disease and who have had previous necrotizing glomerulonephritis, leading to more focal and segmental glomerulosclerosis/fibrosis at the time of presentation. On the other hand, GPA patients with high levels of proteinuria may have a concurrent glomerular disease (e.g., membranous nephropathy) or an atypical histological pattern characterized by glomerular immune complex deposition [32, 33].

Patients with BVAS scores below and above the cohort average did not differ with regard to the frequency of renal involvement. Two patients who developed CKD had low BVAS scores (< 6) at diagnosis, suggesting factors other than kidney damage (possibly old age and late diagnosis and treatment) contributed to the poor prognosis in these cases.

Our ANCA positivity rate (87.5%) was compatible with international reports (85%) [4]. All patients presenting with the limited form of the disease were ANCA-positive. This is higher than previously published rates (up to 40% ANCA negativity) [4]. The fact that only 4 ANCA-positive patients were submitted to anti-PR3 ELISA (c-ANCA $n = 3$;

p-ANCA $n = 1$) was an unfortunate limiting factor in our clinical and epidemiological analysis of the anti-PR3 profile of GPA patients from Northeastern Brazil. The infrequent use of anti-PR3 ELISA in our sample prevented the adoption of GPA classification criteria based specifically on this assay (e.g., modified ACR) [34]. On the other hand, the use of the EMA algorithm offered the possibility of detecting ANCA by indirect immunofluorescence in settings with little or no access to anti-PR3 ELISA [19]. The EMA algorithm uses the 1990 criteria of the American College of Rheumatology (ACR) and the definition of the Chapel Hill Consensus Conference, in addition to the criteria of positive serology for ANCA [19, 35, 36].

ANCA-positive patients with high titers (1:640) (7/7) had low BVAS scores at diagnosis. While there is no consensus on the role of ANCA positivity in the prognosis of GPA patients, Finkielman and colleagues concluded that high ANCA titers were not predictive of disease activity, activity score or organ system affected at the time of recurrence [37].

The observed differences in the frequency of certain types of clinical manifestations (e.g., ENT and pulmonary) between Northeastern Brazil and other regions in the northern and southern hemispheres may be explained by the influence of environmental and latitudinal factors on clinical phenotype. One study showed an inverse relation between GPA incidence and the intensity of UV radiation at specific latitudes, implying Vitamin D synthesis is a major determining factor of the observed gradients [12]. The fact that only 30% of our cohort was Caucasian (the remainder being of primarily indigenous race) should be taken into account when interpreting our findings.

The cohorts of most European studies consist almost exclusively of Caucasians [9, 38]. Likewise, in a U.S. cohort study, over 90% of GPA patients were Caucasian while only 4% were Afro-American, Hispanic or Asian [1].

Improvement in kidney function after combination therapy with glucocorticoids and cyclophosphamide is well documented and is known to revert kidney damage in patients presenting with kidney failure [39]. In the present study, half the patients (4/8) treated endovenously with cyclophosphamide due to glomerulonephritis with creatinine clearance < 50 mL/min at the time of diagnosis recovered kidney function. The other 4 developed CKD, 3 (38%; 3/8) of whom requiring permanent dialysis. Based on its successful use in ANCA-positive vasculitis and its greater likelihood of effectiveness against recurrence (compared to cyclophosphamide) and greater effectiveness at maintenance (compared to azathioprine), rituximab was administered to 32% of our patients, three quarters of whom presented renal involvement [7, 8, 40].

The incidence of infection (including two cases in which infection contributed to the fatal outcome) was low in our cohort. Physicians in Northeastern Brazil are advised to include tuberculosis (a granulomatous disease highly prevalent in the region, with clinical manifestations not unlike those of GPA) in the differential diagnosis of GPA [41]. Despite the fact that some of our patients had a history of contact with, or treatment for, or chest x-rays suggesting tuberculosis (e.g., cavitations and tree-in-bud), no active tuberculosis was observed. However, few patients in our cohort were submitted to the Mantoux test, especially those diagnosed in the five years preceding the study. This is partly due to a lack of supplies in the Brazilian public health care system (SUS) nationwide and partly due to limited access to testing for lymphocyte response against *M. tuberculosis* (interferon-γ release assay). In addition, the frequency of ANCA positivity among patients diagnosed with tuberculosis can introduce a bias in the investigation of suspected cases (10–33% of patients with this condition are ANCA-positive) [42].

Two early deaths (within one year of diagnosis) occurred during the study period (8%). This is compatible with other studies reporting 6–11% early mortality from GPA [43, 44].

The study has a number of limitations as a result of the retrospective design, the inclusion of multiple centers and the extensive period sampled. Thus, the collected information was not always homogenous and complete. The lack of serial follow-up made it impossible to evaluate renal survival and compare clinical and prognostic factors. Possible loss to follow-up associated with difficulties in the diagnosis of the limited form of GPA and high mortality rates among patients with the diffuse form may have led to underreporting.

Conclusions

In this study from Northeastern Brazil, most patients were female, had the generalized form of the disease, presented nephritic syndrome during the evolution of the disease and were diagnosed late. Overall, the frequency of clinical manifestations was comparable to that reported in the international literature, with some differences in relation to the northern hemisphere (pulmonary and renal involvement) and the southern hemisphere (ENT involvement), suggesting the existence of a Northeast Brazilian clinical and epidemiological profile and adding to our knowledge of this rare condition.

Funding
The authors declare that there is no funding sources regarding the publication of this paper.

Authors' contributions
FVAA collected the study data, analyzed the results and wrote the paper. FOL analyzed the results. JFC interpreted the patient data regarding the clinical and laboratory characteristics. ARSM analyzed the results and CEMR was a major contributor in writing the manuscript. All authors contributed to the preparation of this manuscript, read and approved the final manuscript.

Competing interests
The authors declare that they have no competing interests.

Author details
[1]Post-Graduate Program in Medical Sciences, University of Fortaleza (UNIFOR), Fonseca Lobo 560 apto. 1202, Aldeota, Fortaleza, Ceará CEP 60175020, Brazil. [2]Division of Rheumatology, Federal University of Bahia, Salvador, Bahia, Brazil. [3]Division of Rheumatology, University of Fortaleza (UNIFOR), Fortaleza, Brazil.

References
1. Hoffman GS, Kerr GS, Leavitt RY, Hallahan CW, Lebovics RS, Travis WD, et al. Wegener granulomatosis: an analysis of 158 patients. Ann Intern Med. 1992;116(6):488–98.
2. Hagen EC, Daha MR, Hermans J, Andrassy K, Csernok E, Gaskin G, et al. Diagnostic value of standardized assays for anti-neutrophil cytoplasmic antibodies in idiopathic systemic vasculitis. EC/BCR project for ANCA assay standardization. Kidney Int. 1998;53:743–53.
3. Hoffman GS, Specks U. Antineutrophil cytoplasmic antibodies. Arthritis Rheum. 1998;41:1521–37.
4. Koldingsnes W, Nossent H. Epidemiology of Wegener's granulomatosis in northern Norway. Arthritis Rheum. 2000;43:2481–7.
5. Falk RJ, Hogan S, Carey TS, Jennette JC. Clinical course of anti-neutrophil cytoplasmic autoantibody-associated glomerulonephritis and systemic vasculitis. The Glomerular Disease Collaborative Network. Ann Intern Med. 1990;113:656–63.
6. Nachman PH, Hogan SL, Jennette JC, Falk RJ. Treatment response and relapse in antineutrophil cytoplasmic autoantibody-associated microscopic polyangiitis and glomerulonephritis. J Am Soc Nephrol. 1996;7(1):33–9.
7. Besada E, Koldingsnes W, Nossent JC. Long-term efficacy and safety of pre-emptive maintenance therapy with rituximab in granulomatosis with polyangiitis: results from a single center. Rheumatology. 2013;52:2041–7.
8. Guillevin L, Pagnoux C, Karras A, Khouatra C, Aumaître O, Cohen P, et al. Rituximab versus azathioprine for maintenance in ANCA associated vasculitis. N Engl J Med. 2014;371:1772–80.
9. Watts R, Lane S, Scott D, Koldingsnes W, Nossent H, Gonzalez-gay m, et al. Epidemiology of vasculitis in Europe. Ann Rheum Dis. 2001;60:1156–7.
10. Catanoso M, Macchioni P, Boiardi L, Manenti L, Tumiati B, Cavazza A, et al. Epidemiology of granulomatosis with polyangiitis (Wegener's granulomatosis) in Northern Italy: a 15-year population-based study. Semin Arthritis Rheum. 2014;44:202–7.
11. Gibson A, Stamp LK, Chapman PT, O'Donnel JL. The epidemiology of Wegener's granulomatosis and microscopic polyangiitis in a Southern hemisphere region. Rheumatology. 2006;45:624–8.
12. Gatenby PA, Lucas RM, Engelsen O, Ponsonby AL, Clements M. Antineutrophil cytoplasmic antibody-associated vasculitides: could geographic patterns be explained by ambient ultraviolet radiation? Arthritis Rheum. 2009;61:1417–24.

13. Souza FHC, Halpern ASR, Barbas CSV, Shinjo SK. Wegener's granulomatosis: experience from a Brazilian tertiary center. Clin Rheumatol. 2010;29:855–60.

14. Rodrigues CEM, Callado MRM, Nobre CA, Moura FEA, Vieira RMRA, Albuquerque LAF, et al. Prevalência das manifestações clínicas iniciais da granulomatose de Wegener no Brasil – Relato de seis casos e revisão da literatura. Rev Bras Reumatol. 2010;50:150–64.

15. Cisternas M, Soto L, Jacobelli S, Marinovic MA, Vargas A, Sobarzo E, et al. Características clínicas de granulomatosis de Wegener y poliangeítis microscópica em pacientes chilenos. Rev Med Chil. 2005;133:273–8.

16. Gamron S, Muscellini EM, Onetti L, Menso E, Martelloto G, Barberis G, et al. Wegener's granulomatosis: its prevalence in a ten-year period in the rheumatology service of the Clinic Hospital, Cordoba, Argentina. Rev Fac Ciên Méd Univ Nac Cordoba. 2006;63:53–6.

17. Gamarra AI, Coral P, Quintana G, Toro CE, Flores LF, Matteson EL, et al. History of primary vasculitis in Latin America. Med Sci Monit. 2010;16(3):58–72.

18. Instituto Brasileiro de Geografia e Estatística (IBGE). Síntese Dados Demográficos Estados: Ceará, Brasil, 2016. Disponível em: <https://cidades.ibge.gov.br/brasil/ce/fortaleza/panorama> . Acesso em 28 de dezembro de 2016.

19. Watts R, Lane S, Hanslik T, Hauser T, Hellmich B, Koldingsnes W, et al. Development and validation of a consensus methodology for the classification of the ANCA-associated vasculitides and polyarteritis nodosa for epidemiological studies. Ann Rheum Dis. 2007;66:222–7.

20. Mukhtyar C, Guillevin L, Cid MC, Dasgupta B, de Groot K, Gross W, European Vasculitis Study Group, et al. EULAR recommendations for the management of primary small and medium vessel vasculitis. Ann Rheum Dis. 2009;68:310–7.

21. Mukhtyar C, Lee R, Brown D, Carruthers D, Dasgupta B, Dubey S, et al. Modification and validation of the Birmingham Vasculitis activity score (version 3). Ann Rheum Dis. 2009;68:1827–32.

22. Levey AS, Stevens LA, Schmid CH, Zhang YL, Castro AF 3rd, Feldman HI, et al. A new equation to estimate glomerular filtration rate. Ann Intern Med. 2009;150:604–12.

23. Exley AR, Bacon PA, Luqmani RA, Kitas GD, Carruthers DM, Moots R, et al. Examination of disease severity in systemic vasculitis from the novel perspective of damage using the vasculitis damage index (VDI). Br J Rheumatol. 1998;37:57–63.

24. Hogan SL, Falk RJ, Chin H, Cai J, Jennette CE, Jennette JC, et al. Predictors of relapse and treatment resistance in antineutrophil cytoplasmic antibody-associated small-vessel vasculitis. Ann Intern Med. 2005;143:621–31.

25. Fujimoto S, Watts RA, Kobayashi S, Suzuki K, Jayne DR, Scott DG, et al. Comparison of the epidemiology of anti-neutrophil cytoplasmic antibody-associated vasculitis between Japan and the UK. Rheumatology. 2011;50:1916–20.

26. Ormerod AS, Cook MC. Epidemiology of primary systemic vasculitis in the Australian Capital Territory and south-eastern New South Wales. Intern Med J. 2008;38(11):816–23.

27. Gonzalez-Gay MA, Garcia-Porrua C, Guerrero J, Rodriguez-Ledo P, Llorca J. The epidemiology of the primary systemic vasculitides in Northwest Spain: implications of the Chapel Hill consensus conference definitions. Arthritis Care Res. 2003;49:388–93.

28. Watts RA, Lane SE, Bentham G, Scott DG. Epidemiology of systemic vasculitis: a ten-year study in the United Kingdom. Arthritis Rheum. 2000;43:414–9.

29. Reinhold-Keller E, Beuge N, Latza U, DeGroot K, Rudert H, Nolle B, et al. An interdisciplinary approach to the care of patients with Wegener's granulomatosis: long-term outcome in 155 patients. Arthritis Rheum. 2000;43:1021–32.

30. Hazebroek MR, Kemna MJ, Schalla S, Wijk SS, Gerretsen SC, Dennert R, et al. Prevalence and prognostic relevance of cardiac involvement in ANCA-associated vasculitis: eosinophilic granulomatosis with polyangiitis and granulomatosis with polyangiitis. Int J Cardiol. 2015;199:170–9.

31. Neumann I, Kain R, Regele H, Soleiman A, Kandutsch S, Meisl FT. Histological and clinical predictors of early and late renal in ANCA-associated vasculitis. Nephrol Dial Transplant. 2005;20:96–104.

32. Haas M, Eustace JA. Immune complex deposits in ANCA-associated crescentic glomerulonephritis: a study of 126 cases. Kidney Int. 2004;65(6):2145–52.

33. Neumann I, Regele H, Kain R, Birck R, Meisl FT. Glomerular immune deposits are associated with increased proteinuria in patients with ANCA-associated crescentic nephritis. Nephrol Dial Transplant. 2003;18(3):524–31.

34. The WGET Research Group. Design of the Wegener's granulomatosis Etanercept trial (WGET). Control Clin Trials. 2002;23:450–68.

35. Leavitt RY, Fauci AS, Bloch DA, Michel BA, Hunder GG, Arend WP, et al. The American College of Rheumatology 1990 criteria for the classification of Wegener's granulomatosis. Arthritis Rheum. 1990;33:1101–7.

36. Jennette JC, Falk RJ, Andrassy K, Bacon PA, Churg J, Gross WL, et al. Nomenclature of systemic vasculitides. Proposal of an international consensus conference. Arthritis Rheum. 1994;37:187–92.

37. Finkielman JD, Merkel PA, Schroeder D, Hoffman GS, Spiera R, St Clair EW, WGET Research Group, et al. Antiproteinase 3 antineutrophil cytoplasmic antibodies and disease activity in Wegener granulomatosis. Ann Intern Med. 2007;147:611–9.

38. Mahr A, Guillevin L, Poissonnet M, Aymé S. Prevalences of polyarteritis nodosa, microscopic polyangiitis, Wegener's granulomatosis, and Churg-Strauss syndrome in a French urban multiethnic population in 2000: a capture-recapture estimate. Arthritis Rheum. 2004;15(51):92–9.

39. Haubitz M, Schellong S, Göbel U, Schurek HJ, Schaumann D, Koch KM, et al. Intravenous pulse administration of cyclofosfamide versus daily oral treatment in patients with antineutrophil cytoplasmic antibody-associated vasculitis and renal involvement: a prospective, randomized study. Arthritis Rheum. 1998;41:1835–44.

40. Jones RB, Tervaert JW, Hauser T, Hauser T, Luqmani R, Morgan MD, et al. Rituximab versus cyclophosphamide in ANCA-associated renal vasculitis. New England J Med. 2010;363(3):211–20.

41. Ceará. Secretaria De Saúde Do Estado. Boletim epidemiológico da tuberculose no Ceará, março 2016. Brasil. Disponível em:< http://www.saude.ce.gov.br/index.php/boletins >. Acessado em 06 de março de 2016.

42. Teixeira L, Mahr A, Jaureguy F, Noel L-H, Nunes H, Lefort A, et al. Low seroprevalence and poor specificity of antineutrophil cytoplasmic antibodies in tuberculosis. Rheumatology. 2005;44:247–50.

43. Pettersson EE, Sundelin B, Heigl Z. Incidence and outcome of pauci-immune necrotizing and crescentic glomerulonephritis in adults. Clin Nephrol. 1995;43:141–9.

44. Westman KW, Bygren PG, Olsson H, Ranstam J, Wieslander J. Relapse rate, renal survival, and cancer morbidity in patients with Wegener's granulomatosis or microscopic polyangiitis with renal involvement. J Am Soc Nephrol. 1998;9:842–5.

5

Virtual reality therapy for rehabilitation of balance in the elderly

Juleimar Soares Coelho de Amorim[1,4*], Renata Cristine Leite[2], Renata Brizola[2] and Cristhiane Yumi Yonamine[3]

Abstract

Virtual reality therapy (VRT) has clinical indications in rehabilitation programs for the elderly; however, there is still no consensus on the recovery of body balance. The objective of this review was to summarize the effects of physical therapy interventions with VRT in the rehabilitation of balance in the elderly. The studies were identified via a systematic search in the databases PubMed, SciELO, LILACS and PEDro from 2010 onward. Clinical trials with interventions that involved VRT in the elderly were included in the study and were subjected to methodological quality analysis using the PEDro scale. A random effects meta-analysis of the studies that analyzed balance using the Berg Balance Scale and the Timed Up and Go (TUG) test was performed. Ten articles met the inclusion criteria, which presented variability in relation to the types of interventions used (70%) and the outcomes analyzed (60%). The mean duration of the interventions was 13.90 (± 5.08) weeks, with at least two weekly sessions (± 0.73). There were positive results in relation to improvements in both dynamic and static balance (70% of the studies), mobility (80%), flexibility (30%), gait (20%) and fall prevention (20%). A summary of the meta-analysis showed mean effects on the Berg scale (standardized mean difference [SMD]: -0.848; 95% CI: -1.161; − 0.535) and the TUG test (SMD: 0. 894; 95% CI: 0.341; 1.447). Individually, virtual reality is promising in rehabilitation programs for the elderly. The overall measures were sufficient to show beneficial effects of the therapy on balance in the elderly.

Keywords: Virtual reality exposure therapy, Postural balance, Rehabilitation, Physiotherapy modalities, Elderly

Background

The speed of population aging has led to challenges for the health system, especially with regard to interventions to maintain functional capacity and independence and to broaden the framework of rehabilitation professionals. Mobility, body balance (static and dynamic), gait, joint and lower limb muscle flexibility are indicated as musculoskeletal attributes that support functional capacity in the elderly [1]. The loss or decline of balance results in a major public health problem: falls. The imbalance results from interactions of the musculoskeletal, visual, and sensorimotor systems and related functional tasks that undergo changes with senescence, such as sarcopenia, proprioceptive alterations, joint stiffness, postural alignment, latency and temporal incoordination of muscle activation [1–4].

Orthopedic, rheumatologic and neurological diseases are responsible for compromising postural control and mobility, implying greater body oscillation. Similarly, healthy individuals may also suffer from balance disorders due to their own senescence, such as reduced neuromuscular response speed, motor planning, joint degeneration, bone density and sarcopenia. However, these changes should not result in bone fractures, soft tissue injuries or traumatic brain injury due to the occurrence of falls. Therefore, preventive and rehabilitative measures are necessary for the maintenance of the joint and musculoskeletal system [2–4].

Scientific evidence from the scope of physiotherapeutic rehabilitation points to kinesiotherapy for motor coordination, balance training, stretching, muscle strengthening and functional training as approaches capable of preventing functional capacity declines in the

* Correspondence: juleimar@yahoo.com.br
[1]Ciências da Reabilitação, Instituto Federal de Educação, Ciência e Tecnologia do Rio de Janeiro – IFRJ, Rio de Janeiro, RJ, Brasil
[4]Colina, Manhuaçu, Brazil
Full list of author information is available at the end of the article

elderly [5]. However, technological advances, including Virtual Reality Therapy (VRT), which employs games as a resource to help individuals with balance deficits through the use of electronic devices experienced by the "human-machine interface", have modernized the clinical practices of rehabilitation professionals [6–8].

VRT rehabilitation has received increasing attention from researchers and clinicians who recognize its benefits because of its therapeutic potential regarding falls prevention and balance rehabilitation [8, 9]. The easy applicability, the stimuli to the sensory and motor systems and the playful character of the therapy offer a high degree of motivation, pleasure and instantaneous feedback on the execution of the tasks. Thus, VRT stimulates functional activities, promotes social interaction when administered collectively and may encourage the adherence of the elderly to rehabilitation programs [8–10].

The patient's movements are captured by a sensor bar or camera and are similar to those performed in daily life activities, facilitating motor recovery. These movements generally simulate sports practices, and to effectively perform the game, the patient is challenged to perform movements that strengthen the muscles, stimulate brain activity, improve sensory response and increase concentration, balance, motor coordination, motor control and gait efficiency [10].

Contradictory results have been reported in the literature, and VRT dissemination is still incipient [6, 7]. Evidence of the positive and negative effects of virtual reality can prod physiotherapists to broaden their scope of action in the provision of care during rehabilitation of the elderly. Therefore, a literature review can provide information on which domains of functional rehabilitation have demonstrated effective interventions using VRT. This therapy has not yet received a structured critique for improving body balance. Therefore, the objective of this review was to evaluate and synthesize the effects of physiotherapeutic interventions with VRT in balance rehabilitation of the elderly.

Materials and methods

The systematic review identified and selected studies published in Portuguese, English and/or Spanish. Four search themes were combined using the Boolean operators "AND" and "OR". The first search was on virtual reality therapy, combined in the title/abstract from the key words *"Virtual Reality Exposure Therapy"* or *"Video Game"* and *"Rehabilitation"* or *"Physical Therapy"* or *"Physiotherapy Modalities"*. Next, we identified the studies with samples of elderly individuals using the term *"Elderly"*. The third search included the outcomes *"Postural Balance"* and/or *"Proprioception"*. Finally, *"Clinical Trial"* studies were selected as the type of publication. All the keywords were extracted from the Health Descriptors (Descritores em Saúde - DeCS), and the search adopted its equivalents in English and Spanish. The search was performed in the electronic databases MEDLINE via PubMed, EMBASE, SciELO, LILACS and PEDro. The search ended in August 2016.

Clinical trial and controlled or randomized clinical trial articles published from 2010 onward with sample compositions that contained elderly subjects and that used VRT as a method of balance rehabilitation were included. Studies with interventions that were not specific to physical therapy or that presented preliminary data, pilot studies, interventions for vestibular rehabilitation (dizziness, labyrinthitis, vertigo), review articles, case studies, theses and dissertations were excluded.

The materials were selected by two independent reviewers who analyzed the title, the abstract and then the text in full, in this sequence; in cases of disagreement, a third reviewer was asked for consensus. To analyze the methodological quality of the studies, the PEDro scale was used. This scale is a *checklist* widely used in the area of rehabilitation, elaborated by the database *Physiotherapy Evidence Database Research*, which is specific for studies that investigate the effectiveness of interventions in physical therapy [11]. The scale has a total score of 10 points, with scores ≥5 considered to be of high quality.

The following data were extracted from the studies from a form that was specifically developed to analyze the data, adjusted by authors' interest as recommended by the *Cochrane Library* [12]: information about the author, year of publication, research objective, sample composition (size, diagnoses and age group), evaluation instruments, intervention measures (combined VRT or VRT alone), comparison, randomization process, intention-to-treat analysis, loss control and sample calculation, blinding process, number of sessions, weekly frequency, mean duration of therapy and the main results found. The final evaluation of the quality of the evidence was verified by the GRADE (*Grading of Recommendations Assessment, Development and Evaluation*) System, which establishes a consensus about the quantification of the quality of the evidence and of the recommendation strength in high, moderate, low or very low levels [13].

Articles that presented complete data regarding the evaluation and results (means and standard deviations) of the body balance construct and that presented homogeneity in the outcome measure were combined to perform the random effects meta-analysis using Stata13.1 software (StataCop 2013. College Station, TX: StatCopLP). The standardized mean difference (SMD), its 95% confidence intervals and the effect size (Overall Z) were used to estimate the effectiveness of the VRT intervention, with a value of $p < 0.05$ being considered statistically significant. The heterogeneity of the studies was evaluated by the value of the I^2 statistics, the p-value obtained by the Cochran Q test, the tau-square estimate and the difference between means, and those with p values > 0.05 were considered homogeneous.

Results

The search resulted in 486 articles in the MEDLINE, EMBASE, SciELO, LILACS and PEDro databases, of which only 24 met the inclusion and exclusion criteria for reading in full. The final sample of studies consists of 10 articles, as summarized in Fig. 1.

The characteristics of the selected articles regarding the intervention and the outcomes and results are presented in Table 1. There was variability in relation to the type of intervention used and the outcomes analyzed, in which seven different types of interventions were verified (proprioceptive training, aerobic training, static and dynamic balance, muscle flexibility, yoga and strengthening). The mean sample size was 31.40 (± 13.75) participants, with a minimum age of 62.22 (± 4.41) years old and a maximum of 87.40 (± 6.02) years old; eight (80%) studies performed interventions with the elderly without reporting specific diseases (healthy), one study (10%) was on Parkinson's disease, and one study (10%) was on diabetes mellitus. The mean duration of the sessions was 13.90 (± 5.08) weeks, with a mean weekly frequency of

2.10 (± 0.73) times and an average duration of 37 (± 10.85) minutes.

Two studies (20%) analyzed the results by intention to treat, and 30% of the articles had post-intervention follow-up for a mean time of 4.66 weeks (± 1.15). In all studies, there was randomization with a control group; 20% ($N = 2$) had a blinded evaluator, 30% ($N = 3$) used combination therapy, 80% referred to sample calculation ($N = 8$), and the mean score in the PEDro scale equal was to 6.80 (± 1.135) points. The main instruments for measuring the outcomes were the Berg balance scale (60%, $N = 6$), *Timed Up and Go* (TUG) (60%, N = 6), unipedal support (40%, $N = 4$) and functional range (30%, $N = 3$) (Table 2).

The effectiveness of the intervention was present in 70% of the individuals who performed VRT, the main effects being improvements in balance (dynamic and static) (80%, $N = 8$), mobility and flexibility (30%, $N = 3$) and gait (20%, $N = 2$) and a reduction in falls (20%, N = 2). Table 2 shows the variation in the choice of instruments for measuring these outcomes. To systematize the results in relation to the main domains of balance and based on the proportion of studies that adopted specific instruments to assess the efficacy of the therapy, the balance and mobility outcomes were measured, respectively, using the Berg Balance Scale and the TUG

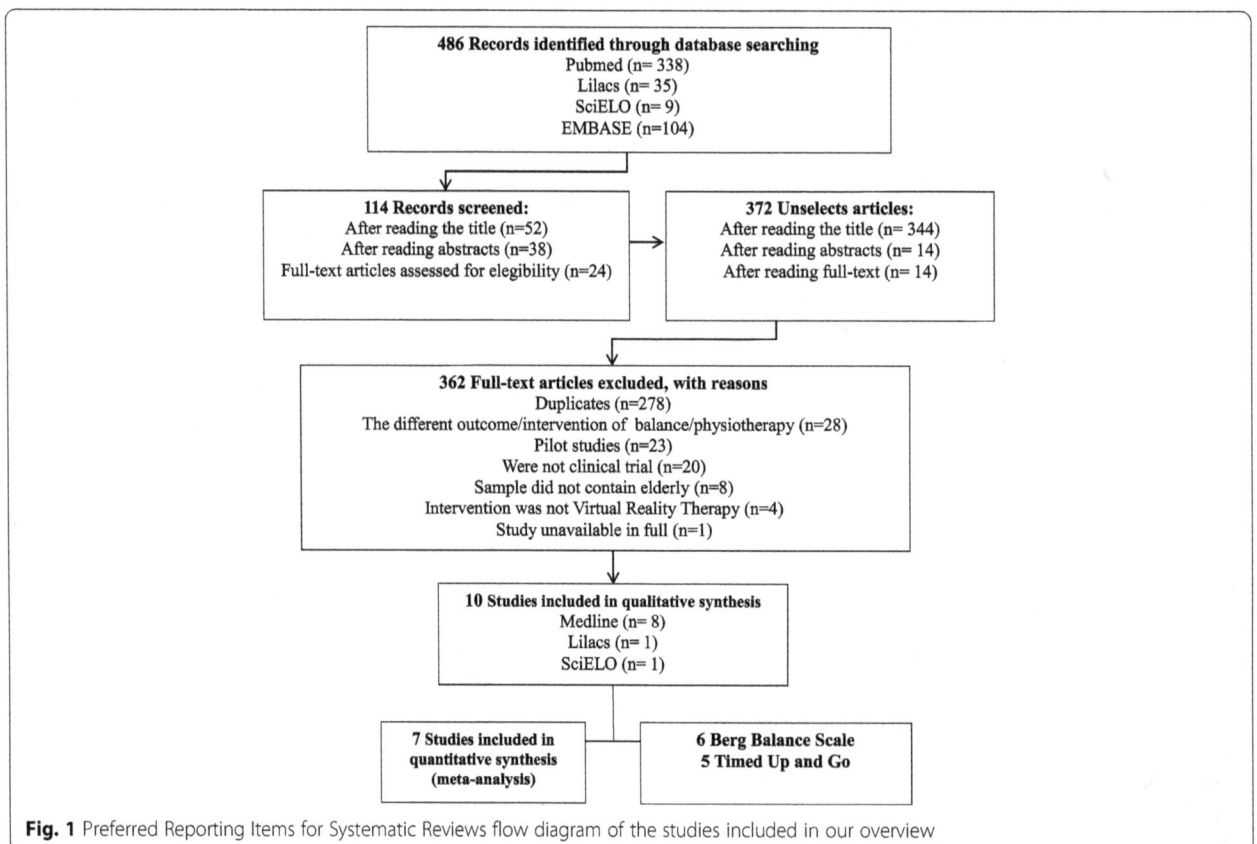

Fig. 1 Preferred Reporting Items for Systematic Reviews flow diagram of the studies included in our overview

Table 1 Characteristics of the articles included in the systematic review

Author/Year	Participants N (mean age)	Diagnosis	Outcomes	Intervention	Result	Conclusion
TREML, 2012 [15]	N = 32 CG = 16 (67.63 years old)EG = 16 (66.88 years old)	Healthy Elderly	Balance, mobility, flexibility and number of falls.	CG: proprioceptive training EG: proprioceptive training and Wii Fit Plus Games. Duration: 2 times a week, 10 sessions of 30 min.	POMA: p = 0.018 Unipedal support: p = 0.018 Anterior functional range: p = 0.012 Lateral functional range: p = 0.012 Berg Balance Scale: p = 0.068	VRT has been shown to be more efficient at conventional proprioceptive training in mobility, static balance and range.
RENDON, 2012 [8]	N = 40 CG = 20 (83.3 years old) EG = 20 (85.7 years old)	Elderly with risk of falls	Dynamic balance	CG: no intervention EG: stationary bicycle warm up and Wii Fit games. Duration: 3 times a week, 18 sessions of 35–45 min.	Balance confidence scale: p = 0.04	Authors reported improved dynamic balance, greater postural stability in the elderly and reduced risk of falls.
YEN, 2011 [18]	N = 42 CG = 14 (71.6 years old) GTC = 14 (70.1 years old) EG = 14 (70.4 years old)	Elderly with Parkinson's balance		CG: no intervention CTG: stretching and conventional balance training protocol EG: stretching, VRT balance board and games. Duration: 2 times per week, 12 sessions of 30 min.	Computerized posturography: p > 0.05	Both CTG and EG improved sensory integration for postural control. However, the demand for attention to postural control did not change after any VR or conventional treatment.
MUSSATO, 2012 [9]	N = 10 CG = 5 (65.6 years old) EG = 5 (66 years old)	Healthy Elderly	Balance and functional capacity	CG: no intervention EG: training with Nintendo Wii Fit accompanied by Balance Board and games. Duration: once a week, 10 sessions of 30 min.	Stabilometric platform variables after training with Wii Fit: p > 0.05 Unipedal support: p = 0.01 TUG: p = 0.004 (comparison between the pre- and post-intervention results of the EG) TUG: p = 0.704 (comparison between EG and CG)	The results did not show changes in stabilometric variables after treatment with Wii Fit. There was a significant difference between the pre- and post-intervention for the experimental group for both the Unipedal Support test and the TUG, but there was no statistical difference when compared with the control group.
LEE, 2013 [10]	N = 55 CG = 28 (74.29 years old) EG = 27 (73.78 years old)	Diabetes Mellitus	Balance anc gait	CG: health education guidelines on diabetes EG: virtual reality and games. Duration: 2 times per week, 20 sessions of 50 min.	Unipedal support: p = 0.001 Gait cadence speed: p = 0.001 Falls efficacy scale: p = 0.002	After the training, the intervention group showed improvement in balance, decreased sitting and standing time, increased gait cadence and perceived falls.
SZTURM, 2011 [16]	N = 27 CG = 14 (81 years old) EG = 13 (80.5 years old)	Deficit of balance and mobility	Balance ard gait	CG: conventional physiotherapy program for strengthening and balance sitting and standing. EG: rehabilitation with exercises of dynamic balance associated to games. Duration: 2 times per week, 16 sessions of 45 min	Berg Balance Scale: p < 0.001 Balance Confidence Scale: p < 0.02 Timed Up and Go: p < 0.01 Gait speed: p = 0.20	Improvement of the dynamic standing balance control (EG) compared with the conventional exercise program (CG). However, there was no statistically significant effect on gait.
BIERYLA, 2013 [17]	N = 10 CG = 5 (80.5 years old) EG = 5 (82.5 years old)	Healthy Elderly	balance	CG: no intervention EG: series of exercises and activities with games Duration: 3 times per week, 9 sessions of 30 min	Berg Balance Scale: p = 0.037 Fullerton Advanced Balance Scale: p = 0.529 Functional Reach Test: p = 0.779 Timed Up and Go: p = 0.174	Better balance results, with delayed effect for 1 month post-intervention on the Berg Balance Scale. No effects on the Advanced Balance Scale, range tests or TUG.
LAI, 2013 [20]	N = 30 CG = 15 (74.8 years old) EG = 15 (70.6 years old)	Healthy Elderly	Balance	CG: no intervention EG: VR therapy in the Xavix Measured Step System (XMSS) Duration: 3 times per week, 18 sessions of 30 min.	Berg Balance Scale: p = 0.001 Timed Up and Go: p = 0.046 Modified Falls Efficacy Scale: p = 0.001 Bipedal balance test on force platform: Eyes open: p = 0.052 Eyes closed: p = 0.092	Improved balance after 6 weeks of training; effects persisted partially after 6 weeks without intervention.

Table 1 Characteristics of the articles included in the systematic review (Continued)

Author/Year	Participants N (mean age)	Diagnosis	Outcomes	Intervention	Result	Conclusion
FRANCO, 2012 [14]	N = 32 CG = 10 (76.9 years old) GTP = 11 (77.9 years old) EG = 11 (79.8 years old)	Healthy Elderly	Balance	WFG: Guidance for balance and flexibility home exercises and intervention in Nintendo Wii Fit with games. MOB: group exercise sessions. CG: no intervention Duration: GTP: 2 times per week, 6 sessions of 10–15 min active play EG: 2 times per week, 6 sessions of 30–45 min	Berg's Balance Scale: $p = 0.837$ Tinetti's Balance Scale: $p = 0.913$ Quality of Life (SF-36): $p = 0.058$	No significant increase in balance in any outcome measures.
TOULOTTE, 2012 [19]	N = 36 G1 = 9 84.2 years old) G2 = 9 (72.2 years old) G3 = 9 (76.4 years old) G4 = 9 (71.8 years old)	Healthy Elderly	Balance	G1: Physical activities - strengthening exercises, proprioception, flexibility and static and dynamic balance. G2: Training with Wii Fit - Games. G3: Physical activities associated with Wii Fit training. G4: control group - watched television and board games Duration: once a week, 20 sessions of 60 min.	Tinetti scale: $p < 0.05$ for G1, G2 and G3 Unipedal support: $p < 0.05$ for G1 and G3. Modified position of center of gravity: $p < 0.05$ for G2 and G3.	Improvement in static balance. G1 and G3 improved dynamic balance.

*CG Control Group, EG Experimental Group, WFG Wii Fit Group, MOB Matter of Balance, TUG Timed Up and Go Group

Table 2 Studies included in the systematic review: analysis of the methodological quality, instruments and equipment to perform the therapy

Author/Year	PS	Outcome evaluation tools	Virtual Reality Therapy
TREML, 2012 [15]	7	Berg Balance Scale; Functional Range; Performance Oriented Gait and Balance Assessment; Unipedal Support	Nintendo Wii console associated with Balance Board and Wii Fit games
RENDON, 2012 [8]	6	TUG; Balance of Confidence Scale; Geriatric Depression Scale	Nintendo Wii console associated with Balance Board and Wii Fit games
YEN, 2011 [18]	7	Dynamic computerized posturography: Standing sensory organization test, sitting cognitive test and sensory organization test and standing cognitive test	Balance board, LCD monitor and a personal computer
MUSSATO, 2012 [9]	7	Stabilometric Platform (Baropodometry), Unipedal Support and TUG.	Nintendo Wii console associated with Balance Board and Wii Fit games
LEE, 2013 [10]	7	Unipedal Support, Berg Balance Scale, Functional Range, TUG, Sitting and standing up, Gait Rite System, Falls Efficacy Scale	PlayStation 2 with the EyeToy accessory: Play 1.2, 3″ (Sony Computer Entertainment)
SZTURM, 2011 [16]	8	Gait Rite System, Berg Balance Scale, TUG, Balance Confidence Scale, modified version of the Clinical Test of Sensory Interaction and Balance	Pressure mat associated with computer games
BIERYLA, 2013 [17]	4	Berg Balance Scale; Fullerton Advanced Balance Scale; Functional Range and TUG	Nintendo Wii console associated with Balance Board and Wii Fit games
LAI, 2013 [20]	8	Berg Balance Scale; Falls Efficacy Scale, TUG and Force Platform for Static Balance	Xavix Measured Step System (XMSS)
FRANCO, 2012 [14]	7	Berg Balance Scale; Tinetti's Scale; Quality of Life Questionnaire - SF36	Nintendo Wii console associated with Balance Board and Wii Fit games
TOULOTTE, 2012 [19]	7	Unipedal Support; Tinetti's Scale and Wii Fit test	Nintendo Wii console associated with Balance Board and Wii Fit games

*PS PEDro Scale. TUG Timed Up and Go test

test. The study included 86 elderly subjects, with a difference of 3.76 (± 1.83) points in the scale; 64 individuals achieved an improvement of 2.16 (± 1.13) seconds in the test.

The meta-analysis for effectiveness of the intervention in improving the scores of the Berg Balance Scale was performed based on six articles [9, 10, 13–17] because the data were missing in 30%. The SMD of the studies was − 0.848, contained in a 95% CI of − 1.161 to − 0.535. The result refutes the null hypothesis and shows the efficacy in the rehabilitation of balance in the elderly through VRT.

Regarding the outcome of the Berg Balance Scale, the difference between means ($p = 0.000$) shows that there is a significant statistical difference in the final score of the scale between the pre- and post-intervention measures with VRT. There was no evidence of heterogeneity ($I^2 = 0.0\%$, $p = 0.666$, Chi^2: 3.03) between the studies. Table 3 presents the results with the synthetic measure of each study by comparing VRT with other therapies or placebo and shows the summary measure (SMD: -0.858; 95% CI:-1.161; − 0.535), which indicates improvement by 5.31 points in the final score (Z: 5.31, $p = 0.000$).

Likewise, five studies [9, 10, 15–17] analyzed the time of the TUG test using VRT in the experimental group. As measured by the meta-analysis summary measure (0.894) and its respective confidence interval (95% CI: 0.341, 1.447), the value of the I^2 statistics (46.4%, $p = 0.114$) and the tau-squared result (0.1715), the improvement obtained showed an absence of heterogeneity, low variability between studies and evidence of a statistically significant difference in test execution speed (Z: 3.17 s; $p = 0.002$) (Table 4). The evaluation of the quality of the evidence, performed through the GRADE System, showed low and very low recommendation of the VRT based on improvements in the parameters of the Berg Scale and the TUG test, respectively (Table 5).

Discussion

This systematic review shows a shortage of intervention studies in the elderly using VRT, likely related to the great challenges of working with technological tools that have a playful character, the novelty of these products in the therapeutic market, the low knowledge of physiotherapists about the benefits of VRT, the preferences of professionals and users, the development and standardization of games

Table 3 Standardized mean difference (95% CI) for the effect of virtual reality therapy on the Berg Balance Scale score, grouping data from six studies ($N = 174$)

Author, year	Therapy	Pre-Intervention			Post-Intervention			SMD (95% CI)	Study weight (%)	SMD, Random Effect Model, 95% CI
		Mean	SD	Total	Mean	SD	Total			
Treml, 2013	VRT vs proprioception	52.75	4.37	16	55.5	1.07	16	-0.864 (-1.591;-0.138)	18.57	
Lee, 2013	VRT vs health education	51.67	2.48	27	53.41	1.89	27	-0.791 (-1.341;-0.241)	32.45	
Szturm, 2011	VRT vs kinesiotherapy	47.0	13.8	13	53.2	12.4	13	-0.474 (-1.240;0.293)	16.70	
Bieryla, 2013	VRT vs placebo	50.0	2.82	4	53.0	1.4	5	-1.410 (-2.918;0.098)	4.31	
Lai, 2013	VRT vs placebo	50.53	4.75	15	53.87	3.56	15	-0.796 (-1.541;-0.050)	17.64	
Franco, 2011	VRT vs placebo	48.0	3.7	11	52.0	0.8	10	-1.460 (-2.434;-0.486)	10.33	
Total				86			86	**-0.848 (-1.161;-0.535)**	**100.0**	

Heterogeneity: $I^2 = 0.0\%$ ($p = 0.696$; $tau^2 = 0.000$)

Overall effect size (overall Z): $Z = 5.31$ ($p = 0.000$)

VRT: virtual reality exposure therapy; SD: standard deviation; SMD: standardized mean difference; CI: confidence interval. The mean of the measure used for evaluation refers to the score obtained (maximum 56 points).

to train functional tasks such as balance, gait and range and the design of clinical trials of high methodological quality [7].

Among the articles analyzed, the forms of intervention differed even in the presence of a similar outcome. Some studies were conducted with a more pragmatic therapeutic approach, with protocols varying according to the individual evaluation of the elderly [14, 18, 19]; others have established systematic, segmented and progressive protocols, including warm-up and isolated or combined exercises [8, 9, 15–17, 20]. Another study had a protocol associating practice at home with the clinical environment [10].

The beneficial effects of VRT presented by the studies included in this systematic review extended to the outcomes of the balance variables, including mobility, flexibility [15], gait cadence and fear of falls [10]. There seems to be agreement among the authors about the positive results in these components; however, the meta-analysis evidenced possible discrepancies in the sample composition and the interventions.

Table 4 Standardized mean difference (95% CI) for the effect of virtual reality therapy on the time (in seconds) of the *Timed Up and Go* (TUG) test, grouping data from five studies ($N = 131$)

Author, year	Therapy	Pre-Intervention			Post-Intervention			SMD (95% CI)	Study weight (%)	SMD, Random Effect Model, 95% CI
		Mean	SD	Total	Mean	SD	Total			
Mussato, 2012	VRT vs placebo	8.2	0.4	5	6.8	0.5	5	3.092 (1.135;5.050)	6.82	
Lee, 2013	VRT vs health education	11.48	2.31	27	9.78	1.58	27	0.862 (0.308;1.416)	31.72	
Szturm, 2011	VRT vs kinesiotherapy	8.0	1.0	13	5.1	3.7	13	1.052 (0.243;1.861)	23.30	
Bieryla, 2013	VRT vs placebo	12.8	1.9	4	11.2	2.61	4	0.686 (-0.677;2.049)	12.17	
Lai, 2013	VRT vs placebo	9.54	3.52	15	8.54	2.85	15	0.312 (-0.408;1.033)	26.00	
Total				64			64	**0.894 (0.341;1.447)**	**100.0**	

Heterogeneity: $I^2 = 46.4\%$ ($p = 0.114$; $tau^2 = 0.1715$)

Overall effect size (overall Z): $Z = 3.17$ ($p = 0.002$)

VRT: virtual reality exposure therapy; SD: standard deviation; SMD: standardized mean difference; CI: confidence interval. The mean of the measurement used to perform the test was in seconds.

Table 5 GRADE system quality of evidence analysis for the Berg Balance Scale and the Timed Up and Go (TUG) test

Quality assessment							Quality	Importance
Number of studies	Design	Serious limitations (risk of bias)?	Inconsistency of results (heterogeneity)?	Indirect evidence?	Inaccuracy?	Publishing bias?		
Berg Scale								
6	Quasi-experimental studies and RCTs	No	No	No	Very important	Sim	++ / ++++ Low	Critical
TUG Test								
5	Quasi-experimental studies and RCTs	No	Low	No	Very important	Sim	+++ / ++++ Very Low	Critical

TUG Timed Up and Go
GRADE Grading of Recommendations Assessment, Development and Evaluation

The study by Holden [7] systematically reviewed the literature on interventions using VRT for balance and motor skills specifically for neurological disorders in individuals over 45 years of age. The authors note that for body balance, the three studies reported significant improvements in performance. Another important meta-analysis reported no significant effect of VRT [21] compared with traditional physical therapy or no intervention. However, the authors' review did not include the electronic databases SciELO and LILACS as a search source on the use of games in balance recovery.

Specifically concerning the interventions with emphasis on the improvement of static balance, Mussato and collaborators [9] have noted that the effect is more sensitive to detection in the baropodometry test since it measures maximum peaks and not the mean oscillation amplitude of the body balance. The games selected for this study offered medial-lateral and anteroposterior imbalances, thus stimulating the recruitment of motor strategies and allowing greater variability in the displacements of the pressure center in the orthostatic posture [22].

For gait training, Lobo [23] points out games for the rehabilitation of weight transfer abilities between limbs, unipedal support, triple flexion and load acceptance during initial support. However, other important aspects, such as dissociation of waists, impulsion and continuous anterior displacement of the center of mass, are not possible through VRT since the step change occurs in a stationary manner, which would justify the fact that Szturm [16] did not obtain a positive effect on the gait speed. In conventional rehabilitation, the stimuli are offered by the equipment through active dynamic training, and the proprioceptive *inputs* are produced by the efferent route [15]. Visualization of the action on the display (visual *feedback*) and interaction with the game stimulate proprioceptive *inputs* in a static manner.

The benefits noted in the aspects of static balance, gait components and sensorimotor integration show that the games provide training conditions that favor an integration between cognitive and motor stimulation. More complex training involving dual tasks, such as cognition and motor activity, requires automatic control during movements since the focus of attention is on the game shown on the display, thus promoting motor function improvement when compared with conventional training [15, 24].

Regarding falls, the training approaches of the articles included in this review aimed to increase or restore the self-confidence of the elderly. Individually, studies showed the superiority of VRT in recovering body balance when compared with conventional interventions, with impacts on the self-efficacy of post-intervention falls and not necessarily on the reduction in the number of falls.

Based on the health problems, it was noted that the designs aimed at prevention of falls and other conditions were evaluated in patients with Parkinson's disease. The study by Yen [18] resulted in improved sensory integration for postural control; however, the demand for attention was not altered after any VRT. Santana [25] and Loureiro [26], in experimental studies without a comparison group, concluded that training using the Nintendo Wii Fit Plus platform proved to be useful for the rehabilitation of degenerative diseases regarding motor performance, flexibility, lower limb joint stiffness and functional independence, in addition to improving the motor learning ability due to the cognitive stimuli provided by the videogame. The activation of neural circuits and structures by virtual games can play a key role in transferring the immediate effects of games to long-term effects. Lai [20] did not attribute maintenance of improvement to VRT per se; after the end of the interventions, the elderly improved their balance and felt confident to engage in physical activity, which justifies maintaining good results regarding balance.

Some methodological aspects were observed in the included clinical trials that reduce the risk of bias and allow better measurements when systematically adopted by the studies. All of them reported randomization, with well-established selection criteria for the participants, to increase the significance of the data, restricting populations with similar characteristics and guaranteeing homogeneity of the samples. Only two of the studies analyzed blinded one of the evaluators, an important item to be considered since this principle is used to avoid systematic errors in the research. Another aspect is intention-to-treat analysis, which also avoids distortions caused by a loss of participants, which may interrupt the equivalence established by randomized selection, reflecting non-adherence to treatment and potential benefits in individuals receiving the treatment established by the study.

The studies sought to guarantee homogeneity of the samples from systematic methods of development of clinical trials, in which the absence of heterogeneity in the articles was confirmed in the meta-analysis. However, we emphasize that there was a discrepancy in the individual results, which can be attributed to the size of the sample, the intensity of the intervention and differences in the participants' baseline risks. It is observed that the sample size and the number of sessions in the studies that were not effective in the balance of the elderly showed lower averages than those of effective studies. In relation to statistical power, only three articles [8, 10, 18] performed the calculation, and it is not possible to state whether the absence of significant improvement due to the interventions in some studies occurred because of the lack of efficacy of the technique or because of the small sample size. The intervention protocol presented great variety regarding the number of sessions, weekly frequency, intervention time and isolated and/or combined exercises, and caution in decision making is required.

The literature evidenced dissent, and the dissemination of VRT was still incipient, which can also be demonstrated by the analysis of the quality of the evidence. According to evaluation criteria for recommending GRADE System evidence, the data selected to compose the meta-analysis may be influenced by publication bias, a tendency for published results to be systematically different from reality, as well as imprecision of the outcome measure and the sample size. Although there is a large body of literature on the role of physiotherapy in rehabilitating balance in the elderly and although studies published using VRT show positive results, the power of generalization is limited due to the samples sizes of the articles included in this review. Therefore, the results reflect a promising tool that requires more scientific investigations about the outcome to improve confidence in estimates of its effects. Future studies should specifically evaluate the types of protocol, as the need for advances in expanding the therapeutic armamentarium for rehabilitation practitioners is highlighted. To increase data reliability, new studies with sufficient sample size, better levels of evidence and methodological rigor are recommended in clinical trials demonstrating blinding techniques, intention-to-treat analysis, sample size and

number of sessions to establish specific protocols of treatment. As a limitation of this study, we highlight the difficulty in exploring other domains of balance rehabilitation of the elderly, given the limited number of clinical trials included limiting the subgroup analysis, in addition to restriction to literature in English, Spanish and Portuguese.

Systematic review of clinical research on physiotherapeutic interventions with VRT in the rehabilitation of balance in the elderly emphasized relevance through the scenario of population aging resulting in unfavorable structural and functional changes predisposing elderly people to falls. Therefore, the therapeutic approach based on virtual reality is another alternative, which may, in addition to promoting motor control stimuli, help in gait efficiency and body balance. Because VRT is a playful method, it can encourage the participation of these individuals in activities of balance rehabilitation. Evidence of the results of virtual reality can awaken physiotherapists to broaden the scope of action in the provision of care during the rehabilitation of the elderly.

Conclusion

This review synthesized the effects of virtual reality therapy. Individually, there was concordance in the analyzed clinical trials regarding the improvements of static balance, gait components, sensorimotor integration and self-efficacy of falls, with no significant relevance for dynamic balance, gait speed and reduction in the number of falls. The data set evaluated in the meta-analysis and the quality of evidence analysis indicate the effectiveness of VRT in the treatment of balance and mobility in the elderly, but further studies are needed. Implications for clinical practice require caution in decision making because of sample profiles, intervention protocols and outcome measures. Regarding implications for the research, due to the lack of homogeneity in the methodologies, interventions and study outcomes in the studies, systematic positive effects were demonstrated for the mobility outcomes. The findings on using virtual reality therapy for recovery and balance training seem promising. However, to make assertions regarding effectiveness, adjustments are still needed for future studies.

Authors' contributions
The individual contributions of authors should be specified following: JSCdA made substantial contributions to conception and design, analysis and interpretation of data; been involved in drafting the manuscript or revising it critically for important intellectual content; given final approval of the version to be published. RCL made substantial contributions to conception and design, acquisition of data and interpretation of data; been involved in drafting the manuscript or revising it critically for important intellectual content; given final approval of the version to be published. RB made substantial contributions to conception and design, acquisition of data and interpretation of data; been involved in drafting the manuscript or revising it critically for important intellectual content; given final approval of the version to be published.

CYY made substantial contributions to conception and design and interpretation of data; been involved in drafting the manuscript or revising it critically for important intellectual content; given final approval of the version to be published.

Competing interests

The authors declare that they have no competing interests.

Author details

[1]Ciências da Reabilitação, Instituto Federal de Educação, Ciência e Tecnologia do Rio de Janeiro – IFRJ, Rio de Janeiro, RJ, Brasil. [2]Centro Universitário Filadélfia – UNIFIL, Londrina, PR, Brasil. [3]Saúde Coletiva, Centro Universitário Filadélfia – UNIFIL, Londrina, PR, Brasil. [4]Colina, Manhuaçu, Brazil.

References

1. Bruniera CAV, Rodacki ALF. Respostas estabilométricas de jovens e idosos para recuperar o equilíbrio após uma perturbação inesperada controlada. Rev Educ Fis UEM. 2014;25(3):345–51.
2. Meireles AE, Pereira LVS, Oliveira TG, Christofoletti G, Fonseca AL. Alterações neurológicas fisiológicas ao envelhecimento afetam o sistema mantenedor do equilíbrio. Rev Neurocienc. 2010;18(1):103–8.
3. Pícoli TS, Figueiredo LL, Patrizzi LJ. Sarcopenia e envelhecimento. Fisioter Mov. 2011;24(3):455–62.
4. Teixeira INAO, Guariento ME. Biologia do envelhecimento: teorias, mecanismos e perspectivas. Ciênc Saúde Coletiva 2010. 2016;15(6):2845–57.
5. Gontijo RW, Leão MRC. Eficácia de um programa de fisioterapia preventiva para idosos. Rev Méd Minas Gerais. 2013;23(2):173–80.
6. Keshner EA. Virtual reality and rehabilitation: a new toy or a new research and rehabilitation tool? J Neuroeng Rehabil 2004. 2016;3(1):8.
7. Holden MK. Virtual environments for motor rehabilitation: review. Cyberpsychol Behav. 2005;8(3):187–211.
8. Rendon AA, Lohman EB, Thorpe D, Johnson EG, Medina E, Bradley B. The effect of virtual reality gaming on dynamic balance in older adults. Age Ageing. 2012;41(4):549–52.
9. Mussato R, Brandalize D, Brandalize M. Nintendo Wii® e seu efeito no equilíbrio e capacidade funcional de idosos saudáveis. Rev Brasil Ciência Mov 2012. 2016;20(2):68–75.
10. Lee S, Shin S. Effectiveness of virtual reality using video gaming. Diabetes Technol Ther. 2013;15(6):489–96.
11. Shiwa SR, Costa LOP, Moser ADL, Aguiar IC, Oliveira LVF. PEDro: a base de dados de evidências em fisioterapia. Fisioter Mov. 2011;24(3):523–33.
12. Higgins JPT, Green S. Cochrane handbook for systematic reviews of interventions 4.2.6 [updated September 2006]. In: The Cochrane Library, Issue 4. Chichester: John Wiley & Sons, Ltda; 2006.
13. Brasil. Ministério da Saúde. Diretrizes metodológicas: elaboração de pareceres técnicos-científicos. 3rd ed. Brasília: Ministério da Saúde; 2011. 80p.: il.
14. Franco JR, Jacobs K, Inzerillo C, Kluzik J. The effect of the Nintendo Wii fit and exercise in improving balance and quality of life in community dwelling elderls. Technol Health Care. 2012;20(2):95–115.
15. Treml CJ, Kalil Filho FA, Ciccarino RFL, Wegner RS, Saita CYS, Corrêa AG. O uso da plataforma Balance Board como recurso fisioterápico em idosos. Rev bras geriatr gerontol. 2012;16(4):759–68.
16. Szturm T, Betkler AL, Moussavi Z, Desai A, Goodeman V. Effects of an interactive computer game exercise regimen on balance impairment in frail community-dwelling older adults: a randomized controlled trial. Phys Ther. 2011;91(10):1449–62.
17. Bieryla KA, Dold NM. Feasibility of Wii fit training to improve clinical measures of balance in older adults. Clin Interv Aging. 2013;8:775–81.
18. Yen CY, Lin KH, Hu MH, Wu RM, Lu Tw LCH. Effects of virtual reality-augmented balance training on sensory organization and attentional demand for postural control in people with Parkinson disease: a randomized controlled trial. Phys Ther. 2011;91(6):862–74.
19. Toulotte C, Toursel C, Olivier N. Wii fit® training vs. adapted physical activities: which one is the most appropriate to improve the balance of independent senior subjects? A randomized controlled study. Clin Rehabil. 2012;26(9):827–35.
20. Lai CH, Peng CW, Chen YL, Huang CP, Hsiao YL, Chen SC. Effects of interactive video-game based system exercise on the balance of the elderly. Gait Posture. 2013;37(4):511–8.
21. Booth V, Masud T, Connell L, Bath-Hextall F. The effectiveness of virtual reality intervention in improving balance in adults with impaired balance compared with standard or no treatment: a systematic review and meta-analysis. Clin Rehabil. 2014;28(5):419–31.
22. Ricci NA, Gazzola JM, Coimbra IB. Sistemas sensoriais no equilíbrio corporal de idosos. Arq Bras Ciên Saúde. 2009;34(2):94–100.
23. Lobo AM. Efeito de um Treinamento em Ambiente Virtual Sobre o Desempenho da Marcha e Funções Cognitivas em Idosos Saudáveis. 2013. 112 f. São Paulo: Dissertação (Mestrado em Psicologia) - Universidade de São Paulo; 2013.
24. Silva, K. G. Efeito de um Treinamento com o Nintendo Wii® Sobre o Equilíbrio Postural e Funções Executivas de Idosos Saudáveis – Um Estudo Clinico Longitudinal, Controlado e Aleatorizado. 2013. 128 f. Dissertação (Mestrado em Psicologia) - Universidade de São Paulo, São Paulo, 2013.
25. Santana CMF, Lins OG, Sanguinetti DCM, Silva FP, Angelo TDA, Cariolano MGWS, Câmara SB, Silva JPA. Efeitos do tratamento com realidade virtual não imersiva na qualidade de vida de indivíduos com Parkinson. Rev bras gerontol. 2015;18(1):49–58.
26. Loureiro APC, Ribas CG, Zotz TGG, Chen R, Ribas F. Viabilidade da terapia virtual na reabilitação de pacientes com doença de Parkinson: estudo-piloto. Fisioter. Mov. 2012;25(3):659–66.

6

Human immunodeficiency virus in a cohort of systemic lupus erythematosus patients

Vanessa Hax[1]* ⓘ, Ana Laura Didonet Moro[1], Rafaella Romeiro Piovesan[2], Luciano Zubaran Goldani[3], Ricardo Machado Xavier[1] and Odirlei Andre Monticielo[1]

Abstract

Background: Systemic lupus erythematosus (SLE) and acquired immunodeficiency syndrome (AIDS) share many clinical manifestations and laboratory findings, therefore, concomitant diagnosis of SLE and human immunodeficiency virus (HIV) can be challenging.

Methods: Prospective cohort with 602 patients with SLE who attended the Rheumatology Clinic of the Hospital de Clínicas de Porto Alegre since 2000. All patients were followed until 01 May 2015 or until death, if earlier. Demographic, clinical and laboratory data were prospectively collected.

Results: Out of the 602 patients, 11 presented with the diagnosis of AIDS (1.59%). The following variables were significantly more prevalent in patients with concomitant HIV and SLE: neuropsychiatric lupus (10.9% vs. 36.4%; $p = 0.028$) and smoking (37.6% vs. 80%; $p = 0.0009$) while malar rash was significantly less prevalent in this population (56% vs. 18.2%; $p = 0.015$). Nephritis (40.5% vs. 63.6%; $p = 0.134$) and hemolytic anemia (28.6% vs. 54.5%; $p = 0.089$) were more prevalent in SLE patients with HIV, but with no statistical significance compared with SLE patients without HIV. The SLICC damage index median in the last medical consultation was significantly higher in SLE patients with HIV (1 vs. 2; p = 0,047).

Conclusions: Our patients with concomitant HIV and SLE have clinically more neuropsychiatric manifestations. For the first time, according to our knowledge, higher cumulative damage was described in lupus patients with concomitant HIV infection. Further studies are needed to elucidate this complex association, its outcomes, prognosis and which therapeutic approach it's best for each case.

Keywords: Systemic lupus erythematosus, Human immunodeficiency virus, Acquired immunodeficiency syndrome, Neuropsychiatric lupus, Opportunistic infections

Background

Concomitant diagnosis of systemic lupus erythematosus (SLE) and acquired immunodeficiency syndrome (AIDS) can be intriguing and challenging. SLE and human immunodeficiency virus (HIV) infection share many clinical manifestations, including musculoskeletal symptoms such as myalgia, arthralgia/arthritis, skin rashes, lymphadenopathy and organ involvement, such as kidneys, heart, lungs and central nervous system [1]. They also have several common laboratory findings such as anemia, leukopenia, lymphopenia, thrombocytopenia and hypergammaglobulinemia [1].

There are few studies assessing the clinical and laboratory manifestations in SLE patients with HIV infection, as well as patient's profile and their evolution. Furthermore, there are no studies assessing the prognosis of this association until now. Therefore, the present study aimed to demonstrate the profile of these patients in our center, appointing their clinical and laboratory features, the significant differences between the patients with or without HIV, the treatment offered and their evolution considering infections, other diseases and mortality.

Methods

Study population

This prospective cohort consisted of 602 SLE patients who attended the Rheumatology Clinic of the Hospital de Clínicas de Porto Alegre since 2000. All patients

* Correspondence: vanessahax@gmail.com.br; vanessahax@gmail.com
[1]Division of Rheumatology, Hospital de Clínicas de Porto Alegre, Universidade Federal do Rio Grande do Sul, 2350 Ramiro Barcelos St, Room 645, Porto Alegre, RS 90035-903, Brazil
Full list of author information is available at the end of the article

fulfilled the American College of Rheumatology (ACR) revised criteria for the classification of SLE [2] and an informed consent form was obtained from all participants. The patients were followed until 01 May 2015 or until death, if earlier. The demographic, clinical and laboratory data were prospectively collected.

Clinical and laboratory variables

The following variables were recorded: age, gender, age at diagnosis of SLE and HIV (when the last was positive) , smoking status (current or previous), cardiovascular diseases, dyslipidemia, other autoimmune diseases and treatment performed. Clinical manifestations of SLE included the presence of photosensitivity, malar rash, discoid rash, oral or nasal ulcers, arthritis, serositis (pleuritis or pericarditis), nephritis and neurological disease, defined as seizures or psychosis. The assessment of the group of patients with concomitant HIV included infections, as well as CD4 and viral load at the diagnosis and the last count available. The laboratory evaluation included the presence of hematological disorders (hemolytic anemia, leukopenia, lymphopenia or thrombocytopenia), positive antinuclear antibody (ANA) (titer> 1:80) or other autoantibodies such as anti-dsDNA, anti-Sm, anti-RNP, anti-Ro, anti-La, anticardiolipin (aCL), lupus anticoagulant and false positive VDRL. The patients were also evaluated in regard to secondary antiphospholipid syndrome and secondary Sjogren's syndrome, according to the classification criteria for both diseases [3, 4]. The SLEDAI and the SLICC damage index of the last medical consultation were recorded too, as a measurement of disease activity and cumulative damage, respectively [5]

Statistical analyses

A descriptive analysis of data through calculation of mean and standard deviation (SD) for quantitative variables was performed while the frequency and percentage were calculated for categorical variables. The median and interquartile range were calculated to quantitative variables with asymmetrical distribution. We used the chi square test or Fisher's exact test to compare categorical variables, and continuous variable were analyzed with Mann-Whitney test. All statistical analyses were performed using SPSS 20.0. All tests were performed at the 0.05 level of significance and were two-sided.

Results

Our study consisted of 602 SLE patients, 75.2% European derived, 92% female and 11 (1.59%) of these patients presented with HIV. The patients mean age was 42.8±12.7 years and the mean SLE diagnostic age was 29.9±13.9 years. Demographic, clinical and laboratory profile were showed in Table 1. The following variables were significantly more

prevalent in patients with concomitant HIV and SLE: neuropsychiatric lupus (10.9% vs. 36.4%; $p = 0.028$) and smoking (37.6% vs. 80%; $p = 0.0009$) while malar rash was significantly less prevalent in this population (56% vs. 18.2%; $p = 0.015$). The following features were more prevalent in SLE patients with HIV, but without to reach statistical significance compared with SLE patients without HIV: nephritis (40.5% vs. 63.6%; $p = 0.134$), hemolytic anemia (28.6% vs. 54.5%; $p = 0.089$), presence of anti-Ro (39.4% vs. 63.6%; $p = 0.125$) and anti-La (13.1% vs. 27.3%; $p = 0.172$), cardiovascular disease (18.1% vs. 36.4%; $p = 0.126$) and diabetes mellitus (7.7% vs. 18.2%; $p = 0.212$). Regarding the autoantibodies, in our cohort, amongst SLE patients with HIV, 72.7% had positive Coomb's test, 45.5% anti-dsDNA, 9.1% anti-Sm, 63.6% anti-Ro, 27.3% anti-La, 27.3% anti-RNP and 9.1% antiphospholipid antibodies. Hypergammaglobulinemia and hypocomplementenemia were observed in 81.8% of SLE patients with HIV.

The survival rate was 96.6% and 93.5% in 5 and 10 years, respectively, in SLE patients without HIV. Meanwhile, the survival rate was 90% in 5 and 10 years in SLE patients with HIV. There was no significant difference between the two groups. The SLICC damage index median in the last medical consultation was significantly higher in SLE patients with HIV (1 vs. 2; $p = 0.047$). The median of the last SLEDAI did not reach significant difference between groups (0 vs. 1; $p = 0.55$). In the HIV group, infections occurred in 54.5%, predominantly human papillomavirus infection, followed by tuberculosis and herpes zoster infection. Coinfection with C hepatitis virus occurred in two patients (18%).

Simultaneous diagnosis of SLE and HIV infection was done in one patient, while HIV following SLE was diagnosed in eight patients and HIV infection preceded SLE in two patients. All the patients were female and at diagnosis of HIV the mean CD4 count was 296 cells/μL and HIV-RNA 60.000 copies/ml. Antiretroviral therapy (ART) was taken by all the patients and, considering SLE, seven were treated with hydroxychloroquine (HCQ), two with azathioprine (AZA), two with cyclophosphamide (CYC), one with methotrexate (MTX) and one with mycophenolate mofetil (MMF), according to the severity of each case (Table 2).

Discussion

The coexistent infection of HIV and SLE is unusual and intriguing, because both diseases are characterized by multisystem involvement and immune dysfunction related to T lymphocytes, cytokine production alterations and polyclonal activation of B lymphocytes [6]. Despite these similarities, several theories have been formulated to explain the reason of the unexpectedly lower prevalence of concomitant diagnosis of HIV and SLE. SLE may prevent HIV infection as a result of polyclonal

Table 1 Demographic, clinical, and laboratory features of SLE patients with and without HIV infection

Patients features	All patients ($n = 602$)	SLE patients without HIV ($n = 591$)	SLE patients with HIV ($n = 11$)	P value[a]
Females	92% (602)	91.9% (591)	100% (11)	1.000
European derived	75.2% (584)	75.4% (573)	63.6% (11)	0.479
Smoking[b]	38.3% (582)	37.6% (215)	80% (11)	0.009
Obesity	25.3% (502)	25.9% (127)	0% (11)	0.074
Age (years)	48.2±14.9(597)	48.3±14.9 (586)	43.1±12.7 (11)	0.245
SLE age at diagnosis (years)	33.5±14.2 (591)	33.6±14.2 (580)	29.9±13.9 (11)	0.390
Malar rash	55.3% (597)	56% (586)	18.2% (11)	0.015
Photosensitivity	72.1% (598)	72.4% (587)	54.5% (11)	0.191
Oral ulcers	35.6% (598)	35.6% (587)	36.4% (11)	1.000
Arthritis	72.4% (597)	74.4% (586)	63.6% (11)	0.486
Serositis	25.2% (595)	25% (585)	36.4% (11)	0.482
Nephritis	40.9% (596)	40.5% (585)	63.6% (11)	0.134
Neurologic disorders	11.4% (596)	10.9% (585)	36.4% (11)	0.028
Psychosis	6.5% (597)	6.3% (586)	18.2% (11)	0.158
Seizures	6% (597)	6% (586)	9.1% (11)	0.498
Hematologic disorders	75.8% (598)	75.8% (587)	72.7% (11)	0.773
Hemolytic anemia	29.1% (598)	28,6% (587)	54,5% (11)	0.089
Leukopenia/Lymphopenia	55.9% (598)	56% (587)	45.5% (11)	0.549
Thrombocytopenia	21.4% (598)	21.5% (587)	18.2% (11)	1.000
Anti-dsDNA	46% (567)	46% (556)	45.5% (11)	1.000
Anti-Sm	20.8% (549)	21% (538)	9.1% (11)	0.474
Anticardiolipin	27.3% (550)	27.6% (539)	9.1% (11)	0.304
Lupus Anticoagulant	10% (548)	10.1% (537)	9.1% (11)	1.000
Anti-Ro	39.9% (516)	39.4% (505)	63.6% (11)	0.125
Anti-La	13.4% (515)	13.1% (504)	27.3% (11)	0.172
Anti-RNP	31.1% (515)	31.2% (504)	27.3% (11)	1.000
SLEDAI (median)[c]	1 (415)	1 (407)	0 (11)	0.550
SLICC damage index (median)[c]	1 (559)	1 (551)	2 (11)	0.047

Abbreviations: *SLE* systemic lupus erythematosus, *SLEDAI* systemic lupus erythematosus disease activity index, *SLICC* systemic lupus international collaborating clinics, *HIV* human immunodeficiency virus
[a]Chi square test for qualitative variables and Mann-Whitney test for quantitative variables
[b]Current or past smoker
[c]Median (interquartile interval)

antibody stimulation [7] and treatment with antimalarials [8]. Patients with SLE have higher levels of interleukin (IL)-16 and IL-16 inhibits HIV infection in vitro, representing a possible protective role against HIV in SLE patients [9]. Likewise, SLE cannot develop in the setting of CD4 cell depletion seen in HIV [10]. Zandman-Goddard and Shoenfeld proposed that autoimmune manifestations in patients with HIV occur after the restoration of immunological competence (CD4 count > 500 cells/µL and low viral load) using ART or during the first stage of HIV (the acute HIV infection), when the immune system is intact and, hence, autoimmune diseases may present [11].

Kopelman and Zolla-Pazner published in 1988 the first report of a patient with HIV infection and SLE [12].

Since then, there have been several case reports or small case series of patients with concomitant SLE and HIV. Literature review has identified a total of 58 patients reported until 2014, some of which did not fulfill the criteria for SLE [1]. Then, in 2014, Mody et al. published a relatively large case series of 13 patients with coexistent HIV infection and SLE evaluated in a hospital of Durban, South Africa [1].

Kopelman and Zolla-Pazner have tested 151 consecutive patients with HIV and found that 19 had positive ANA, most of it in low titers, which usually is not associated with clinical manifestations of SLE [12]. Medina-Rodriguez et al. also found a significant number of HIV-positive patients with positivity for aCL IgG (94%), and aCL IgM (44%) [13].

Table 2 Demographic, clinical and laboratory features, treatment and outcome of SLE patients with HIV

Case	Gender	First DX	Clinical features	Autoantibodies	SLE treatment	ART	CD4 at DX[a]	Last CD4	Outcome
1	F	SLE	Discoid lupus, photosensitivity, oral ulcers and arthritis	ANA and anti-Ro	CS	Yes	434	337	Good health condition, but loss of follow-up in the Rheumatology Clinic
2	F	SLE	Raynaud, arthritis and vasculitis	ANA, anti-dsDNA, anti-Ro and anti-La	CS	Yes	572	205	Disseminated TB at 2015, follow-up in the Infectious Diseases Clinic
3	F	SLE	Arthritis, leucopenia, lymphopenia, alopecia, Raynaud and photosensitivity	ANA	HCQ	Yes	424	1056	SLE in remission, HIV controlled
4	F	SLE	Discoid lupus, photosensitivity, nephritis, leucopenia and lymphopenia	ANA	HCQ	Yes	149	524	HCV coinfection SLE in remission and HIV controlled
5	F	SLE	Photosensitivity, oral ulcers, arthritis and nephritis	ANA, anti-Ro and anti-La	CS, AZA ➔ MMF and tacrolimus	Yes	273	991	Pulmonary TB in 2008, kidney transplantation in 2011
6	F	SLE	Photosensitivity, serositis and arthritis	ANA	None	Yes	172	391	HCV coinfection, SLE in remission and HIV controlled
7	F	SLE	Alopecia, arthritis, nephritis, hemolytic anemia and hypergammaglobulinemia	ANA, anti-dsDNA and anti-Ro	HCQ, CYC ➔ AZA	Yes	321	165	Good initial response, poor adherence to treatment with posterior reactivation of nephritis and CD4 count drop
8	F	HIV	Hemolytic anemia, serositis, oral ulcers and arthritis	ANA, anti-Sm and anti-RNP	HCQ, MTX	Yes	NA	477	CMV Retinitis in 2006, SLE in remission and HIV controlled
9	F	HIV	Hemolytic anemia and nephritis	ANA and anti-dsDNA	CS, HCQ CYC ➔ AZA	Yes	235	252	Complete response to CYC, posterior poor adherence and loss of follow-up due to drug addiction
10	F	SLE	Hemolytic anemia, serositis, leucopenia, lymphopenia, oral ulcers, arthritis and nephritis	ANA and anti-dsDNA	HCQ	Yes	203	323	SLE in remission and HIV controlled
11	F	Both	Alopecia, hemolytic anemia, nephritis, thrombocytopenia, leucopenia and lymphopenia	ANA	CS, HCQ ➔AZA	Yes	111	NA	Both diagnosed in hospital stay, progressing to death from sepsis

Abbreviations: ACL IgG anti-cardiolipin IgG, ACL IgM anti-cardiolipin IgM, ANA anti-nuclear antibody, ART active antiretroviral therapy, AZA azathioprine, CMV cytomegalovirus, CS corticosteroids, CYC cyclophosphamide, dsDNA anti-double-stranded DNA, DX diagnosis, F female, HCQ hydroxychloroquine, HIV human immunodeficiency virus, M male, MMF mycophenolate mofetil, MTX methotrexate, NA not available, SLE systemic lupus erythematosus, TB tuberculosis
[a]CD4 cell count at diagnosis of HIV-infection: cells/mm^3

However, Petrovas et al. in a case-control study that compared the prevalence of antiphospholipid antibodies in patients with HIV infection, SLE with or without antiphospholipid syndrome (APS) and in primary antiphospholipid syndrome (PAPS), also evaluating the reactivity of these antibodies with β2-glicoprotein (GPI). It was demonstrated that the prevalence of aCL antibodies in HIV-infection was 36%. However, anti-β2-GPI occurred in only 5% of HIV, which seems to reduce its thrombogenic potential [14]. Therefore, antiphospholipid antibodies occur in HIV-1 infection, but are not associated with thrombosis [14]. In our cohort, prevalence of

antiphospholipid antibodies did not differ between patients with and without infection by HIV.

Additional studies evaluated the presence of other autoantibodies in HIV-positive patients and found multiple autoimmune phenomena HIV-associated, many of those seen in SLE, including besides the presence of ANAs, antiplatelet antibodies, antilymphocyte antibodies and antineutrophil cytoplasmic antibodies (ANCA), as well as Coomb's positivity, circulating immune complexes, rheumatoid factor and cryoglobulins [7, 13, 15, 16]. Furthermore, the presence of antibodies to extractable nuclear antigens (ENA) has also been described, although with controversial findings. Muller et al. have tested the presence of ENA by enzyme-linked immunosorbent assay (ELISA) in 100 HIV-positive patients, detecting anti-dsDNA, anti-histone, anti-Sm, anti-RNP and anti-Ro in 45% to 90% of these patients [17]. In its turn, Lafeuillade et al. in a study including 119 HIV-positive patients, found a lower frequency of those autoantibodies (4% had ANAs, 1% anti-dsDNA, 4% anti-Sm and 6% anti-histone) [18]. Thus, the presence of these autoantibodies in HIV patients is still controversial. Variations in the studied populations and in the analysis techniques employed explain, in part, these discrepancies [19]. In one study, the positivity for autoantibodies was significantly associated with lower CD4 lymphocyte counts and with increased mortality, which can indicate a prognostic implication of the autoimmunity in the context of HIV infection [15].

In patients with coexistence of HIV infection and diagnosis of SLE, three patterns of disease occurrence have been described: HIV following SLE diagnosis, SLE following the diagnosis of HIV infection and simultaneous diagnosis of HIV and SLE [20]. In our cohort, the most prevalent pattern was the one in which patients with established SLE were subsequently diagnosed with infection by HIV. Some studies suggest that HIV infection can attenuate the natural history of SLE [10, 21–23]. On the other hand, the impact of SLE in patients with pre-existing HIV infection is not well known. Some authors propose that SLE may contribute to a worst outcome of the HIV infection, keeping in mind that there are some reports describing a shorter time span until the development of AIDS in patients with concomitant SLE [23]. Nonetheless, this data is unavailable in many cases and there are some reports in which patients with coexistence of HIV infection and SLE did not developed AIDS even after long periods of observation [19]. Furthermore, some authors believe the immunologic effects of SLE and HIV may antagonize each other, contributing to the uncertainty regarding the clinical impact of this association [23].

Many of the clinical features of SLE overlap with either the primary features or secondary complications of HIV infection [24]: dermatologic findings such as alopecia, oral ulcers and facial rash; constitutional symptoms, including fever and malaise; musculoskeletal involvement such as arthralgias, arthritis and myalgias; renal abnormalities, including hematuria and proteinuria; central nervous system disorders, such as seizures and psychosis; hematologic alterations, including anemia, leucopenia, lymphopenia and thrombocytopenia; and immunologic features such as hypergammaglobulinemia and positive ANA [21, 25]. The term *pseudolupus* has been used to describe patients with HIV infection that present with rheumatic manifestations similar to SLE. In our cohort, nephritis, neuropsychiatric lupus, hemolytic anemia, hypergammaglobulinemia, presence of anti-Ro and anti-

La were the most prevalent features amongst the SLE patients infected by HIV.

Besides, false positive HIV on ELISA tests have also been described in SLE patients, making the diagnosis even more difficult, and making it necessary to perform other confirmatory tests for HIV [26]. In these cases, viral RNA PCR assays were superior than the p24 antigen assay (less sensitive) to exclude the possibility of a false positive HIV on ELISA test [27]. Low complement due to HIV infection has not been reported. Therefore, hypocomplementenemia may be a helpful test to differentiate lupus activity from HIV-related manifestations [24]. In our cohort the majority of patients with AIDS presented with hypocomplementenemia and this finding contributed not only to assess the disease activity, but also to establish the diagnosis of SLE.

The treatment of patients with coexistent SLE and HIV infection is challenging and there aren't well established therapeutic guidelines thus far. Immunosuppressive medications may have a negative impact in patients with preexistent impaired immunity [25]. However, with the adequate suppression of the HIV viral load, it is postulated that the treatment of SLE would not anticipate the development of AIDS [19]. Associated to ART, HCQ seems to be a reasonable and safe approach, considering it also has antiviral properties in HIV patients [28] and that its anti-inflammatory effect doesn't appear to be associated with an increased risk of opportunistic infections [29]. Low-dose corticosteroids may be considered with caution for those with severe immunosuppression by AIDS [25]. Relative safety of using MMF in HIV-positive patients has been confirmed by its successful use in the solid organ transplantation in HIV patients on ART [30]. Therefore, the risks and benefits have to be considered carefully when deciding the therapeutic approach that is more adequate to each patient with concomitant HIV infection and SLE [20]. Patients of our cohort that used CYC for the induction treatment of nephritis, followed by maintenance with AZA, developed a complete response with no major infectious complications.

It is well known that there is an increased risk of opportunistic infection in SLE patients, as well as in patients infected by HIV and this is the leading cause of morbidity and mortality in both diseases [6]. In our cohort, survival in 5 and 10 years was similar in SLE patients with or without AIDS. Even though we emphasized a statistically significant difference in the SLICC, indicating a greater cumulative damage in patients with concomitant AIDS, the clinical and prognostic relevance of this finding is uncertain thus far, once there was no significant difference in the survival rate between the groups in our study population.

Special attention must also be paid to infections caused by Mycobacterium tuberculosis, due to its high prevalence in HIV patients [31] as well as SLE, especially in developing countries [32]. Patients with lupus and HIV seems to have a higher risk of developing tuberculosis as shown by the largest case series available on the subject, in which 7 out of 13 patients were diagnosed with tuberculosis [1]. In our cohort, only 2 patients infected by HIV developed tuberculosis, probably reflecting the demographic differences and the regional prevalences of this disease.

Conclusion

Patients with concomitant HIV and SLE presented with neuropsychiatric manifestations more often. Therefore, it is essential to pay attention to the early diagnosis of HIV, especially in the scenario of this severe manifestation and in light of the need to intensify the immunosuppression. Moreover, there was a higher prevalence of hypergammaglobulinemia and hypocomplementenemia, which in turn, can be an useful tool to identify disease activity. For the first time, higher cumulative damage was described in lupus patients with concomitant HIV infection, which can contribute to a worst life quality and reduction of the survival rates, although further studies are needed to elucidate this complex association, its outcomes and prognosis.

Abbreviations
aCL: Anticardiolipin; ACR: AMERICAN College of Rheumatology; AIDS: Acquired immunodeficiency syndrome; ANA: Antinuclear antibody; ANCA: Antineutrophil cytoplasmic antibodies; APS: Antiphospholipid syndrome; ART: Antiretroviral therapy; AZA: Azathioprine; CYC: Cyclophosphamide; ds-DNA: Anti-double-stranded DNA; ELISA: Enzyme-linked immunosorbent assay; ENA: Extractable nuclear antigens; GPI: Glicoprotein; HCQ: Hydroxychloroquine, IL: Interleukin; MMF: Mycophenolate mofetil; MTX: Methotrexate; PAPS: Primary antiphospholipid syndrome; SD: Standard deviation; SLE: Systemic lupus erythematosus; SLEDAI: Systemic Lupus Erythematosus Disease Activity Index; SLICC: Systemic Lupus International Collaborating Clinics

Authors' contributions
All the authors collaborated in the analysis and in writing the manuscript. All authors read and approved the final manuscript.

Competing interests
The authors declare that they have no competing interests.

Author details
[1]Division of Rheumatology, Hospital de Clínicas de Porto Alegre, Universidade Federal do Rio Grande do Sul, 2350 Ramiro Barcelos St, Room 645, Porto Alegre, RS 90035-903, Brazil. [2]Medical School Student, Universidade Federal do Rio Grande do Sul, Porto Alegre, Brazil. [3]Division of Infectious Diseases, Hospital de Clínicas de Porto Alegre, Universidade Federal do Rio Grande do Sul, Porto Alegre, Brazil.

References
1. Mody GM, Patel N, Budhoo A, Dubula T. Concomitant systemic lupus erythematosus and HIV: case series and literature review. Semin Arthritis Rheum. 2014;44(2):186–94.
2. Hochberg MC. Updating the American College of Rheumatology revised criteria for the classification of systemic lupus erythematosus. Arthritis Rheum. 1997;40(9):1725.
3. Vitali C, Bombardieri S, Jonsson R, et al. Classification criteria for Sjögren's syndrome: a revised version of the European criteria proposed by the American-European consensus group. Ann Rheum Dis. 2002;61(6):554–8.
4. Miyakis S, Lockshin MD, Atsumi T, et al. International consensus statement on an update of the classification criteria for definite antiphospholipid syndrome (APS). J Thromb Haemost. 2006;4(2):295–306.
5. Griffiths B, Mosca M, Gordon C. Assessment of patients with systemic lupus erythematosus and the use of lupus disease activity indices. Best Pract Res Clin Rheumatol. 2005;19(5):685–708.
6. Sekigawa I, Okada M, Ogasawara H, et al. Lessons from similarities between SLE and HIV infection. J Inf Secur. 2002;44(2):67–72.
7. Kaye BR. Rheumatologic manifestations of HIV infections. Clin Rev Allergy Immunol. 1996;14:385–416.
8. Tsai WP, Nara PL, Kung HF, Oroszlan S. Inhibition of immunodeficiency virus infectivity by chloroquin. AIDS Res Hum Retrovir. 1990;6:481–9.
9. Sekigawa I, Lee S, Kaneko H, et al. The possible role of interleukin-16 in the low incidence of HIV infection in patients with systemic lupus erythematosus. Lupus. 2000;9:155–6.
10. Furie RA. Effects of human immunodeficiency virus infection on the expression of rheumatic illness. Rheum Dis Clin North Am. 1991;17:177–88.
11. Zandman-Goddard G, Shoenfeld Y. HIV and autoimmunity. Autoimmun Rev. 2002;1(6):329–37.
12. Kopelman RG, Zolla-Pazner S. Association of human immunodeficiency virus infection and autoimmune phenomena. Am J Med. 1988;84:82–8.
13. Medina-Rodriguez F, Guzman C, Jara LJ, et al. Rheumatic manifestations in human immunodeficiency virus positive and negative individuals: a study of 2 populations with similar risk factors. J Rheumatol. 1993;20:1880–4.
14. Petrovas C, Vlachouyiannopoulos PG, Kordossis T, Moutsopoulos M. Anti-phospholipid antibodies in HIV infection and SLE with or without anti-phospholipid syndrome: comparisons of phospholipid specificity, avidity and reactivity with B2-GPI. J Autoimmun. 1999;13:347–55.
15. Massabki PS, Accetturi C, Nishie IA, da Silva NP, Sato EI, Andrade LEC. Clinical implications of autoantibodies in HIV infection. AIDS. 1997;11:1845–50.
16. Stimmler MM, Quismorio FP Jr, McGehee WG, Boylen T, Sharma OP. Anticardiolipin antibodies in acquired immunodeficiency syndrome. Arch Intern Med. 1989;149:1833–5.
17. Muller S, Richalet P, Laurent-Crawford A, et al. Autoantibodies typical of non-organ-specific autoimmune disease in HIV-seropositive patients. AIDS. 1992;6:933–42.
18. Lafeuillade A, Ritter J, Pellegrino P, Qiulichini R, Monier JC. Lack of anti-nuclear antibodies during HIV infection (correspondence). AIDS. 1993;7:893.
19. Daikh BE, Holyst MM. Lupus-specific autoantibodies in concomitant human immunodeficiency virus and systemic lupus erythematosus: case report and literature review. Semin Arthritis Rheum. 2001;30:18–25.
20. Gindea S, Schwartzman J, Herlitz LC, et al. Proliferative glomerulonephritis in lupus patients with human immunodeficiency virus infection: a difficult clinical challenge. Semin Arthritis Rheum. 2010;40:201–9.
21. Molina JF, Citera G, Rosler D, et al. Coexistence of human immunodeficiency virus infection and systemic lupus erythematosus. J Rheumatol. 1995;22:347–50.
22. Byrd VM, Sergent JS. Suppression of systemic lupus erythematosus by the human immunodeficiency virus. J Rheumatol. 1996;23:1295–6.
23. Fox RA, Isenberg DA. Human immunodeficiency virus infection in systemic lupus erythematosus. Arthritis Rheum. 1997;40:1168–72.
24. Gould T, Tikly M. Systemic lupus erythematosus in a patient with human immunodeficiency virus infection – challenges in diagnosis and management. Clin Rheumatol. 2004;23:166–9.
25. López-López L, González A, Vilá LM. Long-term membranous glomerulonephritis as the presenting manifestation of systemic lupus erythematosus in a patient with human immunodeficiency virus infection. Lupus. 2012;21:900–4.
26. Gul A, Inanc M, Yilmaz G, et al. Antibodies reactive with HIV-1 antigens in systemic lupus erythematosus. Lupus. 1996;5:120–2.
27. UNAIDS/WHO Working Group on Global HIV/AIDS/STI Surveillance 2001 Guidelines for using HIV testing technologies in surveillance: selection, evaluation and implementation. Available at. http://www.who.int/hiv/pub/epidemiology/pub4/en/

28. Sperber K, Kalb TH, Stecher VJ, Banerjee R, Mayer L. Inhibition of human immunodeficiency virus type 1 replication by hydroxychloroquine in T cells and monocytes. AIDS Res Hum Retrovir. 1993;9:91–8.

29. Sperber K, Ornstein MH. The anti-inflammatory effect of hydroxychloroquine in two patients with acquired immunodeficiency syndrome and active inflammatory arthritis. Arthritis and Rheum. 1996;39:157–61.

30. Stock PG, Roland ME, Carlson L, et al. Kidney and liver transplantation in human immunodeficiency virus-infected patients: a pilot safety and efficacy study. Transplantation. 2003;76:370–5.

31. World Health Organization. TB/HIV Facts. Factsheet. Geneva: World Health Organization; 2013. Available at http://www.who.int/tb/challenges/hiv/factsheets/en

32. Zandman-Goddard G, Shoenfeld Y. Infections and SLE. Autoimmunity. 2005; 38:473–85.

7

Relevance of serum angiogenic cytokines in adult patients with dermatomyositis

Thiago Costa Pamplona da Silva, Marilda Guimarães Silva and Samuel Katsuyuki Shinjo[*]

Abstract

Background: Until now, there are few studies evaluating serum levels of angiogenic cytokines in dermatomyositis (DM). Therefore, the aims of the present study were: (a) to analyze systematically and simultaneously serum levels of angiogenin (ANG), angiopoietin (ANGPT)-1, vascular endothelial growth factor (VEGF), fibroblast growth factor (FGF)-1 and − 2, platelet derived growth factor (PDGF)-AA and -BB in DM; (b) to correlate the serum level of these cytokines with the DM clinical and laboratory features.

Methods: This is a cross sectional study, in which 48 patients with DM aged 18 to 45 years were gender-, age- and ethnicity-matched with 48 healthy individuals (control group). The serum levels of cytokines analyses were performed by multiplex immunoassay. The parameters of DM activity were based on the scores established by the International Myositis Assessment & Clinical Studies Group.

Results: The mean ages, gender frequencies and ethnicities were comparable between the patients with DM and the control group. A significantly higher serum FGF-1 and FGF-2 levels ($P < 0.001$ and $P < 0.001$, respectively), lower VEGF and PDGF-AA levels ($P = 0.009$ and $P = 0.022$), and comparable ANG, ANGPT-1 and PDGF-BB levels were observed in DM patients compared to controls. There was a tendency for cytokines (with the exceptions of VEGF and PDGF-BB) to correlate positively with the DM activity parameters, whereas FGF-2 correlated inversely. Moreover, FGF-1 strongly correlated with DM cutaneous manifestations.

Conclusions: The present data provide the relevance of different serum angiogenic cytokines in patients with DM. Additional studies will be needed to validate the data obtained in this work.

Keywords: Angiogenesis, Cytokines, Dermatomyositis, Idiopathic inflammatory myopathies, Myositis

Background

Dermatomyositis (DM) is an autoimmune inflammatory myopathy characterized by a subacute onset and progressive skeletal muscle weakness. The disease is associated with typical cutaneous manifestations, including heliotrope and/or Gottron's papules [1–7]. The cornerstone of DM physiopathogenesis involves vascular disturbances and a primarily humoral immune response [4–6], and can involve multiple cytokines related to mechanisms ranging from inflammation to angiogenesis.

Several serum angiogenic cytokines have been described in the literature, including: angiogenin (ANG), angiopoietin-1 (ANGPT-1), vascular endothelial growth factor (VEGF), fibroblast growth factor (FGF) types 1 and 2, and platelet-derived growth factor (PDGF-AA e PDGF-BB). However, these serum angiogenic cytokines have been scarcely assessed in DM [8–14]. For instance, Kuwahara [8] observed high ANG mRNA expression in the skin tissue of patients with active DM but no significant increase in the serum ANG level. Nevertheless, the authors described a positive correlation between the serum ANG and aldolase levels.

High serum VEGF levels have been noted in DM and polymyositis (PM) [9–11]. However, as a limitation, these data are based on a series of cases, involving individuals mostly ≥40 years of age with no detailed treatment information.

Kadono et al. [13] observed an elevated serum FGF-2 level in DM patients that correlated with the serum creatine phosphokinase (CPK) level and pulmonary fibrosis.

* Correspondence: samuel.shinjo@gmail.com
Division of Rheumatology, Faculdade de Medicina FMUSP, Universidade de Sao Paulo, Av. Dr. Arnaldo, 455, 3° andar, sala 3150 - Cerqueira César, Sao Paulo CEP: 01246-903, Brazil

However, this study assessed only 7 untreated female patients ≥50 years of age.

The serum ANGPT-1 levels were normal in patients with DM in a unique study in the literature [12]; however, although additional information concerning the association between values and clinical or laboratory parameters was provided, no date concerning the serum FGF-1 and PDGFs, there are no data evaluating serum levels were available for these patients.

Therefore, the aim of the present research was to assess simultaneously and systematically the serum ANG, ANGPT-1, VEGF, FGF (types 1 and 2), PDGF-AA and PDGF-BB levels in DM patients. Additionally, we sought to correlate the serum levels of these cytokines with demographic, clinical, laboratory, and therapeutic factors and comorbidities of patients with DM.

Methods

A cross-sectional study was performed at a single centre. The study included 60 consecutive patients with DM (age ≥ 18 and ≤ 45 years) enrolled from 2012 to 2014 who fulfilled all of the Bohan and Peter criteria items [1, 2] and were regularly followed at our outpatient myopathy unit. Patients with cancer-associated myositis, clinically amyopathic DM and overlapped myositis were not included in the study.

The study was approved by the local ethics committee (HCFMUSP - CAPPesq number 1.545.393) and all patients signed the informed consent form.

To avoid possible factors that could interfere with serum cytokine analysis, patients with > 10 years of DM disease ($n = 8$) and tobacco habits ($n = 4$) were excluded. Moreover, no cases of acute and/or chronic infections, liver and renal diseases, menopause, diabetes mellitus, non-controlled chronic systemic arterial hypertension, myocardial infarction, ischemic stroke, alcohol consumption and claudication vascular symptoms were included. Therefore, 48 patients with DM were assessed, and 48 age, gender and ethnicity-matched healthy volunteers were recruited as a control group during the same period.

All participants underwent a clinical evaluation that included a standardized interview, and their charts were extensively reviewed.

Demographic data were collected, including the current age, gender, ethnicity, waist circumference, weight and body mass index [BMI, weight/height^2 (kg/m^2)]. The clinical and laboratory data included the age at disease onset, disease duration, muscle enzyme serum levels [CPK: reference value 26–308 U/L, aldolase: < 7.5 U/L, alanine aminotransferase (ALT): < 41 U/L, aspartate aminotransferase (AST): < 37 U/L, lactate dehydrogenase (LDH): 240–480 U/L)], and clinical manifestations [articular (arthralgia or arthritis), pulmonary (moderated or

severe subjective dyspnea associated simultaneously with confirmed "ground-glass" on high-resolution chest computed tomography) activity, and cutaneous (Gottron's papules, heliotrope rash, ulcers, vasculitis, "shawl" sign, "V-neck" sign, facial rash, Raynaud's phenomenon, and calcinosis].

The disease status was evaluated using the following questionnaires and scores: global assessment of the disease (by the physician and the patient) through the visual analogue scale (VAS) [15–17], Manual Muscle Testing (MMT-8) [18], Health Assessment Quality (HAQ) [19].

Therapy data included the use of immunosuppressives and, glucocorticoids (current and cumulative doses).

Cytokine assessment. A blood sample (10 mL of blood) obtained from each participant after a 12-h overnight fast was immediately (< 30 min) centrifuged at 3000 rpm for 10 min at 4 °C. The serum was stored at – 80 °C prior analysis of the cytokines ANG, ANGPT-1, VEGF, FGF-1, FGF-2, PDGF-AA and PDGF-BB. The analysis was performed using the Luminex 200- xMAP Technology (Millipore, USA), as described elsewhere [20].

Statistical analysis. The Kolmogorov-Smirnov test was used to evaluate the distribution of each parameter. The demographic and clinical features were expressed as the mean ± standard deviation (SD) for continuous variables or as frequencies and percentages (%) for categorical variables. The median (25th - 75th interquartile range) was calculated for continuous variables that were non-normally distributed. Comparisons between the patient and control parameters were made using Student's t-test or the Mann-Whitney test for continuous variables, whereas the Chi-square test or Fisher's exact test was used to evaluate categorical variables. The correlations among the parameters were analysed by Spearman's correlation. All of the analyses were performed using the SPSS 15.0 statistical software (Chicago, USA). A $P < 0.05$ was considered to indicate statistical significance.

Results

Forty-eight patients with DM and 48 controls were evaluated. As expected, the mean age, gender frequency and ethnicity were similar between the groups (Table 1). The mean age at disease onset was 30.9 years, with 5.0 months of symptoms prior to diagnosis and median disease duration of 1.0 year.

The articular, pulmonary and cutaneous involvements were present in 29.2, 35.4 and 100% of the cases, respectively.

The disease status parameters are shown in Table 1. As expected, all muscle enzymes were significantly higher in the patients with DM than in the controls.

Table 1 General features of patients with dermatomyositis and health individuals

Parameters	DM (n = 48)	Control (n = 48)	P value
Age (years)	33.3 ± 7.6	35.8 ± 8.2	1.000
White ethnicity	36 (75.0)	32 (66.7)	0.501
Female gender	36 (75.0)	36 (75.0)	1.000
Age at disease onset (years)	30.9 ± 7.4	–	–
Duration: diagnosis - symptoms (months)	5.0 (2.3–8.5)	–	–
Disease duration (years)	1 (0–4)	–	–
Clinical cumulative manifestations			
Articular involvement	14 (29.2)	–	–
Pulmonary involvement	17 (35.4)	–	–
Cutaneous involvement	48 (100.0)	–	–
Gottron's papules	47 (97.9)	–	–
Heliotrope rash	40 (83.3)	–	–
Facial rash	30 (62.5)	–	–
Raynaud' phenomenon	24 (50.0)	–	–
"V-neck" sign	15 (31.3)	–	–
Ulcers	10 (20.8)	–	–
Vasculitis	10 (20.8)	–	–
"Shawl" sign	8 (16.7)	–	–
Calcinosis	0	–	–
MMT-8 (0–80)	78 (71–80)		
HAQ (0.00–3.00)	0.36 (0.00–2.00)	–	–
Patient VAS (0–10 mm)	5 (1–6)	–	
Physician VAS (0–10 mm)	4 (1–5)	–	–
Creatine phosphokinase (U/L)	200 (93–960)	100 (81–161)	0.002
Aldolase (U/L)	5.9 (4.1–12.9)	3.6 (3.1–4.3)	< 0.001
Lactic dehydrogenase (U/L)	412 (347–597)	323 (296–381)	< 0.001
Alanine aminotransferase (U/L)	25 (16–60)	17 (13–21)	< 0.001
Aspartate aminotransferase (U/L)	25 (19–52)	19 (16–22)	< 0.001
Prednisone			
Current use	34 (70.8)	–	–
Current dose (mg/day)	20.0 (3.1–50.0)	–	–
Cumulative dose[a] (mg)	645 (90–2103)	–	–
Cumulative dose[b] (g)	15.5 (5.8–27.8)	–	–
Immunosupressive/imunmodulatory[c]			–
None	20 (41.7)	–	–
One	11 (22.9)	–	–
Two	17 (35.4)	–	–

Results expressed as percentage (%), mean ± standard deviation, median (25th - 75th interquartile range)
DM dermatomyositis, HAQ Health Assessment Questionnaire, MMT Muscle Manual Testing, VAS visual analogue score
[a] Last 3 months; [b] since the begin of treatment; [c] imunossupressive / imunomodulatory: azathioprine (2–3 mg/kg/day), methotrexate (15–25 mg/week), cyclosporine (1.5–2.5 mg/kg/day), mycophenolate mofetil (2–3 g/day), rituximab (1 g, intravenous, at baseline and after one month - first cycle - and this schema was repeated after six months), cyclophosphamide (0.5–1.0 g/m² body surface), leflunomide (20 mg/day) and/or intravenous human immunoglobulin (2 g/kg, daily, two consecutive days)

Regarding drug treatment, 70.8% of the patients were using prednisone with a mean dose of 20.0 mg/day. The median cumulative dose of prednisone was 645 mg (over the last three months of blood collection) and 15.5 g (since the onset of disease symptoms). Approximately half of the patients were using at least one immunosuppressive or immunomodulatory drug, including azathioprine (2–3 mg/kg/day), methotrexate (15–25 mg/week), cyclosporine (1.5–2.5 mg/kg/day), mycophenolate mofetil (2–3 g/day), rituximab [1 g, intravenous, at baseline and after one month (first cycle); this scheme was repeated after six months], cyclophosphamide (0.5–1.0 g/m^2 body surface), leflunomide (20 mg/day) and/or human intravenous immunoglobulin (2 g/kg, daily, two consecutive days) (Table 1).

The serum levels of the angiogenic cytokines (ANG, ANGPT-1 and PDGF-BB) were comparable between the groups (Table 2). The FGF-1 and FGF-2 levels were elevated, whereas the VEGF and PDGF-AA levels were decreased in the patients with DM compared to the control group.

Table 3 shows only the significant correlations between the angiogenic cytokines analysed in the present study and the demographic, clinical, laboratory and therapeutic parameters shown previously in Table 1. Moreover, the correlations between the cytokines themselves were also analysed. All data refer to patients with DM.

The FGF-1 serum levels were moderately correlated with the cutaneous clinical manifestations (facial rash, "V-neck" sign and "shawl" sign) as well as some disease activity parameters (patient and physician VAS, and muscle enzymes) and were inversely correlated with the disease duration and cumulative prednisone dose. Additionally, the serum FGF-1 levels positively correlated with the serum ANG, ANGPT-1 and PDGF-AA levels and negatively correlated with the FGF-2 levels.

FGF-2 tended to be inversely correlated with the disease activity parameters (patient and physician VAS, MMT-8, and muscle enzymes) and serum FGF-1, ANG, ANGPT-1, PDGF-AA and PDGF-BB levels. A positive correlation was found between the serum FGF-2 levels and the cumulative prednisone dose.

Low serum PDGF-AA and VEGF levels were observed in patients with DM. No correlation was found between the VEGF level and the disease activity parameters or treatment data. However, the serum PDFG-AA, and FGF-1 levels were positively correlated with the DM disease parameters (physician VAS, MMT-8, HAQ, and muscle enzymes) and inversely correlated with the disease duration and cumulative prednisone dose. A positive correlation between the PDGF level and the serum ANG, ANGPT-1 and PDGF-AA levels and a negative correlation with the FGF-2 level were also observed.

ANG, ANGPT-1 and PDGF-BB were not elevated in DM. However, the correlations among the serum levels of these cytokines and the other parameters generally followed the same profiles observed for FGF-1 and PDGF-AA.

Discussion

This study is the first to systematically and simultaneously analyse the serum levels of several angiogenic cytokines in patients with DM.

The great advantage of the present study was its use of rigorous selection criteria for patients. Additionally, we excluded confounding factors that could interfere with the evaluation and interpretation of the angiogenic cytokines.

FGF-1 was positively correlated with the cutaneous clinical manifestations and some disease activity parameters, which was in contrast with FGF-2. We also observed lower FGF-1 levels in the patients with longer disease duration and a cumulative utilization of prednisone.

Both FGF-1 and -2 act in several cellular processes and specifically, in angiogenesis, they induce cell proliferation and the physical organization of endothelial cells into tubular structures [21–24]. Due to their specific biological functions and roles, FGFs have the potential for application to induce the regeneration of a wide spectrum of tissues [24].

By combining these known actions of FGF-1 with our findings, we propose that this cytokine may be involved in the physiopathogenesis of cutaneous manifestations in active DM patients, because patients with more cutaneous lesions, a shorter duration of disease or long-term treatment have higher serum FGF-1 levels. Further studies of cutaneous biopsies to evaluate local levels of FGF-1 or its genic expression could corroborate this hypothesis.

FGF-2 has a more powerful healing action than FGF-1. Indeed, blockage of FGF-2 activity is almost completely impairs wound angiogenesis [25]. Moreover, some in vitro and in vivo studies have demonstrated that FGF-2 promotes stem cell recruitment during the muscle regeneration process [26].

Table 2 Serum levels of angiogenic cytokines in patients with dermatomyositis and healthy individuals

Parameters	DM (n = 48)	Control (n = 48)	P value
ANG (ng/mL)	4383 (3588–7251)	3931 (2735–5397)	0.138
ANGPT-1 (ng/mL)	8576 (4964–13,060)	8080 (5785–9609)	0.224
VEGF (ng/mL)	28.6 (5.8–49.3)	38.6 (21.3–72.6)	0.009
FGF-1 (ng/mL)	3.1 (1.8–14.9)	0.7 (0.4–1.8)	< 0.001
FGF-2 (ng/mL)	1.6 (0.6–3.1)	0.3 (0.0–0.9)	< 0.001
PDGF-AA (ng/mL)	545 (304–797)	654 (411–1083)	0.022
PDGF-BB (ng/mL)	2039 (1539–2506)	2107 (1752–2465)	0.358

Results expressed as median (25th - 75th interquartile range)
ANG angiogenin, *ANGPT-1* angiopoietin-1, *DM* dermatomyositis, *FGF* fibroblast growth factor, *PDGF* platelet-derived growth factor, *VEGF* vascular endothelial growth factor

Table 3 Spearman's correlation between angiogenic cytokines and diferent disease parameters

	ANG		ANGPT-1		FGF-1		FGF-2		VEGF		PDGF-AA		PDGF-BB	
	rho	P	rho	P	rho	P	rho	P	rho	P	rho	P	rho	P
Current age			0.289	0.018							0.399	0.018		
Age at disease onset			0.401	0.005	0.295	0.042					0.416	0.003		
Disease duration			−0.448	0.001	−0.394	0.006					−0.326	0.024	−0.411	0.004
Body mass index									0.317	0.028				
Facial rash	0.387	0.021			0.367	0.010								
"V-neck" sign					0.338	0.019								
"Shawl" sign			0.355	0.013	0.343	0.017								
Pulmonary involvement	0.435	0.009												
Patient VAS	0.410	0.014	0.326	0.024	0.351	0.014	−0.364	0.012						
Physician VAS	0.476	0.004	0.387	0.007	0.341	0.018	−0.385	0.007			0.324	0.025		
MMT-8			−0.470	0.001			−0.413	0.004			−0.457	0.001	−0.382	0.008
HAQ			0.400	0.005							0.338	0.019		
Creatine phosphokinase			0.315	0.035										
Aldolase			0.537	< 0.001	0.397	0.009	−0.344	0.028			0.469	0.002	0.478	0.002
Lactic dehydrogenase					0.339	0.023								
Aspartate aminotransferase					0.429	0.004	−0.398	0.008			0.363	0.016	0.324	0.034
Alanine aminotransferase					0.379	0.010								
Cyclosporin			−0.309	0.032										
Prednisone (current use)			0.463	0.001	0.342	0.017					0.478	0.001	0.510	< 0.001
Prednisone (cumulative[a])			−0.390	0.006	−0.399	0.005	0.301	0.040			−0.315	0.029		
ANG	1.000		0.366	0.001	0.512	< 0.001	−0.594	< 0.001			0.408	0.004		
ANGPT-1	0.360	0.034	1.000		0.502	< 0.001	−0.453	0.001			0.820	< 0.001	0.725	< 0.001
FGF-1	0.344	0.034	0.502	< 0.001	1.000		−0.376	0.009			0.437	0.002		
FGF-2			−0.543	0.001	−0.376	0.009	1.000				−0.459	0.001	−0.391	0.007
VEGF									1.000					
PDGF-AA			0.820	< 0.001	0.437	0.002	−0.459	0.001			1.000		0.720	< 0.001
PDGF-BB			0.725	< 0.001			−0.391	0.007			0.720	< 0.001	1.000	

ANG angiogenin, *ANGPT-1* angiopoietin-1, *FGF* fibroblast growth factor, *HAQ* Health Assessment Questionnaire, *MMT* Muscle Manual Testing, *P* P value, *PDGF* platelet-derived growth factor-AA and BB; *Rho*: Spearmen's correlation, *VAS* visual analogue scores, *VEGF* vascular endothelial growth factor
[a]Since the disease onset symptoms

A negative correlation between the serum FGF-2 level and the disease activity parameters and a positive correlation with the cumulative prednisone dose were noted. One possible explanation for this finding is that FGF-1 and FGF-2 are continuously released into the bloodstream by muscle and endothelial tissues due to myofibrillar necrosis. Alternatively, the muscle regeneration process and fibrosis that occur during the evolution of disease or its treatment may maintain the elevated FGF-2 level due to its potent cure and regeneration actions. This phenomenon would make FGF-2 a marker of the muscular healing process in DM patients.

We found an inverse pattern of correlation between FGF-1 and -2 (positive and negative, respectively) and the other angiogenic cytokines evaluated. We conclude that there are mechanisms that up and down-regulate

FGF-1 and FGF-2 during the different stages of disease progression with a more established counter-regulation in chronic or adequately treated cases.

PDGF-AA and PDGF-BB promote the maturation of blood vessels through the recruitment and adhesion of mural cells by specific interactions with their receptors PDGF-Rαα (positive mitotic signals) and PDGF-Rββ (positive and negative mitotic signals). Both cytokines can promote and inhibit chemotaxis and cell growth [27], and their behavior depends on the context.

In this study, the correlations between the PDGF-AA level and the clinical and laboratory parameters in DM patients had the same pattern as FGF-1 with the exception of the cutaneous manifestations. FGF-1 has been shown to induce the expression of PDGF-AA in endothelial cells through an unknown mechanism [28]. Thus, in active DM, these cytokines may interact in a synergistic manner to potentiate their angiogenic actions through interactions with their receptors.

One possible explanation for the reduction in the VEGF serum levels in DM patients is that most of our patients were in an early stage of the disease, were well treated and were controlled symptomatically; therefore, little inflammatory infiltration was present and the capillary efficiency was more established. Another probable hypothesis is that the release of this cytokine by endothelial and inflammatory cells occurred initially at sites of greater inflammation, such as the muscle and/or skin, without the need for blood transport [10]. Thus, local measurement of VEGF in these tissues and an analysis of its gene expression patterns are needed in future studies.

The serum PDGF- BB, ANG and ANGPT-1 levels were correlated with the DM disease parameters, similar to FGF-1.

As discussed above, the PDGFs interact with specific receptors, and PDGF-BB has an affinity for all PDGF-R heterodimers [27]. Similarly, other cytokines, such as FGF-2, have an activation/inhibition relationship with PDGF [29]. The cytokine profile found in this study shows an increase of FGF-2 in DM patients, which may have inhibitory effects on PDGF-BB.

In agreement with our results, only one study evaluated the serum ANG levels in DM patients [8] and found no significant difference in the ANG levels between groups. However, the authors observed high gene expression of ANG in the analysed skin biopsies which suggests in situ inflammatory activity control more than a systemic control.

ANGPT-1 also interacts with other cytokines, such as VEGF, on endothelial cells to inhibit leukocyte adhesion the expression of some specific cell adhesion molecules [30]. Another important antagonist of ANGPT-1 is ANGPT-2 [31]. The interaction with inhibitory factors, such as ANGPT-2, may allow the serum levels to remain similar the levels observed in healthy people, as shown in our results.

Considering that the cytokines with the highest serum levels evaluated in this work were FGF-1 and FGF-2 and the correlation of these cytokine levels with the treatment received, we cannot exclude the possibility that the immunosuppressive treatment may have influenced the results by interfering with the inflammatory and angiogenic processes.

Among the limitations of the present study were the transversal nature and the analysis of the serum levels of the cytokines performed in a single measurement, because the serum profiles could have changed during the evolution of the disease and the establishment of treatment.

Conclusions

In summary, we found an increase in the serum FGF-1 and FGF-2 levels, a decrease in the VEGF and PDGF-AA levels, and comparable ANG, ANGPT-1 and PDGF-BB levels in patients with DM and the healthy controls. The FGF-1, PDGF-AA, ANG and AGPT-1 levels showed a positive correlation with the disease activity parameters, which was in contrast to the FGF-2 level. Moreover, FGF-1 and FGF-2 correlated positively with the cutaneous DM manifestations and cumulative prednisone dose, respectively. These data provide the possible involvement of angiogenic cytokines in DM disease.

Abbreviations
ALT: Alanine aminotransferase; ANG: Angiogenin; ANGPT: Angiopoietin; AST: Aspartate aminotransferase; BMI: Body mass index; CPK: Creatine phosphokinase; DM: Dermatomyositis; FGF: Fibroblast growth factor; HAQ: Health Assessment Quality; LDH: Lactate dehydrogenase; MMT: Manual muscle testing; PDGF: Platelet derived growth factor; SD: Standard deviation; VAS: Visual analogue scale; VEGF: Vascular endothelial growth factor

Support
Federico Foundation; Fundação Faculdade de Medicina; Fundação de Amparo à Pesquisa do Estado de São Paulo (FAPESP) (#2012/07101–4 and #2012/09633–3) to SKS; Coordenação de Aperfeiçoamento de Pessoal de Nível Superior (CAPES) to MGS.

Authors' contributions
All authors contributed equally to write and review the manuscript. All authors read and approved the final manuscript.

Competing interests
All authors declare that they have no conflicts of interest.

References
1. Bohan A, Peter JB. Polymyositis and dermatomyositis (first of two parts). N Engl J Med. 1975;292:344–7.
2. Bohan A, Peter JB. Polymyositis and dermatomyositis (second of two parts). N Engl J Med. 1975;292:403–7.
3. Dimachkie MM, Barohn RJ, Amato A. Idiopathic inflammatory myopathies. Neurol Clin. 2014;32:595–628.
4. Dalakas MC. Inflammatory muscle diseases. N Engl J Med. 2015;373:393–4.
5. Dalakas MC. Pathophysiology of inflammatory and autoimmune myopathies. Presse Med. 2011;40:e237–47.
6. Dalakas MC. Review: an update on inflammatory and autoimmune myopathies. Neuropathol Appl Neurobiol. 2011;37:226–42.
7. Orlandi M, Barsotti S, Cioffi E, Tenti S, Toscano C, Baldini C, et al. One year in review 2016: idiopathic inflammatory myopathies. Clin Exp Rheumatol. 2016;34:966–74.
8. Kuwahara A. Angiogenin expression in the sera and skin of patients with rheumatic diseases. Biosci Trends. 2012;6:229–33.
9. Kikuchi K, Kubo M, Kadono T, Yazawa N, Ihn H, Tamaki K. Serum concentrations of vascular endothelial growth factor in collagen diseases. Br J Dermatol. 1998;139:1049–51.
10. Grundtman C, Tham E, Ulfgren AK, Lundberg IE. Vascular endothelial growth factor is highly expressed in muscle tissue of patients with polymyositis and patients with dermatomyositis. Arthritis Rheum. 2008;58:3224–38.
11. Volpi N, Pecorelli A, Lorenzoni P, Di Lazzaro F, Belmonte G, Agliano M, et al. Antiangiogenic VEGF isoform in inflammatory myopathies. Mediat Inflamm. 2013;2013:219313.

12. Ishikawa A, Okada J, Nishi K, Hirohata S. Efficacy of serum angiopoietin-1 measurement in the diagnosis of early rheumatoid arthritis. Clin Exp Rheumatol. 2011;29:604–8.

13. Kadono T, Kikuchi K, Kubo M, Fujimoto M, Tamaki K. Serum concentrations of basic fibroblast growth factor in collagen diseases. J Am Acad Dermatol. 1996;35:392–7.

14. Carvalho JF, Blank M, Shoenfeld Y. Vascular endothelial growth factor (VEGF) in autoimmune diseases. J Clin Immunol. 2007;27:246–56.

15. Rider LG, Giannini EH, Harris-Love M, Joe G, Isenberg D, Pilkington C, et al. Defining clinical improvement in adult and juvenile myositis. J Rheumatol. 2003;30:603–17.

16. Miller FW, Rider GL, Chung YL, Cooper R, Danko K, Farewell V, et al. Proposed preliminary core set measures for disease outcome assessment in adult and juvenile idiopathic inflammatory myopathies. Rheumatology (Oxford). 2001;40:1262–73.

17. Isenberg DA, Allen E, Farewell V, Ehrenstein MR, Hanna MG, Lundberg IE, et al. International myositis and clinical studies group (IMACS). International consensus outcome measures for patients with idiopathic inflammatory myopathies. Development and initial validation of myositis activity and damage indices in patients with adult onset disease. Rheumatology (Oxford). 2004;43:49–54.

18. Rider LG, Koziol D, Giannini EH, Jain MS, Smith MR, Whitney-Mahoney K, et al. Validation of manual muscle testing and a subset of eight muscles for adult and juvenile idiopathic inflammatory myopathies. Arthritis Care Res. 2010;62:465–72.

19. Bruce B, FrieS JF. The Stanford health assessment questionnaire: dimensions and practical applications. Health Qual Life Outcomes. 2003;1:20.

20. Sada KE, Yamasaki Y, Maruyama M, Sugiyama H, Yamamura M, Maeshima Y, et al. Altered levels of adipocytokines in association with insulin resistance in patients with systemic lupus erythematosus. J Rheumatol. 2006;33:1545–52.

21. Dignass AU, Tsunekawa S, Podolsky DK. Fibroblast growth factors modulate intestinal epithelial cell growth and migration. Gastroenterol. 1994;106: 1254–62.

22. Holland EC, Varmus HE. Basic fibroblast growth factor induces cell migration and proliferation after glia- specific gene transfer in mice. Proc Nat Acad Sci USA. 1998;95:1218–23.

23. Hossain WA, Morets DK. Fibroblast growth factors (FGF-1. FGF-2) promote migration and neurite growth of mouse cochlear ganglion cells in vitro: immunohistochemistry and antibody perturbation. J Neurosci Res. 2000;62: 10–55

24. Yun YR, Won JE, Jeon E, Lee S, Kang W, Jo H, et al. Fibroblast growth factors: biology, function and application for tissue regeneration. J Tissue Eng. 2010;218142:2010.

25. Broadley KN, Aquino AM, Hicks B, Ditesheim JA, McGee GS, Demetriou AA, et al. The diabetic rat as an impaired wound healing model: stimulatory effects of transforming growth factor-beta and basic fibroblast growth factor. Biotechnol Ther. 1989;1:55–68.

26. Yablonka-Reuveni Z, Seger R, Rivera AJ. Fibroblast growth factor promotes recruitment of skeletal muscle satellite cells in young and old rats. J Histoch Cytoch. 1999;47:23–42.

27. Tengood JE, Ridenour R. BrodskYR, Russell AJ, little SR. sequential delivery of basic fibroblast growth factor and platelet-derived growth factor for angiogenesis. Tissue Eng. Part. 2011;7:1181–9.

28. Delbridge GJ, Khachigian LM. FGF-1 induced platelet-derived growth factor-a chain gene expression in endothelial cells involves transcriptional activation by early growth response factor-1. Circ Res. 1997;81:282–8.

29. Facchiano A, De Marchis F, Turchetti E, Facchiano F, Guglielmi M, Denaro A, et al. The chemotactic and mitogenic effects of platelet-derived growth factor-BB on rat aorta smooth muscle cells are inhibited by basic fibroblast growth factor. J Cell Sci. 2000;113:2855–63.

30. Fukuhara S, Sako K, Noda K, Zhang J, Minami M, Mochizuki N. Angiopoietin-1/Tie2 receptor signaling in vascular quiescence and angiogenesis. Histol Histopathol. 2010;25:387–96.

31. Kim I, Moon SO, Park SK, Chae SW, Koh GY. Angiopoietin-1 reduces VEGF-stimulated leukocyte adhesion to endothelial cells by reducing ICAM-1. VCAM-1 and E-selectin expression. Circ Res. 2001;89:477–9.

8

A cross-sectional study of associations between kinesiophobia, pain, disability, and quality of life in patients with chronic low back pain

Josielli Comachio[*] [iD], Mauricio Oliveira Magalhães, Ana Paula de Moura Campos Carvalho e Silva and Amélia Pasqual Marques

Abstract

Background: Low back pain is a significant health problem condition due to high prevalence among the general population. Emotions and physical factors are believed to play a role in chronic low back pain. Kinesiophobia is one of the most extreme forms of fear of pain due to movement or re-injury.

The purpose of this study was to investigate the association between kinesiophobia and pain intensity, disability and quality of life in people with chronic low back pain.

Methods: The study included 132 individuals with chronic back pain, with ages between 18 and 65 years old. Kinesiophobia was assessed using the Tampa Scale of Kinesiophobia, pain intensity was measured using the Numeric Rating Scale with a cut-off more than 3 for inclusion in the study, disability was assessed using the Roland Morris questionnaire, quality of pain was assessed using the McGill questionnaire, and quality of life was assessed using the Quality of Life questionnaire SF-36.

Results: The results are statistically significant, but with weak associations were found between kinesiophobia and pain intensity ($r = 0.187$), quality of pain (sensory, $r = 0.266$; affective, $r = -0.174$; and total $r = 0.275$), disability ($r = 0.399$) and physical quality of life (emotional $r = -0.414$).

Conclusion: Kinesiophobia is an important outcome to assess in patients with chronic low back pain. The results suggest that correlations between kinesiophobia and disability and quality of life are statistically significant.

Keywords: Kinesiophobia, Low back pain and fear of movement

Background

Nonspecific low back pain (LBP) refers to pain and discomfort localized in the lumbosacral region, with or without radiating leg pain. The patient often show pain between the costal margins and the inferior gluteal folds, and it is usually accompanied by painful limitation of movement [1]. The prevalence of low back pain in the general population is reported to be up to 18%, increasing to 31% of the population reporting low back pain in the last 30 days, 38% in the last 12 months, and 39% at any point in life [2]. A prognosis of low back pain is directly related to the duration of the symptoms [3–5].

It is estimated that 73.3% of patients with chronic low back pain suffer from depression [6, 7]. In addition, psychosocial factors (e.g. anxiety, fear, stress, somatization, and socioeconomic problems) have negative impacts on patients with chronic low back pain. One psychological factor that has received much attention in the case of chronic pain is fear in association with disability, related to the intensity and persistence of pain [8]. Kinesiophobia is one of the most extreme forms of fear of pain due to movement or re-injury [9, 10].

According to cognitive-behavioral models such as fear-avoidance [11], painful experiences can cause a fear of movement and injury in certain individuals, which

* Correspondence: josiellicomachio@usp.br
Department of Speech, Physical and Occupational Therapy, School of Medicine, University of Sao Paulo, Cipotânea, n 51, Cidade Universitária, Sao Paulo, Brazil

often leads to behavioral agitation and, in the long-run, depression, and increased levels of functional disability. Furthermore, fear avoidance beliefs and kinesiophobia are relevant factors regarding chronic pain complaints in the general population. Therefore, it is necessary to develop strategies for prevention so that kinesiophobia does not development in patients with low back pain [11]. For low back pain, these prevention initiatives would change in beliefs and attitudes about low back pain [12, 13] once the impact on patients' fear of movement about biomechanics to protect the spinal structures has not been well defined [14].

Therefore, the objective of this study was to evaluate kinesiophobia, pain, and functional disability in patients with chronic low back pain and to determine if there are associations of kinesiophobia with any of the measures.

Methods

This cross-sectional study involved 132 patients with chronic nonspecific low back pain and was approved by the ethics committee of the xxxxxxxxxxxxxx (Protocol XXXXX). We contacted the participants using study flyers, newspaper advertisements, and a list of patients with low back pain at the Specialized Rehabilitation Center. All the participants were confirmed as having chronic nonspecific low back pain, as diagnosed by an orthopedist through a detailed evaluation and imaging (x-ray), to exclude associated diseases. After the evaluation by a physician, the participants were contacted the patients by phone and invited to participate in the study. Participants gave their informed consent before participation. A blind evaluator, a physiotherapist who was trained to evaluate kinesiophobia, pain intensity, functional disability, quality of pain and quality of life, assessed the participants.

The inclusion criteria were: nonspecific chronic low back pain for more than 3 months, an age between 18 and 65 years old, and a minimum pain intensity score of 3 on the Numerical Rating Scale (NRS) [15]. Subjects who had any history of malignancy or spinal fracture, had undergone any surgical procedure in the previous 6 months, had orthopedic or neurological diseases affecting ambulation, or did not understand written and spoken Portuguese were excluded from the study. All the instruments used to assess the outcome measures had previously been translated and adapted to Brazilian-Portuguese versions, and had adequate psychometrical properties [16–20].

Kinesiophobia was assessed using the Tampa Scale of Kinesiophobia, which it was developed to measure the fear of movement due to chronic low back pain. It is a self-report questionnaire of 17 items, and it was used to assess the kinesiophobia of the subjects. Each question has four response options (strongly disagree, disagree, agree, or strongly agree) with scores ranging from 1 to 4 points, respectively. The total score is calculated after inversion of the individual scores of items 4, 8, 12, and 16. The total score ranges between 17 and 68. Increased scores reflect an increased fear of movement [18]. Vlaeyen et al. defined a cut off score of 37 as a high degree of kinesiophobia [21].

Pain intensity was assessed using the numeric pain rating scale (NPRS). This is an 11-point numeric pain scale, ranging from 0 to 10, on which 0 indicates "no pain" and 10 the "worst possible pain" at the time of the assessment [22].

Quality of pain was assessed using the McGill Pain Questionnaire, a multidimensional assessment of pain. It consists of 77 descriptors of the quantity and quality of pain, grouped into four major domains: sensory, affective, evaluative, and miscellaneous. The domains have 20 sub-domains represented by words that qualify the feelings of pain of a subject, for which intensity values, on a scale of 1 to 5, are assigned. The questionnaire is used to describe the pain experienced by a subjects and the score is the sum of the aggregate values. Maximum scores for each domain are: sensory = 41, affective = 14, evaluative = 5, and miscellaneous = 17, with a total possible score of = 77. The index of the pain assessment of each domain is the sum of the scores of the sub-domains, and each option chosen in domain in questionnaire for represented the pain was the maximum score for each category [17].

Quality of life was assessed using the Short Form Health Survey Questionnaire SF36 to assess health related qualify of life. The Sf36 consists of 36 questions, grouped in eight domains: vitality (4 items), physical functioning (10 items), bodily pain (2 items), general health (5 items), physical role limitation (2 items), emotional role limitation (3 items), social functioning (2 items), and mental health (5 items). For each section, the score ranges from 0 to 100, and higher scores reflect better quality of life. In is study, the focus was on the physical and emotional role limitation domains [19].

For disability, the Roland Morris Disability Questionnaire was used to assess functional disability due to low back pain. This questionnaire consists of 24 questions that focus on regular activities in daily living. Each affirmative answer is awarded 1 point and the final score is determined as the total number of points. Total scores range from 0 to 24, with higher scores reflecting increased disability. Scores above 14 indicate severe impairment [16].

All analyses were conducted using SPSS version 22.0 (IBM Corporation, USA). One-way fixed effects analysis of variance (ANOVA) was used. A statistical power of 80% (1 β error probability) with an α error level probability of 0.05 was chosen to detect between-group differences in the primary outcome measures. A medium effect size of 0.35 was used. Thus, it was estimated the study needed a minimum number of 132 subjects.

In statistical analysis, mean ± standard deviation (SD) values were calculated for the quantitative variables and percentages were calculated for qualitative variables. Pearson correlation coefficients and a multiple linear regression model were used to analyze of the associations of the clinical variables (pain intensity, disability, quality of life and pain duration) with kinesiophobia. The following indices were used to rank the correlations: < 0.49 = low; 0.50−0.69 = good; > 0.7 = excellent [23]. Significance was accepted for values of $p \leq 0.05$.

Results

This study evaluated 132 patients (40 males, 92 females) with chronic low back pain lasting on mean 43 months who reported a mean (SD) of pain and 43.9 (6.6) points of kinesiophobia. Table 1 shows the demographic characteristics the population of is study, and their self-reported levels of kinesiophobia, pain intensity, disability and quality of life.

The Table 2 shows the associations between kinesiophobia and the clinical variables. Kinesiophobia correlated with pain intensity, disability, and physical and emotional roles limitation of quality of life. However, the

Table 1 Demographic and clinical characteristics of the participants

Variable	Mean (SD) ($n = 132$)
Age (years)	47.4 ± 9.4
Weight (kg)	71.4 ± 12.8
Height (cm)	1.62 ± 0.9
BMI (kg/m^2)	27.2 ± 4.5
Sex (Male/Female)	40(30%)/ 92(69%)
Marital Status	
Single	35 (26%)
Married	79 (59%)
Divorced	13 (9%)
Widow	5 (3%)
Use of medication	96 (73%)
Kinesiophobia (17−68)	43.9 ± 6.6
Intensity of pain (0−10)	7.7 ± 1.7
Quality of pain (0−100)	
Sensory (0−41)	20.4 ± 7.7
Affective (0−14)	5.4 ± 3.4
Disability (0−24)	14.0 ± 5.1
Quality of life (0−100)	
Physical roles limitation	38.0 ± 40.6
Emotional roles limitation	51.2 ± 44.4
Duration of low back pain (months)	43.8 ± 32.2

Categorical variables are expressed as n (%) and the continuous variable are expressed as mean ± SD. $p \leq 0.05$

Table 2 Correlation between kinesiophobia and the measured clinical variables

	Kinesiophobia ($n = 132$)	
	R	Coefficients (95% CI)
Intensity of pain (0−10)	0.187*	(−0.002 to 0.364)
Quality of pain (0−77)		
Sensory	0.266**	(0.112 to 0.406)
Affective	0.174*	(0.024 to 0.331)
Total	0.275**	(0.117 to 0.433)
Disability (0−24)	0.399*	(0.254 to 5.30)
Quality of life (0−100)		
Physical roles limitation	0.111	(−0.062 to 0.276)
Emotional roles limitation	−0.414**	(− 0.560 to − 0.258)
Duration of low back pain (months)	0.105	(− 0.065 to 0.258)

*significant, $p < 0.05$ **significant, $p < 0.01$

correlations between kinesiophobia and physical role limitations and the duration of pain were not significant.

Similarly, when the kinesiophobia scores were adjusted for possible confounding variables, (duration of pain, pain intensity, quality of life and disability), no association with the severity of symptoms was observed, except for the emotional role limitation component of quality of life (Table 3).

Discussion

The objectives of this study were to evaluate kinesiophobia, pain, and functional disability in patients with chronic low back pain and to determine if there were associations of kinesiophobia with the other measured variables. The patients of this study demonstrated weak but statistically significant associations of kinesiophobia with pain intensity, quality of pain, disability and quality of life in the emotional domain. However, there was no association with the duration of symptoms.

The patients of this study scored an average 43.9 points on the scale of kinesiophobia, which is considered a moderate level for patients with chronic nonspecific low back pain [12]. Furthermore, they had other symptoms such as high intensity of pain, low quality of pain and life, frequent use of drugs and another characteristic's. Although the correlations were weak, the results corroborate those of other studies [5, 24−26], supporting the hypothesis that low back pain patients show a worsening prognosis due to the fear of moving, negative thoughts, and sick leave for low back pain.

Some authors [11, 25] have attempted to explain the exact mechanisms and factors related to chronic low back pain, and have reported that a model based on clinical signs and symptoms suggests that intensity and quality of pain are proportional to the extent of tissue injury, which eventually evolves into high levels of

Table 3 Multiple linear regression model of the comparison between kinesiophobia scores and the clinical variables

	Kinesiophobia ($n = 132$)	
	Standardized coefficients	Std. Error
Intensity of pain (0–10)	0.249	0.326
Quality of pain (0–77)		
Sensory	0.086	0.084
Affective	−0.114	0.194
Disability (0–24)	0.272	0.125
Quality of life (0–100)		
Physical roles functional	0.018	0.128
Emotional roles functional	−0.042*	0.013
Duration of low back pain	0.003	0.008

Significant, $p \leq 0.05$

disability [27]. However, there is also evidence that the persistence of symptoms of pain cannot be explained by objective clinical findings; therefore, a specific approach based on a biomedical model may prove insufficient due to the complexity of factors that are related to low back pain (e.g. unhelpful beliefs, catastrophizing, maladaptive coping strategies, poor self-efficacy, and depression) [28–30]. It is our opinion that the present study presents weak but confirmatory evidence, that kinesiophobia and low back pain are associated.

According to the biopsychosocial model, some individuals with musculoskeletal pain develop a chronic pain syndrome, the *"cognitive model of fear of movement/(re) injury"* suggested by Vlaeyen [31], which is based on fear of pain, or more specifically, the fear that physical activity may cause pain and/or recurrence of injury. Two opposing behavioral responses are postulated: 1) individuals choose to face pain in an attempt to improve, believing that the presence of pain does not justify the limitation of their functional activities, or 2) people maintain a fear of movement and believe that the activity is directly related to the presence of pain [32].

According by Sions [27], when beliefs and fear of movement are present in patients with low back pain, kinesiophobia must be considered in the management of patients with LBP. Patients need to be aware that pain may be misinterpreted as being more severe than it is, causing them to be excessively cautious in their actions, thereby causing disability. Our findings regarding kinesiophobia in patients with chronic LBP were significant statistically. The pain intensity and the quality of pain were high in our patients with low back pain and consequently, the emotional quality of life had decreased. The pain intensity and higher levels of kinesiophobia in our low back pain group may also have been associated with low quality of life.

This study was representative of the general population with low back pain in Brazil. A possible limitation of this study was that we did not investigate the relationships between functional outcome tests and kinesiophobia. Moreover, this was a cross-sectional study; therefore, it is not possible to establish causal relationships proving the existence of a temporal sequence between an exposure factor and the subsequent development of the disease. However, cross sectional studies could be carried out as the first step of a cohort study.

Conclusion

The results of the study of kinesiophobia levels was present, weak to moderate negative correlations existed between kinesiophobia and health-related quality of life at emotional, pain, disability. Even so, it is believed that the results can be useful in the scientific base of professionals Involved in clinical assessment and rehabilitation of people affected by low back pain and kinesiophobia.

Our findings indicate that the kinesiophobia is associated with pain intensity, disability, and quality of life and should be taken into consideration when planning preventive and curative physical therapy programs for patients with low back pain.

Abbreviations
LBP: Nonspecific low back pain; NRS: Numerical Rating Scale; SD: Standard deviation; SF36: Short Form Health Survey Questionnaire

Acknowledgements
We thank to patients who contributed for do the study and the SER - Center of Rehabilitation, Taboão da Serra, SP.

Authors' contributions
JC, had the idea of study, wrote, analyzed and interpreted the patient data regarding the low back pain and kinesiophobia. MM, helped analyzed and contributed with the recruited of patients. APMC, statistical analyses. AP, supervised the study. All authors read and approved the final manuscript.

Competing interests
The authors declare that they have no competing interests.

References
1.	Airaksinen O, Brox JI, Cedraschi C, Hildebrandt J, Klaber-Moffett J, Kovacs F, et al. Chapter 4 - European guidelines for the management of chronic nonspecific low back pain. Eur Spine J. 2006;15:192–S300.
2.	Nascimento PRC, Costa LOP. Low back pain prevalence in Brazil: a systematic review. Cadernos de Saúde Pública. 2015;31:6.
3.	Tulder MW. Chapter I. European guidelines. Eur Spine J. 2006;15:134–5.
4.	Costa LDM, Maher CG, McAuley JH, Hancock MJ, Herbert RD, Refshauge KM, et al. Prognosis for patients with chronic low back pain: inception cohort study. Br Med J. 2009;339–82.
5.	Ulug N, Yakut Y, Alemdaroglu I, Yilmaz O. Comparison of pain, kinesiophobia and quality of life in patients with low back and neck pain. J Phys Ther Sci. 2016;28(2):665–70.
6.	Rush A, Polatin P, Gatchel R. Depression and chronic low back pain establishing priorities in treatment. Spine J. 2000;25(20):2566–71.
7.	Fanian H, Ghassemi G, Jourkar M, Mallik S, Mousavi M. Psychological profile of Iranian patients with low-back pain. East Mediterr Health J. 2007;13(2):335–46.

8. Currie S, Wang J. Chronic back pain and major depression in the general Canadian population. Pain. 2004;107(1–2):54–60.

9. Kori S, Miller R, Todd D. Kinesiophobia: a new view of chronic pain behavior. Pain Manager. 1990;3:35–43.

10. Pincus T, Vogel S, Burton A, Santos R, Field A. Fear avoidance and prognosis in back pain: a systematic review and synthesis of current evidence. Arthritis Rheum. 2006;54(12):3999–4010.

11. Leeuw M, Goossens MEJB, Linton SJ, Crombez G, Boersma K, Vlaeyen JWS. The fear-avoidance model of musculoskeletal pain: current state of scientific evidence. J Behav Med. 2007;30:77–94.

12. Picavet HS, Vlaeyen JW, Schouten JS. Pain catastrophizing and kinesiophobia: predictors of chronic low back pain. Am J Epidemiol. 2002; 156(11):1028–34.

13. George SZ, Calley D, Valencia C, Beneciuk JM. Clinical investigation of pain-related fear and pain catastrophizing for patients with low back pain. Clin J Pain. 2011;27(2):108–15.

14. Atalay A, Arslan S, Dinçer F. Psychosocial function, clinical status, and radiographic findings in a group of chronic low back pain patients. Rheumatol Int. 2001;21(2):65–2.

15. Childs JD, Piva SR, Fritz JM. Responsiveness of the numeric pain rating scale in patients with low back pain. Spine (Phila Pa 1976). 2005;30(11):1331–4.

16. Nusbaum L, Natour J, Ferraz MB, Goldenberg J. Translation, adaptation and validation of the Roland-Morris questionnaire-Brazil Roland-Morris. Braz J Med Biol Res. 2001;34(2):203–10.

17. Costa LDM, Maher CG, McAuley JH, Hancock MJ, Oliveira WD, Azevedo DC, et al. The Brazilian-Portuguese versions of the McGill pain questionnaire were reproducible, valid, and responsive in patients with musculoskeletal pain. J Clin Epidemiol. 2011;64(8):903–12.

18. Souza FS, Marinho CD, Siqueira FB, Maher CG, Costa LOP. Psychometric testing confirms that the Brazilian-Portuguese adaptations, the original versions of the fear-avoidance beliefs questionnaire, and the Tampa scale of Kinesiophobia have similar measurement properties. Spine. 2008;33(9):1028–33.

19. Ciconelli RM, Feraz MB, Santos W. Tradução para a língua portuguesa e validação do questionário genérico de avaliação de qualidade de vida SF-36. Rev Bras Reumatol. 1999;39:143–9.

20. Costa LO, Maher CG, Latimer J, Ferreira PH, Ferreira ML, Pozzi GC, et al. Clinimetric testing of three self-report outcome measures for low back pain patients in Brazil: which one is the best? Spine. 2008;33(22):2459–63.

21. Vlaeyen JW, Kole-Snijders AM, Boeren RG, van Eek H. Fear of movement/(re)injury in chronic low back pain and its relation to behavioral performance. Pain. 1995;62(3):363–72.

22. George S, Fritz J, McNeil D. Fear-avoidance beliefs as measured by the fear-avoidance beliefs questionnaire: change in fear-avoidance beliefs questionnaire is predictive of change in self-report of disability and pain intensity for patients with acute low back pain. Clin J Pain. 2006;22:197–203.

23. Fleiss JL. The design and analysis of clinical experimental. New York: Wiley Classics Library Edition Published; 1999.

24. Gomes JL, Kingma M, Kamper SJ, Maher CG, Ferreira PH, Marques AP, et al. The association between symptom severity and physical activity participation in people seeking care for acute low back pain. Eur Spine J. 2015;24:452–7.

25. Boersma K, Linton S. Psychological processes underlying the development of a chronic pain problem prospective study of the relationship between profiles of psychological variables in the fear-avoidance model and disability. Clin J Pain. 2006;22(2):160–6.

26. Kasdan AS, Kasdan ML. The RN assistant in hand surgery. Todays OR Nurse. 1987;9(5):28–32.

27. Sions JM, Hicks GE. Fear-avoidance beliefs are associated with disability in older American adults with low back pain. Phys Ther. 2011;91(4):525–34.

28. Sloan TJ, Gupta R, Zhang W, Walsh DA. Beliefs about the causes and consequences of pain in patients with chronic inflammatory or noninflammatory low back pain and in pain-free individuals. Spine (Phila Pa 1976). 2008;33(9):966–72.

29. Darlow B, Fullen BM, Dean S, Hurley DA, Baxter GD, Dowell A. The association between health care professional attitudes and beliefs and the attitudes and beliefs, clinical management, and outcomes of patients with low back pain: a systematic review. Eur J Pain. 2012;16(1):3–17.

30. Shorthouse FM, Roffi V, Tack C. Effectiveness of educational materials to prevent occupational low back pain. Occup Med (Lond). 2016; 66(8); 623–29.

31. Vlaeyen J, Linton S. Fear-avoidance and its consequences in chronic musculosketal pain: a state of the art. Pain. 2000;85:317–32.

32. McKilligin HR. Letter: Women's lib. Can Med Assoc J. 1973;109(7):573–4.

9

Hand strength in patients with RA correlates strongly with function but not with activity of disease

Graziela Sferra da Silva[*] ⓘ, Mariana de Almeida Lourenço and Marcos Renato de Assis

Abstract

Background: Rheumatoid arthritis (RA) is a systemic autoimmune disease characterized by chronic inflammation of the joints, especially of the hands. The evaluation of handgrip strength (HS) and pinch strength can be useful to detect reduction in hand function in RA patients. The aim of the study was to compare HS and pinch strength between RA patients (RA Group - RAG) and a non-RA control group (CG) and to relate HS and pinch strength to functional capacity, duration and disease activity in the RAG.

Methods: A cross-sectional case control study. The RAG was assessed for disease activity by the Disease Activity Score (DAS-28); for functional capacity by the Health Assessment Questionnaire (HAQ), the Cochin Hand Functional Scale (CHFS) questionnaire, and the Disability of the Arm, Shoulder, and Hand (DASH) questionnaire; and for HS and pinch strength (2-point tip-to-tip, lateral or key, and 3-point) using Jamar® and pinch gauge dynamometers, respectively. Associations were analyzed by Pearson and Spearman tests, and groups were compared by the independent samples t test, with a significance level of $P < 0.05$.

Results: The convenience sample included 121 rheumatoid patients and a control group matched by age, sex, and body mass index. The RAG showed lower strength values compared with the CG in all measurements ($P < 0.01$, 95% CI) and these values were associated with worse performance in the functional questionnaires and greater disease activity and duration. There was a strong correlation among the functional assessment instruments.

Conclusions: The decrease in grip and pinch strength, easily measured by portable dynamometers, is a strong indicator of functional disability in RA patients.

Keywords: Rheumatoid arthritis, Hand strength, Pinch strength, Muscle weakness, Disability evaluation

Background

Rheumatoid arthritis (RA) is a chronic inflammatory joint disease that preferentially affects the hands, resulting in reductions in muscle strength and mobility and deformities associated with considerable functional impairment [1, 2]. Loss of muscle strength, made worse by lack of use [3], can impair the basic grip and pinch functions of the hands. Some studies conducted with portable dynamometers have shown reductions in hand strength in patients with RA compared with healthy controls and correlated with functional ability [4–8]. However, such studies exhibit several limitations, such as small sample size, lack of control groups, and poor description of the measurement protocols.

The aims of the present study were to measure the hand grip strength (HS) and pinch strength of individuals with RA, compared with a control group, and to correlate hand strength with functional ability and length and activity of disease.

Methods

This cross-sectional, case-control study was conducted with individuals with RA (RA group - RAG) followed up at the rheumatology outpatient clinic, School of Medicine of Marilia, interior of the state of São Paulo, Brazil. Controls (Control group - CG), matched by sex, age, and body mass index (BMI), were selected among escorts of

[*] Correspondence: gra_sferra@hotmail.com
Faculty of Medicine of Marilia (Famema), Marília, SP, Brazil

patients at the rheumatology outpatient clinic and at the internal medicine, obstetrics, and otorhinolaryngology outpatient clinics.

The Institutional Ethics Committee, under Certificate of Presentation for Ethical Appraisal (CAAE) 45,124,815.0000.5413, approved the study. Participants were included in the study after signing an informed consent form. The study was conducted from September 2015 to September 2016.

Sample size was calculated using a two-tailed test with the significance level set to 5, 90% power, standard deviation 9.8 kgf [9] for handgrip strength, and a clinically significant difference of 4.5 kgf. To compensate for eventual losses, the calculated sample size was increased by 20%, resulting in 121 participants per group.

Individuals 18 years old or older were included. RAG members had to meet the classification criteria formulated by the American College of Rheumatology in 1987 (ACR 1987) or the criteria formulated by the American College of Rheumatology and the European League Against Rheumatism in 2010 (ACR/ EULAR 2010) [10, 11]. Exclusion criteria for both groups were understanding, cognition, or sensory deficits hindering participation in interviews; skin or neurological lesions impairing the grip and pinch functions; and amputation of the upper limbs. Individuals with hand joint complaints were excluded from CG.

Patients with RA were subjected to assessment of activity of disease. All participants were subjected to measurements of body mass and height (Filizola mechanical scale with stadiometer, 100-g and 0.1-cm precision), functional ability questionnaires, and hand dynamometry.

Disease activity was assessed by means of the Disease Activity Score (DAS28) and the measurement of C-reactive protein (CRP; immunoturbidimetric method) [12–14]. The DAS28 final score was interpreted according to the following classification: remission ≤2.4; low disease activity ≤3.2; moderate activity ≤5.5; and high activity > 5.5, and according to the Boolean definition of remission (2010 ACR/EULAR remission criteria): tender and swollen joint count < 1, CRP ≤ 1 mg/dl, and visual analog scale (VAS) score ≤ 1 or Simplified Disease Activity Index (SDAI) ≤ 3 [15, 16].

Functional ability was assessed by means of 3 questionnaires: a) the Health Assessment Questionnaire (HAQ), one of the most widely used for patients with RA and that was translated to and validated for the Portuguese language [17–19]; b) the Cochin Hand Functional Scale (CHFS), developed in France initially for assessment of patients with RA and then extended to other conditions, and translated and adapted for Brazilian populations [20, 21]; and c) the Disability of the Arm, Shoulder, and Hand (DASH) questionnaire, developed for assessment of the upper limb functional ability in various

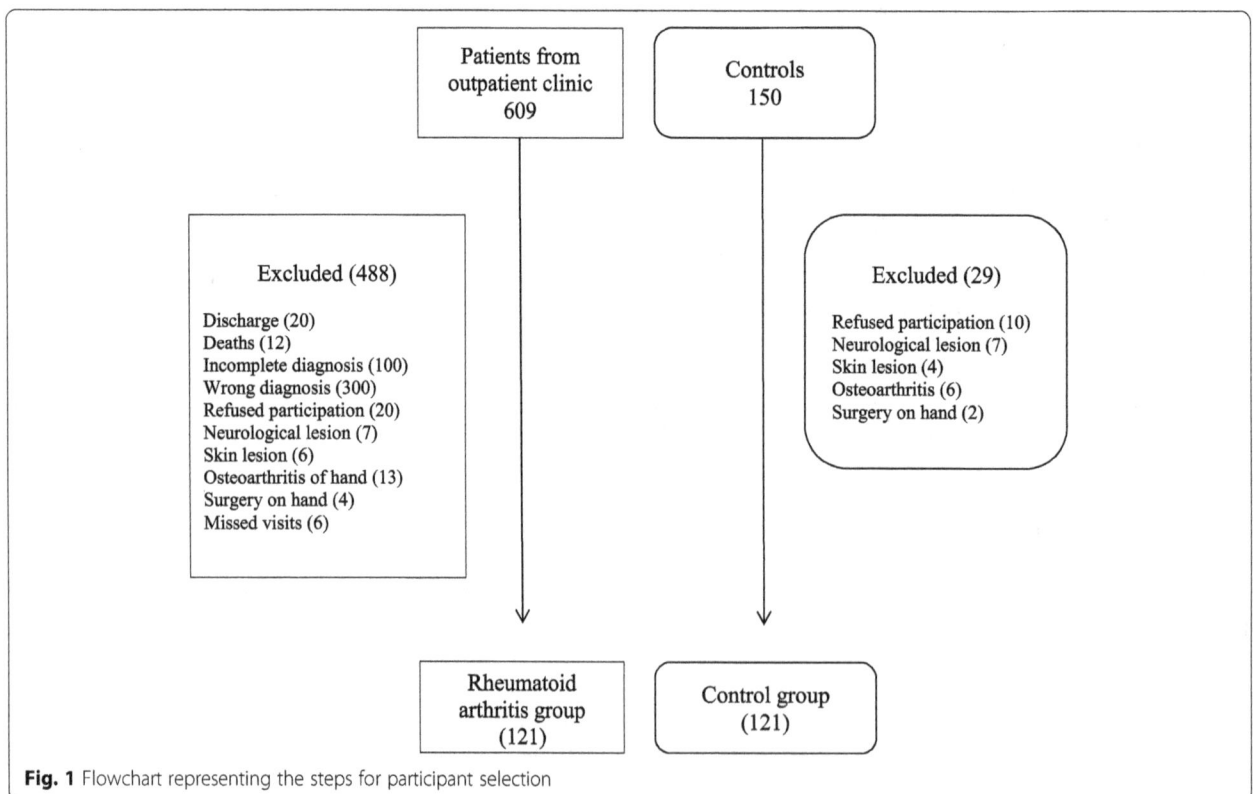

Fig. 1 Flowchart representing the steps for participant selection

Table 1 Characteristics of the rheumatoid arthritis group (RAG) and the control group (CG)

Variables	RAG n = 121	CG n = 121
Age (years)	57.50 ± 10.75	57.48 ± 10.48
BMI (kg/m ^{2})	28.26 ± 5.84	29.74 ± 6.08
Sex (%)		
Male	14 (11.6)	14 (11.2)
Female	107 (88.4)	107 (88.4)
Ethnicity (%)		
White	81 (66.9)	67 (55.4)
Black	3 (2.5)	12 (9.9)
Brown skin	36 (29.8)	42 (34.7)
Indian	1 (0.8)	–
Educational level (%)		
None	8 (6.6)	5 (4.1)
Incomplete elementary school	49 (40.5)	52 (43.0)
Complete elementary school	17 (14.0)	15 (12.4)
Incomplete secondary school	22 (18.2)	5 (4.1)
Complete secondary school	18 (14.9)	37 (30.6)
Higher education	7 (5.8)	7 (5.8)
Marital status (%)		
Single	19 (15.7)	10 (8.3)
Married	65 (53.7)	72 (59.5)
Divorced	19 (15.7)	14 (11.6)
Widowed	14 (11.6)	18 (14.9)
Stable union	4 (3.3)	7 (5.8)
Dominant hand (%)		
Right	114 (94.2)	115 (95.0)
Associated diseases (%)		
Systemic arterial hypertension	71 (58.7)	74 (61.2)
Osteoporosis	31 (25.6)	3 (2.5)
Diabetes	18 (14.9)	32 (26.4)

SD: standard deviation; kg/m ^{2}: kilograms per square meter

conditions and translated, validated, and adapted for the Portuguese language in 2005 [22, 23].

Hand strength was assessed with the participants sitting on an armless chair, with 90° elbow flexion, forearms in a neutral position, and 0 to 30° wrist extension. Maximum strength was assessed after a 3-s sustained contraction; the average of 3 attempts at 1-min intervals was considered for analysis. During the tests, all participants received verbal feedback by means of the sentence "strength, strength, strength" [24, 25]. Measurements included a) handgrip strength (HS) measured with a Jamar® hydraulic dynamometer at handle position 2, as established by the *American Society of Hand Therapists* (ASHT); results were recorded in kilogram-force (kgf) [24], and b) pinch strength measured using a B&L *Engineering®* PG-30 pinch gauge, including 2-point tip-to-tip pinch strength (classic, between the thumb and index finger), lateral or key pinch strength (between the pad of the thumb and the lateral surface of the middle phalanx of the index finger), and 3-point pinch strength (between the thumb, index, and middle fingers) [26].

The data were subjected to descriptive statistics; normality was assessed by means of the Kolmogorov-Smirnov test. Groups were matched 1:1 by sex, age, and BMI and were compared with the t-test. Correlations were investigated using Pearson's and Spearman's tests, and the strength of correlation was categorized as follows: 0.0 to 0.3, non-significant; 0.3 to 0.5 weak; 0.5 to 0.7 moderate; 0.7 to 0.9 strong; and 0.9 to 1.0 very strong [27]. Intergroup comparisons were performed by means of the independent t-test, with significance level $P < 0.05$. Analyses were performed with software Statistical Package for the Social Sciences (SPSS version 24) - US.

Results

Figure 1 most participants in the groups were female, married, and white (self-reported ethnicity) with a low educational level, reported arterial hypertension, and

Table 2 Hand strength of participants in the rheumatoid arthritis group (RAG) and the control group (CG)

Strength test	RAG Mean ± SD (kgf)	CG	CG-RAG difference (%)	P
Handgrip R	17.74 ± 9.23	25.94 ± 8.33	30	< 0.01
Handgrip L	17.34 ± 8.87	25.85 ± 8.32	31	< 0.01
2-point tip-to-tip pinch R	3.47 ± 1.56	5.24 ± 1.49	32	< 0.01
2-point tip-to-tip pinch L	3.33 ± 1.58	4.98 ± 1.39	31	< 0.01
3-point R	4.55 ± 1.99	6.87 ± 2.10	32	< 0.01
3-point L	4.50 ± 2.05	6.57 ± 1.95	30	< 0.01
Lateral pinch R	6.02 ± 2.40	7.79 ± 1.96	21	< 0.01
Lateral pinch L	5.60 ± 2.31	7.26 ± 1.86	21	< 0.01

kgf: kilogram-force; R: right; L: left. Independent t-test

Table 3 Length and activity of disease and functional ability of participants in the rheumatoid arthritis group (RAG)

Variables (n = 121)	Mean (±SD)	Median [P25-P75]
Length of disease (years)		10 [5–16]
DAS28	2.98 (±1.32)	
HAQ		0.87 [0.31–1.75]
Cochin Hand Functional Score		8 [1–27]
DASH		20 [7.50–43.33]

N: sample; SD: standard deviation; P25-P75: 25th and 75th percentiles; DAS28: Disease Activity Score; HAQ: Health Assessment Questionnaire; DASH: Disability of Arm, Shoulder, and Hand

were right-handed for writing and performing activities of daily living (ADL). Details on the characteristics of the participants from both groups are described in (Tables 1 and 2).

Rheumatoid factor tested positive in 78.5% (*n* = 95) of participants in the RAG; data on anti-citrullinated protein antibodies (ACPAs) were missing for 43 patients. The drug most widely used by patients was methotrexate, 71.9% (*n* = 87), followed by leflunomide, 52.9% (*n* = 64), and hydroxychloroquine, 38% (*n* = 46) (Tables 3 and 4).

Length of disease did not exhibit any significant correlations with activity of disease, scores on questionnaires, or functional ability.

In a separate analysis by age range (10-year interval) in the RAG, we found that HS decreased after 35 years of age and was more accentuated after 65 years of age. In the CG, the highest strength level was exhibited by G2, with a gradual decline with age (Table 5).

The scores on the functional ability scales showed strong mutual correlations: HAQ and CHFS 0.789 (*P* < 0.01), HAQ and DASH 0.825 (P < 0.01), and CHFS and DASH 0.820 (P < 0.01), but weak correlations with activity of disease.

There was no correlation of hand strength and functional ability with RA Boolean remission (Table 6).

Discussion

The handgrip strength and pinch strength were lower among the patients with RA compared with the controls.

Handgrip strength and pinch strength were lower among patients with poorer functional ability but showed weak correlations with activity and length of disease.

The average age of the participants was 58 years; age did not exhibit a correlation with HS, as has been described in the literature [1, 18, 28–31].

A study conducted with healthy individuals found that the peak HS occurred in the age range of 25 to 39 years; pinch strength remained stable until age 59 years, followed by a gradual decline together with age [32]. In another study performed with healthy Brazilians, peak HS occurred in the age range of 35 to 39 years, followed by a gradual decline with age [33]. A study that analyzed patients with RA did not find a difference in 2-point pinch after 5-year follow up [34]. However, the meta-analysis conducted by Beenakker et al. [31] showed a decline of HS before age 50 years, suggesting that the disease might cause premature aging. In our study, we did not find a clear-cut strength reduction gradient, but strength declined in the groups with patients older than 35 years, similar to previous studies; this variation might be attributed to the expected loss of muscle mass and strength that occurs after age 40. The group with patients older than 65 years old showed additional HS reduction, which is consistent with the frailty developed by older seniors [35].

There is controversy regarding hand strength and dominance. Some studies conducted with healthy individuals found significant differences, with the dominant hand being the strongest [36]. Two studies simultaneously analyzed patients with RA and healthy individuals. In one study, the dominant hand was 20% weaker than the non-dominant one among patients with RA and 8% stronger among healthy individuals [37]. The other study found differences among the healthy participants only [38]. In our study, we did not find a correlation between strength and dominance in either group; in addition, dominance might be influenced by several factors, such as work and leisure demands [39].

Regarding associated diseases, systemic arterial hypertension was the most prevalent in the analyzed sample. Use of cardiovascular medications has been associated

Table 4 Negative correlations among hand strength, functional ability, activity, and duration of disease in the rheumatoid arthritis group (RAG)

Variables	Handgrip		2-point tip-to-tip pinch		3-point pinch		Lateral pinch	
	D	E	D	E	D	E	D	E
HAQ	0.585*	0.528*	0.446*	0.472*	0.505*	0.501*	0.470*	0.555*
DASH	0.606*	0.559*	0.453*	0.444*	0.484*	0.486*	0.444*	0.535*
CHFS	0.606*	0.512*	0.452*	0.448*	0.496*	0.474*	0.474*	0.509*
Length of disease	0.168	0.196**	0.171	0.204**	0.189**	0.217**	0.187**	0.238*
DAS28	0.431*	0.401*	0.473*	0.436*	0.467*	0.424*	0.341*	0.336*

HAQ: *Health Assessment Questionnaire*; DASH: *Disabilities Arm, Shoulder, and Hand*; CHFS: *Cochin Hand Functional Scale*. Pearson's correlation test for DAS28; Spearman's correlation test for all others; * *P* < 0.01, ** *P* < 0.05

Table 5 Handgrip strength per age range in the rheumatoid arthritis group (RAG) and the control group (CG)

| Age range | RAG | | CG | |
	HS R Mean ± SD	HS L Mean ± SD	HS R Mean ± SD	HS L Mean ± SD
26–35 - G1	25.53 ± 14.89	20.67 ± 14.26	30.17 ± 11.49	32.33 ± 10.54
36–45 - G2	16.37 ± 8.22	18.54 ± 7.94	34.13 ± 8.51	33.75 ± 9.66
46–55 - G3	17.55 ± 8.13	17.39 ± 7.86	27.54 ± 8.20	27.67 ± 7.07
56–65 - G4	18.18 ± 9.77	18.30 ± 9.52	24.96 ± 8.44	24.90 ± 9.49
+ 65 - G5	14.75 ± 11.52	13.61 ± 10.22	22.46 ± 5.66	21.93 ± 4.45

HS R: right handgrip strength; HS L: left handgrip strength

with HS reduction in a cohort of older adults [40]. In our study, neither hypertension nor use of medications – with similar prevalence rates in both groups – showed a relationship with hand strength.

There was no difference in hand strength according to the use of synthetic drugs for disease control. An isolated correlation was detected between pinch strength and the use of a biological agent, without sufficient consistency to infer a causal relationship.

Rheumatoid factor – related to poor prognosis in RA – tested positive in 78.5% of the RAG, somewhat above the average of 70% reported in the literature [18]; however, positive rheumatoid factor was not associated with hand strength. Data on ACPAs were missing for 43 patients; therefore, we did not investigate their correlation with hand strength.

A meta-analysis performed in 2010 [31] found that the average HS of patients with RA was 17.68 kgf. Although the analyzed studies had excluded individuals with diabetes mellitus, chronic obstructive pulmonary disease, and testosterone and/or growth hormone deficiencies, the abovementioned value is similar to the one we found in the present study, in which patients with such conditions were not excluded. Alomari et al. [41] found a 30% reduction in HS among patients with RA compared with healthy individuals recruited from the local community

without ischemia, systemic arterial hypertension, angina, diabetes mellitus, anemia, dyslipidemia, kidney failure, obesity, or higher cardiovascular risk and who were non-smokers. Even without excluding participants with any of these conditions, in our study, we found a similar difference between patients and controls.

The study by Dedeoğlu et al., which correlated hand strength with pain, activity of disease, functional ability, and joint lesions in RA, found average values of 24.6 kgf for HS, 4.4 kgf for tip-to-tip pinch strength, 5.65 kgf for 3-point pinch strength, and 6.65 kgf for lateral pinch strength. These values are higher than those found in the present study; however, Dedeoğlu et al. excluded individuals with diabetes mellitus, hypo- or hyperthyroidism, and cervical disc disease [9], constituting a sample with a profile different from the one met in clinical practice. In addition, their study did not include a control group.

The data described above show that there is wide variability among studies, with the issue of the inclusion of control groups being crucial. When designing our study, we took special care to include a control group with a profile similar to the one of patients seen in clinical practice, who have several associated diseases, and to match the groups according to variables with potentially strong influences on hand strength. We believe that one strength of our study is that it has satisfactory internal quality without any impairment of its external validity.

In their study, Poole et al. [42] found that among patients with RA, HS, 2-point tip-to-tip, and 3-point pinch strength were lower with lower hand functional ability, as measured by means of the CHFS. Another study assessed HS, 2-point tip-to-tip, 3-point pinch strength, and lateral pinch strength and found the same correlations with functional ability [9]. Although utilizing a small sample of 36 patients with RA, Adams et al. [4] found that DASH showed a strong correlation with HS and 3-point pinch strength and suggested that DASH is the best instrument to discriminate the functional ability of the upper limbs. Similarly, the study by Nampei et al.

Table 6 Hand strength of patients with rheumatoid arthritis (RA) and Boolean remission or active disease

Hand strength	RA in remission (n = 8) Mean ± SD (kgf)	RA in activity (n = 113)	P
Handgrip R	18.44 ± 5.71	17.69 ± 9.44	> 0.05
Handgrip L	19.63 ± 5.88	17.18 ± 9.04	> 0.05
2-point tip-to-tip pinch R	4.03 ± 1.20	3.43 ± 1.58	> 0.05
2-point tip-to-tip pinch L	4.10 ± 1.50	3.28 ± 1.57	> 0.05
3-point R	4.82 ± 0.99	4.54 ± 2.05	> 0.05
3-point L	5.44 ± 2.14	4.43 ± 2.03	> 0.05
Lateral pinch R	6.46 ± 1.62	5.99 ± 2.45	> 0.05
Lateral pinch L	6.98 ± 1.99	5.50 ± 2.30	> 0.05

kgf: kilogram-force; R: right; L: left; Independent t-test

[43] concluded that there were significant correlations of 2-point tip-to-tip, 3-point pinch strength, and lateral pinch strength with loss of hand function among patients with RA. This is the only study that also described associations with thumb and index deformities. In addition, our study showed associations with hand function, but we did not record deformities.

The DAS28 score (2.98 ± 1.32) showed a weak correlation with grip and pinch strength. A recent study found a moderate negative correlation between DAS28 score and grip and pinch strength, as measured with a dynamometer coupled to a smartphone; the authors concluded that HS might contribute to the assessment of disease activity in the outpatient setting [44]. In addition, a recent pilot study reported a reduction of HS among patients with RA and high disease activity and a negative correlation of HS with pain and swelling [38].

In contrast, in our study, we observed a weak correlation between strength and disease activity, which was not expected because the hand joints have considerable weight on the DAS28 scores. There were correlations for some of the hand strength parameters, but those correlations were below 0.3 in all cases, i.e., they were clinically insignificant.

There was not any significant difference between patients with Boolean remission and active RA; however, the low representation of the former, just 8 patients, makes drawing robust conclusions difficult [38, 45].

Like ours, one study observed a strong correlation between CHFS and HAQ [9], which reinforces the fact that RA hand involvement impairs functional ability in a global manner [46].

In the validation study of CHFS for the Brazilian population, it showed moderate correlation with DASH. Conversely, in our study, these two instruments showed a strong correlation, which might be accounted for by the fact that RA affects not only the small but also the large joints of the upper limbs. There is considerable overlap among the items assessed with the HAQ, CHFS, and DASH, rendering their simultaneous use unnecessary. However, there is a wide diversity of parameters cited in the literature; thus, we chose to apply all three instruments to enable comparisons with other studies.

Length of disease had a significant, albeit, weak correlation with functional activity, as was the case of the study by Dedeoğlu et al., who used CHFS [9], and Toyama et al. [34], who employed DASH, which must be quite variable as a function of disease aggressiveness, early diagnosis, and intensity of treatment in each patient.

We believe that our study provides a relevant reference for the measurement of hand strength in patients with RA, as the sample size was larger compared with the studies available in the literature [37, 38, 41, 45, 47]. In addition, we used a control group composed of individuals with sociocultural profiles similar to those of the RA patients and matched per sex, age, and BMI; therefore, both the internal and external validity are satisfactory. Nevertheless, we admit some limitations, such as not having recorded radiological deformities of the hands and fingers, which might be associated with measurements of strength.

Several issues still need to be elucidated. Our sample did not have a sufficient number of patients for assessment of the hand strength impairment at baseline, which might contribute to discriminating the roles that inflammation and sequelae play in loss of strength. The sample size was also restricted for the purpose of drawing conclusions on male patients. What is the correlation between hand strength and lower limb strength and risk of falls? What are the impacts of rehabilitation programs and physical exercise on hand strength among patients with RA? These data will contribute to elucidate the potential of hand strength measurement along the follow-up of patients with RA as an additional parameter for therapeutic decision-making to contribute to improve the functional ability and quality of life of patients and disease control.

We conclude that handgrip and pinch strength were lower in patients with RA compared with individuals without disease. Grip and pinch strength were inversely correlated with global functional ability and hand and upper limb function; however, they showed weak correlations with activity and length of disease.

Acknowledgements
Jamil Natour and Anamaria Jones from the Spine, Procedures, and Rehabilitation in Rheumatology Sector at Rheumatology Division, UNIFESP, Brazil for their support and for making dynamometers available.

Funding
To the Coordination for the Improvement of Higher Education Personnel (CAPES) for the assistance of research through the scholarship awarded.

Authors' contributions
GSS: Main author and acted in data collection, literature review and author of the manuscript. MAL: Acted in data collection. MRA: He acted as counselor and critically reviewed the manuscript for key intellectual content. All authors read and approved the final manuscript.

Authors' information
Graziela Sferra da Silva.
Specialization in physiology of physical exercise and resitance training in health, disease and aging. Main author and acted in data collection, literature review and author of the manuscript.
Mariana de Almeida Lourenço.
PhD stundent in the Human Development and Technologies Program at Unesp Rio Claro Campus, MSc in Health and Aging at Marilia School of Medicine (Famema). Acted in data colletion.
Marcos Renato de Assis.
PhD in Sciences by the Rehabilitation Program. He acted as advisor and reviewer of the manuscript.

Competing interests

The authors declare that they have no competing interests.

References

1. Louzada-Júnior P, Souza BDB, Toledo RA, Ciconelli RM. Análise descritiva das características demográficas e clínicas de pacientes com artrite reumatóide no estado de São Paulo. Brazil Rev Bras Reumatol. 2007;47(2): 84–90.
2. Sociedade Brasileira de Reumatologia. Artrite reumatoide: diagnóstico e tratamento. In: Associação Médica Brasileira e Comissão Federal. São Paulo: Projeto Diretrizes; 2002.
3. Helliwell PS, Jackson S. Relationship between weakness and muscle wasting in rheumatoid arthritis. Ann Rheum Dis. 1994;53(11):726–8.
4. Vargas A, Chiapas-Gasca K, Hernández-Díaz C, Canoso JJ, Saavedra MÁ, Navarro-Zarza JE, et al. Clinical anatomy of the hand. Reumatol Clin. 2013; 8(2):25–32.
5. Bodur H, Yilmaz O, Keskin D. Hand disability and related variables in patients with rheumatoid arthritis. Rheumatol Int. 2006;26(6):541–4.
6. Adams J, Burridge J, Mullee M, Hammond A, Cooper C. Correlation between upper limb functional ability and structural hand impairment in an early rheumatoid population. Clin Rehabil. 2004;18(4):405–13.
7. Santana FS, Nascimento DC, Freitas JPM, Miranda RF, Muniz LF, Santos Neto L, et al. Avaliação da capacidade funcional em pacientes com artrite reumatoide: implicações para a recomendação de exercícios físicos. Rev Bras Reumatol. 2014;54(5):378–85.
8. Oku EC, Pinheiro GRC, Araújo PMP. Hand functional assessment in patients with rheumatoid arthritis. Fisioter Mov. 2009;22(2):221–8.
9. Dedeoğlu M, Gafuroğlu Ü, Yilmaz Ö, Bodur H. The relationship between hand grip and pinch strengths and disease activity, articular damage, pain and disability in patients with rheumatoid arthritis. Turk J Rheumatol. 2013; 28(2):69–77.
10. Villeneuve E, Nam J, Emery P. ACR-EULAR classification criteria for rheumatoid arthritis. Rev Bras Reumatol. 2010;50(5):481–3.
11. Aletaha D, Neogi T, Silman AJ, Funovits J, Felson DT, Bingham CO 3rd, et al. 2010 rheumatoid arthritis classification criteria: an American College of Rheumatology/European league against rheumatism collaborative initiative. Arthritis Rheum. 2010;62(9):2569–81.
12. Wells G, Becker JC, Teng J, Dougados M, Schiff M, Smolen J, et al. Validation of the 28-joint disease activity score (DAS28) and European league against rheumatism response criteria based on C-reactive protein against disease progression in patients with rheumatoid arthritis, and comparison with the DAS28 based on erythrythrocyte sedimentation rate. Ann Rheum Dis. 2009; 68(6):954–60.
13. Pinheiro GRC. Instrumentos de medida da atividade da artrite reumatóide - Por que e como empregá-los. Rev Bras Reumatol. 2007;47(5):362–5.
14. Prevoo ML, Van't Hof MA, Kuper HH, van Leeuwen MA, van de Putte LB, Van RP. Modified disease activity scores that include twenty-eight-joint development and validation in a prospective longitudinal study of patients with arthritis, rheumatoid. Arthritis Rheum. 1995;38(1):44–8.
15. Felson DT, Smolen JS, Wells G, Zhang B, Van LHD, Funovits J, et al. American College of Rheumatology / European league against rheumatism provisional Defi nition of remission in rheumatoid arthritis for clinical trials. Ann Rheum Dis [Internet]. 2011;70(3):404–13.
16. Bykerk VP, Massarotti EM. The new ACR/EULAR remission criteria: rationale for developing new criteria for remission. Rheumatol (United Kingdom). 2012;51(SUPPL. 6):16–20.
17. Corbacho MI, Dapueto JJ. Avaliação da capacidade funcional e da qualidade de vida de pacientes com artrite reumatoide. Rev Bras Reum. 2010;50(1):31–43.
18. Mota LMH, Cruz BA, Brenol CV, Pereira IA, Fronza LSR, Bertolo MB, et al. Consenso da Sociedade Brasileira de Reumatologia 2011 para o diagnóstico e avaliação inicial da artrite reumatoide. Rev Bras Reumatol. 2011;51(3):199–219.
19. Bruce B, Fries JF. The health assessment questionnaire (HAQ). Clin Exp Rheumatol. 2005;23(5 Suppl 39):S14–8.
20. Chiari A, Sardim CC, Natour J. Translation, cultural adaptation and reproducibility of the cochin hand functional scale questionnaire for Brazil. Clinics (Sao Paulo). 2011;66(5):731 6.
21. Lefevre-Colau MM, Poiraudeau S, Fermanian J, Etchepare F, Alnot JY, Le Viet D, et al. Responsiveness of the cochin rheumatoid hand disability scale after surgery. Rheumatology. 2001;40(8):843–50.
22. Aktekin LA, Eser F, Başkan BM, Sivas F, Malhan S, Öksüz E, et al. Disability of arm shoulder and hand questionnaire in rheumatoid arthritis patients: relationship with disease activity, HAQ, SF-36. Rheumatol Int. 2011;31(6):823–6.
23. Orfale AG, Araújo PMP, Ferraz MB, Natour J. Translation into Brazilian Portuguese, cultural adaptation and evaluation of the reliability of the disabilities of the arm, shoulder and hand questionnaire. Brazilian J Med Biol Res. 2005;38(2):293–302.
24. Shiratori AP, Iop R, Borges Júnior NG, Domenech SC, Gevaerd MS. Protocolos de avaliação da força de preensão manual em indivíduos com artrite reumatoide: uma revisão sistemática. Rev Bras Reum. 2014;54(2):140–7.
25. Kapandji AI. Fisiologia articular: esquemas comentados de mecânica humana: membro superior. 5 ed. Panamericana São Paulo. 2000;1:140–298.
26. Häkkinen A, Kautiainen H, Hannonen P, Ylinen J, Mäkinen H, Sokka T. Muscle strength, pain, and disease activity explain individual subdimensions of the health assessment questionnaire disability index, especially in women with rheumatoid arthritis. Ann Rheum Dis. 2006;65(1):30–4.
27. Mukaka MM. Statistics corner: a guide to appropriate use of correlation coefficient in medical research. Malawi Med J. 2012;24(3):69–71.
28. Vaz AE. Perfil epidemiológico e clínico de pacientes portadores de artrite reumatóide em um hospital escola de medicina em Goiânia, Goiás, Brasil. Med (Ribeirão Preto). 2013;46(2):141–53.
29. Alamanos Y, Drosos AA. Epidemiology of adult rheumatoid arthritis. Autoimmun Rev. 2005;4(3):130–6.
30. Goeldner I, Skare T, Reason I, Utiyama S. Artrite reumatoide: uma visão atual. J Bras Patol Med Lab. 2011:495–503. [cited 2015 Feb 9]; Available from: http://www.scielo.br/pdf/jbpml/v47n5/v47n5a02.pdf
31. Beenakker KG, Ling CH, Meskers CG, de Craen AJ, Stijnen T. Westendorp RGet al. Patterns of muscle strength loss with age in the general population and patients with a chronic inflammatory state. Ageing Res Rev. 2010;9(4):431–6.
32. Mathiowetz V, Kashman N, Volland G, Weber K, Dowe M, Rogers S. Grip and pinch strength: normative data for adults. Arch Phys Med Rehabil. 1985; 66(2):69–74.
33. Caporrino FA, Faloppa F, Santos JBG, Réssio C, Soares FHC, Nakachima LR, et al. Estudo populacional da força de preensão palmar com dinamômetro Jamar. Rev Bras Ortop. 1998;33(2):150–4.
34. Toyama S, Tokunaga D, Fujiwara H, Oda R, Kobashi H, Okumura H, et al. Rheumatoid arthritis of the hand: a five-year longitudinal analysis of clinical and radiographic findings. Mod Rheumatol. 2014;24(1):69–77.
35. Lenardt MH, Binotto MA, Carneiro NHK, Cechinel C, Betiolli SE, Lourenço TM. Handgrip strength and physical activity in frail elderly. Rev Esc Enferm USP. 2016;50(1):86–92. https://doi.org/10.1590/S0080-623420160000100012.
36. Nicolay CW, Walker AL. Grip strength and endurance: influences of anthropometric variation, hand dominance, and gender. Int J Ind Ergon. 2005;35(7):605–18.
37. Fraser A, Vallow J, Preston A, Cooper RG. Predicting 'normal' grip strength for rheumatoid arthritis patients. Rheumatology. 1999;38(6):521–8.
38. Iop RR, Shiratori AP, Ferreira L. Borges Júnior, Domenech SC, Gevaerd MS. Capacidade de produção de força de preensão isométrica máxima em mulheres com artrite reumatoide : um estudo piloto. Fisioter Pesq. 2015; 22(1):11–6.
39. Figueiredo IM, Sampaio RF, Mancini MC, Silva FCM, Jamar SMAPT d f d p u o d. Acta Fisiátrica. 2007;14:104–10.
40. Ashfield TA, Syddall HE, Martin HJ, Dennison EM, Cooper C, Aihie Sayer A. Grip strength and cardiovascular drug use in older people: findings from the Hertfordshire cohort study. Age Ageing. 2009;39(2):185–91.
41. Alomari MA, Keewan EF, Shammaa RA, Alawneh K, Khatib SY, Welsch MA. Vascular function and handgrip strength in rheumatoid arthritis patients. Sci World J. 2012;2012:1–6.
42. Poole JL, Santhanam DD, Latham AL. Hand impairment and activity limitations in four chronic diseases. J Hand Ther. 2013;26(3):232–6.
43. Nampei A, Shi K, Hirao M, Murase T, Yoshikawa H, Hashimoto J. Association of pinch strength with hand dysfunction, finger deformities and contact points in patients with rheumatoid arthritis. Clin Exp Rheumatol. 2011;29(6):1061.
44. Espinoza F, Le Blay P, Coulon D, Lieu S, Munro J, Jorgensen C, et al. Handgrip strength measured by a dynamometer connected to a

smartphone: a new applied health technology solution for the self-assessment of rheumatoid arthritis disease activity. Rheumatology. 2016; 55(5):897–901.

45. Sheehy C, Gaffney K, Mukhtyar C. Standardized grip strength as an outcome measure in early rheumatoid arthritis. Scand J Rheumatol. 2013;42(4):289–93.

46. Birtane M, Kabayel DD, Uzunca K, Unlu E, Tastekin N. The relation of hand functions with radiological damage and disease activity in rheumatoid arthritis. Rheumatol Int. 2008;28(5):407–12.

47. Cima SR, Barone A, Porto JM, de Abreu DC. Strengthening exercises to improve hand strength and functionality in rheumatoid arthritis with hand deformities: a randomized, controlled trial. Rheumatol Int. 2013;33(3):725–32.

10

Survey on joint hypermobility in university students aged 18–25 years old

Darcisio Hortelan Antonio and Claudia Saad Magalhaes*

Abstract

Background: Joint hypermobility is defined as a wide range of movements beyond the physiological limits, it has been recognized in healthy people, gymnasts, acrobats, and carriers of genetic affections of connective tissue. A survey among young adults was conducted to describe the frequency of joint hypermobility, estimating its impact on function and quality of life.

Methods: Volunteer university students aged 18 to 25 years old who answered a valid 5-item questionnaire about hypermobility, a physical activity questionnaire, and the Brazilian version of the Medical Outcome Survey Short Form 36 (SF-36) were included. Hypermobility was also assessed by a guided self-examination, with Beighton's criteria being scored and scores greater than or equal to 4 or less than 4 being discriminated.

Results: A total of 388 subjects were included, of which 299 were women (77.06%) and 89 were men (22.94%); the median age was 23 years old. Generalized joint hypermobility (Beighton score ≥ 4) was observed in 104 individuals (26.8%). Localized hypermobility (Beighton score 1–3) was observed in 135 (34.79%) individuals, where the hypermobility of the 5th finger was the most frequent in 165 (57.47%) individuals, followed by hypermobility of the thumb in 126 (32.56%) individuals, hypermobility of the elbows and knees each in 72 (18.6%) individuals, and hypermobility of the spine in 69 (17.79%) individuals. The descriptive observation of physical activity indicated regular practice. The correlation coefficients between the SF-36 domains and hypermobility scores were very low and statistical comparison not significant.

Conclusion: In this population of youngsters, predominantly women, localized hypermobility was more frequent than generalized hypermobility; however, with low impact on health domains and quality of life scores, estimated in each domain of the SF-36, the physical and mental component scores, and the time dedicated to physical activity.

Keywords: Joint hypermobility, Generalized hypermobility, Localized hypermobility, SF-36 health questionnaire

Background

Hypermobility is defined as the wider range of movements beyond the limits considered physiological. It has been recognized as a phenomenon frequently observed in healthy people, acrobats, gymnasts, and ballerinas [1–5]. Hypermobility is also part of the syndromic presentation of certain genetic diseases, [6] such as Ehler-Danlos Syndrome, Marfan Syndrome, Down Syndrome, Osteogenesis imperfecta, and Stickler Syndrome, among others.

The concept of benign joint hypermobility, as a rheumatic condition leading to chronic musculoskeletal symptoms, emerged in the 1970s with several case series and population studies identifying the association with chronic musculoskeletal pain [7, 8] and, more recently, with dysautonomia and gastrointestinal dysmotility [7–9].

The incidence and prevalence of hypermobility vary greatly among populations, with marked differences according to age, gender, ethnicity, physical activity, or sports and athletic abilities. Approximately 25–50% of children younger than 10 years old have some degree of hypermobility [10–17]. There is a higher prevalence in populations of Asian origin, followed by populations of African and European origins [10, 12, 14, 15, 17–26]. However,

* Correspondence: claudi@fmb.unesp.br
Pediatrics Department, Botucatu Medical School, Graduate Program in Public Health of UNESP, Sao Paulo State University UNESP, Avenida Prof. Mario Rubens Guimarães Montenegro SN, Campus da Unesp, Rubião Junior, CEP, Botucatu, SP 18618-687, Brazil

comparisons among different populations have been hampered by the use of different criteria and methodologies for the evaluation of hypermobility.

Most clinicians recognize joint hypermobility in routine practice and by the use of the range of motion scale assessment proposed by Beighton [20]. The presence or absence of hypermobility in the joints is categorized, signaling the flexibility of five areas of the body with extension beyond the physiological limits. The maneuvers that make up the Beighton scale represented in Fig. 1 are 1) extension of 5th metacarpal phalangeal joint by placing the 5th finger parallel to the forearm, 2) extension of the thumb touching the flexor side of the forearm, 3) extension greater than 10° beyond the limit of 180° of the elbow, 4) extension greater than 10° beyond the limit of 180° in the knee, and 5) flexion and elongation of the spine by placing the hands flat on the floor with the knees in maximum extension. These maneuvers are individually scored on each side of the body and spine, to a total of 9 points. Scores greater than or equal to 4 are classified as generalized joint hypermobility, and scores 1–3 are classified as localized joint hypermobility [1, 4, 27].

Physiotherapists are trained to identify reduced range of motion and its clinical repercussions, associating it with several conditions of inflammatory origin. Greater ranges of movement are interpreted as variations of the normality of individual characteristics. Intervention with physical exercises still does not result in consistent evidence because a systematic review of intervention with exercises for those with functional repercussions was not conclusive regarding the effectiveness of the intervention with exercises or physical activity on hypermobility and its functional repercussions [28].

A wide spectrum of extra-articular clinical manifestations has been progressively recognized in association with musculoskeletal symptoms [29], such as predisposition to ecchymosis, poor wound healing, early onset of osteoarthritis, valvulopathy, osteoporosis, vesicoureteral reflux, inguinal hernia, and changes in intestinal motility [5, 6, 26, 30–33]. There are also other manifestations, such as fatigue, anxiety, and depression, negatively affecting social function and well-being [34].

The main musculoskeletal manifestation is chronic and generalized pain [7, 9, 17, 26, 35]. Proprioceptive functions may also be adversely affected, possibly due to damage to mechanical connective tissue receptors. Failure to recognize extreme joint range of movement can lead to joint instability and traumas to repetitive stress [36–38]. Decreased muscle strength can occur in children with limb pain and joint hypermobility [39]. There is evidence that hypermobility syndrome is a multisystemic manifestation, incorporating three main components: chronic pain, autonomic dysfunction, and dysfunction of gastrointestinal motility [6, 8, 26, 30, 32, 39, 40].

There have been few population studies on the impact of hypermobility among young adults. The frequencies of generalized and localized hypermobility have been widely studied in several populations, including the Brazilian pediatric population of pre-schoolers and schoolchildren [10, 14, 21]; however, studies on adolescents and young adults are scarce in the global literature [11, 16] and have not been referred to our population.

Objective

To investigate the frequency of joint hypermobility among university students 18 to 25 years old through survey and self-examination, estimating its functional impact and its impact on quality of life through the Medical Outcome Survey Short Form 36 (SF-36) questionnaire.

Methods

Volunteers between 18 and 25 years of age from medical and physiotherapy courses were invited to participate in this study after the work team provided explanations about the study.

The project obtained institutional ethics committee approval (CEP-457/2010) and agreement from the course councils; the subjects who agreed were included in the study by signing the Terms of Free and Informed Consent. The research was conducted in accordance with the Helsinki Declaration for research on humans beings.

Participants completed the self-administered questionnaires on hypermobility, including a valid five-item questionnaire adapted by Moraes et al. [41] and a survey on multisystemic associations of hypermobility syndrome [26]. The Brazilian version of the SF-36 [42] was completed by the subjects, and their records were identified by alpha-numerical code without personal identification. The self-examination was observed and recorded in case report forms by three trained observers, and the data were transferred to analysis worksheets.

The SF-36 is a widely used measure of health-related quality of life. The purpose of this questionnaire is to detect clinically and socially relevant differences in the health conditions of both the general population and individuals affected by certain diseases, along with any changes in health status over time through a small number of statistically efficient dimensions. The SF-36 consists of 36 items in 8 domains: Physical Functioning (CF), Role-Physical (RF), Bodily Pain (BP), General Health (GH), Vitality (VT), Social Functioning (SF), Role-Emotional (RE), and Mental health (MH), resulting in two summary components, the Physical Component (PCo) and the Mental Component (MCo). The score ranges from 0 to 100 points, where 0 represents the worst state of health and 100 the best state of health in the last 4 weeks.

A single evaluation was performed; there was no gender selection, and participation was voluntary, with consecutive inclusion of participants until reaching the sample size estimated by means of statistical calculation. The specific musculoskeletal examination, which includes hypermobility maneuvers, was instructed and conducted according to the scheme outlined in Fig. 1.

The sample size was calculated considering the prevalence of hypermobility in this specific age group as unknown ($p = 0.50$), with a reliability of 95% and a margin of error of 5%. The minimum size calculated for the sample was 385 subjects, and the maximum was 400 subjects.

The descriptive analysis of the frequency of signs and symptoms of the joint hypermobility survey and of the Beighton scale score was performed. Qualitative variables were described by absolute and percentage frequencies. Quantitative variables were described by medians and variation ranges (minimum-maximum) or means and standard deviations when appropriate. SF-36 scores on valid questionnaires (< 5% lost data) were calculated using SAS for Windows software version 9.3.

The frequency of hypermobility was scored individually by determining the frequency of joints scored and compared by gender. The comparison of hypermobility areas in men and women was performed using Student's *t* test (two categories). The categorization of generalized hypermobility by means of the limit of 4 or more joints scored using the Beighton criteria was also estimated according to the frequencies and possible associations explored.

The association tests between the hypermobility parameters and the SF-36 domain scores with the respective summary scores were performed using the Pearson Correlation Test. The association is represented by the Pearson r, and the significance is expressed by the values of $p < 0.05$. Correlations < 0.4 were considered weak or with no association, those between 0.4 and 0.7 were considered moderate, and those > 0.7 were considered strong.

Results

The participants of the research were volunteers who agreed to participate in the study through signing the Terms of Informed Consent. There was no refusal to participate. The sample consisted of 388 subjects, of which 28 were from the Medicine course and 360 were from the Physiotherapy course. The evaluation period was from February 2013 to April 2014.

A total of 388 subjects were recruited, including 299 women (77%) and 89 men (23%), with a minimum age of 18 years and a maximum age of 25 years (median 23), with the following anthropometric characteristics: mean weight (64.5 ± 15.7), median weight 60 kg, mean height (1.66 ± 0.09), and median height 1.65 m. The mean body mass index (BMI) was (23 ± 4), and the median BMI was 22.

The self-evaluation of physical activity, by means of estimating the number of hours per week of practice of leisure activities, sports, and competitions, was compiled. The descriptive analysis was as follows: 165 declared a mean leisure activity practice time of (1.7 ± 2.9) hours/week; 124 subjects declared a mean sports practice time of (1.6 ± 3.2)

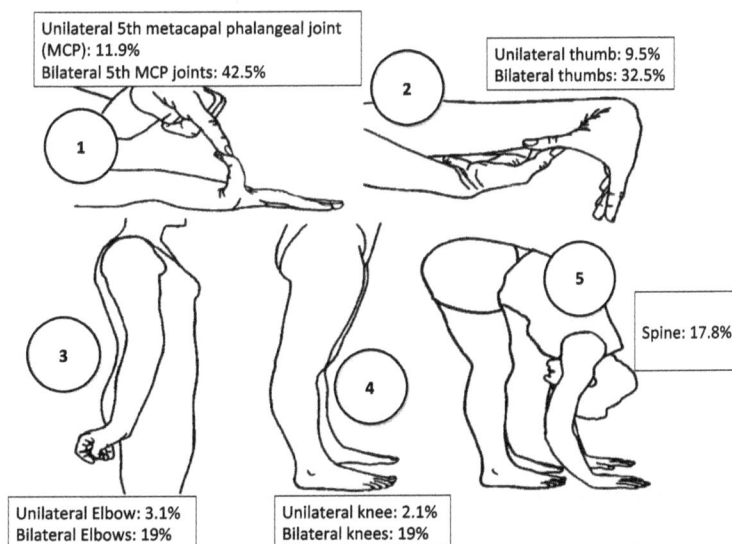

Fig. 1 Percentage frequencies of unilateral or bilateral signs of hypermobility identified through 5 maneuvers in the Beighton scale: 1) extension of the 5th metacarpal phalangeal joint by placing the 5th finger parallel to the forearm, 2) extension of the thumb touching the flexor side of the forearm, 3) extension greater than 10° beyond the limit of 180° of the elbow, 4) extension greater than 10° beyond the limit of 180° in the knee, and 5) flexion and elongation of the spine by placing the hands flat on the floor with knees in maximum extension

Table 1 Frequencies of responses on hypermobility, described in a 5-item questionnaire for joint hypermobility [41]

	Yes	No	Do not know
1. Can you or have you managed to get your hands placed flat on the floor without bending your knees?	187 (48.2%)	188 (48.4%)	13 (3.4%)
2. Can you or have you been able to turn your thumb until it touches your forearm?	101 (26%)	278 (71.7%)	9 (2.3%)
3. When you were a kid, did you amuse your friends by twisting your body in strange positions OR did you open your legs completely?	153 (39.4%)	229 (59%)	6 (1.6%)
4. As a child or teenager have you dislocated your shoulder or patella more than once?	29 (7.5%)	348 (89.7%)	11 (2.8%)
5. Do you consider your joints supple? Do you think your joints bend as much as those of a contortionist?	31 (8%)	337 (86.9%)	20 (5.1%)

hours/week, and 23 subjects declared a mean competition practice time of (0.2 ± 1.2) hours/week.

The responses to the 5-item hypermobility questionnaire, estimating the presence or absence of joint hypermobility, are presented in Table 1. Among the most scored items, the highest was the spine (48.2%).

The survey on musculoskeletal and extra-articular or systemic complaints associated with joint hypermobility and their respective frequencies is presented in Table 2. The most frequently reported problem was low back pain, present in 176 (45.4%) of the subjects.

The classification of hypermobility was established using the instructed self-examination recorded by three trained observers, using the criteria of Beighton [20], with a limit of 4 or more joints (≥ 4) to determine generalized hypermobility and a 3-joint limit (≥ 1 and ≤ 3) for localized hypermobility [43].

Generalized joint hypermobility was observed in 104 (26.8%) individuals. The frequency of generalized joint hypermobility in women was 27.8%, and that of the male

population was 23.6%. The locations of the hypermobility signs and their respective frequencies and distributions are shown in Fig. 1, with the paired signs being independently and bilaterally scored in the majority.

The 5th finger hypermobility sign was the most frequent, being described in 165 (42.52%) individuals, followed by the thumb in 126 (32.56%) individuals, elbows and knees in 72 subjects each (18.6%), and spine in 69 (17.79%) individuals. There were no statistically significant differences in gender for any of the signs (Table 3).

In the SF-36 questionnaire, the results were comparable with the normative data in adults of the Brazilian population. No significant differences were observed in the results of each domain and in the physical and mental indices among those with generalized hypermobility, localized hypermobility, or absence of hypermobility (Table 4).

The following correlations were found between each SF-36 domain and the generalized hypermobility condition (score ≥ 4): Vitality (VT) $r = -0.05284$, $p = 0.2991$; Mental Health (MH) $r = -0.10007$, $p = 0.05$; Physical Functioning (PF) $r = -0.04907$, $p = 0.3350$; Role-Physical (RP) $r = -0.03178$, $p = 0.5325$; Bodily Pain $r = 0.07304$, $p = 0.1510$; General Health (GH) $r = -0.11050$, $p = 0.03$; Role-Emotional (RE) $r = -0.02224$, $p = 0.6623$; Social Functioning (SF) $r = -0.05410$, $p = 0.2878$; Physical Component (PCo) $r = -0.06839$, $p = 0.1789$; and Mental Component (MCo) $r = -0.02491$, $p = 0.6248$. All correlations were weak (0.1 to 0.3), although they were significant for Mental Health and General

Table 2 Frequencies of valid responses in the inquiry of signs and symptoms, musculoskeletal and systemic, related to joint hypermobility

Signs and symptoms	Yes	No
Contortionist tricks	54 (15%)	328 (85%)
Ankle sprain	118 (32%)	255 (68%)
Other ligament injuries	55 (15%)	309 (85%)
Arthralgia	122 (33%)	252 (67%)
Arthritis	18 (5%)	356 (95%)
Frequent cramps	143 (37%)	243 (63%)
Pain in the knees	102 (27%)	278 (73%)
Cervical pain	107 (28%)	270 (72%)
Dorsal pains	111 (29%)	268 (71%)
Lower back pain	176 (46%)	206 (54%)
Shoulder dislocations	29 (8%)	355 (92%)
Patella dislocations	16 (4%)	362 (96%)
Poor wound healing	28 (7%)	351 (93%)
Fractures	79 (20%)	304 (80%)

Table 3 Comparison of the frequencies of joint hypermobility signs scored in the Beighton Scale according to gender (Student's t-test)

Sign Manouver	Men	Women	Total	p
1) 5th Finger	32/89 (35.95%)	133/299 (44.48%)	165 (42.52%)	NS*
2) Thumb	24/89 (26.96%)	102/299 (34.11%)	126 (32.56%)	NS*
3) Elbow	9/89 (10.11%)	63/299 (21.07%)	72 (18.6%)	NS*
4) Knee	11/89 (12.35%)	61/299 (20.40%)	72 (18.6%)	NS*
5) Spine	14/89 (15.73%)	55/299 (18.39%)	69 (17.79%)	NS*

*NS - not significant

Table 4 Comparison of the SF-36 scores in the total sample of volunteers, without hypermobility (Beighton score = 0) or with localized hypermobility (1–3) and generalized hypermobility (≥ 4)

Variable	n	Total Sample	Median	N (%)	Localized hypermobility (1–3) Without hypermobility (0)	Median	N (%)	Generalized hypermobility (≥ 4)	Median
PF	388	88.2 ± 12.4	90	284 (73.2%)	88.3 ± 12.7	90	104 (26.8%)	87.7 ± 11.5	90
RP	388	72.4 ± 31	75	284 (73.2%)	73.9 ± 30	75	104 (26.8%)	68 ± 33.3	75
BP	388	51.7 ± 8.1	50	284 (73.2%)	51.3 ± 8.5	50	104 (26.8%)	52.6 ± 7	50
GH	388	60.8 ± 15.5	65	284 (73.2%)	61.7 ± 15.3	65	104 (26.8%)	58.4 ± 15.8	60
VT	388	54.8 ± 19.7	57.5	284 (73.2%)	55.4 ± 19.3	60	104 (26.8%)	53.1 ± 20.7	55
SF	388	64 ± 11.5	65.1	284 (73.2%)	64.4 ± 11.5	65	104 (26.8%)	62.8 ± 11.3	64.8
RE	388	67.2 ± 38.2	100	284 (73.2%)	67.5 ± 37.7	100	104 (26.8%)	66.4 ± 39.6	100
MH	388	65 ± 19.4	68	284 (73.2%)	66 ± 19.7	68	104 (26.8%)	62 ± 18.3	64
PCo	388	65.5 ± 11	67	284 (73.2%)	66.1 ± 10.9	67.5	104 (26.8%)	64 ± 11	65.5
MCo	388	61.3 ± 16.3	64.2	284 73.2%	61.6 ± 16.2	64.6	104 26.8%	60.7 ± 16.6	61.7

Physical Functioning (PF), Role-Physical (RP), Bodily Pain (BP), General Health (GH), Vitality (VT), Social Functioning (SF), Role-Emotional (RE), and Mental Health (MH); Physical Component (PCo), and Mental Component (MCo)

Health. There was no association between the SF-36 score and hypermobility, indicating a minimal impact on the health, physical, and psychosocial aspects of volunteers.

Discussion

The primary objective was to estimate the frequency of hypermobility among young university students and the possible repercussions on their health condition as evaluated using objective methods. Women were predominantly included in an unselected population, as students of both genders were invited. We found a frequency of 27% generalized joint hypermobility and an interesting result of 35% localized hypermobility. Localized signs of hypermobility predominated on the hands and secondarily on the elbows, knees, and spine. The selection of volunteers in medical and physiotherapy schools was aimed at achieving a homogeneous sample of the healthy population with regular physical activity.

The frequency of generalized hypermobility found in our study in young people was similar to that of English adolescents reported by Clinch et al. 2011 [16] using the same threshold of more than 4 points in the Beighton scale found in the cohort up to 14 years old, with proportions of 27.5% in girls and 10.6% in boys. Accordingly, 45% of the girls had finger hypermobility compared with 29% of boys with finger hypermobility. These authors also did not describe any associations between hypermobility and physical activity, body mass index, or maternal education level.

A recent study among Korean girls and women [44] described the presence of generalized hypermobility in 50% of respondents, 59% in girls and 36.5% in adult women, with the number of signs inversely proportional to age. Significant differences of localized hypermobility in the thumb and 5th finger were found in both groups. The lower frequency of hypermobility according to age

occurred symmetrically on both thumbs but it was more pronounced in the fifth finger of the dominant hand, more often on the right hand.

Based on anthropometric data including weight, height, and body mass index, overweight was occasional, and physical activity was relatively regular, with a higher proportion of patients with localized hypermobility, especially in the hands. Population studies are described in the pediatric literature, but data on their frequency, effects, and consequences in the young adult population have been infrequent. Musculoskeletal pain is a sign often related to hypermobility and obesity; sedentary lifestyle may play a relevant role [45, 46], as there is a two-fold increased risk in adolescents with hypermobility.

Although the Bodily Pain domain had minimum impact or correlation with hypermobility in the SF-36 investigation, the frequency of musculoskeletal pain was relevant, mainly due to the proportions of low back pain, frequent cramps, arthralgia, and sprains. Long-term studies on sequelae, including the risk of osteoarthritis, are still inconclusive. Conditions such as tendinitis, bursitis, fasciitis, and fibromyalgia correspond to 25% of referrals to rheumatologists. The association with generalized and localized joint hypermobility, repetitive strain activities, and pain in areas of localized hypermobility [47], has been explored in professional artistic activities such as ballet, gymnastics, and acrobatics [48, 49], predisposing to pain and injury due to associated mechanical trauma,.

In a Brazilian study, the prevalence of hypermobility in academic ballet activity was 58%, with a higher frequency among teachers compared with students [49]. It is also interesting to observe the performance of flute players, who have particularly greater range of motion in the hands, and even finger hypermobility, presenting more accurate proprioception through training, which is an ideal model to study the interaction between localized flexibility and joint proprioception [50].

Questions about the practice of music or dance activities were not part of our inquiry; we questioned only the number of hours practicing leisure physical activities and sports activities. The options for the Beighton criteria may have some criticism due to variability and divergence in the cutoff scores. The higher scores, such as ≥4, ≥ 5, ≥ 6, and ≥ 7 hipermobile joints could also be considered; however, the score ≥ 4 was the most widely reported in the literature as the most frequent cutoff point [1, 2, 11–13, 17, 20, 21, 39, 49, 50].

For the diagnosis of generalized joint hypermobility in children and adolescents, at least 5 of the 9 criteria on the Beighton scale are recommended; the difference between the conditions of generalized joint hypermobility and joint hypermobility syndrome is the presence of symptoms. Associated symptoms including predominant musculoskeletal conditions, such as joint pain and instability [26], are more frequently observed in adults and are possibly related to mechanical impact or repeated strain activity.

However, dysfunctional gastrointestinal manifestations [32, 40], such as constipation, vesicoureteral reflux [3], or inguinal hernia [31], are more frequently described in pediatric age. Our survey was limited in the approach of other systems involved. Among the systemic manifestations, poor wounds healing, which had a low frequency of responses, was questioned. In the recall survey about pain in the lumbar spine region and arthralgia, these complaints were the most frequent, involving 319 reports in total, but without repercussions on quality of life and health status. Our data are consistent with Ruperto et al. 2004 [25], who used the CHQ-PF 50 questionnaire among healthy schoolchildren with hypermobility and also did not identify repercussions in their physical and psychosocial components.

Musculoskeletal pain can be triggered by physical activity in the absence of adequate physical conditioning, intense physical exercise, an accident, or a traumatic event or may develop without any apparent reason; its association with hypermobility mmay be of mere chance. There are also associations of chronic pain with fatigue, dysautonomia, and negative impacts on quality of life scores due to anxiety and depression [28], which require intervention. However, these associations have been reported in samples of symptomatic hypermobile individuals who seek clinical treatment, comprising approximately 1% of men and 5% of women.

More comprehensive population studies including healthy individuals are still needed to estimate the magnitude of the problem and the generalization of our results.

Conclusion

In conclusion this young population sample with a predominance of women, localized hypermobility was more frequent than generalized hypermobility; however, there was minimum impact on either health or quality of life.

Acknowledgments

Darcisio Hortelan Antonio attended the Public Health Graduate Course, Sao Paulo State University (Universidade Estadual Paulista - UNESP), accredited by the Brazilian Federal Agency for the Support and Evaluation of Graduate Education (CAPES). Claudia Saad Magalhães MD, graduate mentor was funded by CNPq Scholarship (301644-2010, 301479/2015). The students Fabricio Lopes Stafussi, Juliana de Freitas, and Susan Nawaly collaborated in the data collection and Prof. José Eduardo Corrente (UNESP) perfomed the statistical analysis.

Authors' contributions

Both authors contributed equally to the paper development. It was developed as master's thesis under the Public Health Graduate Programme at UNESP.

Authors' information

No other than the above disclosure and acknowledgement.

Competing interests

There is no other competing interest than the academic research.

References

1. Kirk JA, Ansell BM, Bywaters EG. The hypermobility syndrome. Musculoskeletal complaints associated with generalized joint hypermobility. Ann Rheum Dis. 1967;26:419–25.
2. Jessee EF, Owen DS Jr, Sagar KB. The benign hypermobile joint syndrome. Arthritis Rheum. 1980;23:1053–6.
3. Klemp P, Stevens JE, Isaacs SA. Hypermobility study in ballet dancers. J Rheumatol. 1984;11:692–6.
4. Scheper MC, Engelbert RH, Rameckers EA, Verbunt J, Remvig L, Juul-Kristensen B Children with generalised joint hypermobility and musculoskeletal complaints: state of the art on diagnostics, clinical characteristics, and treatment. Biomed Res Int 2013:12105 [http://dx.doi.org/ https://doi.org/10.1155/2013/121054].
5. Murray KJ. Hypermobility disorders in children and adolescents. Best Pract Res Clin Rheumatol. 2006;20:329–51.
6. Grahame R. Joint hypermobility and genetic collagen disorders: are they related? Arch Dis Child. 1999;80:188–91.
7. Simmonds JV, Keer RJ. Hypermobility and the hypermobility syndrome. Man Ther. 2007;12:298–309.
8. Fikree A, Aziz Q, Grahame R. Joint hypermobility syndrome. Rheum Dis Clin N Am. 2013;39:419–30.
9. Simmonds JV, Keer RJ. Hypermobility and the hypermobility syndrome, part 2: assessment and management of hypermobility syndrome: illustrated via case studies. Man Ther. 2008;13:e1–11.
10. Santos MC, Azevedo ES. Generalized joint hypermobility and black admixture in school children of Bahia, Brazil. Am J Phys Anthropol. 1981;55:43–6.
11. Larsson LG, Baum J, Mudholkar GS. Hypermobility: features and differential incidence between the sexes. Arthritis Rheum. 1987;30:1426–30.
12. Rikken-Bultman DG, Wellink L, van Dongen PW. Hypermobility in two Dutch school populations. Eur J Obstet Gynecol Reprod Biol. 1997;73:189–92.
13. Jansson A, Saartok T, Werner S, Renstrom P. General joint laxity in 1845 Swedish school children of different ages: age- and gender-specific distributions. Acta Paediatr. 2004;93:1202–6.
14. Lamari NM, Chueire AG, Cordeiro JA. Analysis of joint mobility patterns among preschool children. Sao Paulo Med J. 2005;12:119–23.
15. Hasija RP, Khubchandani RP, Shenoi S. Joint hypermobility in Indian children. Clin Exp Rheumatol. 2008;26:146–50.
16. Clinch J, Deere K, Sayers A, Palmer S, Riddoch C, Tobias JH, Clark EM. Epidemiology of generalized joint laxity (hypermobility) in fourteen-year-old children from the UK: a population-based evaluation. Arthritis Rheum. 2011; 63:2819–27.

17. Abujam B, Aggarwal A. Hypermobility is related with musculoskeletal pain in Indian school-children. Clin Exp Rheumatol. 2014;32:610–3.
18. Remvig L, Jensen DV. Ward RC are diagnostic criteria for general joint hypermobility and benign joint hypermobility syndrome based on reproducible and valid tests? A review of the literature. J Rheumatol. 2007; 34:798–803.
19. Ohman A, Westblom C, Henriksson M. Hypermobility among school children aged five to eight years: the hospital del mar criteria gives higher prevalence for hypermobility than the Beighton score. Clin Exp Rheumatol. 2014;32:285–90.
20. Beighton P, Solomon L, Soskolne CL. Articular mobility in an African population. Ann Rheum Dis. 1973;32:413–8.
21. Forleo LH, Hilario MO, Peixoto AL, Naspitz C, Goldenberg J. Articular hypermobility in school children in Sao Paulo, Brazil. J Rheumatol. 1993;20: 916–7.
22. Subramanyam V. Janaki KV joint hypermobility in south Indian children. Indian Pediatr. 1996;33:771–2.
23. El-Garf AK, Mahmoud GA. Mahgoub EH hypermobility among Egyptian children: prevalence and features. J Rheumatol. 1998;25:1003–5.
24. Qvindesland A, Jonsson H. Articular hypermobility in Icelandic 12-year-olds. Rheumatology (Oxford). 1999;38:1014–6.
25. Ruperto N, Malattia C, Bartoli M, Trail L, Pistorio A, Martini A, Ravelli A. Functional ability and physical and psychosocial well-being of hypermobile schoolchildren. Clin Exp Rheumatol. 2004;22:495–8.
26. Adib N, Davies K, Grahame R, Woo P, Murray KJ. Joint hypermobility syndrome in childhood. A not so benign multisystem disorder? Rheumatology (Oxford). 2005;44:744–50.
27. Pacey V, Tofts L, Wesley A, Collins F, Singh-Grewal D. Joint hypermobility syndrome: a review for clinicians. J Paediatr Child Health. 2015;51:373–80.
28. Palmer S, Bailey S, Barker L, Barney L, Elliott A. The effectiveness of therapeutic exercise for joint hypermobility syndrome: a systematic review. Physiotherapy. 2014;100:220–7.
29. Mishra MB, Ryan P, Atkinson P, Taylor H, Bell J, Calver D, et al. Extra-articular features of benign joint hypermobility syndrome. Brit J Rheumatol. 1996;35: 861–6.
30. Beiraghdar F, Rostami Z, Panahi Y, Einollahi B, Teimoori M. Vesicoureteral reflux in pediatrics with hypermobility syndrome. Nephrourol Mon. 2013;5: 924–7.
31. Nazem M, Mottaghi P, Hoseini A. Khodadadi HA benign joint hypermobility syndrome among children with inguinal hernia. J Res Med Sci. 2013;18:904–5.
32. Kovacic K, Chelimsky TC, Sood MR, Simpson P, Nugent M, Chelimsky G. Joint hypermobility: a common association with complex functional gastrointestinal disorders. J Pediatr. 2014;165:973–8.
33. Roberto AM, Terreri MT, Szejnfeld V, Hilario MO. Bone mineral density in children. Association with musculoskeletal pain and/or joint hypermobility. J Pediatr. 2002;78:523–8.
34. Albayrak I, Yilmaz H, Akkurt HE, Salli A, Karaca G. Is pain the only symptom in patients with benign joint hypermobility syndrome? Clin Rheumatol. 2015;34:1613–9.
35. Engelbert RH, Bank RA, Sakkers RJ, Helders PJ, Beemer FA, Uiterwaal CS. Pediatric generalized joint hypermobility with and without musculoskeletal complaints: a localized or systemic disorder? Pediatrics. 2003;111:e248–54.
36. Cameron KL, Duffey ML, De Berardino TM, Stoneman PD, Jones CJ, Owens BD. Association of generalized joint hypermobility with a history of glenohumeral joint instability. J Athlet Train. 2010;45:253–8.
37. Kavuncu V, Sahin S, Kamanli A, Karan A, Aksoy C. The role of systemic hypermobility and condylar hypermobility in temporomandibular joint dysfunction syndrome. Rheumatol Int. 2006;26:257–60.
38. Azma K, Mottaghi P, Hosseini A, Abadi HH. Nouraei MH benign joint hypermobility syndrome in soldiers; what is the effect of military training courses on associated joint instabilities? J Res Med Sci. 2014;19:639–43.
39. Marcolin ALV, Cardin SP, Magalhaes CS. Muscle strength assessment among children and adolescents with growing pains and joint hypermobility. Rev Bras Fisiot. 2009;13:110–5.
40. Farmer AD, Fikree A, Aziz Q. Addressing the confounding role of joint hypermobility syndrome and gastrointestinal involvement in postural orthostatic tachycardia syndrome. Clin Autonom Res. 2014;24:157–8.
41. Moraes DA, Baptista CA, Crippa JA, Louzada-Junior P. Translation into Brazilian Portuguese and validation of the five-part questionnaire for identifying hypermobility. Rev Bras Reumatol. 2011;51:53–69.
42. da Mota Falcao D, Ciconelli RM. Ferraz MB translation and cultural adaptation of quality of life questionnaires: an evaluation of methodology. J Rheumatol. 2003;30:379–85.
43. Remvig L, Jensen DV. Ward RC epidemiology of general joint hypermobility and basis for the proposed criteria for benign joint hypermobility syndrome: review of the literature. J Rheumatol. 2007;34:804–9.
44. Kwon JW, Lee WJ, Park SB, Kim MJ, Jang SH, Choi CK. Generalized joint hypermobility in healthy female koreans: prevalence and age-related differences. Ann Rehab Med. 2013;37:832–8.
45. Tobias JH, Deere K, Palmer S, Clark EM, Clinch J. Joint hypermobility is a risk factor for musculoskeletal pain during adolescence: findings of a prospective cohort study. Arthritis Rheum. 2013;65:1107–15.
46. Sperotto F, Balzarin M, Parolin M, Monteforte N, Vittadello F, Zulian F. Joint hypermobility, growing pain and obesity are mutually exclusive as causes of musculoskeletal pain in schoolchildren. Clin Exp Rheumatol. 2014;32:131–6.
47. Hudson N, Fitzcharles MA, Cohen M, Starr MR, Esdaile JM. The association of soft-tissue rheumatism and hypermobility. Brit J Rheumatol. 1998;37:382–6.
48. McCormack M, Briggs J, Hakim A, Grahame R. Joint laxity and the benign joint hypermobility syndrome in student and professional ballet dancers. J Rheumatol. 2004;31:173–8.
49. Sanches SB, Oliveira GM, Osorio FL, Crippa JA, Martin-Santos R. Hypermobility and joint hypermobility syndrome in Brazilian students and teachers of ballet dance. Rheumatol Int. 2015;35:741–7.
50. Artigues-Cano I, Bird HA. Hypermobility and proprioception in the finger joints of flautists. J Clin Rheumatol. 2014;20:203–8.

11

Vitamin D receptor gene polymorphisms and susceptibility for primary osteoarthritis of the knee in a Latin American population

Norma Celia González-Huerta[1], Verónica Marusa Borgonio-Cuadra[1], Eugenio Morales-Hernández[2], Carolina Duarte-Salazar[3] and Antonio Miranda-Duarte[1]* ⓘ

Abstract

Background: Primary Osteoarthritis (OA) of the knee is a multifactorial disease that has an important genetic component, and several genes have been associated with its development. The vitamin D receptor has a role in skeletal metabolism that suggests a relationship with OA. The aim of this study was to analyze the association of Vitamin D receptor gene (*VDR*) polymorphisms in Mexican Mestizo patients.

Methods: A case-control study was conducted in which 107 cases with primary OA of the knee and 114 controls were included. Cases were patients > 40 years of age with a Body mass index (BMI) of ≤27 and a radiological score for OA of the knee of ≥2. Controls were subjects > 40 years of age with a radiological score of < 2. *VDR* polymorphisms rs1544410, rs7975232, and rs731236 were analyzed by means of restriction endonucleases, and logistic regression was developed to evaluate risk magnitude.

Results: A significantly increased risk was found of nearly two-fold for the allele T and TT genotypes of rs731236, independently of other well recognized risk factors.

Conclusions: The rs731236 polymorphism is associated with the risk of primary OA of the knee in Mexican Mestizo population.

Keywords: Osteoarthritis, Vitamin D receptor gene, Polymorphism, Mexican Mestizo population, Association study

Background

Osteoarthritis (OA) is the most frequent form of arthritis and is a leading cause of musculoskeletal disability worldwide. The World Health Organization (WHO) estimates that approximately 10% of the world's population aged ≥60 years have symptomatic OA and that it is the fourth leading cause of Years lived with disability (YLD) [1, 2]. OA can occur in any joint, but the knee is the most common site involved; in fact, it is considered that 6% of adults can be affected and that this is one of the most common reasons for total joint replacement [3–5]. OA is characterized by progressive degeneration of articular cartilage in synovial joints, resulting in joint space narrowing, osteophyte formation, and subchondral sclerosis, which is clinically translated as pain and joint stiffness [4, 5].

OA is a multifactorial disease in which genetics and environmental factors, such as aging, gender, obesity, significant trauma, occupation, and sports activities, among others, are strongly related with its development [4, 5]. It is classified as primary when no discernible cause is evident and secondary when a triggering factor is apparent. Primary OA possess a strong genetic component, as demonstrated by several twin and family studies, which have demonstrated 39–65% heritability (h^2) and an increased risk for OA of up to 14-fold in first-degree relatives of probands with OA [6, 7]. On the other hand, genetic association studies have demonstrated that primary OA is associated with several genes related to different molecular pathways or classes of molecules such as inflammation, Extracellular matrix

* Correspondence: fovi01@prodigy.net.mx
[1]Departments of Genetics, Instituto Nacional de Rehabilitación "Luis Guillermo Ibarra Ibarra", Calzada México-Xochimilco No. 289, Arenal Guadalupe, Tlalpan, CP 14389 México City, Mexico
Full list of author information is available at the end of the article

(ECM) molecules, Wnt signaling, Bone morphogenetic proteins, proteases or their inhibitors, and genes related with modulation of osteocyte or chondrocyte differentiation [6, 7].

The Vitamin D receptor plays an important role in skeletal metabolism because this acts as an important regulator of calcium metabolism and bone cell function; therefore, its abnormalities are probably related with OA [8]. The vitamin D receptor gene (VDR) is located on chromosome 12q13.11, contains 11 exons, and spans approximately 75 kb. The gene contains several polymorphisms, and three have been frequently studied for determining an association in OA: rs1544410 and rs7975232 in intron 8, and the synonymous variant rs731236 in exon 9 [9–11]. With regard to primary OA of the knee, some reports have shown an association in the presence of these VDR polymorphisms [12–14], however, this has not always been confirmed [15–18]. A meta-analysis on the three most frequently studied VDR polymorphisms in OA analyzed Asian and European studies; however, the results showed no association in all study subjects, as well as by stratification by ethnicity [19]. An updated meta-analysis, showed a significant association between the A allele and AA genotype of the rs7975232 with OA in Asian population, but not in the whole population [20]. Because genetic associations could vary among populations and because there are no association studies on VDR and OA in Latin-American populations, our aim was to analyze the association of the three VDR polymorphisms in Mexican Mestizo patients.

Methods

Subjects

We conducted a case-control study whose protocol was approved by the Ethics and Investigation Committee of the National Rehabilitation Institute, a tertiary-care referral center in Mexico City. All of the participants were recruited at the Articular Rehabilitation Clinic and were of Mexican Mestizo origin, the latter defined as a person born in Mexico, with a Spanish-derived last name, and with a family of Mexican ancestors back to the third generation [21]. Cases included persons aged > 40 years with a clinical diagnosis of OA and a radiologic score of ≥2 for OA of the knee, with a Body mass index (BMI, kg/m^2) of ≤27, with no history of serious injuries or knee surgeries, and with no other articular diseases. Controls were subjects aged > 40 years without a clinical diagnosis of OA of the knee, with a radiologic score of < 2, and with no history of serious knee injuries or diseases of the joints. All controls arrived at the clinic mainly due to orthopedic problems, such as shoulder lesions or fractures, or orthopedic problems not involving serious knee damage. Radiological evaluation of all participants was performed by a sole trained observer who

was blinded to the patients' diagnosis. Grading of OA was assessed using a 5-point scale according to the Kellgren-Lawrence radiographic-classification grading method in anteroposterior weight-bearing and lateral x-rays of the knees [22]. To perform a more efficient classification of cases and controls and to identify possible co-variables or confounders, all study subjects were interviewed by application of a questionnaire designed specifically for this study in order to collect information regarding general, occupational, and sports activities, possible knee injuries, and clinical manifestations of OA, among others.

Genotyping

After obtaining signed informed consent, a 5-ml blood sample was drawn from each patient into tubes containing EDTA. Peripheral blood mononuclear cells were isolated, and DNA was extracted utilizing a salting out method. The genotype for three polymorphisms of the VDR was determined by Polymerase-chain-reaction (PCR) amplification and enzymatic digestion of the products using the primer pair listed previously [23]. The forward primer was the same for all three polymorphisms: 5′-CAACCAAGACTACAAGTACCGCGTCAGTGA-3′. For rs7975232 and rs731236 polymorphisms, the reverse primer was 5′-CACTTCGAGCACAAGGGGCGTTAGC-3′; and for rs1544410 was 5′-AACCAGCGGGAAGAGGT-CAAGGG-3′. PCR was performed with a Gene Amp PCR system 9700 PE Applied Biosystems under standard conditions. Briefly, for fragment amplification 1X buffer solution was used (KCl 50 mM, Tris-HCl 20 mM pH 8.4), 0.6 mM DNTP, 0.5 μM of each primer, 4 mM MgCl2, 2.5 U Taq polymerase, and 250 ng genomic DNA, for a final volume reaction of 50 μL. A thermal profile was optimized as follows: 94 °C for 5 min for initial denaturation, followed by 28 cycles at 94 °C for 1 min, at 65 °C for 1 min, at 72 °C for 1 min, and 5 min at 72 °C for final extension. Subsequently, one microgram of the PCR product was digested with an excess of the endonucleases under conditions specified by the supplier (New England Biolabs, Inc., Beverly, MA, USA) and was electrophoresed on 1.5% ethidium- stained agarose gels. Information of Single Nucleotide Polymorphism (SNP) and product size after digestion with endonucleases is shown in Table 1.

Statistical analysis

Comparisons of continuous variables were tested by the Student t test, and corrected chi-squared statistics (x^2) were applied for categorical variables. Uni- and multivariate nonconditional logistic regression analyses were conducted to estimate probability for developing OA, comparing genotypes as main effect; Odds ratios and 95% Confidence intervals [OR (95% CI)] were reported. Alpha level was 0.05. Hardy-Weinberg equilibrium (HWE) was assessed for VDR polymorphisms by means of the chi-squared test, and the

Table 1 Information of the three single nucleotide polymorphisms of VDR gene

SNP	Alleles	Location	Change	Enzyme	Fragments (bp)		Frequencies Cases, controls	HWE
rs1544410	A/G	Intron 8	None	BsmI	G: 650/175	A: 825	0.615, 0.576	< 0.05
rs7975232	A/C	Intron 8	None	ApaI	C: 1700/300	A: 2000	0.528, 0.500	< 0.05
rs731236	C/T	Exon 9	Ile352=	TaqI	C: 1800/200	T: 2000	0.835, 0.759	0.28

SNP: rs numbers were taken from NCBI dbSNP (http://www.ncbi.nlm.nih.gov/SNP)
HWE p value in the control group

STATA ver.10.0 statistical software package and Haplo View 4.0 were utilized for calculations.

Results

The characteristics of the study population are shown in Table 2. We observed statistically significant differences in mean age and in previous sport-activity frequency ($p = 0.00001$ and 0.004; respectively).

The SNPs rs1544410 and rs7975232 were not in HWE (Table 1) and their allelic and genotypic frequencies did not showed significant differences between the study groups (Tables 1 and 3). Only rs731236 was in HWE, and its C and T alleles showed statistically significant differences [OR (95% CI) = 0.6 (0.4–1.0) and 1.6 (1.0–2.6); respectively]. In regard to its genotypes, CT genotype suggested a protective factor [OR (95%CI) = 0.5 (0.3–0.9)], and TT genotype exhibited an increased risk with an OR (95%CI) of 1.96 (1.1–3.4) (Table 3). For multivariate analysis two models were constructed, and the risk trends for CT and TT genotypes were maintained when

these results were adjusted for gender, age, BMI, and previous sport activity (Table 4).

Discussion

VDR polymorphisms are probably among those most studied for a genetic association in OA; however, there is no consistency in the results [12–18]. Even in the meta-analyses, there is no agreement in their findings [19, 20]. Those studies could entertain some limitations, because of the absence of analysis by OA site, since it is important to

Table 2 General characteristics of the study population

	Cases (n = 107)	Controls (n = 114)	p
Age (mean ± SD years)	57.6 ± 8.9	51.7 ± 8.7	0.00001
BMI (mean ± SD kg/m²)	26.4 ± 2.8	25.7 ± 3.4	0.08
Gender, females (n, %)	86 (81.1)	95 (83.3)	0.66
Smoking (n, %)	21 (26.9)	11 (26.83)	0.9
Alcoholism (n, %)	22 (28.2)	10 (24.4)	0.6
Occupational activity (n, %)			
Current (n, %)	9 (8.4)	11 (9.6)	0.7
Previous (n, %)	11 (10.3)	14 (12.3)	0.6
Sports activity			
Current (n, %)	18 (16.8)	29 (25.4)	0.12
Previous (n, %)	51 (47.7)	76 (66.7)	0.004
Kellgren-Lawrence grading			
Grade 0, n (%)	0	70 (61.4)	
Grade 1, n (%)	0	44 (38.6)	
Grade 2, n (%)	38 (35.5)	0	
Grade 3, n (%)	46 (42.9)	0	
Grade 4, n (%)	23 (21.5)	0	

Table 3 Allelic and genotype association testing results of rs1544410, rs7975232, and rs731236 in VDR for Mexican cases with osteoarthritis of the knee and controls

SNP	Cases (n = 107) n (%)	Controls (n = 114) n (%)	OR (CI 95%)[a]	p
rs1544410				
Allele				
A	82 (38.0)	97 (43.0)	0.8 (0.6–1.2)	0.4
G	132 (62.0)	131 (57.0)	1.1 (0.8–1.8)	0.4
Genotype				
AA	4 (3.7)	9 (7.9)	0.4 (0.1–1.5)	0.2
GA	74 (69.2)	79 (69.3)	0.9 (0.5–1.8)	0.9
GG	29 (27.1)	26 (22.8)	1.2 (0.6–2.3)	0.5
rs7975232				
Allele				
G	112 (52.0)	115 (50.0)	1.1 (0.7–1.6)	0.7
T	102 (48.0)	113 (50.0)	0.9 (0.6–1.4)	0.7
Genotype				
GG	17 (15.9)	16 (14.0)	1.1 (0.5–2.4)	0.7
GT	78 (72.9)	83 (72.8)	1.0 (0.5–1.8)	0.9
TT	12 (11.2)	15 (13.2)	0.8 (0.3–1.9)	0.7
rs731236				
Allele				
C	35 (16.0)	55 (24.0)	0.6 (0.4–1.0)	0.04
T	179 (84.0)	173 (76.0)	1.6 (1.0–2.6)	0.04
Genotype				
CC	3 (2.8)	3 (2.6)	1.1 (0.2–5.4)	0.9
CT	29 (27.1)	49 (42.9)	0.5 (0.3–0.9)	0.01
TT	75 (70.1)	62 (54.4)	1.9 (1.1–3.4)	0.02

[a]Unadjusted Odds ratios and 95% Confidence intervals [OR (95% CI)]

Table 4 Multivariate analysis results of rs731236 for Mexican cases with osteoarthritis of the knee and controls

Genotype	OR (CI 95%)[a]	p	OR (CI 95%)[b]	p
CC	0.9 (0.1–6.0)	0.9	1.1 (0.2–6.7)	0.9
CT	0.5 (0.3–0.9)	0.03	0.5 (0.3–0.9)	0.03
TT	1.9 (1.1–3.4)	0.03	1.8 (1.02–3.3)	0.04

[a]adjusted by gender, age, BMI
[b]adjusted by gender, age, BMI, previous sport activities

consider that associations in OA appear to be joint-specific, as suggested by association studies [6, 24] and supported by functional analyses [25]. Therefore, the genetic associations in OA of the knee should be analyzed independently of other anatomic sites. Our findings suggest that there is an association between the rs731236 polymorphism and knee OA in this Mexican Mestizo population, conferring an increased risk of nearly two-fold in the presence of T allele and TT genotype independently of other well recognized risk factors such as age, gender, BMI, and sport activities.

The rs731236 is a synonymous polymorphism located in the coding sequence and exerts no effect in the encoded protein [10, 11]. However, a functional effect of this polymorphism is suggested by studies in which homozygous TT were associated with low *VDR* messenger RNA (mRNA) levels, and with low serum vitamin D level in some types of cancer [26, 27]. Interestingly, Subjects with low serum levels of vitamin D had a 3-fold increased risk for progression of OA of the knee [28]. Moreover, the activity of Matrix metalloproteinases (MMP) in the growth plate chondrocyte is regulated by vitamin D [29], and low levels of vitamin D increase MMP activities [30], which contributes to cartilage degradation, the hallmark in OA [4, 5].

On the other hand, it is possible that the rs731236 reflects a real association with other genes located in the same chromosomal region, such as Collagen type II alpha 1 chain (*COL2A1*), which is localized at a distance of 20 kb upstream [31]. Indeed, previously an association of *COL2A1* polymorphisms with knee OA was observed [32]. Or Histone deacetylase 7 (*HADC7*), at 10 kb downstream, which although there are not association studies with *HDAC7* polymorphisms, its increased expression in the cartilage of patients with OA suggests that it may contribute to cartilage degradation [33].

VDR polymorphisms have been analyzed in different ethnic groups and differences in allele frequencies have been noted [11]; this could be due to population stratification and could explain the inconsistency in the results. For case-control genetic-association studies, this is a matter of concern because it has been suggested that the existence of genetic subgroups in a population may lead to spurious associations [34]. To control this genetic confounder, ancestry informative markers are suggested

to be analyzed to avoid bias [35]. Mexican Mestizos are an admixed population [36], therefore, a possible weakness in this work is that ethnicity was determined only by self-reported family ancestry and by family history. However, the degree to which population stratification has caused confounding remains controversial [37, 38], and it has been suggested that this should not be a major confounder and that self-reported ethnicity may be sufficient to resolve that bias [38, 39]. In fact, it have been demonstrated that self-identified ethnicity correlate well with ancestral markers [40, 41]. Additionally, it is also important to consider that our controls were originated from the same geographic regions of the country as that of cases, and that the allele associated with primary OA of the knee follows HWE. This may indicate that allele frequency is not affected by inbreeding, mutation, natural selection, migration, or even population stratification [42]. Thus, spurious associations resulting from the presence of genetically different strata in our study sample are unlikely.

We are aware that being a hospital-based case-control study, it is exposed to incurring in selection bias. Therefore, to assess cases with primary OA of the knee as close as possible, the variables considerably associated with the development of secondary OA were strictly controlled during study-subject recruitment. Therefore, we think that the possibility of selection bias in our sample is low. Additionally, other potential confounders were controlled during statistical analyses, through multivariate analysis because this protects against population structure and limits the number of false positives [43]. In that sense, variables with significant differences during univariate analysis did not exhibit an effect on risk magnitude during multivariate analysis.

We recognize that our main limitation comprises sample size. However, we attempted to increase our internal validity by strictly controlling possible confounder variables through selection criteria and multivariate analysis, and we consider that our cases are truly primary OA of the knees. Finally, it is important to consider that association studies in diverse ethnic groups worldwide, especially those with a complex admixture of ancestral populations such as Latin-American populations, are a powerful resource for analyzing the genetic bases of complex diseases [44]; therefore, genetic association studies in Latino Americans would provide a better appreciation of the genetic contributions to primary OA.

Conclusions

According to the findings of this study, the rs731236 polymorphism is associated with the risk of primary OA of the knee in Mexican Mestizo population.

Abbreviations

BMI: Body mass index; COL2A1: Collagen type II alpha 1 chain gene; ECM: Extracellular matrix; HADC7: Histone deacetylase 7 gene; HWE: Hardy-Weinberg equilibrium; MMP: Matrix metalloproteinases; mRNA: messenger RNA; OA: Osteoarthritis; OR (95% CI): Odds ratios (95% Confidence intervals); PCR: Polymerase-chain-reaction; SNP: Single Nucleotide Polymorphism; VDR: Vitamin D receptor gene; WHO: World Health Organization; YLD: Years lived with disability

Authors' contributions

Concept and Study design: NCG-H, VMB-C and AM-D. Data acquisition: NCG-H, VMB-C, EM-H, CD-S. Data analysis, manuscript preparation: AM-D. All authors read and approved the final manuscript.

Competing interests

The authors declare that they have no competing interests.

Author details

[1]Departments of Genetics, Instituto Nacional de Rehabilitación "Luis Guillermo Ibarra Ibarra", Calzada México-Xochimilco No. 289, Arenal Guadalupe, Tlalpan, CP 14389 México City, Mexico. [2]Departments of Radiology, Instituto Nacional de Rehabilitación "Luis Guillermo Ibarra Ibarra", Calzada México-Xochimilco No. 289, Arenal Guadalupe, Tlalpan, CP 14389 México City, Mexico. [3]Departments of Rheumatology, Instituto Nacional de Rehabilitación "Luis Guillermo Ibarra Ibarra", Calzada México-Xochimilco No. 289, Arenal Guadalupe, Tlalpan, CP 14389 México City, Mexico.

References

1. Woolf AD, Pfleger B. Burden of major musculoskeletal conditions. Bull World Health Organ. 2003;81:646–56.
2. Haq SA, Davatchi F. Osteoarthritis of the knees in the COPCORD world. Int J Rheum Dis. 2011;14:122–9.
3. Weinstein AM, Rome BN, Reichmann WM, Collins JE, Burbine SA, Thornhill TS, et al. Estimating the burden of total knee replacement in the United States. J Bone Joint Surg Am. 2013;95:385–92.
4. Michael JW, Schlüter-Brust KU, Eysel P. The epidemiology, etiology, diagnosis, and treatment of osteoarthritis of the knee. Dtsch Arztebl Int. 2010;107:152–62.
5. Johnson VL, Hunter DJ. The epidemiology of osteoarthritis. Best Pract Res Clin Rheumatol. 2014;28:5–15.
6. Valdes AM, Spector TD. Genetic epidemiology of hip and knee osteoarthritis. Nat Rev Rheumatol. 2011;7:23–32.
7. Loughlin J. Genetic contribution to osteoarthritis development: current state of evidence. Curr Opin Rheumatol. 2015;27:284–8.
8. Colombini A, Cauci S, Lombardi G, Lanteri P, Croiset S, Brayda-Bruno M, et al. Relationship between vitamin D receptor gene (VDR) polymorphisms, vitamin D status, osteoarthritis and intervertebral disc degeneration. J Steroid Biochem Mol Biol. 2013;138:24–40.
9. Baker AR, McDonnell DP, Hughes M, Crisp TM, Mangelsdorf DJ, Haussler MR, et al. Cloning and expression of full-length cDNA encoding human vitamin D receptor. Proc Natl Acad Sci U S A. 1988;85:3294–8.
10. Miyamoto K, Kesterson RA, Yamamoto H, Taketani Y, Nishiwaki E, Tatsumi S, et al. Structural organization of the human vitamin D receptor chromosomal gene and its promoter. Mol Endocrinol. 1997;11:1165–79.
11. Uitterlinden AG, Fang Y, Van Meurs JB, Pols HA, Van Leeuwen JP. Genetics and biology of vitamin D receptor polymorphisms. Gene. 2004;338:143–56.
12. Uitterlinden AG, Burger H, Huang Q, Odding E, Duijn CM, Hofman A, et al. Vitamin D receptor genotype is associated with radiographic osteoarthritis at the knee. J Clin Invest. 1997;100:259–63.
13. Keen RW, Hart DJ, Lanchbury JS, Spector TD. Association of early osteoarthritis of the knee with a Taq I polymorphism of the vitamin D receptor gene. Arthritis Rheum. 1997;40:1444–9.
14. Uitterlinden AG, Burger H, van Duijn CM, Huang Q, Hofman A, Birkenhäger JC, et al. Adjacent genes, for COL2A1 and the vitamin D receptor, are

15. associated with separate features of radiographic osteoarthritis of the knee. Arthritis Rheum. 2000;43:1456–64.
15. Loughlin J, Sinsheimer JS, Mustafa Z, Carr AJ, Clipsham K, Bloomfield VA, et al. Association analysis of the vitamin D receptor gene, the type I collagen gene COL1A1, and the estrogen receptor gene in idiopathic osteoarthritis. J Rheumatol. 2000;27:779–84.
16. Huang J, Ushiyama T, Inoue K, Kawasaki T, Hukuda S. Vitamin D receptor gene polymorphisms and osteoarthritis of the hand, hip, and knee: a case-control study in Japan. Rheumatology. 2000;39:79–84.
17. Baldwin CT, Cupples LA, Joost O, Demissie S, Chaisson C, Mcalindon T, et al. Absence of linkage or association for osteoarthritis with the vitamin D receptor/type II collagen locus: the Framingham Osteoarthritis Study. J Rheumatol. 2002;29:161–5.
18. Muraki S, Dennison E, Jameson K, Boucher BJ, Akune T, Yoshimura N, et al. Association of vitamin D status with knee pain and radiographic knee osteoarthritis. Osteoarthr Cartil. 2011;19:1301–6.
19. Lee YH, Woo JH, Choi SJ, Ji JD, Song GG. Vitamin D receptor TaqI, BsmI and ApaI polymorphisms and osteoarthritis susceptibility: a meta-analysis. Joint Bone Spine. 2009;76:156–61.
20. Zhu ZH, Jin XZ, Zhang W, Chen M, Ye DQ, Zhai Y, et al. Associations between vitamin D receptor gene polymorphisms and osteoarthritis: an updated meta-analysis. Rheumatology. 2014;53:998–1008.
21. Gorodezky C, Aláez C, Vázquez-García MN, de la Rosa G, Infante E, Balladares S, et al. The genetic structure of Mexican Mestizos of different locations: tracking back their origins through MHC genes, blood group systems, and microsatellites. Hum Immunol. 2001;62:979–91.
22. Kellgren JH, Lawrence JS. Radiological assessment of osteo-arthrosis. Ann Rheum Dis. 1957;16:494–502.
23. Yokoyama K, Shigematsu T, Tsukada T, Ogura Y, Takemoto F, Hara S, et al. Apa I polymorphism in the vitamin D receptor gene may affect the parathyroid response in Japanese with end-stage renal disease. Kidney Int. 1998;53:454–8.
24. Reynard LN, Loughlin J. The genetics and functional analysis of primary osteoarthritis susceptibility. Expert Rev Mol Med. 2013;15:e2.
25. Xu Y, Barter MJ, Swan DC, Rankin KS, Rowan AD, Santibanez-Koref M, et al. Identification of the pathogenic pathways in osteoarthritic hip cartilage: commonality and discord between hip and knee OA. Osteoarthr Cartilage. 2012;20:1029–38.
26. Carling T, Rastad J, Åkerström G, Westin G. Vitamin D receptor (VDR) and parathyroid hormone messenger ribonucleic acid levels correspond to polymorphic VDR alleles in human parathyroid tumors. J Clin Endocrinol Metab. 1998;83:2255–9.
27. Yaylim-Eraltan I, Arzu Ergen H, Arikan S, Okay E, Oztürk O, Bayrak S, et al. Investigation of the VDR gene polymorphisms association with susceptibility to colorectal cancer. Cell Biochem Funct. 2007;25:731–7.
28. McAlindon TE, Felson DT, Zhang Y, Hannan MT, Aliabadi P, Weissman B, et al. Relation of dietary intake and serum levels of vitamin D to progression of osteoarthritis of the knee among participants in the Framingham study. Ann Intern Med. 1996;125:353–9.
29. Boyan BD, Schwartz Z. 1,25-Dihydroxy vitamin D3 is an autocrine regulator of extracellular matrix turnover and growth factor release via ERp60-activated matrix vesicle matrix metalloproteinases. Cells Tissues Organs. 2009;189:70–4.
30. Dean DD, Schwartz Z, Schmitz J, Muniz OE, Lu Y, Calderon F, et al. Vitamin D regulation of metalloproteinase activity in matrix vesicles. Connect Tissue Res. 1996;35:331–6.
31. Fang Y, van Meurs JB, d'Alesio A, et al. Promoter and 3'-untranslated-region haplotypes in the vitamin d receptor gene predispose to osteoporotic fracture: the Rotterdam study. Am J Hum Genet. 2005;77:807–23.
32. Gálvez-Rosas A, González-Huerta C, Borgonio-Cuadra VM, Duarte-Salazár C, Lara-Alvarado L, de los Angeles Soria-Bastida M, et al. A COL2A1 gene polymorphism is related with advanced stages of osteoarthritis of the knee in Mexican Mestizo population. Rheumatol Int. 2010;30:1035–9.
33. Higashiyama R, Miyaki S, Yamashita S, Yoshitaka T, Lindman G, Ito Y, et al. Correlation between MMP-13 and HDAC7 expression in human knee osteoarthritis. Mod Rheumatol. 2010;20:11–7.
34. Lander ES, Schork NJ. Genetic dissection of complex traits. Science. 1994; 265:2037–48.
35. Cardon LR, Palmer LJ. Population stratification and spurious allelic association. Lancet. 2003;361:598–604.

36. Moreno-Estrada A, Gignoux CR, Fernández-López JC, Zakharia F, Sikora M, Contreras AV, et al. Human genetics. The genetics of Mexico recapitulates native American substructure and affects biomedical traits. Science. 2014; 344:1280–5.
37. Thomas DC, Witte JS. Point: population stratification: a problem for case-control studies of candidate-gene associations? Cancer Epidemiol Biomark Prev. 2002;11:505–12.
38. Wacholder S, Rothman N, Caporaso N. Counterpoint: bias from population stratification is not a major threat to the validity of conclusions from epidemiological studies of common polymorphisms and cancer. Cancer Epidemiol Biomark Prev. 2002;11:513–20.
39. Barnholtz-Sloan JS, McEvoy B, Shriver MD, Rebbeck TR. Ancestry estimation and correction for population stratification in molecular epidemiologic association studies. Cancer Epidemiol Biomark Prev. 2008;17:471–7.
40. Tang H, Quertermous T, Rodríguez B, Kardia SL, Zhu X, Brown A, et al. Genetic structure, self identified race/ethnicity, and confounding in case-control association studies. Am J Hum Genet. 2005;76:268–75.
41. Yaeger R, Ávila-Bront A, Abdul K, Nolan PC, Grann VR, Birchette MG, et al. Comparing genetic ancestry and self-described race in African Americans born in the United States and in Africa. Cancer Epidemiol Biomark Prev. 2008;17:1329–38.
42. Rodríguez S, Gaunt TR, Day IN. Hardy-Weinberg equilibrium testing of biological ascertainment for Mendelian randomization studies. Am J Epidemiol. 2009;169:505–14.
43. Setakis E, Stirnadel H, Balding DJ. Logistic regression protects against population structure in genetic association studies. Genome Res. 2006; 16:290–6.
44. González-Burchard E, Borrell LN, Choudhry S, Naqvi M, Tsai HJ, Rodriguez-Santana JR, et al. Latino populations: a unique opportunity for the study of race, genetics, and social environment in epidemiological research. Am J Public Health. 2005;95:2161–8.

12

Characterization of falls in adults with established rheumatoid arthritis and associated factors

Mariana de Almeida Lourenço*, Flávia Vilas Boas Ortiz Carli and Marcos Renato de Assis

Abstract

Background: Rheumatoid arthritis patients may have an increased risk of falls due to changes caused by the disease such as muscle weakness, joint impairment, reduced mobility and postural instability. The aim of this study was to prospectively analyze the occurrence of falls in RA patients and its risk factors.

Methods: A cohort of 86 RA patients were assessed over 1 year for disease activity using the Disease Activity Score (DAS-28), for functionality using the Health Assessment Questionnaire (HAQ), for the characterization of falls and for the use of medications, and they were subjected to the Berg Balance Scale (Berg), Timed Up and Go (TUG), 6-Minute Walk (6MWT) and Short Physical Performance Battery (SPPB) tests. The Kolmogorov-Smirnov, Spearman's correlation, Student's t, Mann-Whitney and chi-square tests were performed with a significance level of $P \leq 0.05$.

Results: A total of 86 patients were evaluated, of which 48.8% had at least one fall and 75.6% reported having a fear of falling. No association of falls with age, disease duration, functional capacity, disease activity or physical performance was found. Patients with poorer performance in the physical tests had more functional impairment, higher disease activity and more advanced age. No differences in physical or functional performance, disease activity, gender or fear of falling were found between fallers and non-fallers; only a greater amount of medications used was found in the group of fallers.

Conclusions: The occurrence of falls was high and associated with a previous history of falls and polypharmacy, with no association with disease activity or duration, functional capacity, physical performance, age or gender.

Keywords: Postural balance, Physical aptitude, Rheumatoid arthritis, Accidental falls

Background

Falls have a multifactorial etiology in the elderly, mainly due to intrinsic factors such as decreased muscle strength, balance deficits, and gait pattern changes. These age-related changes can also be observed in other diseases [1–3].

Rheumatoid arthritis (RA) is a chronic systemic inflammatory autoimmune disease of joint predominance, with a high prevalence of falls occurring in 14.3 to 54% of patients over a one-year period, which are high values compared to the general population [4–19]. This increased risk of falls may be due to pain, edema, deformities, loss of muscle strength or gait changes, and

prospective studies have shown associations with altered balance, use of psychotropic medications, fear of falling and previous falls [4–8]. However, findings regarding several other risk factors, the characterization of falls and the consequences of falls in RA patients are still scarce or contradictory.

The aim of this study was to prospectively analyze the occurrence of falls in RA patients for 1 year and to investigate whether physical fitness and balance tests, medication use, previous history of falls, disease activity and functionality are associated with falls.

Methods
Sample

A prospective study based on the sample of a previous retrospective study composed of 99 patients diagnosed

---

* Correspondence: maalmeida1@terra.com.br
Marília School of Medicine, R. Pedro Martins, 209. Marília/SP – Brazil, Marília, São Paulo CEP 17519-430, Brazil

with RA was conducted at the Rheumatology outpatient clinic of the Marília School of Medicine [19, 20].

Adults with a diagnosis of RA according to the American College of Rheumatology (ACR) classification criteria of 1987 and/or the 2010 ACR/EULAR (European League Against Rheumatism) RA classification criteria were included [21]. Patients with cognitive impairments precluding them from answering the questionnaires, using a wheelchair or with other physical disabilities that impeded the execution of the tests were excluded.

The study was approved by the Research Ethics Committee of the Marília School of Medicine, protocol CAAE: 22845513.3.0000.5413. All participants signed the informed consent form.

Procedure

The rheumatologist confirmed the RA diagnosis and performed the measurements to assess disease activity, and the nurse collected the blood samples. Next, the anthropometric data were measured, and the functional questionnaires and physical tests were applied by the nurse and the physical therapist.

From the initial evaluation, the patients were followed up for 1 year by quarterly telephone contact to record the occurrence of falls and their characteristics. After 12 months, the disease activity and functionality assessments and physical tests were repeated.

Instruments

Patients were assessed for disease activity using the Disease Activity Score (DAS-28) [21], for functional capacity using the Health Assessment Questionnaire (HAQ) [22, 23] and for the occurrence of falls using a fall characterization questionnaire [19, 20].

The following physical tests were performed:

The Berg Balance Scale was used to determine risk factors for loss of independence and falls in the elderly. The scale has 14 items common to daily life, scored from 0 to 4, with a higher fall risk associated with lower scores. The predictive value of falls in the elderly ranges from 45 to 48 [24–27].

The Short Physical Performance Battery (SPPB) was used to assess standing balance, walking ability and sit-to-stand performance. The three items are scored from 0 to 4, with poorer physical function associated with lower scores. Standing balance is evaluated in three positions with progressive difficulty - feet together, with the hallux leaning against the medial edge of the opposite heel and with the hallux leaning against the posterior edge of the opposite heel. Walking is evaluated by measuring time, in seconds, for a distance of four meters. In the sit-to-stand evaluation using a chair, the action is

performed five times with the arms crossed in front of the chest, and time is also recorded in seconds [28, 29].

The Timed Up and Go Test (TUG) was used to assess body balance and risk of falls, especially in the elderly. The test begins with the patient sitting on a chair, then getting up, walking a three-meter distance, making a 180° turn, returning and sitting on the same chair. The different lengths of time spent indicate the following: ≤10 s - elderly without balance alteration and with low risk of falls; between 10 and 20 s - elderly with no significant balance alteration but presenting some weakness and medium risk of falls; and ≥ 20 s - elderly with a high risk of falls [30]. Other studies consider a higher risk of falls between 10 and 14 s [24, 31, 32].

The 6-Minute Walk Test (6MWT) was used to assess functional capacity and exercise tolerance through the distance an individual is able to walk on a hard, flat surface for 6 min. In healthy adults, the reference values are 580 m for men and 500 m for women [33, 34].

Statistical analysis

The Kolmogorov-Smirnov (KS) test was used to evaluate the normality of the data distribution. Values were expressed as the mean and standard deviation (SD) for variables with normal distribution and as the median and percentages for the others. Correlations were analyzed using Spearman's test, and other analyses were conducted using Student's t-test, the Mann-Whitney U-test and chi-square tests with a significance level of $p < 0.05$. The statistical program used was SPSS v.21 (IBM Armonk, NY, USA, 2012).

Results

A total of 99 patients were included in the study, but 13 were lost – three died, three had medical follow-up unit changes, three were not found, two were bedridden, one refused to participate, and one suffered an ankle sprain – leaving 86 patients. The majority of the sample consisted of white married women with a mean age of 55 ± 11.8 years (Table 1).

There were 67 fall episodes in the one-year follow-up period; 48.8% of these patients fell at least once, and 75.6% reported the fear of experiencing a fall episode. Falls occurred most often at home (58.2%), in the morning (41.8%), while the patients walked (65.7%) and due to tripping and slipping (65.5%), and fracture occurred in three falls (4.4% of the total).

No association was found between the number of falls and age, disease duration, functional capacity, disease activity or physical performance. Patients with poorer performance on the physical tests had more functional impairment, higher disease activity and advanced age. The higher disease activity was associated with poorer

Table 1 Characteristics of the sample of patients with rheumatoid arthritis

Participants, n		86
Women, n (%)		76 (88.4)
Age (years), mean ± SD (min-max)		55 ± 11.8 (23–88)
BMI (kg/m²), mean ± SD (min-max)		27.7 ± 5.3 (15.35–40.04)
Self-reported ethnicity, n (%)	White	54 (62.8)
	Mixed	20 (23.3)
	Black	12 (14)
Marital status, n (%)	Married	52 (62.8)
	Single	14 (16.3)
	Divorced	10 (11.6)
	Widowed	8 (9.3)
Duration of disease (years), median (P25–75) (min-max)		10 (5–16.5); (2–40)
Self-reported associated diseases (%)	HBP	53.5
	Osteoporosis	17.4
	DM	12.6
	Labyrinthitis	11.6
	HF	8.1
	Fibromyalgia	7.0
	Hypothyroidism	7.0
	Depression	3.4
Falls in the previous year (%)		37.4
Walking aids (%)		9.3

n: number; %: percentage; SD: standard deviation; min: minimum; max: maximum; BMI: body mass index; kg: kilogram; m²: square meter; P25–75: 25th percentile and 75th percentile; HBP: high blood pressure; DM: diabetes mellitus; HF: heart failure

physical performance, poorer functional capacity and longer disease duration (Table 2).

There was no significant difference in functional capacity or disease activity in the initial evaluation and after 1 year. However, in the physical tests, better performance was observed in the final evaluation when compared to the initial evaluation (Table 3).

When divided into groups according to the occurrence of falls, considering fallers as patients with at least one fall episode during the follow-up period, no significant differences were found between fallers and non-fallers

regarding physical or functional performance, disease activity, gender or fear of falling (Tables 4 and 5). The number of medications used and history of falls differed significantly between fallers and non-fallers (Table 5).

Discussion

The incidence of falls in this sample of RA patients was high (48.8%) compared to that found in the literature, which shows ranges from 14.3 to 54% in retrospective studies and from 18.8 to 50% in prospective studies [4–9, 11–19]. The incidence of falls

Table 2 Correlations between the number of falls with clinical variables and functional tests

	Number of falls, r (P)	Age, r (P)	HAQ, r (P)	DAS28, r (P)
Age	0.059 (0.592)	–	−0.109 (0.317)	0.034 (0.755)
RA duration	−0.077 (0.483)	0.187 (0.087)	0.066 (0.550)	0.224 (0.039)*
HAQ	0.151 (0.165)	−0.109 (0.317)	–	0.468 (0.000)*
DAS28	0.004 (0.973)	0.034 (0.755)	0.468 (0.000)*	–
Berg	−0.127 (0.244)	−0.367 (0.001)*	−0.541 (0.000)*	−0.422 (0.000)*
6MWT	−0.124 (0.260)	−0.244 (0.024)*	−0.495 (0.000)*	−0.294 (0.006)*
TUG	0.064 (0.558)	0.243 (0.025)*	0.557 (0.000)*	0.363 (0.001)*
SPPB	−0.121 (0.266)	−0.291 (0.007)*	−0.658 (0.000)*	−0.404 (0.000)*

RA: rheumatoid arthritis; HAQ: Health Assessment Questionnaire; DAS28: Disease Activity Score 28; Berg: Berg Balance Scale; 6MWT: 6-min walk test; TUG: Timed Up and Go; SPPB: Short Physical Performance Battery; r: Spearman's correlation; P: significance level

Table 3 Initial and final scores on physical, functional and disease activity tests

	Initial	Final	P
HAQ, median (P25–75)	0.62 (0.12–1.25)	0.62 (0.12–1.37)	0.318
DAS28, mean (±SD)	3.40 (±1.17)	3.58 (±1.32)	0.215
6MWT (meters), mean (±SD)	391.27 (±103.78)	429.52 (±129.01)	0.001
Berg, median (P25–75)	53 (49.75–56)	55 (50.75–56)	0.019
TUG (seconds), median (P25–75)	8.89 (7.59–11.69)	8.75 (7.14–11.28)	0.071
SPPB, median (P25–75)	10 (8–12)	11 (9–12)	0.001

HAQ: Health Assessment Questionnaire; DAS28: Disease Activity Score 28; 6MWT: 6-min walk test; Berg: Berg Balance Scale; TUG: Timed Up and Go; SPPB: Short Physical Performance Battery; P25–75: 25th percentile and 75th percentile; SD: standard deviation; P: t test significance level

observed was also high compared to that of non-institutionalized elderly individuals, which ranges from 15.9 to 56.3% [2]. Although age is an important risk factor for falls, the association between falls and advanced age was not observed in this sample, which is in agreement with previous RA studies [4–6, 12, 15, 35].

Comparing fallers with non-fallers, there was again agreement with other RA studies but a difference from what occurs in the elderly - there was no predominance of falls among females. It is possible that no difference was observed between men and women because both genders have decreased muscle mass and similar patterns of medication consumption [5–7, 15, 35].

The use of several medications may increase the occurrence of falls due to interactions between medications or their side effects. In the present study, we found a significant difference between fallers and non-fallers in relation to polypharmacy. Armstrong et al. [15] reported an association between a higher number of medications and a higher risk of falling, while Stanmore et al. [36] found that using four or more medications more than doubles the risk of falling in RA patients. An association has also been found between falls and the use of medications such as antihypertensives, diuretics, sedatives, antidepressants and antipsychotics [6, 8, 15, 36–39].

The history of falls was associated with the occurrence of new falls, which indicates the need for special attention in the evaluation of RA patients who have already fallen [4, 6, 7, 36].

Most of the sample presented moderate disease activity, which, similar to the study by Bohler et al. [12], was associated with poorer performance in most physical tests, but not the occurrence of falls. Koerich et al. [40] argued that the level of disease activity may influence physical performance (Berg and TUG), suggesting an increased risk of falling or dependence in performing activities of daily life. The lack of association between poor physical performance and disease activity with the presence of falls may be related to the time of evaluation, which usually occurs at the beginning or end of the study and not at the time of the falls. Another reasonable explanation is that the increased disease activity results in restriction of activities and therefore reduces the individuals' exposure to situations with a risk of falls.

Other studies have indicated functional disability as a risk factor for falls, but in our study, although it was associated with poorer performance in physical tests, it was not correlated with falls [4, 9, 12, 13, 19, 20, 35]. In a prospective study with 80 patients in Japan, Hayashibara et al. [6] found no relationship between functional disability and the presence of falls and explained that the

Table 4 Differences between disease activity and physical and functional performance in fallers and non-fallers

	Fallers (n = 42)	Non-fallers (n = 44)	Test	P
HAQ	0.81 (0.22–1.75)	0.50 (0.12–1.34)	U = 763.5	0.164
DAS28	3.70 (±1.49)	3.47 (±1.16)	t = −0.798	0.427
6MWT	376.31 (±100.74)	405.88 (±105.79)	t = 1.320	0.190
Berg	53 (47.75–55.25)	54.5 (50–56)	U = 787	0.229
TUG	9.27 (7.89–11.62)	8.73 (7.35–12.08)	U = 852	0.660
SPPB	10 (7.75–11)	10.5 (9–12)	U = 784.5	0.219

HAQ: Health Assessment Questionnaire; DAS28: Disease Activity Score 28; 6MWT: 6-min walk test; Berg: Berg Balance Scale; TUG: Timed Up and Go; SPPB: Short Physical Performance Battery; P: significance level; t: t test; U: Mann-Whitney U-test
Values are expressed as the mean (± standard deviation) or median (25th - 75th percentile)

Table 5 Differences between number of medications, history of falls, gender and fear of falling between fallers and non-fallers

		Occurrence of falls (n)			
		No	Yes	χ^2	P
Polypharmacy	Up to three medications	20	9	5.55	0.018
	Four or more	24	33		
History of falls	Yes	10	22	8.087	0.004
	No	34	20		
Gender	Female	38	38	0.354	0.552
	Male	6	4		
Fear of falling	Present	31	31	0.120	0.729
	Absent	13	11		

χ^2: chi-square; P: significance level

findings were due to the fact that five of the eight HAQ categories assess the function of the upper limbs.

Although the physical tests used in the present study are aimed at the elderly population, RA patients may present an early decrease in muscle strength, physical activity and balance in a pattern similar to that of elderly individuals, anticipating the risks resulting from the aging process. This may explain the finding that performance on physical tests was correlated with age: the older the patient, the poorer the physical performance. Although the four physical tests were significantly correlated among themselves, no significant association was found between any of the tests and the occurrence of falls. While some studies found an association between poorer performance on physical tests and a greater occurrence of falls or risk of falling, others found no such association [6, 11, 12, 16, 19, 36, 37]. The lack of standardization in the choice of tests for the RA population may be an important factor to be considered when analyzing these results, a gap that was observed by Santana et al. [41].

Several studies suggest that prospective studies be conducted to minimize memory bias [13–15, 19]. Cummings et al. [42], in a prospective, 12-month study of the elderly, found that 13–32% of the participants who fell did not report the episode at the end of the evaluation period. The follow-up strategies used were calendars, journals, fall log cards and self-reports to the researcher at the time of the fall. The present study has a methodological advantage, as it obtained the information quarterly by telephone, which improved the reliability of the report of falls and facilitated detailed clarification regarding the characteristics [4–8, 36].

Conclusions

The occurrence of falls in RA patients is high and is associated with a previous history of falls and polypharmacy, showing no association with disease activity or duration, functional capacity, physical performance, age or gender. In addition, the performances in the physical tests were associated with each other, and a poorer physical condition was related to greater disease activity, poorer functional capacity and older age.

Funding
A Master's degree fellowship from Coordenação de Aperfeiçoamento de Pessoal de Nível Superior (CAPES).

Authors' contributions
The rheumatologist (MRA) confirmed the RA diagnosis and performed the measurements to assess disease activity, and the nurse (FVBOC) collected the blood samples. Next, the anthropometric data were measured, and the functional questionnaires and physical tests were applied by the nurse and the physical therapist (MAL). All authors read and approved the final manuscript.

Competing interests
The authors declare that they have no competing interests

References
1. Pinho TAM, Silva AO, Tura LFR, Moreira MASP, Gurgel SN, Smith AAF, et al. Avaliação do risco de quedas em idosos atendidos em Unidade Básica de Saúde. Rev Esc Enferm USP. 2012;46(2):320-7.
2. Sandoval RA, Sá ACAM, Menezes RL, Nakatani AYK, Bachion MM. Ocorrência de quedas em idosos não institucionalizados : revisão sistemática da literatura. Rev Bras Geriatr Gerontol. 2013;16(4):855-63.
3. Oliveira AS, Trevizan PF, Bestetti MLT, Melo RC. Fatores ambientais e risco de quedas em idosos: revisão sistemática. Rev Bras Geriatr Gerontol. 2014;17(3):637-45.
4. Smulders E, Schreven C, Weerdesteyn V, van den Hoogen FHJ, Laan R, Van Lankveld W. Fall incidence and fall risk factors in people with rheumatoid arthritis. Ann Rheum Dis. 2009 [cited 2013 may 23];68(11):1795-1796. Available from: http://www.ncbi.nlm.nih.gov/pubmed/19822719.
5. Stanmore EK, Oldham J, Skelton DA, O'Neill T, Pilling M, Campbell AJ, et al. Fall incidence and outcomes of falls in a prospective study of adults with rheumatoid arthritis. Arthritis Care Res (Hoboken). 2013;65(5):737-44.
6. Hayashibara M, Hagino H, Katagiri H, Okano T, Okada J, Teshima R. Incidence and risk factors of falling in ambulatory patients with rheumatoid arthritis: a prospective 1-year study. Osteoporos Int. 2010 [cited 2013 may 23];21(11):1825-33. Available from: http://www.ncbi.nlm.nih.gov/pubmed/20119662.
7. Bugdayci D, Paker N, Rezvani A, Kesiktas N, Yilmaz O, Sahin M, et al. Frequency and predictors for falls in the ambulatory patients with rheumatoid arthritis: a longitudinal prospective study. Rheumatol Int. 2013 Apr;33(10):2523-7.
8. Brenton-Rule A, Dalbeth N, Bassett S, Menz HB, Rome K. The incidence and risk factors for falls in adults with rheumatoid arthritis: a systematic review. Semin Arthritis Rheum. 2015;44:389-98.
9. Kaz Kaz H, Johnson D, Kerry S, Chinappen U, Tweed K, Patel S. Fall-related risk factors and osteoporosis in women with rheumatoid arthritis. Rheumatology (Oxford). 2004;43(10):1267-71. Available from: https://academic.oup.com/rheumatology/article-lookup/doi/10.1093/rheumatology/keh304
10. Pereira IA, Mota LMH, Cruz BA, Brenol CV, Fronza LSR, Bertolo MB, et al. Consenso 2012 da Sociedade Brasileira de Reumatologia sobre o manejo de comorbidades em pacientes com artrite reumatoide. Rev Bras Reum. 2012;52(4):474-95.
11. Duyurçakit B, Nacir B, Erdem HR, Karagoz A, Saraçoglu M. Fear of falling, fall risk and disability in patients with rheumatoid arthritis. Turk J Rheumatol. 2011;26(3):217-25.
12. Böhler C, Radner H, Ernst M, Binder A, Stamm T, Aletaha D, et al. Rheumatoid arthritis and falls: the influence of disease activity. Rheumatology (Oxford). 2012 [cited 2013 may 23];51(11):2051-2057. Available from: http://www.ncbi.nlm.nih.gov/pubmed/22879462.
13. Marques WV, Cruz VA, Rêgo J, Silva NA. Influência da capacidade funcional no risco de quedas em adultos com artrite reumatoide. Rev Bras Reum. 2014;54(5):404-8.
14. Fessel KD, Nevitt MC. Correlates of fear of falling and activity limitation among persons with rheumatoid arthritis. Arthritis Care Res. 1997;10(4):222-8.
15. Armstrong C, Swarbrick CM, Pye SR, O'Neill TW. Occurrence and risk factors for falls in rheumatoid arthritis. Ann Rheum Dis. 2005;64(11):1602-4.
16. Jamison M, Neuberger GB, Miller PA. Correlates of falls and fear of falling among adults with rheumatoid arthritis. Arthritis Care Res (Hoboken). 2003;49(5):673-80.
17. Schober HC, Maass K, Maass C, Reisinger EC, Schröder G, Kneitz C. Value of fall-risk tests for patients with rheumatoid arthritis. Z Rheumatol. 2011;70(7):609-14.
18. Sugioka Y, Koike T. Fall risk and fracture. Associated factors for falls in patients with inflammatory polyarthritis. Clin Calcium. 2013;23(5):701-5.
19. Lourenço MA, Roma I, Assis MR. Ocorrência de quedas e sua associação com testes físicos, capacidade funcional e aspectos clínicos e demográficos em pacientes com artrite reumatoide. Rev Bras Reum. 2017;57(3):217-23.
20. Lourenço MA, Roma I, Assis MR. Correlação entre instrumentos de avaliação da funcionalidade e equilíbrio em pacientes com artrite reumatoide. Rev Bras Educ Fís Esporte. 2015;29(3):345-53.

21. Da Mota LMH, Cruz BA, Brenol CV, Pereira IA, Fronza LSR, Bertolo MB, et al. Consenso da Sociedade Brasileira de Reumatologia 2011 para o diagnóstico e avaliação inicial da artrite reumatoide. Rev Bras Reumatol. 2011;51(3):207–19.

22. Bruce B, Fries JF. The Health Assessment Questionnaire (HAQ). Clin Exp Rheumatol. 2005;23(5 SUPPL. 39):S14–8.

23. Ferraz MB, Oliveira LM, Araujo PMP, Atra E, Tugwell P. Crosscultural reliability of the physical ability dimension of the health assessment questionnaire. J Rheumatol. 1990 Jun;17(6):813–7.

24. Figueiredo KMOB, Lima KC, Guerra RO. Instrumentos de avaliação do equilíbrio corporal em idosos. Rev Bras Cineantropom Desempenho Hum. 2007;9(4):408–13.

25. Pimentel RM, Scheicher ME. Comparação do risco de queda em idosos sedentários e ativos por meio da escala de equilíbrio de Berg. Fisioter Pesq. 2009;16(1):6–10.

26. Miyamoto ST, Lombardi Junior I, Berg KO, Ramos LR, Natour J. Brazilian version of the Berg balance scale. Braz J Med Biol Res. 2004 Sep;37(9):1411–21. Available from: https://www.ncbi.nlm.nih.gov/pubmed/15334208.

27. Berg KO, Maki BE, Williams JI, Holliday PJ, Wood-Dauphinee SL. Clinical and laboratory measures of postural balance in an elderly population. Arch Phys Med Rehabil. 1992;73(11):1073–80.

28. Nakano MM, Diogo MJDe, Jacob Filho W. Versão brasileira da Short Physical Performance Battery - SPPB: adaptação cultural e estudo da confiabilidade. UNICAMP; 2007.

29. Sayers SP, Jette AM, Haley SM, Heeren TC, Guralnick JM, Fielding RA. Validation of thelate-life function and disability instrument. J Am Geriatr Soc. 2004;52(9):1554–9.

30. Guimarães LHCT, Galdino DCA, Martins FLM, Vitorino DFM, Pereira KL, Carvalho EM. Comparação da propensão de quedas entre idosos que praticam atividade física e idosos sedentários. Rev Neurociências. 2004;12(2):68–72.

31. Shumway-Cook A, Brauer S, Woollacott M. Predicting the probability for falls in community-dwelling older adults using the timed up & go test. Phys Ther. 2000;80(9):896–903.

32. Podsiadlo D, Richardson S. The timed "Up & Go": a test of basic functional mobility for frail elderly persons. J Am Geriatr Soc [Internet]. 1991 Feb;39(2):142–8. Available from: http://www.ncbi.nlm.nih.gov/pubmed/1991946.

33. Cipriano Junior G, Yuri D, Bernardelli GF, Mair V, Buffolo E, Branco JNR. Avaliação da Segurança do Teste de Caminhada dos 6 Minutos em Pacientes no Pré-Transplante Cardíaco. Arq Bras Cardiol. 2009;92(4):312–9.

34. Rondelli R, Oliveira A, Corso SD, Malaguti C. Uma atualização e proposta de padronização do teste de caminhada de seis minutos. Fisioter Mov. 2009;22(2):249–59.

35. Oswald AE, Pye SR, O'Neill TW, Bunn D, Gaffney K, Marshall T, et al. Prevalence and associated factors for falls in women with established inflammatory polyarthritis. J Rheumatol. 2006 Apr;33(4):690–4. Available from: http://www.ncbi.nlm.nih.gov/pubmed/16482644.

36. Stanmore EK, Oldham J, Skelton D a, O'Neill T, Pilling M, Campbell a J, et al. Risk factors for falls in adults with rheumatoid arthritis: A prospective study. Arthritis Care Res (Hoboken). 2013 Feb;

37. Metlı NB, Kurtaran A, Akyüz M. Impaired balance and fall risk in rheumatoid arthritis patients. Turk J Phys Med Rehab. 2015;61:344–51.

38. Robbins AS, Rubenstein LZ, Josephson KR, Schulman BL, Osterweil D, Fine G. Predictors of falls among elderly people. Results of two population-based studies. Arch Intern Med. 1989;149:1628–33.

39. Furuya T, Yamagiwa K, Ikai T, Inoue E, Taniguchi A, Momohara S, et al. Associated factors for falls and fear of falling in Japanese patients with rheumatoid arthritis. Clin Rheumatol. 2009 Nov [cited 2013 may 23];28(11):1325–30. Available from: http://www.ncbi.nlm.nih.gov/pubmed/19618097.

40. Koerich J, Armanini KK, Iop RR, Borges Júnior NG, Domenech SC, Gevaerd MS. Avaliação do equilíbrio corporal de pacientes com artrite reumatoide. Fisioter e Pesq. 2013;20(4):336–42.

41. De Santana FS, Nascimento DDC, De Freitas JPM, Miranda RF, Muniz LF, Santos Neto L, et al. Avaliação da capacidade funcional em pacientes com artrite reumatoide: implicações para a recomendação de exercícios físicos. Rev Bras Reumatol [Internet]. 2014;4(5):378–85. Available from: http://www.sciencedirect.com/science/article/pii/S0482500414001144

42. Cummings SR, Nevitt MC, Kidd S. Forgetting falls. The limited accuracy of recall of falls in the elderly. J Am Geriatr Soc. 1988;36(7):613–6.

13

Staying in the labor force among patients with rheumatoid arthritis and associated factors in Southern Brazil

Rafael Kmiliauskis Santos Gomes[1,2,5*], Luana Cristina Schreiner[3], Mateus Oliveira Vieira[3],
Patrícia Helena Machado[3] and Moacyr Roberto Cuce Nobre[4]

Abstract

Background: Rheumatoid arthritis primarily affects the working-age population and may cause key functional and work limitations. As the disease progresses, individuals become increasingly unable to conduct daily activities, which has a substantial personal and socioeconomic impact. Fairly recent prior studies showed that patients with RA stop working 20 years earlier than age-matched controls. Factors related to sociodemographic, clinical, care and disease profiles might affect the loss of work capacity. The purpose of this study was to assess the factors associated with the prevalence of working patients with rheumatoid arthritis in the municipality of Blumenau.

Methods: A cross-sectional, population-based study was conducted between July 2014 and January 2015, with 296 individuals aged 20 years or older, male and female, living in Blumenau, Santa Catarina state, Brazil, and diagnosed with rheumatoid arthritis according to the 1987 American College of Rheumatology criteria. The prevalence of working patients with RA was assessed by employment status self-reporting during the interview. The chi-squared test, Wald test and Poisson regression analysis were used to test the possible associations between the independent variables and outcome.

Results: The prevalence of working patients with rheumatoid arthritis was 44.3%. Patients aged 20 to 59 years had a 90% higher prevalence of outcome than subjects aged 60 years or older. The prevalence of working patients was 132% and 73% higher among individuals with low income and high functional disability, measured using the Health Assessment Questionnaire (HAQ), respectively.

Conclusion: The prevalence of working RA patients was highest among adult patients with low income and high functional disability. The first variable is directly related to the individual characteristic, the second reflects the socioeconomic context of the patient, and the third reflects the degree of disability caused by the disease, which may be modifiable by health professionals.

Keywords: Rheumatoid arthritis, Occupation, Job market

Background

Rheumatoid arthritis (RA) is a chronic, autoimmune, and systemic inflammatory disease characterized by symmetrical synovitis of the peripheral joints. Inflammation of the synovial membranes causes pain, edema and stiffness and, if untreated, may lead to joint destruction and a loss of functional capacity [1, 2]. RA occurs in 0.24% to 1% of the population, predominantly among women between the fourth and sixth decades of life [3, 4]. According to a multicenter study, the prevalence of RA in Brazil is similar, ranging from 0.2 to 1% of the population [5].

RA primarily affects the working-age population and may cause key functional and work limitations [6]. As the disease progresses, individuals become increasingly unable to conduct daily activities, which has a substantial personal and socioeconomic impact [7, 8]. Studies report that 40% of patients with early-onset disease and

* Correspondence: gomesmed2002@ibest.com.br
[1]Specialty Center of the City of Blumenau, Blumenau, Santa Catarina State (SC), Brazil
[2]Specialty Center of the City of Brusque, Brusque, SC, Brazil
Full list of author information is available at the end of the article

60% of patients with advanced disease were unable to work [9, 10].

Fairly recent prior studies showed that patients with RA stop working 20 years earlier than age-matched controls [11]. Researchers who conducted a study in Germany concluded that 59% of patients continued working until 12 months after diagnosis, whereas 17% stopped working and received disability payments, and 9% lost their jobs because of RA but received no disability pension [12]. Another study, conducted in the state of São Paulo, showed that 30% of patients were actually employed and that the others were homemakers, on leaves of absence or unemployed [13].

Factors related to sociodemographic, clinical, care and disease profiles might affect the loss of work capacity. Early diagnosis combined with disease-modifying antirheumatic drugs (DMARDs) is the most effective method to reduce the prevalence of disability [13]. Other predictors, such as age, education level, the presence of comorbidities and the use of biopharmaceuticals may also be associated with disease progression [13, 14].

Studies on RA among working-age populations are increasingly conducted in developed countries. However, few studies considering this approach in Brazil were identified. Among them, a study conducted in the state of São Paulo determined that 30% of such patients were actively working, 34% were unemployed, 31% were retirees, and 5% were working retirees [15].

To collect additional data on this subject, the present study aimed to assess the percentage of and the possible factors associated with working patients with RA in Blumenau.

Methods
This cross-sectional, population-based study was conducted between July 2014 and January 2015, with 296 individuals aged 20 years or older, male and female, living in the municipality of Blumenau in the south region of Brazil and diagnosed with rheumatoid arthritis according to the 1987 American College of Rheumatology criteria. According to the United Nations Development Program (UNDP), this municipality had a Human Development Index (HDI) of 0.806 in 2010, ranking 25th among Brazilian municipalities [16]. The number of inhabitants in the study age group corresponded to 221,839 people, which is equivalent to 71.7% of the municipality population [17].

The formula for calculating the sample size required to estimate the prevalence of an event in a simple random sample was used considering the following parameters: 0.5% RA prevalence (1110 patients), 50% prevalence of exposure and unknown outcome, 5% sample error and 95% confidence level. The effective calculated sample size was 286 individuals. The participants

were recruited from all primary care centers (Unidades Básicas de Saúde – UBS), the specialty outpatient clinic and the specialty pharmacy of the municipality.

Sample loss occurred when households were visited twice, once on the weekend and again in the evening, and no resident was at home, the resident had moved or refused to participate in the study on both occasions. The data collection team consisted of a local supervisor docent and 8 medical academics of the Regional University of Blumenau (Universidade Regional de Blumenau – FURB) previously trained to conduct structured interviews at home and, if necessary, by telephone. Quality control was performed in 20% of respondents, who were interviewed for the second time using a short questionnaire.

The dependent variable analyzed was the employment status at the time of the interview, considering the prevalence of working patients with RA, in any type of occupation, the outcome. Conversely, the independent variables were selected based on the sociodemographic, clinical, care and disease profiles. The following sociodemographic variables were analyzed: sex, age in completed years, ranging from 20 to 59 years for adults and 60 years or older for the elderly, in accordance with the status of the elderly/Ministry of Health (Ministério da Saúde – MS), current monthly personal income, ranging from 0 to 2 and greater than 2 minimum wages, education in years of completed study and self-reported skin color, categorized as white, brown, black, yellow or indigenous (IBGE). The clinical variable analyzed was the presence of comorbidities. The care variables analyzed were consultations with another rheumatologist during their treatment, number of consultations with a rheumatologist in the last 12 months, type of medical care classified into two groups, the Unified Health System (Sistema Único de Saúde – SUS; free, public healthcare system) and Public-Private Healthcare (supplementary healthcare system), defined according to the MS, in addition to private healthcare (fee-for-service care), and diagnostic delay in months, which was calculated by subtracting the date of the medical diagnosis by the date of the onset of symptoms. Lastly, the disease-related variables were total disease time in months, current use of DMARDs (methotrexate, sulfasalazine, leflunomide and antimalarial drugs), current use of anti-TNF immunobiologicals (adalimumab, etanercept, infliximab), Health Assessment Questionnaire (HAQ) score, ranging from 0 to 1 (mild disability) and from 1.1 to 3 (moderate and severe disability), presence of rheumatoid factor lower than or equal to 60 (negative or low titer) or higher than 60 (high titer) and, finally, the presence of radiographic changes (joint erosion) in the hands.

The data were entered into a system developed for this study in an Excel file format, and the final file was subsequently exported to the software Stata 10.0 (Stata

Corporation, College Station, United States). The distribution of the variables of interest was analyzed using the mean, standard deviation and median for continuous variables, and the frequency and percentage for categorical variables. To test the association between the employment status and the independent variables, the chi-squared test and, where appropriate, the Wald test were used. Then, crude and Poisson regression analyses were performed to assess the association between the study factors and the dependent variables, estimating the crude and adjusted prevalence ratios (PRs), the respective 95% confidence intervals and the p value.

All variables with p value < 0.20 in the crude analysis were considered for entry into the final model. The variables that maintained a p value ≤0.05 or that fitted the final model remained in the adjusted regression model. The researchers chose to sequentially include sociodemographic, clinical, care and disease-related variables in the regression model.

This research study was submitted to the research ethics committees of the University of São Paulo (Universidade de São Paulo – USP) and of the FURB (protocol numbers 339/13 and 133/12, respectively) and approved; all participants signed the informed consent form.

Results

A total of 336 patients were identified. After excluding deceased patients and those who refused to participate in the study or patients without data for the dependent variable, 296 patients were included in the study. Those individuals who were unemployed, pensioners, housewives or regular or RA-unrelated disability retirees were excluded from the analysis of the dependent variable data, which resulted in an effective final sample of 185 patients (Fig. 1).

In the sociodemographic analysis, females (82.7%) and adults (71.9%) accounted for most individuals, with a mean age of 54.5 years, ranging from 26 to 79 years and with a standard deviation (SD) of 10.4. The mean income was 1.9 minimum wages (SD: 1.4). Approximately one-third of the subjects had education ranging from 0 to 4 years of completed study, with a mean education of 7.9 years (SD: 4.3). Regarding the care variables, the diagnostic delay was longer than or equal to 4 months in 74.1% of the sample and the mean diagnostic delay time was 27.6 months, ranging from 1 to 240 months (SD: 45). Most respondents stated that they visited another rheumatologist (72.4%), with a mean of 3.4 visits in the last 12 months (SD: 2.4). Regarding the type of care, private or public-private healthcare was predominant (55.9%). The analysis of the disease variables showed that most subjects had a disease time longer than or equal to 25 months (89.9%), with a mean of 127.8 months, ranging from 2 to 420 months (SD: 95.8; Table 1).

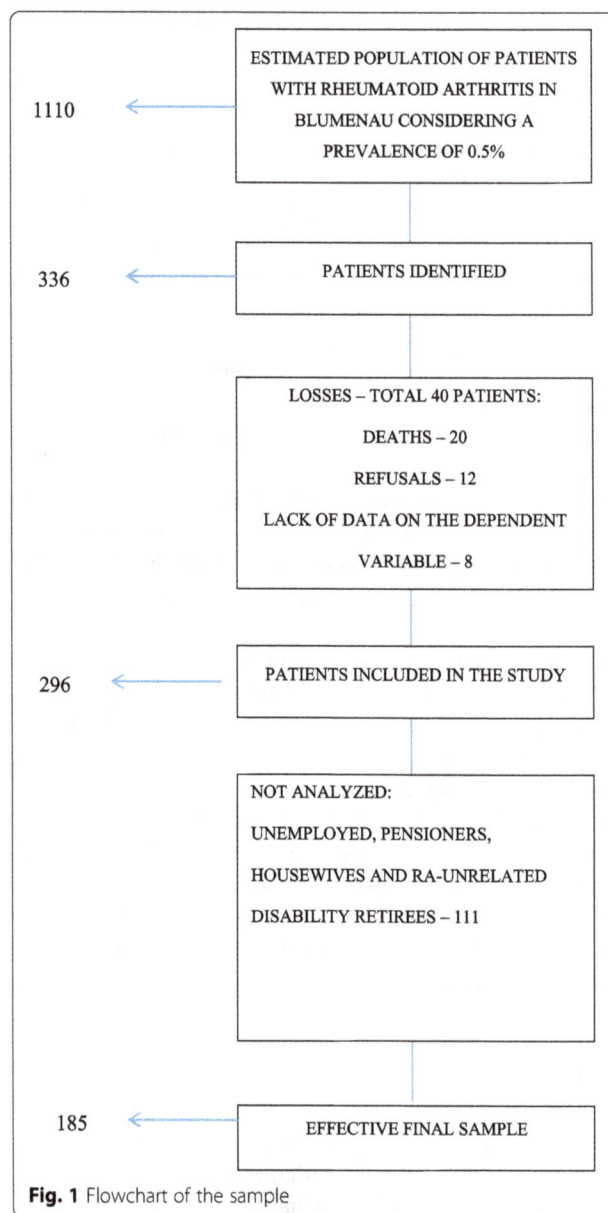

Fig. 1 Flowchart of the sample

The crude analysis showed an increase in outcome with the decrease in age and among low-income individuals. The prevalence of working patients with RA was 64%, 37% and 66% higher among patients with up to 4 years of education, comorbidities and a higher HAQ score, respectively. Due to confounding between education and income in the adjusted analysis, the variables education and comorbidities lost significance and were excluded from the final model, which consisted of age, income and HAQ. The prevalence of working patients was 90% higher among adults than among the elderly. The prevalence of working patients was 132% higher among low-income individuals than among those earning more than 2 minimum wages. The prevalence of working patients was 73% higher among individuals with

Table 1 Description of the sample and of the prevalence of working patients with rheumatoid arthritis in Blumenau, Santa Catarina state, Brazil, according to the independent variables, 2014

Variables	Sample		Working Patients	
	n^*	%	Prevalence (%) 95% CI	p
Total	185	100.0	44.3 (37.0-51.5)	
Sex (n = 185)				0.943**
Male	32	17.3	43.7 (25.5-61.9)	
Female	153	82.7	44.4 (36.4-52.4)	
Age in years (n = 185)				0.025***
20-59 (adults)	133	71.9	48.8 (40.2-57.4)	
≥ 60 (elderly)	52	28.1	32.6 (19.5-45.8)	
Income in minimum wages (n = 154)				0.001***
0-2	117	75.9	34.1 (25.5-42.9)	
> 2	37	24.1	64.8 (48.2-81.0)	
Education in completed years (n = 176)				0.000***
0-4	60	34.1	25.0 (13.7-36.2)	
> 4	116	65.9	54.3 (45.1-63.5)	
Self-reported skin color (n = 178)				0.686**
White	165	92.7	44.2 (36.5-51.9)	
Brown and black	13	7.3	38.4 (7.8-69.0)	
Presence of comorbidities (n = 181)				0.016**
No	87	48.1	52.8 (42.1-63.5)	
Yes	94	51.9	35.1 (25.2-44.9)	
Consultation with another rheumatologist (n = 181)				0.900**
No	50	27.6	44.0 (29.7-58.2)	
Yes	131	72.4	45.0 (36.4-53.6)	
Number of visits in the last 12 months (n = 176)				0.111***
0-2	74	42.1	51.3 (39.6-63.0)	
≥ 3	102	57.9	39.2 (29.5-48.8)	
Type of medical care (n = 163)				0.637**
SUS	72	44.1	40.2 (28.6-51.8)	
Private and Public-Private Partnership	91	55.9	43.9 (33.5-54.3)	
Diagnostic delay in months (n = 178)				0.982***
0-3	46	25.9	45.6 (30.6-60.6)	
≥ 4	132	74.1	45.4 (36.8-54.0)	
Disease time in months (n = 185)				0.681***
0-24	20	10.9	4.0 (16.4-63.5)	
≥ 25	165	89.1	44.8 (37.1-52.5)	
Current use of DMARDs (n = 168)				0.724**
No	46	27.3	45.6 (30.6-60.6)	
Yes	122	72.7	42.6 (33.7-51.5)	
Current use of biologicals (anti-TNF) (n = 172)				0.162**
No	116	67.4	42.2 (33.1-51.3)	

Table 1 Description of the sample and of the prevalence of working patients with rheumatoid arthritis in Blumenau, Santa Catarina state, Brazil, according to the independent variables, 2014 (Continued)

Variables	Sample		Working Patients	
	n*	%	Prevalence (%) 95% CI	p
Yes	56	32.6	53.5 (40.0-67.0)	
HAQ score (n = 110)				0.009***
0-1	45	41.0	62.2 (47.4-76.9)	
1.1-3	65	59.0	36.9 (24.8-48.9)	
Rheumatoid factor (n = 160)				0.873**
0-60 (normal or low titer)	90	56.2	45.4 (35.0-56.0)	
≥ 61 (high titers)	70	43.8	44.2 (32.3-56.2)	
Radiography of hands with joint erosion (n = 151)				0.375**
No	62	41.0	50.0 (37.1-62.8)	
Yes	89	59.0	42.6 (32.2-53.1)	

95% CI 95% confidence interval
*Number of working patients with rheumatoid arthritis who were on sick leave or were disability retirees
**Chi-squared test
***Wald test

high functional disability, assessed using the HAQ (Table 2).

Discussion

The present study showed that job retention among RA patients in the city of Blumenau was 44.3%. Higher percentages of working RA patients were identified among low-income adult RA patients with high functional disability. The first variable is directly related to individual characteristics, the second reflects the socioeconomic context of the patient and the third reveals the degree of disability caused by RA.

Studies conducted in Germany and the Netherlands found 41% and 40% working RA patients, respectively [12, 18]. Furthermore, a systematic review of North American data found rates of working RA patients ranging from 22% to 76% [19]. Regarding the Brazilian data, a study conducted in Sorocaba found a prevalence of 46% working RA patients, similar to that found in the present study [20]. However, another study conducted in São Paulo found a 31% prevalence of such working patients, possibly due to different inclusion criteria and sampling and to the use of secondary data from medical records [13].

Age is a non-modifiable predictive factor of work disability. Our study confirmed this finding because the prevalence of working RA patients among elderly individuals was almost twice as high as that among adults. Synergistically, two systematic reviews of cohort studies on disability also reported the existence of this relationship [21, 22].

A study with 878 patients, conducted in the Netherlands, showed that a low socioeconomic status was related to worsened disease activity, physical and mental health and quality of life [23]. Similarly, a Latin American cohort with 1093 patients from 14 countries, including Brazil, concluded that low and middle incomes were associated with increased disease activity and higher HAQ scores [24]. Notably however, this association has not been consistently reported [25].

In contrast to the aforementioned findings, our study found a prevalence of working RA patients among low-income individuals who was 132% higher than that among individuals with a higher income. This finding suggests social inequality because the prevalence of working RA patients was expected to be higher among individuals with a higher income considering that higher income is usually associated with easier access to information, medical consultations and pharmacological treatments. This finding may be due to circumstances directly related to the individual, such as a lack of access to information, lack of knowledge of the right to disability retirement, limited legal expenses, lack of payment to social security and the need to work to avoid income loss.

Regarding the HAQ, the results showed that the prevalence of working RA patients was 73% higher among individuals with high disability than among individuals with a low HAQ score. This finding may be related to low-income patients with increased inflammatory activity of the disease and, therefore, increased disability [24]. Although this variable had a lower sample number than the others, an association with outcome was observed. An English study of two cohorts, totaling 244 patients, described HAQ as the most important factor of work disability [26].

Regarding education, the prevalence of working RA patients among the group with more than 4 years of study was 64% higher in the crude analysis; however,

Table 2 Crude and adjusted Poisson regression analyses of the prevalence of working patients with rheumatoid arthritis as a function of independent variables in Blumenau, Santa Catarina state, Brazil, 2014

Variables	Crude analysis		Adjusted analysis	
	PRc (95% CI)	p	PRa (95% CI)	p
Sex (n = 185)		0.943[*]		NS
Male	0.98 (0.70-1.38)			
Female	1			
Age in years (n = 185)		0.023		0.001
20-59 (adults)	1.33 (1.04-1.71)		1.90 (1.31-2.75)	
≥ 60 (elderly)	1		1	
Income in minimum wages (n = 154)		0.007		0.008
0-2	1.87 (1.18-2.96)		2.32 (1.24-4.36)	
> 2	1		1	
Education in completed years (n = 176)		0.000		0.676[**]
0-4	1.64 (1.28-2.10)		1.08 (0.74-1.58)	
> 4	1		1	
Self-reported skin color (n = 178)		0.669[*]		NS
White	1			
Black + Brown	1.1 (0.70-1.73)			
Presence of comorbidities (n = 181)		0.019		0.464[**]
No	1		1	
Yes	1.37 (1.05-1.80)		1.08 (0.74-1.58)	
Consultation with another rheumatologist (n = 181)		0.900[*]		NS
No	1			
Yes	0.98 (0.73-1.31)			
Number of visits in the last 12 months (n = 176)		0.121		0.619[**]
0-2	1.03 (0.99-1.08)		0.91 (0.65-1.28)	
≥ 3	1		1	
Type of medical care (n = 103)		0.637[*]		NS
SUS	1.06 (0.81-1.38)			
Private + Public-Private Partnership	1			
Diagnostic delay in months (n = 178)		0.982[*]		NS
0-3	1			
≥ 4	1.01 (0.73-1.36)			
Disease time in months (n = 185)		0.667[*]		NS
0-24	1			
≥ 25	0.91 (0.62-1.35)			
Current use of DMARDs (n = 168)		0.729[*]		NS
No	0.94 (0.69-1.28)			
Yes	1			
Current use of biologicals (n = 172)		0.184		0.481[**]
No	1.24 (0.90-1.71)		1.17 (0.79-1.73)	

Table 2 Crude and adjusted Poisson regression analyses of the prevalence of working patients with rheumatoid arthritis as a function of independent variables in Blumenau, Santa Catarina state, Brazil, 2014 (Continued)

Variables	Crude analysis		Adjusted analysis	
	PRc (95% CI)	p	PRa (95% CI)	p
Yes	1		1	
HAQ (n = 110)		0.017		0.017
0-1	1		1	
1.1-3	1.66 (1.09-2.54)		1.73 (1.10-2.72)	
Rheumatoid factor (n = 160)		0.873**		NS
0-60 (normal or low titer)	1			
≥ 61 (high titers)	1.02 (0.77-1.35)			
Radiography of hands with joint erosion (n = 151)		0.385**		NS
No	1			
Yes	1.14 (0.84-1.55)			

95% CI 95% confidence interval, NS non-significant p value, PRc crude prevalence ratio, PRa adjusted prevalence ratio
*Excluded from the adjusted analysis (p value > 0.20)
**Excluded from the final model (p value > 0.05)

when subjected to adjusted analysis, the variable lost significance. Despite this result, a systematic review of studies on RA found a significant association between higher levels of education and the prevalence of working patients [21]. The same result was found regarding the presence of comorbidities, which was initially 37% higher among working RA patients, although the lack of a significant association was subsequently assessed. A Saudi study also found no significant association between the prevalence of working patients and the presence of comorbidities, although comorbidities were found in 95% of the subjects [27]. Conversely, a longitudinal study conducted in the United States with patients from the National Data Bank for Rheumatic Diseases, a national database for rheumatologic diseases, found progression of work disability, particularly in individuals with cardiovascular disease and a high number of comorbidities [28].

Regarding the sociodemographic profile variables, although sex and self-reported skin color were not significantly associated with the outcome (possibly due to the predominance of white over brown and black individuals in the sample), studies describing significant associations between these variables and the prevalence of working patients have been reported in the literature. A study showed that women had a higher risk for being out of the labor force, whereas men were more likely to continue working and to report negative workplace experiences [29].

Regarding the care variables, a Brazilian study showed that diagnostic delay may increase the prevalence of loss of work capacity and found a mean diagnostic delay of 39 months [20]. Although a lower mean diagnostic delay was found in our study (27.6 months), the importance of this variable for early treatment is noteworthy.

Regarding the disease variables, disease time is directly related to decreased prevalence of working RA patients.

A cohort of Swedish patients with RA followed for 15 years showed that after 5, 10 and 15 years of disease, 65%, 61% and 56% of the individuals were actively working, respectively [30]. The lack of association and the decreased prevalence of outcome in our study may be related to the sample, which predominantly consisted of patients with established RA (> 2 years), to the mean disease time of approximately 10 years and to the fact that most subjects had higher levels of education.

Although the prevalence of working RA patients was not associated with the use of DMARDs or anti-TNF biologicals, several studies showing that these drugs may decrease the number of sick-leave days have been published [31–33]. The work capacity of patients may approximate that of healthy individuals during early treatment [34, 35].

The study limitations might include methodological differences caused by the lack of consistency in defining work disability [10], specific population characteristics, the very high HDI of the municipality of Blumenau (which differs from the rest of the country), the sample losses of some variables such as the HAQ score (which would likely be more significantly associated with the prevalence of working RA patients in a larger sample), possible memory biases of the respondents and reverse causation typical of cross-sectional studies.

The strengths of the study were the representative sample of the population of the municipality where the study was conducted (encompassing all social classes), the interviews conducted through pre-structured questionnaires by trained staff and the quality control of the interviews. The labor market context presumably had no effect on the results because the unemployment rate in Brazil in the study period ranged from 4.3% to 5.3%, in contrast to Blumenau, which had a 2% unemployment rate in 2014. Furthermore, the state of Santa Catarina had the lowest unemployment rate of all Brazilian states in 2015 (IBGE).

Conclusion

This study analyzed the prevalence of RA patients in the labor market in a southern region of Brazil. A higher prevalence of working RA patients was found among adult, low-income individuals with high functional disability. We suggest new population-based studies to improve the consistency of information on the employment status of patients with RA and to signal future budgetary impacts on social security.

Abbreviations
DMARDs: Disease-modifying antirheumatic drugs; FURB: Regional University of Blumenau; HAQ: Health assessment questionnaire; HDI: Human development index; MH: Ministry of Health; PR: Prevalence ratios; RA: Rheumatoid arthritis; SD : Standard deviation; SUS: Unified Health System; UBS: Primary care centers; UNPD: United Nations Development Program

Authors' contributions
RKSG and MRCN contributed to elaboration, literature review, statistical analysis and article writing. LCS, MOV and PHM contributed to writing and literature review. All approved final version for submission in journal.

Competing interests
The authors declare that they have no competing interests.

Author details
[1]Specialty Center of the City of Blumenau, Blumenau, Santa Catarina State (SC), Brazil. [2]Specialty Center of the City of Brusque, Brusque, SC, Brazil. [3]School of Medicine, Regional University of Blumenau (Universidade Regional de Blumenau – FURB), Blumenau, Brazil. [4]Clinical Epidemiology Unit, Heart Institute, University Hospital, School of Medicine, University of São Paulo (Universidade de São Paulo – USP), São Paulo, SP, Brazil. [5]Centro de Referência Policlínica Lindolf Bell, Rua: Dois de Setembro, 1234 - Itoupava Norte, 3° andar, sala 1, Blumenau, SC CEP: 89052-003, Brazil.

References
1. Cheung PP, Dougados M, Andre V, Balandraud N, Chales G, Chary-Valckenaere I, et al. Improving agreement in assessment of synovitis in rheumatoid arthritis. Jt Bone Spine. 2013;80(2):155–9.
2. Mota LMH, Laurindo IMM, Neto LL dos S, FAC L, Viana SL, Mendlovitz PS, et al. Diagnóstico por imagem da artrite reumatoide inicial. Rev Bras Reumatol. 2012;52(5):761–6.
3. Hoy D, March L, Brooks P, Blyth F, Woolf A, Bain C, et al. The global burden of rheumatoid arthritis: estimates from the global burden of disease 2010 study. Ann Rheum Dis. 2014;73(6):968–74.
4. Gabriel SE. The epidemiology of rheumatoid arthritis. Rheum Dis Clin N Am. 2001;27:269–81.
5. Marques WV, Cruz VA, Rego J, da Silva NA. Influência das comorbidades na capacidade funcional de pacientes com artrite reumatoide. Rev Bras Reumatol. 2015;56(1):14–21.
6. Schoels M, Wong J, Scott DL, Zink A, Richards P, Landewé R, et al. Economic aspects of treatment options in rheumatoid arthritis: a systematic literature review informing the EULAR recommendations for the management of rheumatoid arthritis. Ann Rheum Dis. 2010;69(6):995–1003.
7. Kwoh CK, Simms RW, Anderson LG, Erlandson DM, Greene JM, Moncur C, et al. Guidelines for the management of rheumatoid arthritis: American College of Rheumatology ad hoc Committee on clinical guidelines. Arthritis Rheum. 1996;39(5):713 22.
8. Diretrizes P. Projeto Diretrizes Artrite Reumatóide : Diagnóstico e Tratamento Projeto Diretrizes; 2002. p. 1–15.
9. Han C, Smolen J, Kavanaugh A, St. Clair EW, Baker D, Bala M. Comparison of employability outcomes among patients with early or long-standing rheumatoid arthritis. Arthritis Care Res. 2008;59(4):510–4.
10. Verstappen SMM, Bijlsma JWJ, Verkleij H, Buskens E, Blaauw AAM, ter Borg EJ, et al. Overview of work disability in rheumatoid arthritis patients as observed in cross-sectional and longitudinal surveys. Arthritis Rheum 2004; 51(3):488–497.
11. Woolf AD, Pfleger B. Burden of major musculoskeletal conditions. Bull World Health Organ. 2003;81(9):646–56.
12. Merkesdal S, Ruof J, Schffski O, Bernitt K, Zeidler H, Mau W. Indirect medical costs in early rheumatoid arthritis: composition of and changes in indirect costs within the first three years of disease. Arthritis Rheum. 2001;44(3):528–34.
13. Louzada P, Souza BDB, Toledo RA, Ciconelli RM. Análise descritiva das características demográficas e clínicas de pacientes com artrite reumatóide no estado de São Paulo. Brazil Rev Bras Reumatol. 2007;47(2):84–90.
14. Vilsteren van M, Boot CR, Knol DL, van Schaardenburg D, Voskuyl AE, Steenbeek R, et al. Productivity at work and quality of life in patients with rheumatoid arthritis. BMC Musculoskelet Disord. 2015;16(1):107.
15. De Abreu MM, Kowalski SC, Ciconelli RM, Ferraz MB. Avaliação do perfil sociodemográfico, clínico-laboratorial e terapêutico dos pacientes com artrite reumatóide que participaram de projetos de pesquisa na Escola Paulista de Medicina, nos últimos 25 anos. Rev Bras Reumatol. 2006;46(2):103–9.
16. Programa das Nações Unidas - PNUD. Atlas do Desenvolvimento Humano no Brasil 2003. Available from: http://www.pnud.org.br/atlas. [Accessed in 21 Feb 2016].
17. Instituto Brasileiro de Geografia e Estatística-IBGE. Sinopse do Censo Demográfico de 2010/2011. Available from: http://www.ibge.gov.br/home/estatistica/populacao/censo2010/. [Accessed in 21 Feb 2016].
18. Young A, Dixey J, Kulinskaya E, Cox N, Davies P, Devlin J, et al. Which patients stop working because of rheumatoid arthritis? Results of five years' follow up in 732 patients from the early RA study (ERAS). Ann Rheum Dis. 2002;61(4):335–40.
19. Cooper NJ. Economic burden of rheumatoid arthritis: a systematic review. Rheumatology (Oxford). 2000;39(1):28–33.
20. de Melo Jr VA, Aguiar FA, Baleroni TCG, Novaes GS. Análise temporal entre início dos sintomas, avaliação reumatológica e tratamento com drogas modificadoras de doença em pacientes com artrite reumatóide. Revista da Faculdade de Ciências Médicas de Sorocaba. 2008;10(2):12–5.
21. De Croon EM, Sluiter JK, Nijssen TF, Dijkmans BA, Lankhorst GJ, Frings-Dresen MH. Predictive factors of work disability in rheumatoid arthritis: a systematic literature review. Ann Rheum Dis. 2004;63:1362–7.
22. Detaille SI, Heerkens YF, Engels JA, van der Gulden JW, van Dijk FJ. Common prognostic factors of work disability among employees with a chronic somatic disease: a systematic review of cohort studies. Scand J Work Environ Health. 2009;35:261–81.
23. Jacobi CE, Mol GD, Boshuizen HC, Rupp I, Dinant HJ, Van Den Bos GAM. Impact of socioeconomic status on the course of rheumatoid arthritis and on related use of health care services. Arthritis Rheum. 2003;49(4):567–73.
24. Massardo L, Pons-Estel BA, Wojdyla D, Cardiel MH, Galarza-Maldonado CM, Sacnun MP, et al. Early rheumatoid arthritis in Latin America: low socioeconomic status related to high disease activity at baseline. Arthritis Care Res. 2012;64(8):1135–43.
25. Liao KP, Karlson EW. Classification and epidemiology of rheumatoid arthritis. Rheumatology. 2011;5:823–8.
26. Barrett EM, Scott DG, Wiles NJ, et al. The impact of rheumatoid arthritis on employment status in the early years of disease: a UK community-based study. Rheumatology. 2000;39:1403–9.
27. Janoudi N, Almoallim H, Husien W, Noorwali A, Ibrahim A. Work ability and work disability evaluation in Saudi patients with rheumatoid arthritis: special emphasis on work ability among housewives. Saudi Med J. 2013;34(11): 1167–72.
28. Michaud K, Wallenstein G, Wolfe F. Treatment and nontreatment predictors of health assessment questionnaire disability progression in rheumatoid arthritis: a longitudinal study of 18,485 patients. Arthritis Care Res (Hoboken). 2011;63(3):366–72.
29. Kaptein SA, Gignac MA, Badley EM. Differences in the workforce experiences of women and men with arthritis disability: a population health perspective. Arthritis Rheum. 2009;61:605 13.

30. Eberhardt K, Larsson BM, Nived K, Lindqvist E. Work disability in rheumatoid arthritis–development over 15 years and evaluation of predictive factors over time. J Rheumatol. 2007;34:481–7.

31. Augustsson J, Neovius M, Cullinane-Carli C, et al. Patients with rheumatoid arthritis treated with tumour necrosis factor antagonists increase their participation in the workforce: potential for significant long-term indirect cost gains (data from a population-based registry). Ann Rheum Dis. 2010;69: 126–31.

32. Sokka T. Work disability in early rheumatoid arthritis. Clin Exp Rheumatol. 2003;21:S71–4.

33. Puolakka K, Kautiainen H, Möttönen T, Hannonen P, Korpela M, Julkunen H, et al. Impact of initial aggressive drug treatment with a combination of disease-modifying antirheumatic drugs on the development of work disability in early rheumatoid arthritis: a five-year randomized followup trial. Arthritis Rheumatism. 2004;50:55–62.

34. Tiippana-Kinnunen T, Paimela L, Peltomaa R, Kautiainen H, Laasonen L, Leirisalo-Repo M. Work disability in Finnish patients with rheumatoid arthritis: a 15-year follow-up. Clin Exp Rheumatol. 2014;32:88–94.

35. Puolakka K, Kautiainen H, Mattonen T. Predictors of productivity loss in early rheumatoid arthritis: a year follow up study. Ann Rheum Dis. 2005;64:130–3.

14

Physical exercise among patients with systemic autoimmune myopathies

Diego Sales de Oliveira[1], Rafael Giovani Misse[1], Fernanda Rodrigues Lima[2] and Samuel Katsuyuki Shinjo[1*]

Abstract

Systemic autoimmune myopathies (SAMs) are a heterogeneous group of rare systemic autoimmune diseases that primarily affect skeletal muscles. Patients with SAMs show progressive skeletal muscle weakness and consequent functional disabilities, low health quality, and sedentary lifestyles. In this context, exercise training emerges as a non-pharmacological therapy to improve muscle strength and function as well as the clinical aspects of these diseases. Because many have feared that physical exercise exacerbates inflammation and consequently worsens the clinical manifestations of SAMs, it is necessary to evaluate the possible benefits and safety of exercise training among these patients. The present study systematically reviews the evidence associated with physical training among patients with SAMs.

Keywords: Dermatomyositis, Physical exercise, Myositis, Polymyositis

Background

Systemic autoimmune myopathies (SAMs) are a heterogeneous group of rare autoimmune systemic diseases that primarily affect skeletal muscles [1, 2]. Depending on demographic, clinical, laboratory, histopathological, and evolutionary data, SAMs can be subdivided into dermatomyositis (DM), polymyositis (PM), inclusion body myositis (IBM), and others [3].

Patients with SAMs share a common clinical presentation characterized by skeletal muscle weakness, which ultimately leads to functional disability and increased morbidity and mortality [4].

Until the 1960s, absolute rest was recommended for patients with autoimmune rheumatic diseases to help treat the disease [5]. However, this recommendation has changed because sedentary behavior is now known to be associated with increases in triglyceride levels, blood pressure, insulin resistance, and cardiovascular risk [6, 7]. In this context, exercise training emerged as a non-pharmacological therapy for patients with SAMs, thereby contributing to the restoration of the muscle strength and functional capacity of these individuals and improving their clinical condition. Because exercise training among these patients was prohibited for many years, it is necessary to understand the mechanisms through which physical exercise acts to improve these parameters, as well as the safety of recommending exercise training to treat these diseases. Thus, the purpose of this review was to describe the safety of exercise training among patients, particularly those with SAMs.

Methods

For the present study, a bibliographic search was performed using the electronic databases Medline and PubMed.

The descriptors were selected in January 2017 and were defined based on the following keywords (in English): dermatomyositis, inclusion body myositis, polymyositis, idiopathic inflammatory myopathies, aerobic capacity, muscle strength, functional capacity, physical activity, exercise training, resistance training, vascular occlusion training, and resistance training with vascular occlusion. These keywords were combined using the Boolean operators "AND" and "OR" and adapted to each database as needed. In addition, the reference lists of all retrieved articles were manually reviewed.

The following inclusion criteria were adopted: no time limit; published in English; original articles, case reports, case series, controlled clinical trials, or longitudinal experimental studies (with experimental and control groups); exercise/physical training interventions were conducted for

* Correspondence: samuel.shinjo@gmail.com
[1]Division of Rheumatology, Faculdade de Medicina FMUSP, Universidade de Sao Paulo, Av. Dr. Arnaldo, 455, 3° andar, sala 3150 - Cerqueira César, Sao Paulo 01246-903, Brazil
Full list of author information is available at the end of the article

individuals with SAMs; details of the intervention, such as duration, frequency, types of exercise and intensity, were listed; and muscle strength and/or functionality were evaluated and presented as primary or secondary outcomes through physical performance tests.

Abstracts of congresses, monographs, theses and dissertations, articles about other myopathies (e.g., muscular dystrophy, metabolic myopathy, and neuromuscular disease), and letters to the editor that were purely commentary were excluded from this review.

The search identified 26 articles. The concepts used in this study are explained in Table 1.

Literature review

The first studies that evaluated the effect of physical exercise on patients with SAMs were performed in the 1990s by Hicks et al. [8] (Table 2) and Escalante et al. [9] (Table 3). Hicks et al. [8] demonstrated that a 4-week quadriceps and biceps isometric strengthening program for patients with PM effectively increased isometric strength without increasing muscle enzyme serum levels. Escalante et al. [9] were the first to suggest that patients with active SAMs can participate in rehabilitation programs involving strength training. Furthermore, these programs were associated with a clinical improvement in strength without increasing muscle enzyme serum levels.

Wiesinger et al. [10] was the first to conduct a prospective, controlled, and randomized study evaluating the effects of physical training on patients with SAMs. In that study, 14 patients with DM/PM (seven undergoing physical training and seven controls) were prospectively evaluated over a 6-week period. Patients undergoing physical training demonstrated significant improvements in aerobic capacity, isometric muscle strength, activities of

daily living, and quality of life compared with the control group. In addition, patients undergoing physical training showed an elevation in the inflammatory markers of the disease, suggesting that physical training is safe for these patients. Several additional studies have built on those preliminary studies to better understand the effects of physical training among patients with SAMs.

Physical exercise among patients with DM/PM

Patients with DM/PM have decreased aerobic capacity, with a lower peak oxygen consumption (VO_2 peak) [11, 12]. In addition, this decrease in aerobic capacity is positively correlated with a decrease in isometric strength, suggesting that the decrease in muscle strength among these patients impairs aerobic capacity [11].

The impairment in the aerobic capacity of these patients might also be related to elevated levels of blood lactate and the low proportion of type 1 muscle fibers, suggesting that patients with DM/PM show an impaired skeletal muscle oxidative capacity [13, 14]. Because one of the causes of mortality among patients with SAMs is cardiopulmonary diseases [15, 16] and decreases in aerobic capacity are associated with an increased risk of these diseases [17, 18], it is essential to employ strategies that can improve these parameters among these patients.

Based on this assumption, Wiesinger et al. [19] studied eight patients with DM/PM in remission who engaged in a physical training program. These authors observed a 28% improvement in aerobic capacity after 6 months of training, which was considered clinically significant. The same authors [10] demonstrated a significant improvement in aerobic capacity after 6 weeks of physical training among 14 patients with DM/PM (7 in the training group and 7 controls) in a randomized study. Munters

Table 1 Concepts used in physical training

Term	Concept
Aerobic capacity	Maximum capacity of the individual to capture oxygen from the environment, transport it through the bloodstream, and use it in cellular respiration. It can be estimated using peak oxygen consumption (peak VO_2) via ergospirometry
Aerobic training	Training characterized by low and moderate intensity efforts with a prolonged duration (over 150 s). This training predominantly uses oxygen (O_2)-dependent bioenergetic pathways to meet the energy demand required by the activity
1RM	Test used to determine the maximum muscle strength of the individual, determined as the maximum amount of weight lifted in only one repetition during a standardized exercise
MVC	Test used to determine the maximum number of repetitions/contractions that the participant can perform with a preset load
Strength training	Training that uses exercises requiring a level of strength above that used in everyday tasks to increase muscle function. When prescribing this training, the 1RM and/or MVC test is necessary, and the training is based on the percentage of each participant's 1RM (usually between 50 and 80% of 1RM/MVC)
Isometric exercise	During this exercise, the production of muscle tension equals the external load imposed on the muscle. Moreover, this exercise is characterized by the absence of joint movement during its execution
Dynamic exercise	This exercise involves the displacement of the body in time and space, and it is characterized by alternations between eccentric and concentric contractions

1RM 1-repetition maximum test, *MVC* maximum voluntary contraction test

Table 2 Physical exercise in patients with chronic stable dermatomyositis, polymyositis, or both

Author	Patients (n)	Protocol (Exercises)	Time (week)	Evaluated Components	Inflammatory markers	Results
Hicks et al. [8]	1	Isometric strength	4	Isometric strength 3 MVC	↔ CPK	↑ Isometric strength
Wiesinger et al. [10]	14	Aerobic	6	VO₂ peak Isometric strength Activities of daily living	↔ CPK	↑ VO₂ peak ↑ Isometric strength ↑ Activities of daily living
Wiesinger et al. [19]	13	Aerobic	24	VO₂ peak Isometric strength Activities of daily living	↔ CPK	↑ VO₂ peak ↑ Isometric strength ↑ Activities of daily living
Alexanderson et al. [23]	10	Strength Dynamic	12	Muscle function Walking distance Quality of life	↔ CPK ↔ Immune / inflammatory markers	↑ Muscle function ↑ Walking distance ↑ Quality of life
[a]Heikkilä et al. [44]	22	Strength Dynamic	3	Functional capacity Pain	↔ CPK	↑ Muscle function ↔ Pain
[b]Varvu et al. [45]	19	Strength Dynamic	3	Respiratory function (Spirometry) Muscle strength	↔ CPK	↑ Respiratory function ↑ Muscle function
Harris-Love et al. [46]	1	Strength Eccentric	12	Isometric strength	↔ Muscle enzymes	↑ Isometric strength ↑ Concentric strength
Alexanderson et al. [23]	8	Strength Dynamic	7	10–15 MVC Functional capacity	↔ CPK	↑ 10–15 MVC ↔ Disease activity ↔ Functional capacity
Dastmalchi et al. [14]	9	Aerobic Strength	12	Type of muscle fiber Quality of life Functional capacity	Not reported	↑ Type I Fiber ↑ Functional Capacity ↑ Quality of Life
Chung et al. [47]	37	Strength Dynamic Creatine supplementation	20	Functional capacity Muscle strength Quality of life Pain and fatigue Anxiety and depression	↔ CPK	↑ Functional capacity ↑ Muscle strength ↔ Quality of life ↔ Anxiety and depression ↔ Pain and fatigue
Nader et al. [21]	8	Strength Dynamic	7	Genes related to inflammation and fibrosis	↓ CPK	↓ Genes related to inflammation and fibrosis ↓ Tissue fibrosis
Munters et al. [12]	9	Aerobic	12	Aerobic capacity Activity of mitochondrial enzymes	↔ CPK	↑ Aerobic capacity ↑ Activity of mitochondrial enzymes
Munters et al. [20]	11	Aerobic	12	Aerobic capacity Disability Disease activity Quality of life 5 MVC	↔ CPK	↓ Disease activity ↑ Muscle strength ↑ Quality of life ↑ Aerobic capacity ↑ Quality of life
Mattar et al. [25]	13	Strength Dynamic Vascular occlusion	12	Muscle strength Functional capacity Quality of life	↔ CPK↔ Aldolase	↑ Muscle strength ↑ Functional capacity ↑ Quality of life
Munters et al. [22]	15	Aerobic	12	Aerobic capacity Proteomic analysis Molecular profile	↔ CPK	↑ Aerobic capacity ↑ Genes related to capillary growth, mitochondrial biogenesis, protein synthesis, cytoskeletal remodeling and muscular hypertrophy ↑ Genes related to the immune and inflammatory response and sarcoplasmic reticulum stress

CPK creatine phosphokinase, *DM* dermatomyositis, *PM* polymyositis, *MVC* maximum voluntary contraction, *VO₂ peak* oxygen consumption, ↑: increase, ↔: no change, ↓: decrease
[a] included patients with inclusion body myositis
[b] included patients with active disease

Table 3 Physical exercise among patients with dermatomyositis, newly diagnosed polymyositis, clinically active disease, or some combination therein

Author	Patients (n)	Disease activity	Protocol (Exercises)	Time (week)	Evaluated components	Inflammatory markers	Results
Escalante et al. [9]	5	Active	Strength Dynamic	8	Isometric strength	↔ CPK	↑ Isometric strength
Alexanderson et al. [24]	11	Active	Strength Dynamic	12	Muscle function Quality of life	↔ CPK	↑ Muscle function ↑ Quality of life
[a]Varvu et al. [45]	19	Chronic/Active	Strength Dynamic	3	Respiratory function (Spirometry) Muscle strength	↔ CPK	↑ Respiratory function ↑ Muscle function
Mattar et al. [29]	3	Active	Strength Aerobic	12	Muscle strength Functional capacity Quality of life	↔ CPK ↔ Aldolase	↑ Muscle strength ↑ Functional capacity ↑ Quality of life

CPK creatine phosphokinase, DM dermatomyositis, PM polymyositis, ↑: increase, ↔: no change
[a] Active disease but with chronic evolution

et al. [12] corroborated these findings by demonstrating that aerobic training over a 12-week period effectively improved the aerobic capacity of patients with DM/PM and increased the activity of the mitochondrial enzymes in their skeletal muscles. Aerobic training also led to a change in muscle fiber type (increased type I fibers) in these patients as well as an increase in the cross-sectional area of the muscle, which contributed to improvements in aerobic capacity and decreases in muscle fatigue [14]. In addition, Munters et al. [20] demonstrated that aerobic training improves the overall health of patients with DM/PM in a multicenter study; furthermore, improved aerobic capacity through training was associated with reduced disease activity.

Although aerobic training has important benefits for patients with DM/PM, the molecular effects of physical exercise on the skeletal muscles of these patients are unknown. Physical exercise might positively modulate the genetic profile of patients with DM/PM. Nader et al. [21] evaluated the genes related to inflammation and fibrosis in eight patients with DM/PM undergoing strength training. After 7 weeks of training, the expression levels of genes related to skeletal muscle inflammation and fibrosis were reduced, and these changes were accompanied by a reduction in tissue fibrosis among these patients. Similarly, Munters et al. [22] evaluated the effect of a 12-week aerobic training program on the molecular profile of the skeletal muscles of seven patients with DM/PM compared with eight controls. After 12 weeks, the patients undergoing training showed increased expression levels of genes related to capillary growth, mitochondrial biogenesis, protein synthesis, cytoskeletal remodeling, and muscle hypertrophy as well as decreased expression of genes related to inflammation, immune response, and endoplasmic reticulum stress [22]. These data suggest that the training activates an aerobic phenotype and promotes muscle growth as

well as suppresses the inflammatory response in the muscles of these patients.

As with aerobic capacity, patients with DM/PM show a significant decrease in muscle strength, primarily in the proximal muscles, which in turn leads to functional impairment [1, 2]. Several studies have demonstrated that physical training plays an important role in reversing the losses in muscle strength and function in patients with DM/PM [19, 23–25]. Escalante et al. [9] was the first to demonstrate an increase in muscle strength among three patients with DM/PM who engaged in physical training for 2 weeks. Based on these preliminary data, Wiesinger et al. [25] studied eight patients with DM/PM who participated in a physical training program for 6 months and observed increases in isometric strength, which led to improvements in activities of daily living (e.g., sitting down, standing up, and walking) in these patients. Alexanderson et al. [23] corroborated these data when they demonstrated that an intensive 7-week physical training program led to increases in muscle strength, helping to improve the impairments and limitations in daily activities without increasing inflammatory markers.

Strength training with intensities ranging from 70 to 80% of one-repetition maximum (1RM) has been recommended to increase muscle strength and mass [26]. As an alternative to this type of exercise, the practice of low-intensity strength training (20 to 30% of 1RM) combined with partial blood flow restriction likely induces similar improvements in muscle strength and hypertrophy in both healthy individuals and patients with chronic diseases [25–27]. Because patients with SAMs are generally unable to exercise at high intensities, this type of training is an alternative to conventional strength training. Mattar et al. [25] were the first to demonstrate that low-intensity strength training combined with partial blood flow restriction was a safe and effective method of increasing muscle strength, function, and mass and that it could lead to significant improvements in the quality of life of patients with DM/PM. These results suggest that this type of training act as a new non-pharmacological therapy to reverse the clinical manifestations associated with these diseases.

Physical exercise among patients with DM/PM during clinical disease activity

The data presented above lead us to believe that physical exercise is a powerful aid in improving the impaired physical abilities of patients with DM/PM. In addition, because inflammatory markers were not exacerbated in the studies presented, exercise training might be safe for these patients.

However, newly diagnosed patients and those with clinical disease activity are often fearful regarding the use of exercise training. Because patients present with a high degree of inflammation, fear remains about exercising during these periods.

Alexanderson et al. [28] evaluated the effect of intensive physical training performed at home five times per week over a 12-week period on the clinical disease activity of patients with DM/PM. After 12 weeks, significant increases were observed in muscle strength and function, which in turn led to an improvement in the quality of life of these patients. These authors suggested that this physical exercise program was safe because the inflammatory markers did not increase; therefore, exercise training was recommended for the rehabilitation of these patients. Similarly, Mattar et al. [29] conducted a case series study of three patients with clinical DM/PM activity and assessed the safety and effect of aerobic training combined with supervised strength training over a 12-week period. After this period, physical training was well tolerated and safe (i.e., increases in creatine phosphokinase (CPK) and aldolase levels were not found). In addition, specific parameters of aerobic capacity, muscle function, and quality of life improved, suggesting that supervised physical training positively affects these parameters during clinical disease activity.

Alexanderson et al. [24] were the first to demonstrate that physical exercise is safe during this period for patients newly diagnosed with DM/PM. A total of 19 patients newly diagnosed with DM/PM receiving high doses of prednisone were selected. The patients were randomized into a training group ($n = 10$) and a control group ($n = 9$). The patients in the training group were instructed to perform an intensive physical training program (five times per week for 12 weeks); the patients were then evaluated at the 24th, 52nd, 78th and 104th weeks. No significant differences were found between the training and control groups with regard to the parameters evaluated; however, intensive physical training was found to be safe for these patients because it did not exacerbate inflammation

during the evaluated period, suggesting that exercise training is safe even for newly diagnosed patients.

Physical exercise in patients with IBM

Although the effects of physical training on patients with DM/PM have been well described in the literature, few studies have evaluated the effect of physical training on patients with IBM.

Studies comparing the aerobic capacity of these patients with healthy controls are scarce. Because patients with IBM also present with significant impairments in their mitochondrial oxidative capacity [30, 31], studies are necessary to determine whether these patients have impaired aerobic capacity. To date, only one study has evaluated the effect of 12 weeks of stationary bicycle training combined with strength training on the aerobic capacity of seven patients with IBM (Table 4). After 12 weeks of physical training, a 38% increase in aerobic capacity was observed among these patients [32].

Like those with DM/PM, patients with IBM present with an important impairment in muscle strength as a characteristic of the disease [33, 34]. Spector et al. [35] examined five patients with IBM who completed a 12-week progressive strength-training program. These authors did not observe an increase in the cross-sectional area of the muscle; however, a significant increase in muscle strength was shown without the exacerbation of inflammatory markers. Low-intensity strength training combined with partial blood flow restriction is also an important aid when reversing the losses in strength and muscular function as well as stimulating the increase of muscle mass in these patients. Gualano et al. [36] were the first authors to demonstrate that strength training combined with partial blood flow restriction for 12 weeks effectively and safely increased muscle strength (through the 1RM test), balance, and function as well as lead to 15.9, 60, and 4.7% increases in the cross-sectional area of muscle in a case study of a patient with IBM resistant to all types of treatment. In addition, there was an improvement in quality of life, varying from 18 to 600%. In addition to these effects, the same research group [37] demonstrated that strength training combined with the partial restriction of blood flow for 12 weeks decreased the expression of the myostatin gene and increased the expression of endogenous myostatin inhibitors. These data might partially explain the increase in muscle mass observed in the aforementioned case study [36]. Corroborating the previous findings, Jorgensen et al. [38] examined a 74-year-old man with who participated in strength training combined with partial blood flow restriction over a 12-week period. These authors observed substantial increases in mechanical muscle strength and gait speed, suggesting that this type of training reverses the losses in strength and functional capacity associated with these patients.

Table 4 Physical exercise in patients with chronic inclusion body myositis

Author	Patients (n)	Protocol (Exercises)	Time (week)	Evaluated Components	Inflammatory markers	Results
Spector et al. [35]	5	Strength Dynamic	12	Isometric strength 3 MVC	↔ CPK ↔ Immune / inflammatory markers	↑ Isometric strength ↑ 3 MVC ↔ Increased cross-sectional area
Arnardottir et al. [39]	7	Strength Dynamic	12	Isometric strength	↔ CPK ↔ Cytokines ↔ Adhesion molecules	↑ Isometric strength
Johnson et al. [32]	7	Aerobic	12	VO$_2$ peak Functional Capacity	↔ CPK	↑ VO$_2$ peak ↔ Functional capacity
	7	Strength Dynamic	16	Muscle strength Functional capacity	↔ CPK	↑ Muscle strength ↑ Functional capacity
Gualano et al. [36]	1	Strength Dynamic With vascular occlusion	12	Muscle strength Balance Quality of life Cross-sectional area	↔ CPK	↑ Muscle strength ↑ Balance ↑ Quality of life ↑ Cross-sectional area
Santos et al. [37]	1	Strength Dynamic With vascular occlusion	12	Myostatin gene Myostatin inhibitor genes	↔ CPK	↓ Myostatin gene ↑ Myostatin inhibitor genes
Jorgensen et al. [38]	1	Strength Dynamic With vascular occlusion	12	Isometric strength Functional capacity Gait speed	↔ CPK	↑ Isometric strength ↑ Functional capacity ↑ Gait speed

CPK creatine phosphokinase, MVC maximum voluntary contraction, VO$_2$ peak oxygen consumption, ↑: increase, ↔: no change

Physical exercise performed at home is also an important therapy for patients with IBM. Intensive home training (5 days per week for 12 weeks) was also found to be safe (no increase in creatine phosphokinase levels) and effective at increasing the muscle strength and function of these patients [39], suggesting that this practice effectively rehabilitates patients with IBM.

Future prospects and final considerations

SAMs are characterized by periods of clinical activity and remission. During clinical disease activity, patients present with a significant decrease in skeletal muscle strength, which remains lower throughout the lifespan. This decrease in strength leads to functional impairment and consequent decreases in daily activities, resulting in marked sedentary lifestyles among these patients.

The data presented in this review suggest that physical training is an important non-pharmacological tool for increasing muscle strength, improving functional impairment, and improving the quality of life of patients with SAMs. In addition, physical training likely improves the impaired aerobic capacity of patients with SAMs. This effect is likely associated with the ability of physical training to improve the molecular profile (thereby increasing the expression of the genes related to mitochondrial neoangiogenesis and biogenesis) and leading to increases in the activities of mitochondrial enzymes and the type I fibers in the skeletal muscle [12, 21, 22].

Additional studies are needed to better understand how physical exercise acts in the pathogenesis of SAMs. The causes of these diseases are not yet known; however, immune and nonimmune mechanisms are most likely involved [40–43]. Studies that demonstrate how physical exercise affects these parameters might help to understand how exercise training acts toward the clinical improvement of these diseases.

Clinical, controlled, and randomized studies of patients with IBM are necessary to show the real effects of physical exercise among this population. Physical training likely stimulates increases in muscle strength and improves the aerobic capacities of these patients; however, without an increase in the cross-sectional area of the muscle [32, 35, 39]. Strength training with vascular occlusion appears to efficiently increase strength, function, balance, and the cross-sectional area of muscle in these patients [36, 37]. Thus, this type of training is an alternative to conventional training that is capable of stimulating increases in the muscle mass of patients with IBM. Because these patients are generally resistant to drug therapy, the use of strength training with vascular occlusion is an important aid to minimize the clinical manifestations of this disease.

Studies have yet to evaluate the effect of physical exercise among patients with immune-mediated necrotizing myopathy; therefore, future trials should explore this area.

Conclusions

The data presented in this review suggest that physical training is an important cal tool for increasing muscle strength, improving functional impairment, and improving the quality of life of patients with SAMs. In addition, physical training likely improves the impaired aerobic capacity of patients with SAMs.

Abbreviations

CPK: Creatine phosphokinase; DM: Dermatomyositis; IBM: Inclusion body myositis; PM: Polymyositis; RM: repetition maximum; SAMs: Systemic autoimmune myopathies; VO2 peak: Peak oxygen consumption

Support

FAPESP #2017/13109-1 and Fundação Faculdade de Medicina to SKS.

Authors' contributions

All authors contributed equally to write and review the manuscript. All authors read and approved the final manuscript.

Competing interests

The authors declare that they have no competing interests.

Author details

[1]Division of Rheumatology, Faculdade de Medicina FMUSP, Universidade de Sao Paulo, Av. Dr. Arnaldo, 455, 3° andar, sala 3150 - Cerqueira César, Sao Paulo 01246-903, Brazil. [2]Division of Rheumatology, Hospital das Clinicas HCFMUSP, Faculdade de Medicina, Universidade de Sao Paulo, Sao Paulo, Brazil.

References

1. Feldman BM, Rider LG, Reed AM, Pachman LM. Juvenile dermatomyositis and other idiopathic inflammatory myopathies of childhood. Lancet. 2008; 371:2201–12.
2. Greenberg SA. Inflammatory myopathies: evaluation and management. Semin Neurol. 2008;28:241–9.
3. Dalakas MC. Review: an update on inflammatory and autoimmune myopathies. Neuropathol Appl Neurobiol. 2011;37:226–42.
4. Dimanckhie MM, Barohn R, Amato AA. Idiopathic inflammatory myopathies. Neurol Clin. 2014;32:595–628.
5. Partridge RE, Duthie JJ. Controlled trial of the effect of complete immobilization of the joints in rheumatoid arthritis. Ann Rheum Dis. 1963;22:91–9.
6. Lim MS, Park B, Kong IG, Sim S, Kim SY, Kim JH, et al. Leisure sedentary time is differentially associated with hypertension, diabetes mellitus, and hyperlipidemia depending on occupation. BMC Public Health. 2017;17:278–87.
7. Garelnabi M, Veledar E, Abramson J, White-Welkley J, Santanam N, Weintraub W, et al. Physical inactivity and cardiovascular risk: baseline observations from men and premenopausal women. J Clin Lab Anal. 2010;24:100–5.
8. Hicks JE, Miller F, Plotz P, Chen TH, Gerber L. Isometric exercise increases strength and does not produce sustained creatinine phosphokinase increases in a patients with polymyositis. J Rheumatol. 1993;20:1399–401.
9. Escalante A, Miller L, Beardmore TD. Resistive exercise in the rehabilitation of polymyositis/dermatomyositis. J Rheumatol. 1993;41:1124–32.
10. Wiesinger GF, Quittan M, Aringer M, Seeber A, Volc-platzer B, Smolen J, et al. Improvement of physical fitness and muscle strength in polymyositis/dermatomyositis patients by a training programme. Br J Rheumatol. 1998;37:196–200.
11. Wiesinger GF, Quittan M, Nuhr M, Volc-Platzer B, Ebenbichler G, Zehetgruber M, et al. Aerobic capacity in adult dermatomyositis/polymyositis patients and healthy controls. Arch Phys Med Rehabil. 2000;81:1–5.
12. Alemo Munters L, Dastmalchi M, Katz A, Esbjörnsson M, Loell I, Hanna B, et al. Improved exercise performance and increased aerobic capacity after endurance training of patients with stable polymyositis and dermatomyositis. Arthritis Res Ther. 2013;15:83–96.
13. Bertolucci F, Neri R, Dalise S, Venturi M, Rossi B, Chisari C. Abnormal lactate levels in patients with polymyositis and dermatomyositis: the benefits of a specific rehabilitative program. Eur J Phys Rehabil Med. 2014;50:161–9.
14. Dastmalchi M, Alexanderson H, Loell I, Stahlberg M, Borg K, Lundberg IE, et al. Effect of physical training on the proportion of slow-twitch type I muscle fibers, a novel nonimmune-mediated mechanism for muscle impairment in polymyositis or dermatomyositis. Arthritis Rheum. 2007;57:1303–10.
15. Moraes MT, De Souza FH, De Barros TB, Shinjo SK. An analysis of metabolic syndrome in adult dermatomyositis with a focus on cardiovascular disease. Arthritis Care Res. 2013;65:793–9.
16. Limaye V, Hakendorf P, Woodman RJ, Blumbergs P, Roberts-Thomson P. Mortality and its predominant causes in a large cohort of patients with biopsy-determined inflammatory myositis. Intern Med J. 2012;42:191–8.
17. Ladenvall P, Persson CU, Mandalenakis Z, Wilhelmsen L, Grimby G, Svärdsudd K, et al. Low aerobic capacity in middle-aged men associated with increased mortality rates during 45 years of follow-up. Eur J Prev Cardiol. 2016;23:1557–64.
18. Sui X, LaMonte MJ, Laditka JN, Hardin JW, Chase N, Hooker SP, et al. Cardiorespiratory fitness and adiposity as mortality predictors in older adults. JAMA. 2007;298:2507–16.
19. Wiesinger GF, Quittan M, Graninger M, Seeber A, Ebenbichler G, Sturm B, Kerschan K, Smolen J, Graninger W. Benefit of 6 months long-term physical training in polymyositis/dermatomyositis patients. Br J Rheumatol. 1998;37:1338–42.
20. Alemo Munters L, Dastmalchi M, Andgren V, Emilson C, Bergegård J, Regardt M, et al. Improvement in health and possible reduction in disease activity using endurance exercise in patients with established polymyositis and dermatomyositis: a multicenter randomized controlled trial with a 1-year open extension followup. Arthritis Care Res (Hoboken). 2013;65:1959–68.
21. Nader GA, Dastmalchi M, Alexanderson H, Grundtman C, Gernapudi R, Esbjörnsson M, et al. A longitudinal, integrated, clinical, histological and mRNA profiling study of resistance exercise in myositis. Mol Med. 2010;16:455–64.
22. Munters LA, Loell I, Ossipova E, Raouf J, Dastmalchi M, Lindroos E, et al. Endurance exercise improves molecular pathways of aerobic metabolism in patients with myositis. Arthritis Rheumatol. 2016;68:1738–50.
23. Alexanderson H, Dastmalchi M, Esbjornsson-Liljedahl M, Opava CH, Lundberg IE. Benefits of intensive resistance training in patients with chronic polymyositis or dermatomyositis. Arthritis Rheum. 2007;57:768–77.
24. Alexanderson H, Stenström CH, Jenner G, Lundberg I. The safety of a resistive home exercise program in patients with recent onset active polymyositis or dermatomyositis. Scand J Rheumatol. 2000;29:295–301.
25. Mattar MA, Gualano B, Perandini LA, Shinjo SK, Lima FR, Sá-Pinto LA, et al. Safety and possible effects of low-intensity resistance training associated with partial blood flow restriction in polymyositis and dermatomyositis. Arthritis Res Ther. 2014;16:473.
26. Scott BR, Loenneke JP, Slattery KM, Dascombe BJ. Exercise with blood flow restriction: an updated evidence-based approach for enhanced muscular development. Sports Med. 2015;45(3):313–25.
27. Scott BR, Loenneke JP, Slattery KM, Dascombe BJ. Blood flow restricted exercise for athletes: a review of available evidence. J Sci Med Sport. 2016;19:360–7.
28. Alexanderson H, Stenström CH, Lundberg I. Safety of a home exercise programme in patients with polymyositis and dermatomyositis: a pilot study. Rheumatology (Oxford). 1999;38:608–11.
29. Mattar MA, Gualano B, Roschel H, Perandini LA, Dassouki T, Lima FR, Shinjo SK, de Sá Pinto AL. Exercise as an adjuvant treatment in persistent active polymyositis. J Clin Rheumatol. 2014;20:11–5.
30. Lindgren U, Roos S, Hedberg Oldfors C, Moslemi AR, Lindberg C, et al. Mitochondrial pathology in inclusion body myositis. Neuromuscul Disord. 2015;25:281–8.
31. Joshi PR, Vetterke M, Hauburger A, Tacik P, Stoltenburg G, Hanisch F. Functional relevance of mitochondrial abnormalities in sporadic inclusion body myositis. J Clin Neurosci. 2014;21:1959–63.

32. Johnson LG, Collier KE, Edwards DJ, Philippe DL, Eastwood PR, Walters SE, et al. Improvement in aerobic capacity after an exercise program in sporadic inclusion body myositis. J Clin Neuromuscul Dis. 2009;10:178–84.

33. Gallay L, Petiot P. Sporadic inclusion-body myositis: recent advances and the state of the art in 2016. Rev Neurol (Paris). 2016;172:581–6.

34. Needham M, Mastaglia FL. Sporadic inclusion body myositis: a review of recent clinical advances and current approaches to diagnosis and treatment. Clin Neurophysiol. 2016;127:1764–73.

35. Spector SA, Lemmer JT, Koffman BM, Fleisher TA, Feuerstein IM, Hurley BF, et al. Safety and efficacy of strength training in patients with sporadic inclusion body myositis. Muscle Nerve. 1997;20:1242–8.

36. Gualano B, Neves M Jr, Lima FR, Pinto AL, Laurentino G, Borges C, et al. Resistance training with vascular occlusion in inclusion body myositis: a case study. Med Sci Sports Exerc. 2010;42:250–4.

37. Santos AR, Neves MT Jr, Gualano B, Laurentino GC, Lancha AH Jr, Ugrinowitsch C, et al. Blood flow restricted resistance training attenuates myostatin gene expression in a patient with inclusion body myositis. Biol Sport. 2014;31:121–4.

38. Jørgensen AN, Aagaard P, Nielsen JL, Frandsen U, Diederichsen LP. Effects of blood-flow-restricted resistance training on muscle function in a 74-year-old male with sporadic inclusion body myositis: a case report. Clin Physiol Funct Imaging. 2016;36:504–9.

39. Arnardottir S, Alexanderson H, Lundberg IE, Borg K. Sporadic inclusion body myositis: pilot study on the effects of a home exercise program on muscle function, histopathology and inflammatory reaction. J Rehabil Med. 2003;35:31–5.

40. Grundtman C, Malmström V, Lundberg IE. Immune mechanisms in the pathogenesis of idiopathic inflammatory myopathies. Arthritis Res Ther. 2007;9:208–20.

41. Rayavarapu S, Coley W, Kinder TB, Nagaraju K. Idiopathic inflammatory myopathies: pathogenic mechanisms of muscle weakness. Skelet Muscle. 2013;3:13–26.

42. Lightfoot AP, Nagaraju K, McArdle A, Cooper RG. Understanding the origin of non-immune cell-mediated weakness in the idiopathic inflammatory myopathies - potential role of ER stress pathways. Curr Opin Rheumatol. 2015;27:580–5.

43. Ceribelli A, De Santis M, Isailovic N, Gershwin ME, Selmi C. The immune response and the pathogenesis of idiopathic inflammatory myositis: a critical review. Clin Rev Allergy Immunol. 2017;52:58–70.

44. Heikkila S, Viitanen JV, Kautiainen H, et al. Rehabilitation in myositis. Physiother. 2001;87:301–9.

45. Varjú C, Pethö E, Kutas R, Czirják L. The effect of physical exercise following acute disease exacerbation in patients with dermato/polymyositis. Clin Rehabil. 2003;17:83–7.

46. Harris-Love MO. Safety and efficacy of submaximal eccentric strength training for a subject with polymyositis. Arthritis Rheum. 2005;53:471–4.

47. Chung YL, Alexanderson H, Pipitone N, Morrison C, Dastmalchi M, Ståhl-Hallengren C, et al. Creatine supplements in patients with idiopathic inflammatory myopathies who are clinically weak after conventional pharmacologic treatment: six-month, double-blind, randomized, placebo-controlled trial. Arthritis Rheum. 2007;57:694–702.

15

Within and between-days repeatability and variability of plantar pressure measurement during walking in children, adults and older adults

Pedro S. Franco[1,2], Cristiane F. Moro[1], Mariane M. Figueiredo[1], Renato R. Azevedo[1,2], Fernando G. Ceccon[1,2] and Felipe P. Carpes[1,2]* (iD)

Abstract

Background: Previous studies discussed the repeatability and variability in plantar pressure measurement, but a few considered different age groups. Here we determine within and between-days repeatability and variability of plantar pressure measurement during gait in participants from different age groups.

Method: Plantar pressure was recorded in children, young adults and older adults walking at preferred speed in four non-consecutive days within one week. Data from 10 steps from each foot in each day were analyzed considering the different regions of the foot. Mean and peak plantar pressure and data variability were compared between the steps, foot regions and days.

Results: To describe mean and peak pressure during gait in children and adults a single measurement can be enough, but elderly will requires more attention especially concerning peak values. Variability in mean pressure did not differ between age groups, but peak pressure variability differed across foot regions and age groups.

Conclusion: One single observation can be used to describe plantar pressure during gait in children and adults. When the interest concerns older people, it might be pertinent to consider more than one day of assessment, especially when looking at peak pressure.

Keywords: Kinetics, Foot, Gait, Aging, Peak pressure

Background

Plantar pressure analysis concerns the quantification and interpretation of the force applied to the ground and its distribution over the foot plantar surface area. Among the different ways for its quantification is the use of pressure mat systems that allows not only quantification of the pressure distribution but also analysis of the specific foot regions [1–4]. Instrumentation, foot region, and number of steps are factors influencing repeatability and variability of plantar pressure measurement [1–4]. The number of steps required for characterization of

plantar pressure during gait is a source of discussion in the literature [5]. Three steps are commonly assumed in clinical analysis of gait [6], and three to five steps are assumed to be enough to record plantar pressure in adults aged 20 to 35 years old [7].

Plantar pressure variability is also a topic of interest because most of clinical decisions are based in single-day measurement. Considering data from three [4], four [4] and five [1] different days, mean pressure, peak pressure, peak force, and force-time integral showed good repeatability. However, participants of different ages were considered in each of these studies [1, 2, 4]. There is a lack of evidences concerning differences between age groups, which are especially important for studies interested in influence of age on plantar pressure.

* Correspondence: carpes@unipampa.edu.br
[1]Applied Neuromechanics Research Group, Federal University of Pampa,Uruguaiana, BR 472 km 592, Po box 118, Uruguaiana, RS ZIP 97500-970, Brazil
[2]Graduated Program in Physical Education, Federal University of Santa Maria, Santa Maria, Brazil

There are gait characteristics that influence plantar pressure in people of different ages. In children, it includes changes in body mass and contact area of the foot [8] as well the establishment of a heel-strike landing pattern [9, 10]. Children also experience increase in peak pressure, ground reaction forces and foot length that influence center of pressure displacement [11]. Among young adults, magnitudes of pressure become stable and patterns of higher peak pressures in the rearfoot and hallux are observed [12–14]. Among older adults, a change in foot landing pattern may occur and pressure and reaction forces in the rearfoot decrease with a longer contact time [12]. These illustrate the differences between age groups that may influence plantar pressure measurements. Therefore, in this study we determine within and between-days repeatability and variability of plantar pressure measurement in people from different age groups.

Methods

Participants and experimental design

This research was conducted in agreement with the declaration of Helsinki and was approved by the local institution ethics committee. All participants and the parents (for the case of children) signed a consent term. To be included participants should be able to walk independently, be free of lower extremity injuries that limit locomotion and should be able to visit the laboratory on days previously scheduled. Those subjects that missed one evaluation session were excluded from the data analysis. Sixty participants (20 children, 20 young adults, and 20 elderly) from the local community started participation in the study. During the development of the study (see the flowchart; Fig. 1) some participants missed sessions and were excluded. In the end, 37 subjects completed all the procedures, which included 12 children, 13 adults, and 12 older adults. Participants completed four sessions of assessment in non-consecutive days within a period of 7 days for measurement of plantar pressure during walking at preferred speed.

Data acquisition

Plantar pressure was recorded during barefoot walking at preferred gait speed. Participants were requested to walk as they walk in streets. Data were acquired at 400 Hz using a pressure mat system (Matscan, Tekscan Inc., Boston, MA, US) placed halfway in a 9 m walkway. The mat had 5 mm thickness, detection area of 435.9 × 368.8 mm, comprising 2288 resistive sensors (1.4 sensors / cm^2). The system was calibrated before every evaluation for each individual using the individual body mass. Ten steps were randomly recorded for each foot, and data from right foot were considered in the analyses. Gait speed was determined using a chronometer. The evaluation session was

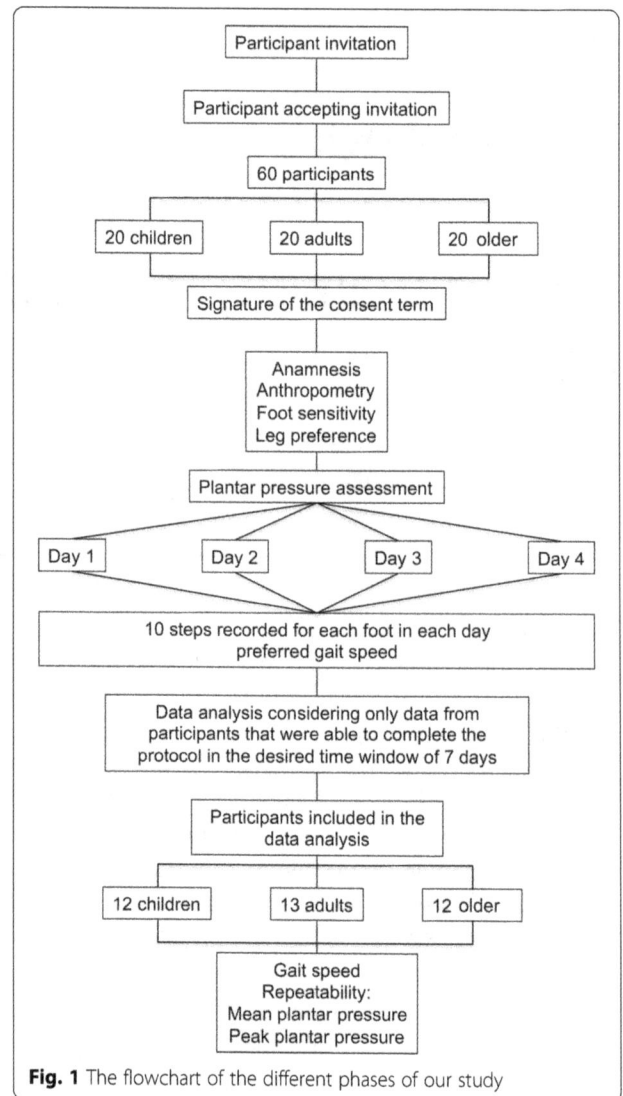

Fig. 1 The flowchart of the different phases of our study

repeated in four non-consecutives days within a period of up to 7 days.

Plantar pressure was analyzed considering the forefoot (FF), midfoot (MF) and rearfoot (RF) regions defined using a software (Research Foot 6.64, Tekscan Inc., Boston, MA, USA) and anatomical aspects determining that the rearfoot comprised 31% of the foot length, the midfoot comprised 19% of the foot length, and the forefoot comprised 50% of the foot length [15]. Data were averaged for each foot region and normalized to the total foot pressure to minimize effects body mass and foot size that differ among the participants [16]. Variables of interested in our study were mean pressure, computed by the average pressure over active sensors, and peak pressure, defined as the highest value observed among the selected active sensors [17]. Data variability was determined by the coefficient of variation that is the ratio between standard deviation and mean values.

Statistical analyses

Data are present considering mean (standard deviation). All data were checked for normality with Shapiro-Wilk test. ANOVA one-way with Tukey post-hoc was used to compare steps and to compare foot regions within a same day of assessment. Similar approach was used to compare the different days of assessment and the different groups. All analyses considered a significance level of 0.05 using a commercial statistical package.

Results

Groups of study included 12 children [8 women; 10 (1) years old, 44 (16) kg, 1.43 (0.1) m, for age, body mass and height, respectively], 13 adults [7 women; 38 (6) years old, 71 (15) kg, 1.65 (0.1) m], and 12 older adults [7 women; 74 (3) years old, 70 (14) kg, 1.59 (0.1) m]. Preferred gait speed in children was 1.21 (0.1) m/s, in adults was 1.56 (0.2) m/s, and in older adults was 0.89 (0.10) m/s. Mean pressure did not differ between the steps in both adults and older adults in within-day comparisons (Fig. 2). Among children, mean pressure differed between some of the steps only for the fourth day (F $_{(9)}$ = 4.389; P = 0.03; Fig. 2). Peak pressure did not differ between the steps in adults and older adults (Fig. 3). Peak pressure in children differed between some of the steps only in the rearfoot for the fourth day (F $_{(9)}$ = 2.688; P = 0.04, Fig. 3).

Regardless of the day of measurement, when comparing the foot regions, adults showed lower peak pressure in the midfoot compared to forefoot and rearfoot (Fig. 4). In children, peak pressure was smaller in the midfoot than forefoot and rearfoot, while forefoot and rearfoot showed similar values. Among older adults, peak pressures were higher in the forefoot and differed between the three regions of the foot (Fig. 4).

To compare pressure between the days we considered the average of mean and peak pressures from each day of measurement (Fig. 4). Mean and peak pressure in children did not differ between the days. Among adults, mean pressure in the midfoot was higher for the fourth day [F $_{(3)}$ = 5.190; P = 0.027], while peak pressure was similar for the different days. In older adults, mean pressure did not differ between the days, but peak pressure differed between all the days [F $_{(3)}$ = 4.717; P = 0.008].

Data on pressure variability were also considered in our analyses (see Table 1 for variability of mean and peak pressure). Mean pressure variability did not differ between the days of measurement in foot regions of children, adults and older adults. However, when mean pressure variability was compared between the foot regions, regardless of the day of measurement, higher variability in the midfoot, and similar variability in the rearfoot and forefoot were observed in children (F $_{(2)}$ = 36.10; P < 0.001), adults (F $_{(2)}$ = 174.1; P < 0.001), and older adults (F $_{(2)}$ = 125.4; P < 0.001). When groups were

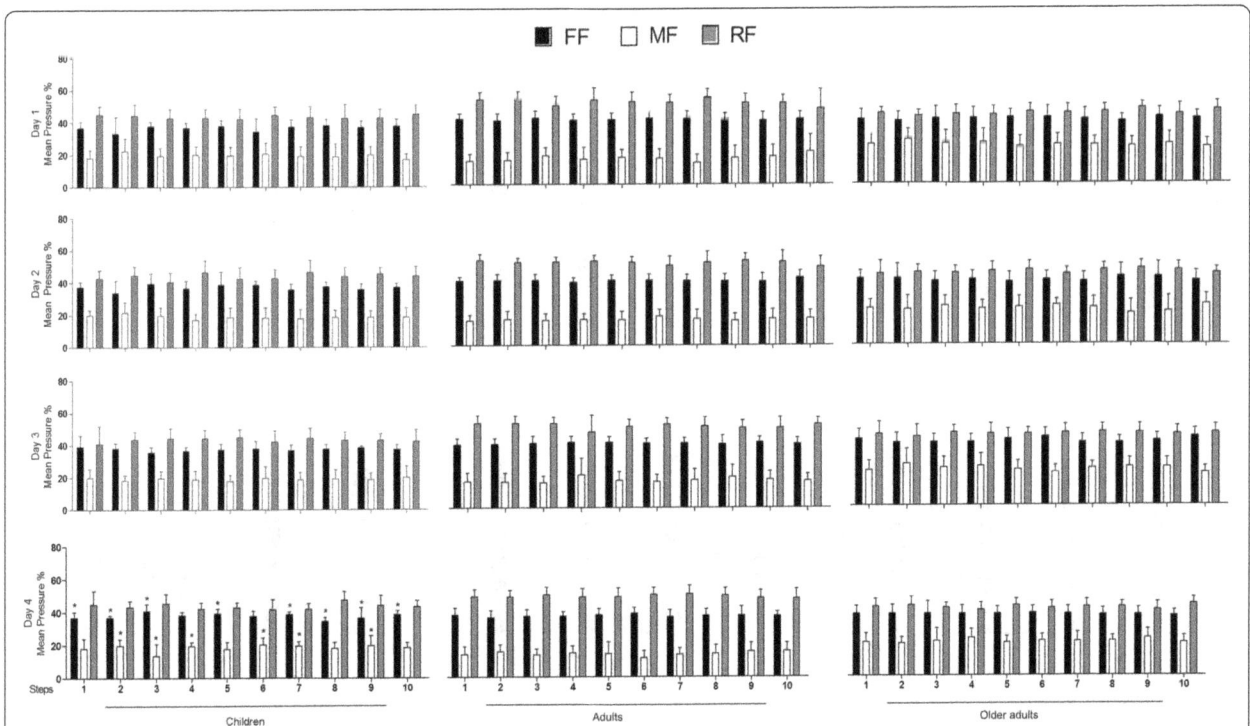

Fig. 2 Mean pressure determined in different foot regions and expressed as a percentage of total foot pressure. Data are presented for each step and group in the four days of measurement. * indicates difference between the steps

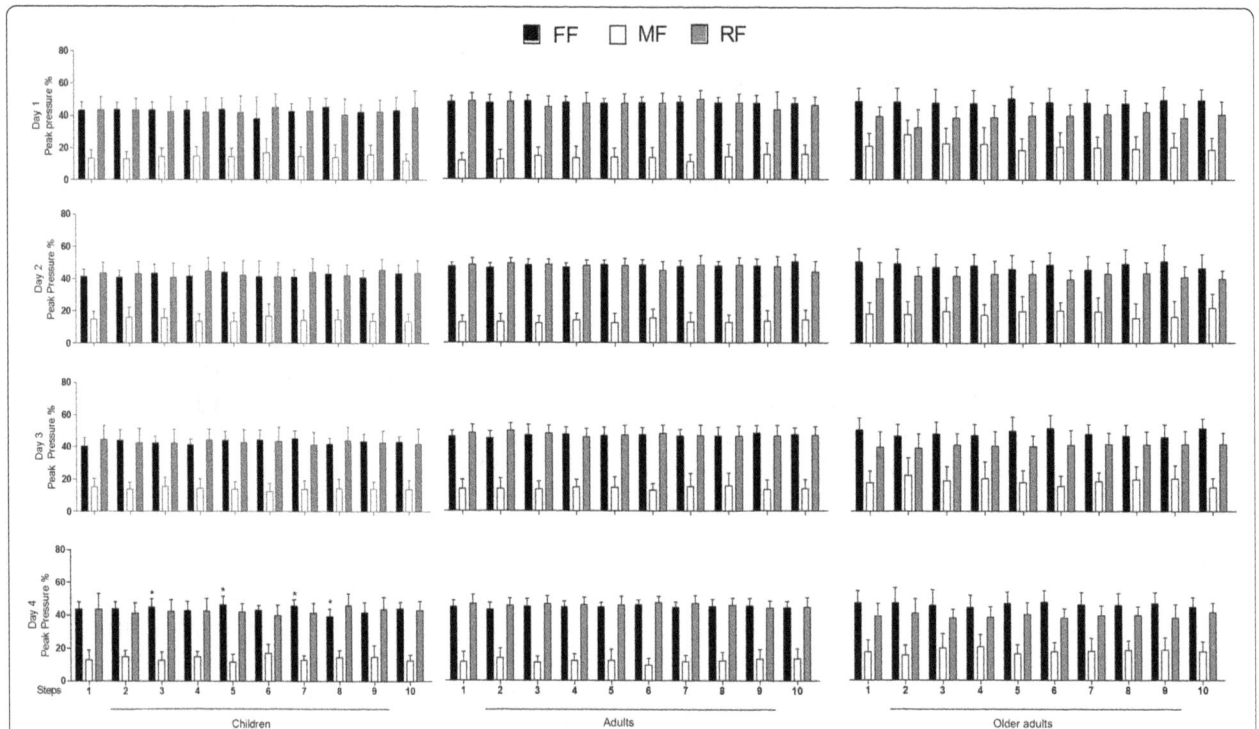

Fig. 3 Peak pressure determined in different foot regions and expressed as a percentage of total foot pressure. Data are presented for each step and group in the four days of measurement. * indicates difference between the steps

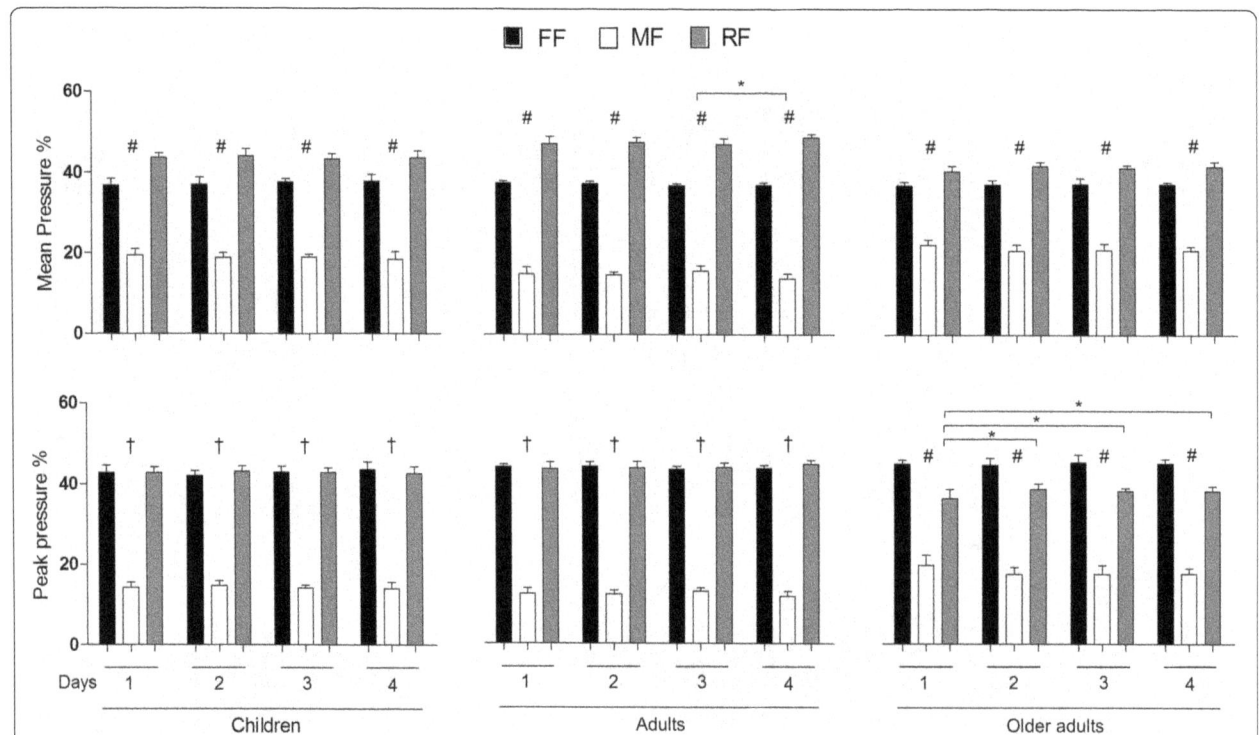

Fig. 4 Mean and peak pressure compared between the four days of measurement for each group and foot region. # indicates difference between all foot regions. † indicate difference in the rearfoot (RF) and forefoot (FF) compared to midfoot (MF) * indicates difference between the days

Table 1 Coefficient of variation determined for each day, foot region and group, considering data of mean and peak pressure. Data are expressed in percentage (%) considering mean and standard deviation data from each foot region. FF: forefoot; MF: midfoot; FR: rearfoot

Variable	Group	Foot region	Day 1 (%)	Day 2 (%)	Day 3 (%)	Day 4 (%)
Mean pressure variability	Children	FF	13.6 (7.6)	12.2 (5.8)	9.1 (3.9)	7.8 (4.0)
		MF	29.5 (5.9)*	27.0 (5.7)*	26.6 (6.1)*	24.6 (12.3)*
		RF	14.3 (2.7)	13.5 (2.5)	14.3 (5.0	11.3 (3.0)
	Adults	FF	10.2 (1.3)	9.3 (1.8)	9.7 (2.0	10.5 (2.2)
		MF	38.4 (8.0)*#	29.9 (5.1)*#	34.1 (7.8)*#	34.1 (7.4)*#
		RF	11.8 (5.0)	9.1 (3.2)	10.4 (4.4)	9.8 (1.4)
	Older adults	FF	14.2 (2.8)	15.9 (3.4)	12.7 (1.7)	12.8 (2.6)
		MF	26.1 (3.9)*	29.5 (10.1)*	25.6 (6.0)*	23.1 (4.7)*
		RF	10.7 (2.5)	10.7 (3.0)	12.4 (3.0)	10.0 (1.8)
Peak pressure variability	Children	FF	14.9 (7.3)$	13.5 (3.7)$	11.3 (2.7)$	10.6 (2.5)$
		MF	41.2 (6.3)*	37.7 (4.0)*	36.8 (4.0)*	32.7 (9.8)*
		RF	20.4 (2.8)+	18.4 (2.1)+	19.5 (2.1)+	16.0 (2.9)+
	Adults	FF	7.9 (1.4)$+	6.8 (1.7)$+	9.9 (1.8)$+	8.4 (1.6)$+
		MF	43.7 (6.9) *	38.8 (5.5) *	42.6 (7.7) *	43.2 (7.8) *
		RF	13.4 (4.5)	10.2 (2.8)	11.9 (1.7)	10.4 (1.4)
	Older adults	FF	17.0 (1.4)$+	18.0 (1.8)$+	15.0 (1.9)$+	16.0 (2.3)$+
		MF	40.8 (4.8)*	44.2 (9.7)*	41.5 (5.1)*	36.3 (4.8)*
		RF	19.3 (5.6)	16.7 (3.8)	19.6 (2.7)	17.1 (3.1)

* different of FF and RF ($P < 0.05$); $ different of RF and MF ($P < 0.05$); # different of children and older adults ($P < 0.05$); + identify days that differed between them ($P < 0.05$)

compared, the only difference relies on the mean pressure variability in the midfoot that showed an effect for age ($F_{(2)} = 8.88$; $P = 0.002$), being higher in adults compared to older adults. Mean pressure variability in other foot regions did not differ between groups.

Peak pressure variability differed between the days in the different groups and foot regions. In children, variability of peak pressure in the rearfoot differed between the days ($F_{(3)} = 4.84$; $P = 0.015$), while in adults ($F_{(3)} = 5.37$; $P = 0.011$) and older adults ($F_{(3)} = 8.12$; $P = 0.002$) differences were observed in the forefoot. No differences were observed in foot regions not mentioned. When peak pressure variability was compared between the regions, regardless of the day of assessment, children showed higher variability in the midfoot, followed by the rearfoot and then forefoot ($F_{(2)} = 67.21$; $P < 0.001$). Among adults, higher variability also was observed in the midfoot, followed by the rearfoot and then forefoot ($F_{(2)} = 177.1$; $P < 0.001$). Older adults showed higher peak pressure variability in the midfoot, while rearfoot and forefoot did not differ ($F_{(2)} = 177.1$; $P < 0.001$).

We compared peak pressure variability between the groups and found that variability in the forefoot was higher in adults and older adults, which differed of children ($F_{(2)} = 11.26$; $P = 0.006$). An age effect was also observed for rearfoot peak pressure variability ($F_{(2)} = 6.21$;

$P = 0.010$), which was higher in children compared to adults and older adults.

Discussion

In this study we set out to determine within and between-days repeatability of plantar pressure in participants from different age groups. Our main findings suggest that plantar pressure in the children and adults can be described by a single-day assessment, but elderly may require assessments in more than one day. Furthermore, foot region showing higher variability in peak pressure differs between age groups. It might be of special interest when analyzing peak pressure, which is frequently associated with sites of foot injuries. Additionally, our data show that measurement of plantar pressure variability is influenced by age and foot region.

The lack of difference between the steps for most of the variables obtained from a single-day assessment has two main implications. One concerns a methodological aspect, in which repeatability of the measurement increases as the number of records increases [18]. In the other hand, the lack of differences in the magnitude of pressure may reflect repeated loading over the foot regions. Is has been suggested that foot injuries depend on the magnitude of load, especially in the rearfoot [19] and the head of the metatarsals [20]. We observed that plantar pressure differed between some of the steps of children in the last day of assessment. However, differences were between a few particular steps and it is possible that after the repeated days of testing children were impatience and it might have affected their gait pattern. Despite of differences observed only in the last day, other possible explanation is the higher within-trials variability in spatial gait parameters, which is know to be higher among children [21].

Differences in mean plantar pressure between the foot regions were similar in children and adults (see Fig. 4). Children and adults showed smaller peak pressure in the midfoot and similar peak pressure in the rearfoot and forefoot. In the older adults higher peak pressure occurred in the forefoot, followed by rearfoot and midfoot. Higher peak of pressure in the forefoot in older adults may rely on altered foot sensitivity in the midfoot and rearfoot. According to a previous research [22], the forward shift in plantar pressure (away from the insensitive heel) constitutes a strategy of older adults to maintain balance. This hypothesis is reinforced by the results of variability in the peak pressure, which was higher in the forefoot of older adults and may be a strategy of older adults to promote propulsion during weight bearing [22].

Assuming that pressure did not differ between steps within each day, we compared the mean values between the fours days of measurement. Children and adults presented similar peak pressure in different days, but in older adults peak values differed between all the days. Children gait suffer continuous adaptations until the adulthood, and therefore some patterns of gait change very fast [23]. However, after reaching the adult age, patterns can be much more stable [14]. We observed that peak pressure varied between the days in older adults. One could argue that variability in the gait speed could determine the variability in peak pressure in older adults. However, gait speed variability in the older adults was 11.23%, which is similar to the 12.80% observed in adults whom showed no differences in the peak pressure between the days. It is possible that variability in the peak pressure rely on tissue characteristics for impact absorption in the elderly, especially stiffness observed in the rearfoot and midfoot [24, 25]. This hypothesis may find support on the higher variability in pressure observed among older adults in comparison to the other groups and the apparent higher dependence on forefoot sensitivity during weight bearing tasks [22].

The age group showed influence on pressure across the regions of the foot. Children and young adults showed similar patterns of plantar pressure distribution with pressure varying between the regions but higher in the rearfoot. In the older adult loading on midfoot was larger than in children and adults. The change in midfoot pressure may rely on increased stiffness in forefoot (hallux and metatarsal I, III and V) as result of aging

[25]. The higher variability in the peak pressure in forefoot among older adults can also be related to the change in foot landing pattern leading to longer contact time during support phase of gait [12].

Our study has inherent limitations. We opted for participants walking at preferred speed. Walking speed may affect plantar pressure and to minimize its effects we considered pressure data normalized to the foot total pressure. Participants were evaluated barefoot, which do not permit to infer on shod walking.

Conclusion

Plantar pressure in children and adults is consistent within and between-days. In other hand, plantar pressure in older adults requires measurements in different days to determine the plantar pressure, especially peak values.

Acknowledgements
PSF, RRA and FGC were supported by student fellowships from CAPES. FAPERGS granted this research to FPC (grant number 1013100).

Funding
FAPERGS granted this research to FPC (grant number 1013100). The agency had no role on the performance of the experiments or writing the paper, just provide financial resources to acquire instrumentation.

Authors' contributions
Experiment design: PSF and FPC.
Data collection and analysis: PSF, CFM, MMF, RAR, FGC.
Manuscript draft and critical review: PSF, CFM, MMF, RAR, FGC and FPC.
Approval of the final version: PSF, CFM, MMF, RAR, FGC and FPC.

Competing interests
All authors declare that they had no financial or personal relationships with other people or organizations that could inappropriately influence their work.

References
1. Gurney JK, Kersting UG, Rosenbaum D. Between-day reliability of repeated plantar pressure distribution measurements in a normal population. Gait & posture. 2008;27:706–9.
2. Franco PS, Silva CB, Rocha ES, Carpes FP. Variability and repeatability analysis of plantar pressure during gait in older people. Rev Bras Reumatol. 2015;55: 427–33.
3. Deepashini H, Omar B, Paungmali A, Amaramalar N, Ohnmar H, Leonard J. An insight into the plantar pressure distribution of the foot in clinical practice: narrative review. Polish Annals of Medicine. 2014;21:51–6.
4. Cousins SD, Morrison SC, Drechsler WI. The reliability of plantar pressure assessment during barefoot level walking in children aged 7-11 years. J Foot Ankle Res. 2012;5
5. Zammit GV, Menz HB, Munteanu SE. Reliability of the TekScan MatScan(R) system for the measurement of plantar forces and pressures during barefoot level walking in healthy adults. J Foot Ankle Res. 2010;3:11.
6. Bus SA, de Lange A. A comparison of the 1-step, 2-step, and 3-step protocols for obtaining barefoot plantar pressure data in the diabetic neuropathic foot. Clin Biomech (Bristol, Avon). 2005;20:892–9.
7. McPoil TG, Cornwall MW, Dupuis L, Cornwell M. Variability of plantar pressure data. A comparison of the two-step and midgait methods. J Am Podiatr Med Assoc. 1999;89:495–501.

8. Hennig EM, Staats A, Rosenbaum D. Plantar pressure distribution patterns of young school children in comparison to adults. Foot & ankle international. 1994;15:35–40.

9. Hennig EM, Rosenbaum D. Pressure distribution patterns under the feet of children in comparison with adults. Foot & ankle. 1991;11:306–11.

10. Bosch K, Gerss J, Rosenbaum D. Preliminary normative values for foot loading parameters of the developing child. Gait & posture. 2007;26:238–47.

11. Bosch K, Gerss J, Rosenbaum D. Development of healthy children's feet– nine-year results of a longitudinal investigation of plantar loading patterns. Gait & posture. 2010;32:564–71.

12. Scott G, Menz HB, Newcombe L. Age-related differences in foot structure and function. Gait & posture. 2007;26:68–75.

13. Menz HB, Zammit GV, Munteanu SE, Scott G. Plantarflexion strength of the toes: age and gender differences and evaluation of a clinical screening test. Foot & ankle international. 2006;27:1103–8.

14. Bosch K, Nagel A, Weigend L, Rosenbaum D. From "first" to "last" steps in life–pressure patterns of three generations. Clin Biomech (Bristol, Avon). 2009;24:676–81.

15. Burns J, Crosbie J, Hunt A, Ouvrier R. The effect of pes cavus on foot pain and plantar pressure. Clin Biomech (Bristol, Avon). 2005;20:877–82.

16. Fernandez-Seguin LM, Diaz Mancha JA, Sanchez Rodriguez R, Escamilla Martinez E, Gomez Martin B, Ramos Ortega J. Comparison of plantar pressures and contact area between normal and cavus foot. Gait & posture. 2014;39:789–92.

17. Shu L, Hua T, Wang YY, Li QA, Feng DD, Tao XM. In-shoe plantar pressure measurement and analysis system based on fabric pressure sensing Array. Ieee T Inf Technol B. 2010;14:767–75.

18. Hughes J, Pratt L, Linge K, Clark P, Klenerman L. Reliability of pressure measurements: the EM ED F system. Clin Biomech (Bristol, Avon). 1991;6:14–8.

19. Wong DW, Niu W, Wang Y, Zhang M. Finite element analysis of foot and ankle impact injury: risk evaluation of calcaneus and talus fracture. PLoS One. 2016;11:e0154435.

20. Zwitser EW, Breederveld RS. Fractures of the fifth metatarsal; diagnosis and treatment. Injury. 2010;41:555–62.

21. Stolze H, Kuhtz-Buschbeck JP, Mondwurf C, Johnk K, Friege L. Retest reliability of spatiotemporal gait parameters in children and adults. Gait & posture. 1998;7:125–30.

22. Machado AS, Bombach GD, Duysens J, Carpes FP. Differences in foot sensitivity and plantar pressure between young adults and elderly. Arch Gerontol Geriatr. 2016;63:67–71.

23. Guffey K, Regier M, Mancinelli C, Pergami P. Gait parameters associated with balance in healthy 2- to 4-year-old children. Gait & posture. 2016;43:165–9.

24. Hsu CC, Tsai WC, Chen CP, et al. Effects of aging on the plantar soft tissue properties under the metatarsal heads at different impact velocities. Ultrasound Med Biol. 2005;31:1423–9.

25. Kwan RL, Zheng YP, Cheing GL. The effect of aging on the biomechanical properties of plantar soft tissues. Clin Biomech. 2010;25:601–5.

16

A case-control study about bite force, symptoms and signs of temporomandibular disorders in patients with idiopathic musculoskeletal pain syndromes

Liete Zwir*[ID], Melissa Fraga, Monique Sanches, Carmen Hoyuela, Claudio Len and Maria Teresa Terreri

Abstract

Background: The purposes of this study were to assess the prevalence of temporomandibular disorders symptoms and signs and the bite force in pediatric patients with idiopathic musculoskeletal pain syndrome and to compare to healthy control individuals paired by gender and age.

Methods: Forty consecutive patients (32 girls) from our outpatient pediatric rheumatology pain clinic with diagnosis of idiopathic musculoskeletal pain syndrome were included in this study. Twenty healthy subjects (16 girls) were considered the control group. All individuals were interviewed according to a standardized questionnaire concerning the presence of orofacial pain and functional impairment, and were submitted to a clinical evaluation following a structured protocol. After that the bite force was measured.

Results: Twelve patients met the ACR criteria for fibromyalgia, and 28 presented the diagnosis of pain amplification syndrome. The mean age of patients was 13.1 years (range, 6–18 years) and of controls was 12.8 years (range, 6–18 years) with no significant difference. Orofacial symptoms occurred in 25 patients (62.5%) and in 3 controls (15%) ($p = 0.0014$). Sixteen (40%) patients and four (20%) controls presented pain during mandibular function with no significant difference. Although both pain groups presented separately more frequently orofacial symptoms and pain on palpation than the controls, maximal voluntary bite force was similar between patients and controls, between both patient groups and between the two pain groups and controls.

Conclusions: Our findings indicate that temporomandibular disorders symptoms were more prevalent in patients with idiopathic musculoskeletal pain syndrome than in healthy controls. However the bite force was not different among the groups.

Background

Chronic musculoskeletal pain in children is common, affecting 10–20% of schoolchildren [1]. Although a serious underlying disease is not the cause in most cases, some may be life-threatening or potentially crippling [2]. A number of children may develop an idiopathic chronic musculoskeletal pain syndrome (IMPS) and become disabled [3]. This syndrome includes three entities: growing pains (limb pain), pain amplification syndrome and fibromyalgia.

Pain amplification syndrome is a condition where patients develop an abnormal pain sensitivity [4]. Fibromyalgia (FM) is currently defined as chronic widespread pain with allodynia or hyperalgesia to pressure pain [5]. FM may coexist with other clinical conditions such as temporomandibular disorders (TMD).

* Correspondence: lfzwir@gmail.com
Universidade Federal de São Paulo (UNIFESP), Rua Guilherme Moura, São Paulo 95, Brazil

TMD is a term that includes clinical disorders involving the masticatory muscles, the temporomandibular joints (TMJ), and associated structures [6]. The most prevalent reported TMD's symptoms in children and adolescents are headaches, TMJ sounds, difficulty in mouth opening, jaw and facial pain, impaired chewing ability and the most common clinical signs of TMD are TMJ and muscle tenderness, limitation of mandibular movements, and TMJ sounds [7].

It has been shown that adult patients with FM have a high prevalence of orofacial signs and symptoms, ranging from 33 to 97% [8–11].

Bite force (BF) is an indicator of the functional state of the masticatory system in children, and can be considered one of the key determinants of the masticatory performance [12, 13]. Signs and symptoms of TMD have been suggested to affect BF measurements [14]. It has been reported that pain in the masticatory muscles and TMJ can cause significant changes in the maximal BF when compared to individuals without such pain [15]. To the best of our knowledge, there is no study addressing BF in pediatric IMPS patients.

The objectives of the present study were to assess the prevalence of TMD symptoms and signs in pediatric patients with IMPS and controls, and to measure the BF in those patients and to compare them to healthy control individuals paired by gender and age.

Methods
Patients
This was a cross-sectional study where sixty-three consecutive patients with diagnosis of IMPS from our outpatient pain clinic in the pediatric rheumatology division were evaluated and forty were included in the final sample. IMPS was defined by the presence of generalized musculoskeletal pain in 3 or more areas of the body for at least 3 months, and these symptoms are not explained by other causes or diseases [3]. FM was characterized by widespread musculoskeletal pain associated with fatigue, sleep, memory and mood issues [5] and pain amplification syndrome was defined as by the presence of musculoskeletal pain without a well-defined organic basis.

Twenty healthy subjects were considered as control group.

The inclusion criteria were patients with IMPS (FM and pain amplification syndrome) as defined in the literature [3, 5]. Healthy subjects who were referred for control orthodontic evaluation were included as control group and were gender and age matched to the patients. Other inclusion criteria for both groups were the presence of the permanent central incisors completed erupted, first permanent molars in occlusion, and the absence of dental related pain. Twenty-three patients

were excluded because they presented problems with their teeth in the areas where the BF was measured.

After informed consent was obtained, demographic and clinical data were collected from the patients' medical records.

Methods
All patients underwent a rheumatologic examination performed by a single pediatric rheumatologist, and an orofacial examination performed by a single dentist. These examinations were scheduled for the same week.

Assessment of subjective symptoms of the TMJ
The subjects were interviewed according to a standardized questionnaire concerning the presence of pain and functional impairment. Patients and their parents answered questions regarding the presence of headaches, abdominal pain, TMJ or masticatory muscle pain at rest or during functional mandibular movements, impaired maximal mouth opening and impaired chewing ability. The questions were answered by categorical (yes/no) responses.

Clinical examination
Only one blind assessor (dentist) performed the clinical evaluation following a structured protocol. The following registrations were made:

- Maximum mouth opening between the incisal edges of the front teeth (in mm) was measured using a millimeter ruler and adjusted for overbite and open bite as necessary. The subjects were asked to open his or her mouth as widely as possible. The patients performed the movements without any help from the examiner. Limitation of opening was defined as a range of movement in the central incisor region of less than 40 mm from the fully occluded to maximal open position [16, 17].
- Presence of pain on palpation on facial sites (6 sites):
  - Presence of tenderness on lateral digital palpation of the TMJ on either side (2 sites);
  - Presence of tenderness on digital palpation of the masseter and temporalis muscles on either side (4 sites);
- Presence of pain on function: during active mandibular movements (open, laterotrusion and protrusion).

Bite force measurement
The BF registration procedure was carefully explained to all participants. Subjects sat in an upright position without head support. The BF was measured unilaterally in the area of the first permanent molars (right and left sides) and central incisors region, using a calibrated dynamometer (Crown DBC, Oswaldo Filizola, São Paulo,

SP, Brazil). The stainless steel rods were 40 mm long X 12.7 mm wide X 13.5 mm thick. A piece of simple disposable foam tape (15 mm long X 13 mm wide X 4 mm tall) covered the BF application site. The peak force measurements were displayed digitally on its screen and recorded for further analysis. The dynamometer was cleaned with alcohol, a piece of sterile latex encased the device and it was replaced after each subject evaluation. Subjects were instructed to bite as hard as possible. The measurements were repeated three times, with one-minute rest between them. The highest value from the three recordings was considered as the maximal BF. The same operator performed all measurements. BF was not taken if the anterior teeth or the first permanent molars were not completely erupted or if they had had extensive restorations. The measured BF was calculated in Newton (N) and displayed digitally.

Written informed consent was obtained from all participants. This study was reviewed and approved by the local Medical Ethics Committee.

Statistical analysis

In order to verify the association between the variables presence of headaches, abdominal pain, and TMD symptoms and signs in the two patient groups, Pearson's chi-square test and Fisher's exact test were used. These tests were also used to evaluate the association between the TMD symptoms and signs in each patient group and the control group. Student's t-test was used to verify the variation of age, maximal mouth opening capacity, and the BF measurements between each patient group and the control group. The STATISTICA 12.7 (Dell®) program was used for the statistical analysis. The level of significance was set to 5% ($p < 0.05$).

Results

This study included 40 patients with IMPS. Twelve met the ACR criteria for FM (11 girls), and 28 (21 girls) presented the diagnosis of pain amplification syndrome. The mean age of patients was 13.1 years (range, 6–18 years) and of controls was 12.8 years (range, 6–18 years) with no significant difference ($p = 0.464$) (Table 1).

TMD symptoms occurred in 25 patients (62.5%) and in 3 controls (15%) ($p = 0.0014$). Sixteen (40%) patients and four (20%) controls presented pain during mandibular function ($p = 0.2081$). During palpation, 36 (90%) patients and only six (30%) controls complained about pain at least in one site ($p < 0.0001$) (Table 1). In addition, the mean measurement of the vertical range of motion of the mandible during maximum unassisted opening was 48.9 mm (ranging from 37 to 50 mm) in patients and 43.4 mm (ranging from 40 to 64 mm) in control group.

Table 1 Demographic and Temporomandibular Disorders (TMD) symptoms and signs and bite force measurement of patients and controls

	Controls	Patients	p
TOTAL (n)	20	40	
Girls (%)	16 (80.0)	32 (80.0)	0.998
Age (mean)	12.8 years	13.1 years	0.464
TMD symptoms (%)	3 (15.0)	25 (62.5)	0.0014*
Pain on palpation (%)	6 (30.0)	36 (90.0)	< 0.0001*
Pain on function (%)	4 (20.0)	16 (40.0)	0.2081
Bite force (mean), in N			
Anterior	143.3	139.7	0.811
Right side	313.2	337.9	0.386
Left side	314.7	353.0	0.107

N Newton, TMD Temporomandibular Disorders
*-statistically significant difference at $p \le .05$

When we compared the two pain groups we observed that the FM group complained more frequently of soft tissue swelling over the TMJ ($p = 0.0175$). We did not find any difference in relation to the frequency of the complaint of headaches or abdominal pain between them. Both pain groups presented similar TMD signs, but there was a statistically difference between the frequency of 4 or more painful sites on palpation in FM patients compared with pain amplification syndrome patients ($p = 0.0375$). All other features did not present significant differences between the two patient groups (Table 2).

Each pain group presented more frequently TMD symptoms and pain on palpation than the controls (Table 3).

Maximal voluntary BF was similar between patients and controls (Table 1), between both patient groups (Table 2) and between the two pain groups and controls (Table 3).

Discussion

TMD symptoms and signs in pediatric patients with idiopathic musculoskeletal pain conditions were evaluated in this study. In this pioneer study, we observed that TMD symptoms and pain on palpation were more frequent in patients than in controls.

In relation to gender we found a greater prevalence of girls in our consecutive sample. It is known that chronic pain in females involves several factors such as behavior, hormones, morphological characteristics, and emotion. Pereira et al. showed that female adolescents are more likely to experience TMD than males [18]. It is important to note that females generally have lower pain thresholds than males [19].

FM and pain amplification syndrome patients presented more pain on palpation when compared to controls. The

Table 2 Temporomandibular Disorders (TMD) symptoms and signs and bite force measurement between the two pain groups

	Fibromyalgia	Pain amplification syndrome	Total %	p value
n (40)	12	28	100%	
TMD symptoms (25)	9	16	62.5	p = 0.4774
Pain in the face (13)	6	6	30	NS
Pain during mastication (7)	1	6	17.5	NS
Tiredness during mastication (18)	6	11	42.5	NS
Soft tissue swelling over the TMJ (7)	5	2	17.5	p = 0.0175*
TMJ sounds (8)	2	6	20	NS
TMD signs				
Pain on function (17)	6	10	40	NS
Opening (14)	4	9	32.5	NS
Protrusion (7)	2	5	17.5	NS
Right laterotrusion (12)	5	6	27.5	NS
Left laterotrusion (7)	3	4	17.5	NS
Pain on palpation (36)	12	24	90	NS
Number of painful sites				
0 (4)	0	4	10	
1 (2)	0	2	5	
2 (0)	0	0	0	
3 (3)	0	3	7.5	
4 (11)	4	7	27.5	
5 (3)	2	1	7.5	
6 (17)	6	11	42.5	
Frequency of 4 or more painful sites (31)	100%	67.80%	77.5	p = 0.0375*
Maximal mouth opening capacity (mean)	51.58 mm	47.85 mm		NS
Bite force (Newton)				
Anterior	154.6	133.3		NS
Right side	344.9	334.9		NS
Left side	343.7	357		NS

N Newton, TMJ Temporomandibular Joint, TMD Temporomandibular Disorders, NS not significant
*statistically significant difference at p ≤ .05

Table 3 Temporomandibular Disorders (TMD) symptoms and signs and bite force measurement of the two patients groups and controls

	Controls	Fibromyalgia	p	Pain Amplification Syndrome	p
TOTAL (n)	20	12		28	
TMD symptoms (%)	3 (15.0)	9(75)	0.001*	16(57.1)	0.003*
Pain on palpation(%)	6 (30.0)	12(100)	0.0001*	24(85.7)	0.0001*
Pain on function(%)	4 (20.0)	6(50)	0.102	10(35.7)	0.252
Bite force (mean) in N					
Anterior	143.3	154.6	0.629	133.3	0.527
Right side	313.2	344.9	0.377	334.9	0.479
Left side	314.7	343.7	0.444	357	0.157

N Newton, TMD Temporomandibular Disorders
*statistically significant difference at p ≤ .05

most important TMD feature is pain, followed by restricted mouth opening capacity and joint sounds as observed by Manfredini [20]. When we compared our findings with this study, we observed a considerable difference, mainly the absence of functional alterations such as restricted mouth opening capacity. Furthermore, we also did not find a difference in BF between patients and controls. These results were unexpected since these patients should have presented the same findings as other patients with TMD symptoms.

BF is an indicator of normal masticatory function, but many factors may influence the values found for this parameter. Facial structure, general muscular force, gender, state of dentition, and signs and symptoms of TMD are some of them [21, 22]. Lower BF was found among adolescents with TMD [23]. Kobayashi et al. did not detect an association between TMD and BF [24]. Similarly, we did not find differences between the pain of patients and controls in relation to BF, even when we compared the two patients groups with the control group and when BF was compared between the two pain conditions.

We found a high prevalence of TMD complaints in our patients with idiopathic musculoskeletal pain, however these complaints did not correspond to the clinical signs. But interestingly, although they presented pain very frequently on palpation they did not present alterations in other clinical parameters such as pain on function, limited mouth opening capacity or lower maximal BF. These findings indicate the need of functional testing for an accurate differential diagnosis with TMD and the appropriate management of those signs and symptoms. One possible explanation for this could be that individuals with idiopathic musculoskeletal pain should be considered as having a somatoform disorder. Somatisation refers to individuals who report symptoms that have no organic cause, or who report symptoms that greatly exceed those expected by the physical condition [2].

The limitations of this study are the small number of patients and the heterogeneity of clinical features that these patients present.

Health professionals who take care of children and adolescents with IMPS should always consider the subjective symptoms related to the orofacial region and the need of an accurate differential diagnosis with TMD; this could provide valuable information for the appropriate conservative management with a multidisciplinary approach.

Conclusions

In conclusion, our findings indicate that TMD symptoms were more prevalent in patients with IMPS than in healthy controls. However, the bite force was not different among the groups.

Authors' contributions

LZ colected the patients data and was the major contributor in writing the manuscript. MF and CL reviewed the manuscript. MS and CH performed the statistical analysis and reviewed the manuscript. MTT analyzed and interpreted the patient data and wrote the manuscript. All authors read and approved the final manuscript.

Competing interests

The authors declare that they have no competing interests.

References

1. Goodman JE, McGrath PJ. The epidemiology of pain in children and adolescents: a review. Pain. 1991;46:247–64.
2. Malleson PN, Beauchamp RD. Diagnosing musculoskeletal pain in children. CMAJ. 2001;165:183–8.
3. Malleson PN, Al-Matar M, Petty RE. Idiopathic musculoskeletal pain syndromes in children. J Rheumatol. 1992;19:1786–9.
4. Sherry DD, Malleson PN. The idiopathic musculoskeletal pain syndromes in childhood. Rheum Dis Clin North Am. 2002;28:669–85.
5. Wolfe F, Smythe HA, Yunus MB, Bennett RM, Bombardier C, Goldenberg DL, et al. The American College of Rheumatology 1990 Criteria for the Classification of Fibromyalgia. Report of the Multicenter Criteria Committee. Arthritis Rheum. 1990;33:160–72.
6. Thilander B, Rubio G, Pena L, Mayorga C. Prevalence of temporomandibular dysfunction and its association with malocclusion in children and adolescents: an epidemiologic study related to specified stages of dental development. Angle Orthod. 2002;72:146–54.
7. Vierola A, Suominen AL, Ikavalko T, Lintu N, Lindi V, Lakka HM, et al. Clinical signs of temporomandibular disorders and various pain conditions among children 6 to 8 years of age: the PANIC study. J Orofac Pain. 2012;26:17-25.
8. Hedenberg-Magnusson B, Ernberg M, Kopp S. Symptoms and signs of temporomandibular disorders in patients with fibromyalgia and local myalgia of the temporomandibular system. A comparative study. Acta Odontol Scand. 1997;55:344–9.
9. Plesh O, Wolfe F, Lane N. The relationship between fibromyalgia and temporomandibular disorders: prevalence and symptom severity. J Rheumatol. 1996;23:1948–52.
10. Salvetti G, Manfredini D, Bazzichi L, Bosco M. Clinical features of the stomatognathic involvement in fibromyalgia syndrome: a comparison with temporomandibular disorders patients. Cranio. 2007;25:127–33.
11. Gui MS, Pimentel MJ, Rizzatti-Barbosa CM. Temporomandibular disorders in fibromyalgia syndrome: a short-communication. Rev Bras Reumatol. 2015;55:189–94.
12. Hatch JP, Shinkai RS, Sakai S, Rugh JD, Paunovich ED. Determinants of masticatory performance in dentate adults. Arch Oral Biol. 2001;46:641–8.
13. Gavião MB, Raymundo VG, Rentes AM. Masticatory performance and bite force in children with primary dentition. Braz Oral Res. 2007;21:146–52.
14. Pereira LJ, Pastore MG, Bonjardim LR, Castelo PM, Gavião MB. Molar bite force and its correlation with signs of temporomandibular dysfunction in mixed and permanent dentition. J Oral Rehabil. 2007;34:759–66.
15. Svensson P, Graven-Nielsen T. Craniofacial muscle pain: review of mechanisms and clinical manifestations. J Orofac Pain. 2001;15:117–45.
16. Sheppard IM, Sheppard SM. Maximal incisal opening—a diagnostic index? J Dent Med. 1965;20:13–5.
17. Agerberg G. Maximal mandibular movements in children. Acta Odontol Scand. 1974;32:147–59.
18. Pereira LJ, Pereira-Cenci T, Del Bel Cury AA, Pereira SM, Pereira AC, Ambosano GM, et al. Risk indicators of temporomandibular disorder incidences in early adolescence. Pediatr Dent. 2010;32:324–8.
19. Buskila D, Press J, Gedalia A, Klein M, Neumann L, Boehm R, et al. Assessment of nonarticular tenderness and prevalence of FS in children. J Rheumatol. 1993;20:368–70.
20. Manfredini D, Guarda-Nardini L, Winocur E, Piccotti F, Ahlberg J, Lobbezoo F. Research diagnostic criteria for temporo-mandibular disorders: a systematic review of axis I epidemiologic findings. Oral Surg Oral Med Oral Pathol Oral Radiol Endod. 2011;112:453–62.

21. Kiliaridis S, Kjellberg H, Wenneberg B, Engstrom C. The relationship between bite force endurance and facial morphology during growth. A cross-sectional study. Acta Odontol Scand. 1993;51:323–31.

22. Sonnesen L, Bakke M. Molar bite force in relation to occlusion, craniofacial dimensions, and head posture in pre-orthodontic children. Eur J Orthod. 2005;27:58–63.

23. Bonjardim LR, Gaviao MB, Pereira LJ, Castelo PM. Bite force determination in adolescents with and without temporomandibular dysfunction. J Oral Rehabil. 2005;32:577–83.

24. Kobayashi FY, Gavião MB, Montes AB, Marquezin MC, Castelo PM. Evaluation of oro-facial function in young subjects with temporomandibular disorders. J Oral Rehabil. 2014;41:496–506.

17

Effects of a health education program on cytokines and cortisol levels in fibromyalgia patients

Andrei Pereira Pernambuco[1,2,3]* (iD), Lucina de Souza Cota Carvalho[1,4], Luana Pereira Leite Schetino[1,5], Janaíne Cunha Polese[6], Renato de Souza Viana[7] and Débora d' Ávila Reis[1]

Abstract

Background: Fibromyalgia (FM) is a syndrome characterized by widespread chronic pain associated to other symptoms, such as: fatigue, anxiety, depression and sleep disorders. Health education programs (HEP) have emerged as good non-pharmacological strategies to treat it. However, it is still not clear if the benefits are only subjective, or it has also objective impacts on immune and or neuroendocrine systems.

Methods: Fifty-eight fibromyalgia women were randomly allocated in experimental group ($n = 27$) or control group ($n = 31$). The experimental group was submitted to HEP treatment for 11 weeks, while control group did not receive intervention at the same period. All data were collected at zero and 11th week by a blinded researcher. The statistical analysis were made in GraphPad Prism software (version 5.0) with significant level adjusted for $\alpha = 0.05$.

Results: Forty-four patients concluded the full study, 21 in the experimental group and 23 in the control group. Intragroup and intergroup analysis revealed that treatment induced significant increases of IL-4 plasma levels, anti-inflammatory cytokine/inflammatory cytokine ratio (AC/IC ratio), salivary cortisol levels, in addition to significant decreases on FIQ scores. Intergroup variation analyses revealed also significant increases of IL-10 plasma levels.

Conclusion: The results presented suggest that this kind of HEP could induce subjective and objective changes (immune and neuroendocrine), that could explain, at least in part the improvement of fibromyalgia patient's health status.

Keywords: Fibromyalgia, Health education program, Treatment, Cortisol, Cytokines

Background

Fibromyalgia (FM) is a syndrome characterized by chronic widespread pain associated to others symptoms such as fatigue, anxiety, depression and sleep disturbances [1]. Some studies have provided evidence of the neuroendocrine and immune systems involvement in FM, [2–5] but its pathophysiology remain unclear despite all studies in the area [6].

FM has been considered a clinical condition derived from disturbances in the stress system, with abnormalities in the hypothalamic-pituitary-adrenal (HPA) axis and in the serotoninergic system [3, 7, 8]. Patients bearing this syndrome present significant abnormalities in the levels of some hormones such as melatonin [5] and cortisol, [3] and of inflammatory cytokines [4]. For the treatment of this chronic condition, a range of pharmacological and non-pharmacological treatments have been used, however, its multifactorial etiology, associated with patients' clinical heterogeneity has turned out extremely difficult to establish efficient therapeutic practices [6].

Regarding the non-pharmacological treatments, health education programs (HEP) have been successfully adopted in some cases. They can induce healthy habits, coping strategies and empowerment, and their benefits have been demonstrated through clinical progress evaluations, that consider subjective variables such as pain level, fatigue, sleep quality, anxiety and depression [9–11].

* Correspondence: pernambucoap@ymail.com
[1]Departamento de Morfologia, Instituto de Ciências Biológicas da Universidade Federal de Minas Gerais (UFMG), Avenida Presidente Antônio Carlos, 6627 - Pampulha, Belo Horizonte, MG CEP 31270-901, Brazil
[2]Centro Universitário de Formiga, MG. Avenida Doutor Arnaldo de Senna, 328. Água, Vermelha, Formiga, MG CEP 35570-000, Brazil
Full list of author information is available at the end of the article

In the current study we aimed to evaluate if HEP could impact on objective immune and neuroendocrine parameters, besides subjective variables. For this purpose, after 11 week of intervention, we evaluated plasma levels of cytokines: IL-2, IL-4, IL-6, IL-10, TNF, and IL-17A, salivary cortisol levels, and general health status of FM patients evaluated through the self-administered Fibromyalgia Impact Questionnaire (FIQ).

Methods
Ethical aspects
The research protocol was approved by Human Research Committee of XXXXX and by the XXXXX (protocol numbers: 0224.0.203.000–10 and 141/2010). All participants were volunteers and provided written informed consent before inclusion in this study.

Sample size calculation
Based on previous studies that has used the similar intervention [10] and outcomes[2,12,13] which included sample sizes varying between 15 and 30 participants per group, it was estimate a minimum of 21 participants for each group. In order to verify the statistical power of the results achieved with that sample size, a posteriori calculation was performed, using the G*Power software (Version 3.1.9.2), [12] considering a 0.05 significance level ($\alpha = 0.05$) and a power of 80% ($\beta = 0.20$). The variable AC/IC ratio values were used for calculation.

Participants
Patient recruitment was done through advertisements in local radio, print newspapers and posters displayed in health facilities of Formiga, Minas Gerais, Brasil. All potential patients were submitted to clinical evaluation for the research physician to confirm the FM diagnosis according to the 1990's American College of Rheumatology (ACR) criteria [13]. The new diagnosis criteria [1] was not used because they were published after submission of the research project to the Ethics Committee. It was included every women with: confirmed FM diagnosis, those aged between 18 and 60 years old, fluent in Portuguese and who that gave written informed consent. It was excluded every woman that: were not literate, have not confirmed the FM diagnosis, those aged under 18 and over 60 years old, who had past or present of chronic inflammatory disease (such as spondyloarthritis and ankylosing spondylitis) or autoimmune diseases (such as systemic lupus erythematosus or rheumatoid arthritis), who had past or present of psychiatric diseases (such as major depression, schizophrenia, bipolar disorder), who presented acute infectious disease at the time of data collect, who had used anti-allergic, antibiotics or anti-inflammatory drugs in the last three months, those who got pregnant or breast-feeding and those who had no pharmacological stability for a period of at least

three months before the beginning of the intervention or who changed medicines during the intervention period [4, 5]. No man was selected for the study because fibromyalgia affects up to nine women for each affected man, [6] in addition the inclusion of men in a sample composed mostly of women could generate interpretation bias.

Study design
It is a randomized clinical trial with parallel group approved by Brazilian Register of Clinical Trials ReBEC-RBR-5tdnbr (full protocol available in http://www.ensaiosclinicos.gov.br/rg/RBR-5tdnbr/). Seventy-five women were enrolled to the study, but only fifty-eight had confirmed FM diagnosis. Those 58 women were randomly allocated by envelope at experimental or control group. The experimental group was submitted to treatment by Inter-relational School of fibromyalgia, while the control group did not receive intervention at the same period. Both groups had collected blood and saliva samples and filled the FIQ questionnaire at zero and 11th week. All data were collected by a blinded researcher regarding the study objectives and groups (Fig. 1).

Intervention
The experimental group was submitted to the HEP based on the "Inter-relational School of Fibromyalgia (ISF), [10] with some modifications. The intervention started in June 2012. The description of the activities is shown at Table 1. The original ISF use predominantly vertical lectures, but we opted for more patient-oriented and interactive approaches. In each meeting day, the monitors briefly presented the general issue to be addressed, and soon after started up a casual conversation that was based on personal questions raised by the attendees. The duration of the intervention was eleven weeks with a face-to-face meeting once a week and a pause of fifteen days between the sixth and seventh week. This pause was considering important to allow the incorporation of the activities to the daily routine of the participants [10]. Each meeting had two health professionals whose formation varied according to the discussed topic [10]. The duration of the intervention, the number of meetings, the break and the topics covered in each meeting were based on the original study by Souza et al. [10].

During the first eleven weeks, the control group was not submitted to any intervention. Patients were kept in hold and they submitted to the HEP treatment only after the completion of the research.

Data collection
A trained professional unknowing the study objectives and groups performed all data collection. All data of interest were collected in both groups at the same time

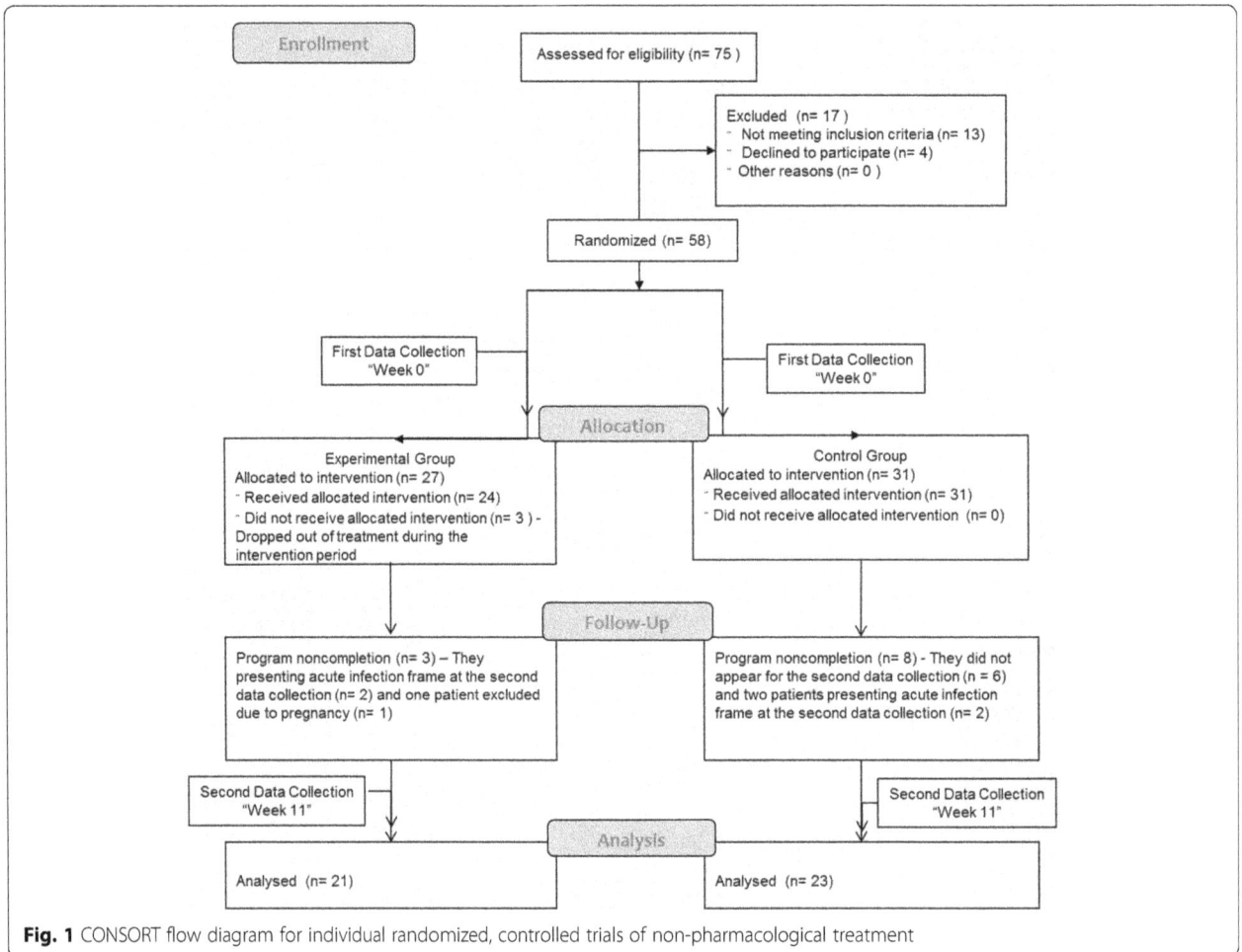

Fig. 1 CONSORT flow diagram for individual randomized, controlled trials of non-pharmacological treatment

and in two moments: a) baseline – before intervention b) after eleven weeks of intervention (Fig. 1).

Cytokines levels

Blood sample was collected in the morning using tubes coated with ethylenediamine tetraacetic acid (EDTA) as the anticoagulant and it was immediately centrifuged for 10 min, at 4 °C and 2000 rpm and the plasma was collected and stored at -80 °C. To measure the cytokine levels it was used the BD™ Cytometric Bead Array kit (CBA) $T_H1/T_H2/T_H17$ according to the manufactory instructions (BD Bioscience, San Jose, CA, USA). The flow cytometer data acquisition was performed using the FACSCalibur (BD Bioscience, San Jose, CA, USA) and the data analyses were done by BD CellQuest Software (BD Bioscience, San Jose, CA, USA). The cytokines levels were calculated by FlowJo 7.6.1 Software (Tree StarTM, Inc., Ashland, OR) and were expressed as pg/ml. The AC/IC ratio was calculated by sum of anti-inflammatory cytokines (IL-4 + IL-10) and the resulted was divided by the sum of inflammatory cytokines (IL-2 + IL-6 + TNF + IL-17A).

Salivary cortisol levels

Salivary cortisol levels were used as an objective marker of HPA axis activity. Saliva samples from patients of experimental and control group were collected using cotton rolls at 8 a.m. at the day before blood sample collected. Subjects were instructed not to intake food nor brush their teeth 30 min before sample collection to avoid contamination of saliva samples, and to store saliva samples at their freezers until completing the experimental protocol and then return the samples to the laboratory. Samples were centrifuged and frozen at −20 °C until the analysis. Free cortisol in saliva was determined using a time-resolved immunoassay according manufactory instructions (DSL-10 67,100 Diagnostic Systems Laboratories, Webster, TX, USA). The sensitivity of this test was 0.071 ng/ml. The intra- and inter-assay coefficients of variation were 5.4 and 9.3% respectively.

Fibromyalgia impact questionnaire – FIQ

It is a self-administered questionnaire designed specifically to analyses the current health status of FM patients [14]. It

Table 1 Description of activities

Meeting topic	Objective
1a – Therapeutic Contract / 1b-Workshop of the senses	Briefly introducing the nine steps of the program and negotiate the therapeutic contract. This contract has an objective to modulate the expectations of patients and consists of: a) define three realistic and measurable personal objectives; b) determine the lowest percentage of improvement in the clinical picture, acceptable (between 5 and 20%). According to the contract, participants also agree to devote 45 min/day, 6 days/week to practice the activities prescribed by the ISF such as relaxation techniques, diaphragmatic breathing, stretching, strengthening and aerobic exercise. Promoting experimentation of sensory organs. Discuss the ways in which people feel and perceive the world and the reality around them. Demonstrating deep diaphragmatic breathing.
2 –Mental Preparation	Demonstrating that the environment perceptions are related to previous experience and so then perception of pain, as well as other symptoms may also be influenced by prior experience. Demonstrate some techniques of mental preparation and coping strategies to deal with the pain. Practice yoga class with emphasis on meditation. The participant will choose a relaxation technique and practice it 3 times a week for 15 to 20 min.
3 – Physical preparation	Discussing the effects of a sedentary lifestyle and physical activity. Demonstrate warm-up, stretching, strengthening and aerobic exercises. Perform calculations to identify heart rate (HR) max. Practice session of Pilates on the ground. Prescribe an exercise program to be held at home: a) exercise routine: 6 times/week, 15 min, with stretching and strengthening; b) walk, moderate 40 to 60% HR max; 3 times/week; 30 min.
4 – Stress and individuality	Studying the hypothalamic-pituitary-adrenal axis, its importance in the homeostatic systems and stress. Discussing coping strategies that contribute to the understanding and improvement of individual levels of energy / disposition (learn to say no when necessary, defer or delegate tasks at moments of suffering, be seen and be valued)
5 – Symptoms	Studying the mechanisms involved in pain, fatigue, muscle stiffness, in sleep disorders, anxiety and depression.
6 – Nutrition	Discussing the basic components of a healthy balanced diet, the benefits of hydration and the dangers provided by foods rich in sugars, fats and or sodium.
PAUSE	2 weeks of self-employment: integration of strategies individually (without meeting with therapists).
7 – Consequence of chronicity	Discussing the influence of chronic pain on the emotional, interpersonal relationships, daily activities and sexuality. Discuss aspects related to suicidal thoughts.
8 – Treatment	Presenting and discuss scientific evidence based on the main types of pharmacological and non-pharmacological treatments currently used to treat fibromyalgia.
9 – Retrospective	Motivate patients to continue the prescribed activities. Presenting a retrospective of the issues addressed.

Adapted from Souza et al., 2008 [10]. All prescribed activities are cumulative and must be maintained throughout the study period. At the end of each meeting the participants were given an activity book that should be performed during the week. The activity book filled was returned to researchers at the beginning of the next meeting. All meetings were held on Saturdays, from 9:00 a.m. to 11:00 a.m. at an University Center

is compound by 19 questions that evaluated the physical functioning, work status (missed days of work and job difficulty) depression, anxiety, morning tiredness, pain, stiffness, fatigue and well-being over the past week. The questions are scored from 0 to 10 wherein the final score could vary from 0 to 100. Higher scores are related to more severe impact in the quality of life [14]. The Brazilian version of the FIQ was used [15].

Statistical analysis

The management of the database and statistical analyzes were performed by an independent researcher, blinded regarding the groups. Professionals responsible for intervention carried out the adherence to the treatment. Descriptive statistics were performed for all outcome measures. The effect of the intervention was analyzed considering only the patients who started and completed the study. The Kolmogorov-Smirnov (with Dallal-Wilkinson Lilliefor p-value) was used to evaluate the distribution of the data. Paired t test was used for comparison between pretreatment and post treatment in both groups. Student's T test or Mann-Whitney test was used to investigate intergroup results. The post treatment data in the experimental group were also

used to perform a linear regression test using the AC/IC as dependent variable. All data were analyzed with GraphPad Prism software (version 5.0) with significance set at 5% level ($\alpha = 0.05$). The results were presented as mean ± standard deviation, and intra-group and inter-group differences were also presented as mean ± standard deviation and 95% confidence interval (95% CI).

Results
Adherence to treatment

Fifth-eight patients were initially enrolled in the study, and forty-four remained until the end o of the research. In the experimental group, three women dropped out during the intervention period (two women claimed they did not have time to participate in activities due to domestic chores and one claimed that she needed to discontinue treatment to travel with her family). Moreover, three patients were excluded close to the end, two of them because of the change in pharmacological treatment, and one because of pregnancy. In the control group, six women dropped out (three of them gave up because of the waiting time, two changed their mind and one moved out). In this group, two patients were excluded because they changed pharmacological treatment (Fig. 1).

Studied groups

The mean age of the 44 women that concluded the study was 49.77 ± 11.13 years old and the body mass index (BMI) was 26.65 ± 4.70 kg/m^2. The mean time of diagnosis was 6.14 ± 5.55 years and mean tender point count was 16.28 ± 1.76. There were no statistical differences between groups considering age, BMI, time of diagnosis and tender point count (Table 2).

Baseline

Table 3 demonstrates that there was not significant difference between groups at the beginning of the study considering the following variables: serum levels of IL-2, IL-4, IL-6, IL-10, TNF, IL-17A, AC/IC ratio, salivary cortisol levels, and FIQ score.

Intervention effects

For intragroup analysis, differences between baseline data and 11th week data were calculated. The group that was submitted to intervention presented increasing of the following parameters analyzed: IL-4 plasma levels **(MD = 0.76; 95%CI = 0.14 to 1.39; p = 0.02)**, AC/IC ratio **(MD = 0.07; 95%CI = 0.01 to 0.13; p = 0.02)**, and salivary cortisol levels **(MD = 0.98; 95%CI = 0.18 to 1.78; p= 0,02)** and significant reduced in the mean FIQ score **(MD = – 30.36; 95%CI = – 39.16 to – 21.56, p < 0.01)**. The other data did not evidence any significant difference during the study period (Fig. 2).

The analysis of difference in the baseline data and at the end of the study in the control group did not show significant differences (Fig. 3).

To evaluate the intergroup analysis, it was calculated the difference between the value of each variable at the 11th week and week zero to every participant to determine the individual variation and followed the means variation of each data. This analysis showed that FM patients from experimental group had significant increased plasma levels of IL-4 **(MD = 1.48; 95%CI = 0.40 to 2.56; p< 0,01)** and IL-10 **(MD =**

0.39; 95%CI = 0.01 to 0.76; p = 0,04), such as significant increase in AC/IC ratio **(MD = 0.10; 95%CI = 0.01 to 0.19; p = 0,03)** and in the salivary cortisol levels **(MD = 1.35; 95%CI = 0.11 to 2.60; p = 0,03)**, in the other hand, it was noticed significant reduced in mean FIQ score **(MD = – 31.42; 95%CI = – 42.96 to – 19.88; p < 0.01)**. No other data presented any significant difference between groups (Table 4).

The regression analysis in the experimental group showed that IL-4 levels at the end of the study explained 51% of the variance on AC/IC ratio **(β = 0.06; 95%CI 0.01 to 0.11; p = 0.02)**.

Discussion

One of the hypotheses that try to explain the pathophysiology of FM is the central sensitization of pain transmission pathways with concomitant increase of neurotransmitters and inflammatory cytokines in the cerebrospinal fluid [16]. Such changes appear to be related to HPA axis dysfunctions, such as decreased release of cortisol, which in turn may influence the metabolic and immune activity of the individual [3]. We believe that the hypocortisolism presented by fibromyalgia patients is responsible for an inflammatory state with increased of inflammatory cytokines [2, 3, 17, 18] that could affected the nociceptors [19, 20].

In this study, we chose to use an RCT for the study of biomarkers in FM patients because most of the research using non-pharmacological treatments for FM uses only subjective variables collected through questionnaires and or interviews [10, 21]. However, here we would like to know if the subjective changes presented by such studies are accompanied by objective changes in biomarkers of immune and neuroendocrine activity. The biomarkers used in this study were selected because they are frequently described as altered in patients with FM [2, 3, 17, 18]. In this sense, the HEP adopted in this study was able to promote reducing of FIQ scores, and, interestingly, it also induces objective changes revealed by changes in salivary cortisol levels, plasma cytokine levels (IL-4 and IL-10) and AC/IC ratio.

Both cytokines, IL-4 and IL-10, are very important in the modulation of immune response [2]. IL-4

Table 2 Studied groups

	Experimental (n = 21)	Control (n = 23)	Mean Difference (MD)		P value
Age (years)	51.43 ± 11.26	48.26 ± 11.03	3.17 ± 3.36	−3.62 a 9.96	0.35
BMI (Kg/cm^2)	26.51 ± 5.18	26.82 ± 4.22	− 0.31 ± 1.53	−3.41 a 2.79	0.84
Time of diagnostic (years)	5.47 ± 5.05	6.74 ± 6.02	− 1.26 ± 1.68	−4.66 a 2.14	0.46
Tender points (number)	16.05 ± 1.79	16.48 ± 1.75	− 0.43 ± 0.54	−1.52 a 0.66	0.43

The above data were collected from both groups during the pre-intervention. It was considered only the data of patients who completed all stages of research. Data expressed were as mean ± standard deviation and 95% confidence interval (95% CI)

Table 3 Baseline data

	Experimental (n = 21)	Control (n = 23)	Mean of difference (MD)	95% CI	P value
IL-2	2.79 ± 1.50	2.59 ± 1.28	0.21 ± 0.43	− 0.66 to 1.07	0.84
IL-4	1.67 ± 1.17	1.93 ± 0.93	− 0.25 ± 0.33	− 0.92 to 0.41	0.25
IL-6	4.13 ± 4.08	4.83 ± 6.40	− 0.70 ± 1.73	−4.21 to 2.81	0.91
IL-10	1.13 ± 0.47	1.14 ± 0.44	− 0.004 ± 0.14	−0.29 to 0.29	0.86
TNF	0.86 ± 0.92	1.11 ± 1.09	−0.25 ± 0.31	−0.87 to 0.37	0.35
IL-17A	11.45 ± 7.26	13.14 ± 8.56	−1.70 ± 2.52	−6.81 to 3.42	0.44
AC/IC ratio	0.13 ± 0.04	0.18 ± 0.11	− 0.04 ± 0.03	−0.10 to 0.01	0.13
Cortisol	5.28 ± 1.67	4.63 ± 1.35	0.64 ± 0.46	− 0.29 to 1.58	0.17
FIQ	72.65 ± 15.10	77.54 ± 8.53	− 4.89 ± 3.83	− 12.65 to 2.87	0.21

The above data were collected from both groups during the baseline. Only the data of 44 patients who completed all stages of the research were considered. Data were expressed as mean ± standard deviation and 95% confidence interval (95% CI)

induces the phosphorylation of the transcription factor STAT6, and thus inhibits the production of some inflammatory cytokines and chemokines such as IL-1β, IL-6, IL-8 and TNF- α by macrophages and monocytes [22, 23]. IL-10 has been considered one of the most powerful anti-inflammatory cytokines, since it blocks NFkB pathway and module JAK-STAT pathway decreasing the synthesis of IL-1, IL-6, TNF and IFNγ by macrophages and Th1 cells [24, 25]. In FM patients, decreased levels of IL- 4 and IL-10 have been described [2, 26]. In this context, the observed HEP induced increasing in both, IL-4 and IL-10 levels, point to the success of such intervention, by inducing a more modulatory immune response. Indeed, IL-4 and IL-10 have been tested in therapeutic interventions in some autoimmune diseases such as psoriasis and rheumatoid arthritis with satisfactory results [27–29]. It is also important to mention that if the inflammatory changes observed in FM are really associated with dysregulation of the HPA axis, [3] it is likely that other health conditions related to psychoemotional stress may benefit from this type of intervention [30–32]. To confirm this hypothesis, further studies should be conducted.

Another important finding in this study was the increased AC/IC ratio presented by HEP treated group that was mainly influenced by the increased levels of IL-4. According to the literature, the imbalance between anti-inflammatory and inflammatory cytokines is one of the responsible for the occurrence and perpetuation of FM symptoms [2, 4, 33–35]. Low levels of IL – 4 and IL-10 have been related to depressive behavior and pain (IL-4), [31] chronic fatigue (IL-10) [36] and hyperalgesia (IL-10) [26]. In the current study, HEP induced increased levels of IL-4 and IL-10 associated with decreased in FIQ score, which in turn is an indicative of an improved clinical status and

quality of life [14, 15]. It is likely that the reduction in FIQ scores is related, at least in part, to the Hawthorne effect. This effect, known as the expectation effect of the individual, consists of positive changes in the behavior of subjects or groups simply because they are receiving attention or interest from others [37, 38]. However, some strategies used in HEP, such as stress management activities and physical activities are able to ameliorate the inflammatory process and improve the health [39–41].

The HEP treatment also induced an enhanced in the salivary morning cortisol levels, which is a clinically important finding. Hypocortisolism in FM, mainly in the morning, has been demonstrated by some studies, [3, 42] and it has been considered to be responsible in part by the claimed pain, fatigue and depression by FM patients [17, 43]. It is important to note that the hypocortisolism presented by FM patients are related to HPA axis dysfunction, also named stress response axis [3]. According to this theory, individuals expose to stress agents (physical or psychoemotional) for long periods could experience a phenomenon called burnout syndrome, characterized by lower cortisol production in response to stress agent [30]. We believe that the increasing of cortisol levels in the experimental group could indicate that the coping strategies taught in the ISF contributed in a positive way to these patients, helping them to live or face more adequately the different types of adversity.

In this study, 78% of those enrolled to treatment remained until the end of the 11th week (the researchers excluded 11% and the other 11% dropped out the study). If we consider only the participants who voluntarily withdrew from the study, the adherence to treatment was 89%. It has been considered that adhesion to treatment is one of the main

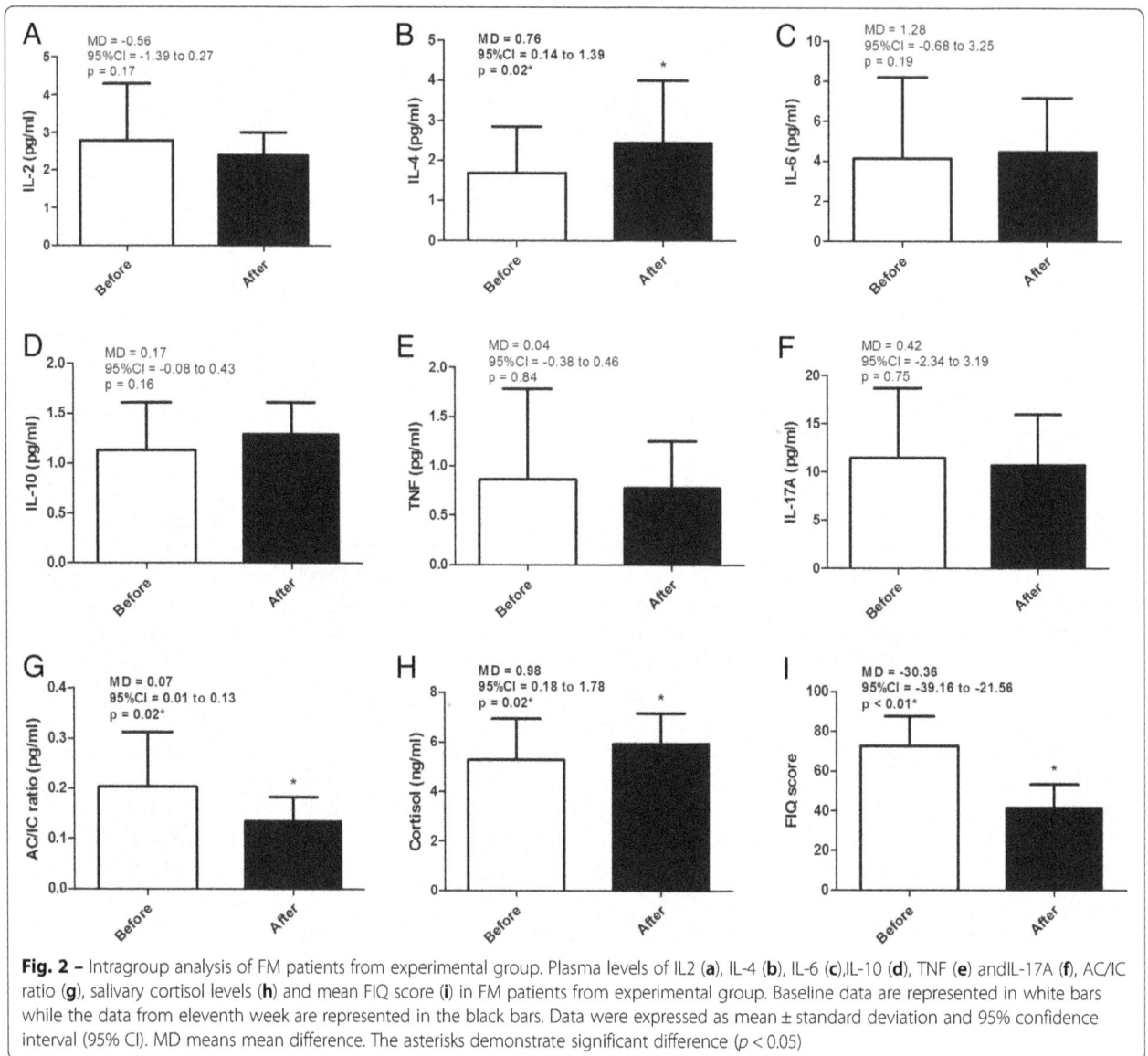

Fig. 2 – Intragroup analysis of FM patients from experimental group. Plasma levels of IL2 (**a**), IL-4 (**b**), IL-6 (**c**),IL-10 (**d**), TNF (**e**) andIL-17A (**f**), AC/IC ratio (**g**), salivary cortisol levels (**h**) and mean FIQ score (**i**) in FM patients from experimental group. Baseline data are represented in white bars while the data from eleventh week are represented in the black bars. Data were expressed as mean ± standard deviation and 95% confidence interval (95% CI). MD means mean difference. The asterisks demonstrate significant difference ($p < 0.05$)

negative points in the HEP [10, 21]. In this study the HEP adherence level could be considered satisfactory, and we think that it could be explained mainly by the use of a patient-centered methodology, instead of using traditional models of HEP, with hierarchical relationships.

Finally, the results from the present study, in conjunction with data from the literature, reinforces the hypothesis that HEP might satisfactorily contribute to FM patients treatment. After all, in this group of FM patients, the HEP like ISF, not only promoted the subjective perception of improvement in the FM patients, but, above all, they were able to promote objective changes in biomarkers of neuroendocrine and

immunological activity. Because of the sample size and clinical variability presented by people with FM, [6] it is not possible to state that this type of intervention will promote the same benefits for all other FM patients. Thus, the use of HEP for FM should be a choice of the health professional in agreement with the patient. We encourage further studies with larger sample size and that seek to analyze other important biomarkers for fibromyalgia.

Conclusion

The HEP like ISF program significantly improved the health status of the participants underwent intervention. This was evidenced by increased plasma levels of IL-4

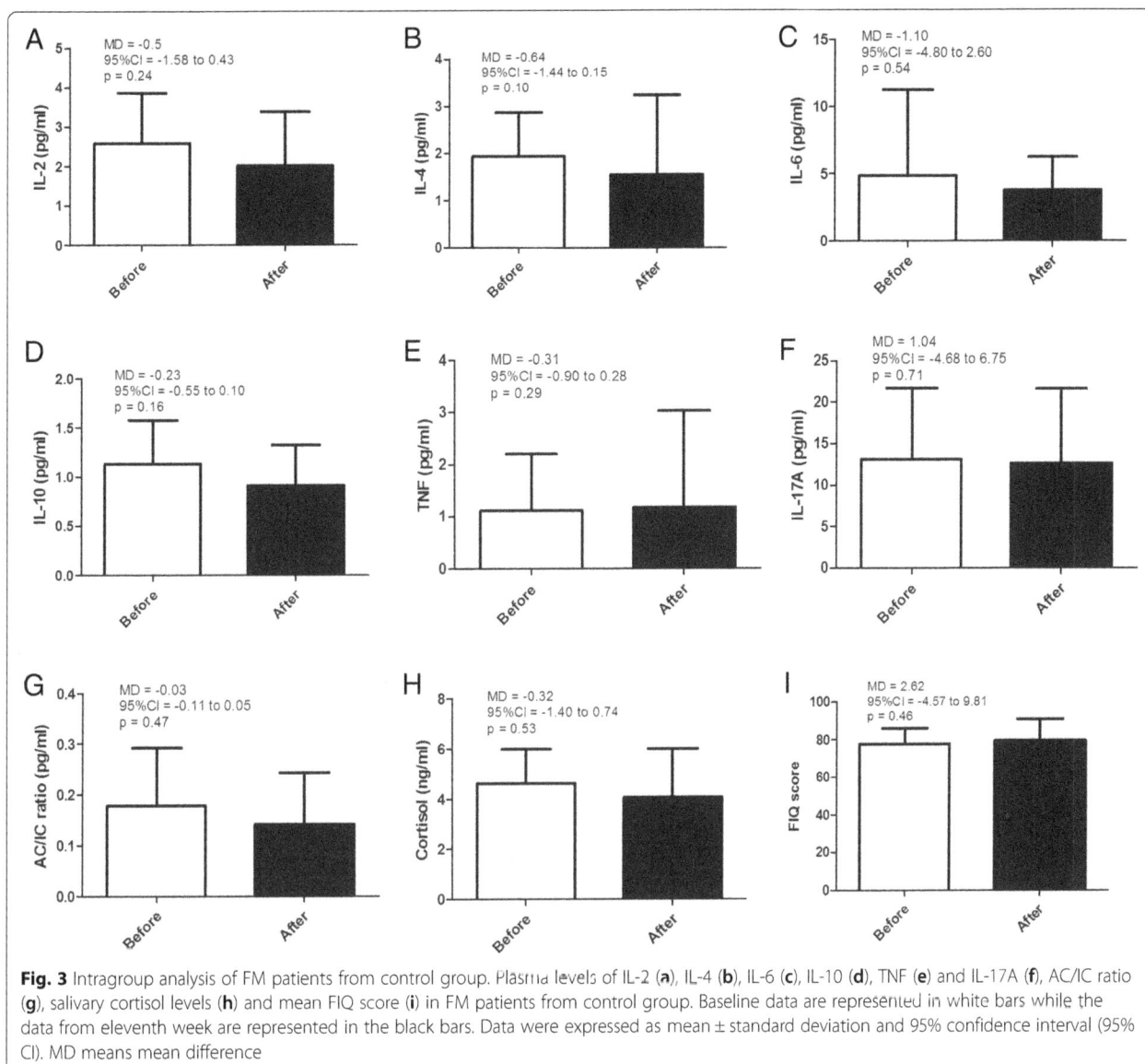

Fig. 3 Intragroup analysis of FM patients from control group. Plasma levels of IL-2 (**a**), IL-4 (**b**), IL-6 (**c**), IL-10 (**d**), TNF (**e**) and IL-17A (**f**), AC/IC ratio (**g**), salivary cortisol levels (**h**) and mean FIQ score (**i**) in FM patients from control group. Baseline data are represented in white bars while the data from eleventh week are represented in the black bars. Data were expressed as mean ± standard deviation and 95% confidence interval (95% CI). MD means mean difference

Table 4 Intergroup analysis at the eleventh week

	VariationEG (EGV)	Variation CG (CGV)	MD (EGV minus CGV)	95%CI	p value
IL2	−0.56	−0.58	0.47 ± 0.77	−1.09 to 2.03	0.54
IL4	0.76	−0.64	*1.48 ± 0.53**	*0.40 to 2.56**	*< 0.01**
IL6	1.28	−1.10	4.98 ± 2.69	−0.46 to 10.42	0.07
IL10	0.17	−0.23	*0.39 ± 0.18**	*0.01 to 0.76**	*0.04**
TNF	0.04	−0.31	0.12 ± 0.32	−0.53 to 0.78	0.70
IL17	0.42	1.04	−2.66 ± 4.09	−10.95 to 5.62	0.51
AC/IC ratio	0.05	−0.04	*0.10 ± 0.04**	*0.01 to 0.19**	*0.03**
Cortisol	0,98	−0.32	*1.35 ± 0.61**	*1.11 to 2.60**	*0.03**
FIQ	−30.36	2.62	*−31.42 ± 5.70**	*− 42.96 to − 19.88**	*< 0.01**

Comparative analysis of variations in the experimental group (EGV) and variations in the control group (CGV) at the end of the 11th week study. To determine the variation within each of the groups was calculated the difference between the value of the variables obtained at the 11th week of the study and the value of the variables obtained at week zero, for every participant. The results were presented as mean ± standard deviation and 95% confidence interval (95%CI). MD refers to the mean of the differences. *Statistically significant results were marked with an asterisk and have been shown in boldface and italic

and IL-10, increase AC/ IC ratio, and the salivary cortisol levels of the participants underwent the intervention in addition to reduced FIQ score. Despite the limited sample size, we recommend the use of HEP like ISF to treat FM patients and we expect that this study may serve as a starting point for further investigations to clarify issues that were not addressed here.

Acknowledgments
We thank the Fundação de Amparo à Pesquisa do Estado de Minas Gerais (FAPEMIG) for the financial support of the Fundação Oswaldo Cruz Foundation (FIOCRUZ) – Instituto René Rachou for laboratory analysis and the Centro Universitário de Formiga - MG (UNIFOR-MG) for logistical support to the project.

Funding
The Fundação de Amparo à Pesquisa do Estado de Minas Gerais (FAPEMIG) financed the PhD scholarship of the APP researcher and the purchase of the reagents for laboratory analysis. The funding agency did not participate in the project's elaboration and did not participate in any stage of project execution or writing of the manuscript.

Declaration
We declare that this research protocol was submitted to the Ethic Committee of Universidade Federal de Minas Gerais and to the Ethic Committee of Centro Universitário de Formiga and that the protocol was approved by both committees according to their respective decisions: ETIC n° 0224.0.203.00–10 and N° 141/210.

We also stated that all participants in the research signed a two-way informed consent form. These and other procedures were based on CNS Resolution 196/96 and the Helsinki Declaration.

Finally, we declare that this randomized clinical trial was protocolized and approved in the Brazilian Registry of Clinical Trials and received the Clinical Trial Registration Number (ReBEC - RBR- 5tdnbr).

Authors' contributions
APP - Planning of the research project, submission to the Ethics Committee, recruitment of participants, initial data collection, intervention, final data collection, laboratory analysis, tabulation of results, article writing, submission to Advances in Rheumatology. LSCC – Co advisor, planning of the research project initial data collection, intervention, final data collection, laboratory analysis, article writing. LPLS - Initial data collection, intervention, final data collection, laboratory analysis, article writing. JCP - Statistical analyzes, article writing. RSV - Selection of participants, confirmation of the diagnosis of fibromyalgia, screening for inclusion and exclusion criteria. DAR – Advisor, planning of the research project, intervention, laboratory analysis, article writing. * All authors read and approved the final manuscript.

Competing interest
All authors declare that there is no conflict of interest related to this article.

Competing interests
We declare that there is no competing interest related to this manuscript, be it financial or otherwise.

Author details
[1]Departamento de Morfologia, Instituto de Ciências Biológicas da Universidade Federal de Minas Gerais (UFMG), Avenida Presidente Antônio Carlos, 6627 - Pampulha, Belo Horizonte, MG CEP 31270-901, Brazil. [2]Centro Universitário de Formiga, MG. Avenida Doutor Arnaldo de Senna, 328. Água, Vermelha, Formiga, MG CEP 35570-000, Brazil. [3]Universidade de Itaúna, MG. Rodovia MG, 431 Km 45, s/n - Campus Verde, Itaúna, MG CEP 35680-142, Brazil. [4]Hospital Mater Dei, Avenida do Contorno, 9000 - Barro Preto, Belo Horizonte, MG CEP 30110-064, Brazil. [5]Universidade Federal do Vale do Jequitinhonha e Mucuri - Campus I. Rua da Glória, n° 187 – Centro, Diamantina, MG CEP 39100-000, Brazil. [6]Pós-Graduação em Ciências da Reabilitação da Universidade Federal de Minas Gerais, Avenida Presidente Antônio Carlos, 6627 - Pampulha, Belo Horizonte, MG CEP 31270-901, Brazil. [7]Santa Casa de Caridade de Formiga, MG. Rua Doutor Teixeira Soares, 335 - Centro, Formiga, MG CEP 35570-000, Brazil.

References
1. Wolfe F, Hauser W. Fibromyalgia diagnosis and diagnostic criteria. Ann Med. 2011;43(7):495–502. Epub 2011/07/21
2. Sturgill J, McGee E, Menzies V. Unique cytokine signature in the plasma of patients with fibromyalgia. J Immunol Res. 2014;2014:938576. Epub 2014/04/18
3. Carvalho LS, Correa H, Silva GC, Campos FS, Baiao FR, Ribeiro LS, et al. May genetic factors in fibromyalgia help to identify patients with differentially altered frequencies of immune cells? Clin Exp Immunol. 2008;154(3):346–52. Epub 2008/11/29
4. Pernambuco AP, Schetino LP, Alvim CC, Murad CM, Viana RS, Carvalho LS, et al. Increased levels of IL-17A in patients with fibromyalgia. Clin Exp Rheumatol. 2013; Epub 2013/09/12
5. Pernambuco AP, Schetino LP, Viana RS, Carvalho LS, d'Avila Reis D. The involvement of melatonin in the clinical status of patients with fibromyalgia syndrome. Clin Exp Rheumatol. 2015;33(1 Suppl 88):S14–9. Epub 2014/02/26
6. Sarzi-Puttini P, Atzeni F, Di Franco M, Buskila D, Alciati A, Giacomelli C, et al. Dysfunctional syndromes and fibromyalgia: a 2012 critical digest. Clin Exp Rheumatol. 2012;30(6 Suppl 74):143–51. Epub 2013/02/27
7. Mease P, Arnold LM, Bennett R, Boonen A, Buskila D, Carville S, et al. Fibromyalgia syndrome. J Rheumatol. 2007;34(6):1415–25. Epub 2007/06/07
8. Cordero MD, Alcocer-Gomez E, Cano-Garcia FJ, de Miguel M, Sanchez-Alcazar JA, Moreno Fernandez AM. Low levels of serotonin in serum correlates with severity of fibromyalgia. Medicina clinica. 2010;135(14):644–6. Epub 2010/07/02. Bajos valores de serotonina en suero se correlacionan con la gravedad de los sintomas de la fibromialgia
9. Lemstra M, Olszynski WP. The effectiveness of multidisciplinary rehabilitation in the treatment of fibromyalgia: a randomized controlled trial. Clin J Pain. 2005;21(2):166–74. Epub 2005/02/22
10. Souza JB, Bourgault P, Charest J, Marchand S. Escola inter-relacional de fibromialgia: aprendendo a lidar com a dor - estudo clínico randomizado. Rev Bras Reumatol. 2008;48:218–25.
11. Mannerkorpi K, Nyberg B, Ahlmen M, Ekdahl C. Pool exercise combined with an education program for patients with fibromyalgia syndrome. A prospective, randomized study. J Rheumatol. 2000;27(10):2473–81. Epub 2000/10/19
12. Faul F, Erdfelder E, Lang AG, Buchner A. G*power 3: a flexible statistical power analysis program for the social, behavioral, and biomedical sciences. Behav Res Methods. 2007;39:175–91.
13. Wolfe F, Smythe HA, Yunus MB, Bennett RM, Bombardier C, Goldenberg DL, et al. The American College of Rheumatology 1990 criteria for the classification of fibromyalgia. Report of the multicenter criteria committee. Arthritis Rheum. 1990;33(2):160–72. Epub 1990/02/01
14. Burckhardt CS, Clark SR, Bennett RM. The fibromyalgia impact questionnaire: development and validation. J Rheumatol. 1991;18(5):728–33. Epub 1991/05/01
15. Marques AP, Santos AMB, Assumpção A, Matsutani LA, Lage LV, Pereira CAB. Validação da versão brasileira do Fibromyalgia Impact Questionnaire (FIQ). Rev Bras Reumatol. 2006;46:24–31.
16. Meeus M, Nijs J. Central sensitization: a biopsychosocial explanation for chronic widespread pain in patients with fibromyalgia and chronic fatigue syndrome. Clin Rheumatol. 2007;26(4):465–73. Epub 2006/11/23

17. Riva R, Mork PJ, Westgaard RH, Lundberg U. Comparison of the cortisol awakening response in women with shoulder and neck pain and women with fibromyalgia. Psychoneuroendocrinology. 2012;37(2):299–306. Epub 2011/07/19

18. Uceyler N, Valenza R, Stock M, Schedel R, Sprotte G, Sommer C. Reduced levels of antiinflammatory cytokines in patients with chronic widespread pain. Arthritis Rheum. 2006;54(8):2656–64. Epub 2006/07/28

19. Pernambuco AP, Schetino LPL, Carvalho LSC, Reis DA. Involvement of oxidative stress and nitric oxide in fibromyalgia pathophysiology: a relationship to be elucidated. Fibromyalgia: Open Access. 2016;1(1):105.

20. Albrecht PJ, Hou Q, Argoff CE, Storey JR, Wymer JP, Rice FL. Excessive Peptidergic sensory innervation of cutaneous arteriole-Venule shunts (AVS) in the palmar glabrous skin of fibromyalgia patients: implications for widespread deep tissue pain and fatigue. Pain Med. 2013;14(6):895–915. Epub 2013/05/23

21. Dobkin PL, Da Costa D, Abrahamowicz M, Dritsa M, Du Berger R, Fitzcharles MA, et al. Adherence during an individualized home based 12-week exercise program in women with fibromyalgia. J Rheumatol. 2006;33(2):333–41. Epub 2006/02/09

22. Albanesi C, Fairchild HR, Madonna S, Scarponi C, De Pita O, Leung DY, et al. IL-4 and IL-13 negatively regulate TNF-alpha- and IFN-gamma-induced beta-defensin expression through STAT-6, suppressor of cytokine signaling (SOCS)-1, and SOCS-3. J Immunol. 2007;179(2):984–92. Epub 2007/07/10

23. Klementiev B, Enevoldsen MN, Li S, Carlsson R, Liu Y, Issazadeh-Navikas S, et al. Antiinflammatory properties of a peptide derived from interleukin-4. Cytokine. 2013;64(1):112–21. Epub 2013/08/27

24. Saraiva M, O'Garra A. The regulation of IL-10 production by immune cells. Nat Rev Immunol. 2010;10(3):170–81.

25. Mosser DM, Zhang X. Interleukin-10: new perspectives on an old cytokine. Immunol Rev. 2008;226:205–18.

26. Üçeyler N, Valenza R, Stock M, Schedel R, Sprotte G, Sommer C. Reduced levels of antiinflammatory cytokines in patients with chronic widespread pain. Arthritis & Rheumatism. 2006;54(8):2656–64.

27. Ren X, Li J, Zhou X, Luo X, Huang N, Wang Y, et al. Recombinant murine interleukin 4 protein therapy for psoriasis in a transgenic VEGF mouse model. Dermatology. 2009;219(3):232–8. Epub 2009/09/05

28. Docke WD, Asadullah K, Belbe G, Ebeling M, Hoflich C, Friedrich M, et al. Comprehensive biomarker monitoring in cytokine therapy: heterogeneous, time-dependent, and persisting immune effects of interleukin-10 application in psoriasis. J Leukoc Biol. 2009;85(3):582–93. Epub 2008/11/29

29. Henningsson L, Eneljung T, Jirholt P, Tengvall S, Lidberg U, van den Berg WB, et al. Disease-dependent local IL-10 production ameliorates collagen induced arthritis in mice. PLoS One. 2012;7(11):16.

30. Cohen M, Granger S, Fuller-Thomson E. The association between bereavement and biomarkers of inflammation. Behav Med. 2013;22:22.

31. Holtzman S, Abbey SE, Chan C, Bargman JM, Stewart DE. A genetic predisposition to produce low levels of IL-10 is related to depressive symptoms: a pilot study of patients with end stage renal disease. Psychosomatics. 2012;53(2):155–61.

32. Hartwell KJ, Moran-Santa Maria MM, Twal WO, Shaftman S, DeSantis SM, McRae-Clark AL, et al. Association of elevated cytokines with childhood adversity in a sample of healthy adults. J Psychiatr Res. 2013;47(5):604–10.

33. Bazzichi L, Rossi A, Massimetti G, Giannaccini G, Giuliano T, De Feo F, et al. Cytokine patterns in fibromyalgia and their correlation with clinical manifestations. Clin Exp Rheumatol. 2007;25(2):225–30. Epub 2007/06/05

34. Iannuccelli C, Di Franco M, Alessandri C, Guzzo MP, Croia C, Di Sabato F, et al. Pathophysiology of fibromyalgia: a comparison with the tension-type headache, a localized pain syndrome. Ann N Y Acad Sci. 2010;1193:78–83. Epub 2010/04/20

35. Rodriguez-Pinto I, Agmon-Levin N, Howard A, Shoenfeld Y. Fibromyalgia and cytokines. Immunol Lett. 2014;161(2):200–3. Epub 2014/01/28

36. Korenromp IHE, Grutters JC, van den Bosch JMM, Zanen P, Kavelaars A, Heijnen CJ. Reduced Th2 cytokine production by sarcoidosis patients in clinical remission with chronic fatigue. Brain Behav Immun. 2011;25(7):1498–502.

37. Paradis E, Sutkin G. Beyond a good story: from Hawthorne effect to reactivity in health professions education research. Med Educ. 2017;51(1):31–9. Epub 2016/09/02

38. Leurent B, Reyburn H, Muro F, Mbakilwa H, Schellenberg D. Monitoring patient care through health facility exit interviews: an assessment of the Hawthorne effect in a trial of adherence to malaria treatment guidelines in Tanzania. BMC Infect Dis. 2016;16:59. Epub 2016/02/05

39. Golzari Z, Shabkhiz F, Soudi S, Kordi MR, Hashemi SM. Combined exercise training reduces IFN-gamma and IL-17 levels in the plasma and the supernatant of peripheral blood mononuclear cells in women with multiple sclerosis. Int Immunopharmacol. 2010;10(11):1415–9. Epub 2010/08/28

40. Bote ME, Garcia JJ, Hinchado MD, Ortega E. Fibromyalgia: anti-inflammatory and stress responses after acute moderate exercise. PLoS One. 2013;8(9): e74524. Epub 2013/09/12

41. Rosenkranz MA, Davidson RJ, MacCoon DG, Sheridan JF, Kalin NH, Lutz A. A comparison of mindfulness-based stress reduction and an active control in modulation of neurogenic inflammation. Brain Behav Immun. 2013;27C:174–84.

42. Kadetoff D, Kosek E. Evidence of reduced sympatho-adrenal and hypothalamic-pituitary activity during static muscular work in patients with fibromyalgia. J rehab med offic j UEMS Europ Board Physic Rehab Med. 2010;42(8):765–72. Epub 2010/09/03

43. Wingenfeld K, Nutzinger D, Kauth J, Hellhammer DH, Lautenbacher S. Salivary cortisol release and hypothalamic pituitary adrenal axis feedback sensitivity in fibromyalgia is associated with depression but not with pain. j pain offic j Am Pain Soc. 2010;11(11):1195–202. Epub 2010/07/16

18

Mycophenolate mofetil in patients with refractory systemic autoimmune myopathies

Pablo Arturo Olivo Pallo, Fernando Henrique Carlos de Souza, Renata Miossi and Samuel Katsuyuki Shinjo[*]

Abstract

Background: Currently, there are only few studies (mostly case reports or case series) on mycophenolate mofetil (MMF) in patients with systemic autoimmune myopathies (SAM). Therefore, the goal of the present study was to evaluate the safety and efficacy of MMF (monotherapy or coadjuvant drug) in a specific sample of patients with refractory SAM: dermatomyositis, polymyositis, anti-synthetase syndrome or clinically amyopathic dermatomyositis.

Methods: A case series including 20 consecutive adult patients with refractory SAM from 2010 to 2016 was conducted. After the introduction of MMF, associated or not with other drugs, the patients were followed for 6 consecutive months.

Results: In 17 out of 20 patients MMF was introduced without any intolerance. The clinical symptoms evaluated in these patients were muscular, cutaneous and/or pulmonary activity. During the 6-month follow-up, 11 out of 17 patients had clinical and laboratory activities response with MMF, allowing significant tapering of the prednisone median dose (15 vs. 5 mg/day, $P=0.005$). On the other hand, in three out of 20 patients; MMF was discontinued in less than two months, because of gastrointestinal intolerance. There were no cases of serious infection or death.

Conclusions: MMF was relatively well-tolerated, safe and effective in patients with refractory SAM. Further studies are needed to confirm the data found.

Keywords: Dermatomyositis, Drugs, Immunomodulator, Immunosuppressive, Myositis, Polymyositis

Background

Systemic autoimmune myopathies (SAM) are a heterogeneous group of rare systemic autoimmune diseases that result in progressive skeletal muscle weakness and disability [1–3]. Depending on the demographic, clinical, laboratory, histological and disease evaluation, SAM can be classified into dermatomyositis (DM), polymyositis (PM), inclusion body myositis, or immune-mediated necrotizing myopathy, among others [2–4].

There are no randomized controlled clinical trials and glucocorticoid has been used as the first-line drug in SAM [5, 6]. Various immunosuppressive or immunomodulatory drugs have been recommended as glucocorticoid-sparing agents, including methotrexate, azathioprine, cyclosporine, cyclophosphamide, tacrolimus and intravenous human immunoglobulin [5–7]. Moreover, the rituximab, an anti-CD20 immunobiological drug, has been administered in refractory SAM cases [7, 8].

Mycophenolate mofetil (MMF) is an agent that inhibits the mitosis and proliferation of T and B lymphocytes and has been successfully used to treat different autoimmune systemic diseases [9]. However, only a few studies in the literature have investigated the use of MMF in adult patients with SAM [10–20]. Furthermore, as limitations, the majority of these studies are case reports or case series [10, 12, 13, 15–18, 20] and analyzed only SAM patients with pulmonary disease activity [15, 19, 20]. Those who used rituximab [10–17, 19, 20] or anti-synthetase syndrome (ASS) patients [10–20] have not been studied.

The aim of the present case series was to evaluate the safety and efficacy of MMF (monotherapy or coadjuvant drug) in refractory SAM (DM, PM, ASS or clinically

* Correspondence: samuel.shinjo@gmail.com
Division of Rheumatology, Faculdade de Medicina FMUSP, Universidade de Sao Paulo, Av. Dr. Arnaldo, 455, 3 andar, sala 3150 - Cerqueira César, CEP 01246-903 Sao Paulo, Brazil

amyopathic DM) as monotherapy or in combination of immunosuppressants.

Methods

This retrospective, case series included 21 consecutive adult patients with refractory SAM: classical DM or PM, according to Bohan and Peter's criteria [21, 22], clinically amyopathic DM, according to Gerami et al. [23], and ASS which was defined as myositis, arthritis, pulmonary disease, positive anti-synthetase antibody, with or without mechanic's hands, fever and/or Raynaud's phenomenon [24].

Refractoriness was defined as primarily cutaneous (worsing heliotrope rash and/or Gottron's sign, new cutaneous lesions attributed to MAS), muscular (objective and progressive limb weakness), articular (arthritis) and/or pulmonary activity (progressive dyspnea), hampering glucocorticoid tapering and/or inadequate response to at least two immunosuppressive or immunomodulatory drugs at full-dose for a minimum period of three months, given sequentially or concomitantly [25].

To improve the homogeneity of the sample under study, only patients followed up at our outpatient clinic between 2010 and 2016 were included.

MMF treatment was defined as effective when the drug promoted over 50% improvement in the initial: cutaneous (evaluated clinically by the rheumatologists from Outgoing clinic); muscular (clinical muscle strength graded according to the Medical Research Council [26]) and/or laboratory parameters (serum creatine phosphokinase level - reference range: 24 - 173 IU/L - assayed by automated kinetic methods)]; articular (arthritis) or pulmonary (subjective dyspnea associated simultaneously with confirmed "ground-glass" on high-resolution chest computed tomography) activity. Comparisons of creatine phosphokinase level values at initial and after 6 months of MMF were considered as expected when variations ranged up to 20%. Moreover, glucocorticoid tapering of over 50% of initial dose was also considered evidence of efficacy of MMF.

All patients were followed for 6 consecutive months after MMF introduction and were examined at baseline and after 6 months by the same examiner.

Myositis overlap syndromes, neoplasia associated myositis, necrotizing myopathies, muscular dystrophy, inclusion body myositis, metabolic myopathies, irregular or doubt treatment adhesions were excluded.

Data were obtained from the ongoing electronic database protocol applied all patients with SAM at 1 - 6 month intervals entailing extensive clinical and laboratory evaluations, including the assessment relevant to this study.

Statistical analysis. The Kolmogorov-Smirnov test was used to evaluate the distribution of each parameter. The demographic and clinical features are expressed as the means ± standard deviations for the continuous variables or as frequencies and percentages for the categorical variables. The medians (25th - 75th percentiles) were calculated for the continuous variables that were not normally distributed. Comparisons between the patients at initial and after 6 months of MMF were performed using Student's t-test or Wilcoxon test for continuous variables, and $P < 0.05$ was considered significant. All of the analyses were performed with the SPSS 15.0 statistics software (Chicago, USA).

Results

Twenty consecutive patients with refractory SAM treated with MMF were initially analyzed. In 7 patients, previous immunosuppressive drugs were exchanged for MMF (monotherapy), whereas in 13, MMF was associated with previous immunosuppressant (Table 1).

Patients #11 used rituximab 12 months before switch to MMF.

As an internal service protocol, the patients were not using antimalarials, except for one patient (#5).

In 17 out of 20 refractory MAS patients (11 DM, three PM, two ASS, one clinically amyopathic DM) (Table 1), MMF was introduced with good tolerance and with 100% of adhesion. The median dose of MMF was 2 g/day. This group comprised patients that were predominantly women, with a mean age of 46.2 ± 12.6 years and median disease duration of 2.0 years. All 17 patients used glucocorticoids (methylprednisolone or prednisone) and received previously a median of three immunosuppressive drugs (Table 1).

Of this group, 8 had muscle activity, three muscular and skin activities, three cutaneous activities, two pulmonary activities, one cutaneous and pulmonary activity and one had muscular, cutaneous and pulmonary activity. No cases had articular activity.

During the 6-month follow-up, prednisone median dose was significant tapering from 15.0 to 5.0 mg/day ($P = 0.005$). Moreover, the prednisone tapering was achieved in 14 out of 17 patients. However, glucocorticoid tapering of more than half occurred in 11 patients, all of whom had good clinical activity response using MMF.

As an additional analysis, the MAS patients with MMF as monotherapy ($n = 6$) were compare to those with MMF in combination therapy ($n = 11$). All clinical, laboratory, therapeutic and outcome parameters were comparable between both groups ($P > 0.05$).

In three out of 20 refractory female patients (one DM, one PM and one ASS) with cutaneous, articular and/or muscular activity, MMF was suspended in less than two month, because of gastrointestinal intolerance. The maximum dose of MMF in these patients was 1.5 g/day.

There were no cases of death or infection during the follow-up of the patients analyzed.

Table 1 General features of 17 refractory idiopathic systemic autoimmune myopathies

No	Disease	Disease (years)	Treatment			Activity		CPK (U/L)		Prednisone (mg/day)*	
			Previous	Immediately Before MMF	Current	Initial	6 months after MMF treatment	Initial	6 months after MMF treatment	Inicial	6 months after MMF treatment
1	PM	2	MP,Pred,Aza,CYC	CP	CP, MMF	P	P	95	130	5.0	20.0
2	DM	2	Pred,Aza,MTX,CYC	AZA	MMF	P	Remission	48	66	15.0	5.0
3	ASS	1	MP,Pred,IVIg,Aza,MTX,CYC	CYC	MMF	Mu,C,P	Mu	242	139	20.0	10.0
4	ASS	2	Pred,Aza,MTX,CYC	MTX	MTX, MMF	Mu,C	Remission	167	200	10.0	5.0
5	DM	8	Pred,AM,Aza,CP,RTX,Tac	AM,Tac	AM, Tac, MMF	Mu,C	C	141	53	15.0	20.0
6	DM	3	Pred,Aza,MTX	AZA	AZA, MMF	Mu,C	Mu	268	148	15.0	7.5
7	DM	2	MP,Pred,Aza,MTX	MTX	MMF	Mu	Mu	40	20	50.0	30.0
8	DM	6	MP,Pred,Aza,MTX,CP	MTX,CP	CP, MMF	Mu	Mu	249	2120	10.0	15.0
9	PM	6	MP,Pred,Aza,MTX	AZA	AZA, MMF	Mu	Mu	1534	3517	5.0	0
10	DM	1	MP,Pred,Aza,CYC,RTX	RTX	RTX, MMF	Mu	Mu	215	255	15.0	2.5
11	PM	1	Pred,Aza,MTX	-	MMF	Mu	Mu	118	205	60.0	5.0
12	DM	1	MP,AM,AZA,MTX	AZA	MMF	Mu	Mu	35	30	40.0	5.0
13	DM	1	MP,Pred,AZA,MTX	MTX	MTX, MMF	Mu	Remission	245	257	10.0	0
14	DM	5	MP,AM,AZA,MTX,CP	AZA,CP	AZA, MMF	Mu	Mu	858	268	10.0	0
15	DM	1	Pred,AZA,CYC	-	MMF	C,P	C	114	138	15.0	5.0
16	DM	1	MP,Pred,MTX	MTX	MTX, MMF	C	Remission	100	80	12.5	5.0
17	CADM	3	Pred,AZA,MTX,LFN,CYC	AZA,LFN	AZA, MMF	C	C	79	95	60.0	2.5
		2.0 (1.0-4.0)								15.0 (10.0-30.0)	5.0 (2.5-12.5)

AM antimalarials, *ASS* anti-synthetase syndrome, *AZA* azathioprine, *CPK* creatine phosphokinase, *CP* cyclosporine, *C* cutaneous, *CADM* clinically amyopathic dermatomyositis, *CYC* cyclophosphamide, *DM* dermatomyositis, *F* female, *IVIg* intravenous human immunoglobulin, *LFN* leflunomide, *M* male, *MP* methylprednisolone pulse therapy, *MTX* methotrexate, *Mu* muscular, *PM* polymyositis, *P* pulmonary, *Pred* prednisone, *RTX* rituximab, *Tac* tacrolymus
*Pred: current *vs.* 6 months: *P* = 0.005

Discussion

This case series showed that MMF, as a monotherapy or coadjunt drug, is relatively safe and effective in patients with refractory SAM.

A strict exclusion in rare diseases criteria was employed in this study, however a sample of 20 consecutive patients with refractory SAM was analyzed based on previously standardized and parameterized data. The protocol was performed at the same service adopting the same standardization of reports, thereby reducing inter-examiner variability. Only patients with refractoriness were included.

MMF has been used in several systemic autoimmune diseases, such as systemic sclerosis, rheumatoid arthritis, Sjögre's syndrome, systemic lupus erythematosus [16, 27–29]. However, there are few studies in the literature investigating the use of MMF in adult patients with SAM [10–20].

Most studies are case reports or case series and MMF was found to promote significant clinical and laboratory improvement in patients with SAM [10, 12–16, 19, 20]. According to the study by Majithia and Harisdangkul [10], 6 out of 7 refractory SAM had marked improvement, with good tolerance, in active myositis using MMF. This response rate was higher than ours, however

in a group with less severity and in previous use of a smaller number of immunosuppressive drugs.

In another study [13], MMF was effective for controlling cutaneous activity in all four patients with SAM analyzed, also resulting in glucocorticoid tapering. In 10 out of 12 patients with recalcitrant DM, Edge et al. [14] observed an improvement in muscular and cutaneous activity after four weeks of treatment with MMF.

Probably we found a smaller rate of success because of all patients of our sample had refractory and severe disease.

The heterogeneity of response evaluation in myopathies in the literature is present. Better criteria have been established [30–33], but in relation to DM, for example, there is still a difficulty in assessing improvement, especially in those with little muscle involvement. The response assessment parameter of the present study was based mainly on the clinical criteria.

Previous study showed that antimalarial could predispose patients with DM/PM to developing herpes zoster, particularly women and DM patients [29]. Therefore, as an internal service protocol, our patients were not using antimalarials (except for one patient) at the time of this study.

Facing the previous refractoriness, in two thirds of the patients, the MMF was introduced as a coadjuvant in the present study. However, during follow-up, there was no difference between this group and those who used MMF as monotherapy for the response parameters analyzed.

In the present study, most frequent side effects of MMF were associated with the gastrointestinal tract (nausea, vomiting, abdominal pain and/or diarrhea). Intolerance was observed in three out of the 20 patients in the present analysis, comparable to findings of other studies [12–14].

Akin to the present study, some investigations have also shown that MMF is safe in patients with SAM [10, 14, 16]. There were no cases of infection or death events in our sample. By contrast, Rowin et al. [11] reported that three out of their 10 DM patients developed opportunistic infections with MMF (pulmonary infections: Blastomycosis, *Mycobacterium xenopi*, legionella).

Limitations of this study include the short follow-up of 6 months. In addition, possible inclusion of more severe cases of the disease due to the characteristics of our tertiary care centre should also be considered. Finally, as this is a review of retrospective cases, tools such as Manual Muscle Testing (MMT)-8 [31], 2016 European League Against Rheumatism / American College of Rheumatology (EULAR/ACR) response criteria [34] were not used and pulmonary involvement was not analyzed with pulmonary function test (at baseline and 6 months of MMF) and high-resolution chest computed tomography (6 months of MMF).

Conclusions
MMF was relatively well-tolerated, safe and effective in patients with refractory SAM, at least in the short follow-up of 6 consecutive months. Further studies are needed to confirm the data found in the present study.

Abbreviations
AM: Antimalarials; ASS: Anti-synthetase syndrome; AZA: Azathioprine; C: Cutaneous; CADM: Clinically amyopathic dermatomyositis; CP: Cyclosporine; CPK: Creatine phosphokinase; CYC: Cyclophosphamide; DM: Dermatomyositis; EULAR/ACR: European League Against Rheumatism / American College of Rheumatology; F: Female; IVIg: Intravenous human immunoglobulin; LFN: Leflunomide; M: Male; MMF: Mycophenolate mofetil; MMT: Manual Muscle Testing; MP: Methylprednisolone pulse therapy; Mu: Muscular; P: Pulmonary; PM: Polymyositis; Pred: Prednisone; RTX: Rituximab; SAM: Systemic autoimmune myopathies; Tac: Tacrolymus

Authors' contributions
All authors contributed equally to write and review the manuscript. All authors read and approved the final manuscript.

Competing interests
All authors declare that they have no competing interest.

References
1. Dalakas MC. Inflammatory muscle diseases. N Engl J Med. 2015;372:1734–47.
2. Dalakas MC. Pathogenesis and therapies of immune-mediated myopathies. Autoimmun Rev. 2012;11:203–6.
3. Nava A, Orozco-barocio G. Approach to the differential diagnosis of inflammatory myopathies. Rheumatol Clin. 2009;5:32–4.
4. Irazoque-Palazuelos F, Barragán-Navarro Y. Inflammatory myopathies: epidemiology, etiology and classification. Rheumatol Clin. 2009;5:2–5.
5. Aggarwal R, Oddis CV. Therapeutic advances in myositis. Curr Opin Rheumatol. 2012;24:635–41.
6. Distad BJ, Amato AA, Weiss MD. Inflammatory myopathies. Curr Treat Options Neurol. 2011;13:19–30.
7. Ernste FC, Reed AM. Idiopathic inflammatory myopathies: current trends in pathogenesis, clinical features, and up-to-date treatment recommendations. Mayo Clin Proc. 2013;88:83–105.
8. Ytterberg SR. Treatment of refractory polymyositis and dermatomyositis. Curr Rheumatol Rep. 2006;8:167–73.
9. Bandelier C, Guerne PA, Genevay S, Finckh A, Gabay C. Clinical experience with mycophenolate mofetil in systemic autoimmune conditions refractory to common immunosuppressant therapies. Swiss Med Wkly. 2009;139:41–6.
10. Majithia V, Harisdangkul V. Mycophenolate mofetil (CellCept): an alternative therapy for autoimmune inflammatory myopathy. Rheumatology. 2005;44: 386–9.
11. Rowin J, Amato AA, Deisher N, Cursio J, Meriggioli MN. Mycophenolate mofetil in dermatomyositis: is it safe? Neurology. 2006;66:1245–7.
12. Tausche AK, Meurer M. Mycophenolate mofetil for dermatomyositis. Dermatology. 2001;202:341–3.
13. Gelber AC, Nousari HC, Wigley FM. Mycophenolate mofetil in the treatment of severe skin manifestations of dermatomyositis: a series of 4 cases. J Rheumatol. 2000;27:1542–5.
14. Edge JC, Outland JD, Dempsey JR, Callen JP. Mycophenolate mofetil as an effective corticosteroid-sparing therapy for recalcitrant dermatomyositis. Arch Dermatol. 2006;142:65–9.
15. Morganroth PA, Kreider ME, Werth VP. Mycophenolate mofetil for interstitial lung disease in dermatomyositis. Arthritis Care Res. 2010;62:1496–501.
16. Saketkoo LA, Espinoza LR. Experience of mycophenolate mofetil in 10 patients with autoimmune-related interstitial lung disease demonstrates promising effects. Am J Med Sci. 2009;337:329–35.
17. Danieli MG, Calcabrini L, Calabrese V, Marchetti A, Loqullo F, Gabrielli A. Intravenous immunoglobulin as add on treatment with mycophenolate mofetil in severe myositis. Autoimmun Rev. 2009;9:124–9.
18. Parziale N, Kovacs SC, Thomas CB, Srinivasan J. Rituximab and mycophenolate combination therapy in refractory dermatomyositis with multiple autoimmune disorders. J Clin Neuromuscul Dis. 2011;13:63–7.
19. Mira-Avendano IC, Parambil JG, Yadav R, Arrossi V, Xu M, Chapman JT, et al. A retrospective review of clinical features and treatment outcomes in steroid-resistant interstitial lung disease from polymyositis / dermatomyositis. Respir Med. 2013;107:890–6.
20. Tsuchiya H, Tsuno H, Inoue M, Takahashi Y, Yamashita H, Kaneko H, et al. Mycophenolate mofetil therapy for rapidly progressive interstitial lung disease in a patient with clinically amyopathic dermatomyositis. Mod Rheumatol. 2014;24:694–6.
21. Bohan A, Peter JB. Polymyositis and dermatomyositis (first of two parts). N Engl J Med. 1975;292:344–7.
22. Bohan A, Peter JB. Polymyositis and dermatomyositis (second of two parts). N Engl J Med. 1975;292:403–7.
23. Gerami P, Schope JM, McDonald L, Alling HW, Sontheimer RD. A systematic review of adult-onset clinically amyopathic dermatomyositis (dermatomyositis sine myositis): a missing link within the spectrum of the idiopathic inflammatory myopathies. J Am Acad Dermatol. 2006;54:597–613.
24. Mahler M, Miller FW, Fritzler MJ. Idiopathic inflammatory myopathies and the anti-synthetase syndrome: a comprehensive review. Autoimmun Rev. 2014;13:367–71.
25. Brandão M, Marinho A. Idiopathic inflammatory myopathies: Definition and management of refractory disease. Autoimmun Rev. 2011;10:720–4.
26. Medical Research Council: Aids to the investigation of peripheral nerve injuries. War Memorandun. No 7, 2. Ed. London: Her Majesty's Stationery Office, 1943.

27. Appel GB, Gerald B, Radhakrishnan J, Ginzler EM. Use of mycophenolate mofetil in autoimmune and renal diseases. Transplantation. 2005;80:S265–71.

28. Iaccarino L, Rampudda M, Canova M, Libera SD, Sarzi-Puttinic P, Doria A. Mycophenolate mofetil: what is its place in the treatment of autoimmune rheumatic diseases? Autoimmun Rev. 2007;6:190–5.

29. Cunha GF, Souza FH, Levy-Neto M, Shinjo SK. Chloroquine diphosphate: a risk factor for herpes zoster in patients with dermatomyositis / polymyositis. Clinics. 2013;68:621–7.

30. Bruce B, Fries JF. The Stanford Health Assessment Questionnaire: dimensions and practical applications. Health Qual Life Outcomes. 2003;1:20.

31. Rider LG, Koziol D, Giannini EH, Jain MS, Smith MR, Whitney-Mahoney K, et al. Validation of manual muscle testing and a subset of eight muscles for adult and juvenile idiopathic inflammatory myopathies. Arthritis Care Research (Hoboken). 2010;62:465–72.

32. Rider LG, Feldman BM, Perez MD, Rennebohm RM, Lindsley CB, Zemel LS, et al. Development of validated disease activity and damage indices for the juvenile idiopathic inflammatory myopathies: I. Physician, parent, and patient global assessments. Juvenile Dermatomyositis Disease Activity Collaborative Study Group. Arthritis Rheum. 1997;40:1976–83.

33. Sultan SM, Allen E, Oddis CV, Kiely P, Cooper RG, Lundberg IE, et al. Reliability and validity of the myositis disease activity assessment tool. Arthritis Rheum. 2008;58:3593–9.

34. Rider LG, Ruperto N, Pistorio A, Erman B, Bayat N, Lachenbruch PA, et al. International Myositis Assessment and Clinical Studies Group and the Paediatric Rheumatology International Trials Organisation. 2016 ACR-EULAR adult dermatomyositis and polymyositis and juvenile dermatomyositis response criteria-methodological aspects. Rheumatology (Oxford). 2017;56:1884–93.

19

Adipokines in rheumatoid arthritis

Elis Carolina de Souza Fatel[1,5]* ⓘ, Flávia Troncon Rosa[2], Andréa Name Colado Simão[3] and Isaias Dichi[4]

Abstract

Rheumatoid arthritis affects millions of people worldwide and is considered a chronic multisystem disease whose causes are unknown. In general, the main objective of rheumatoid arthritis treatment is to improve the quality of life of patients by relieving pain, maintaining or improving functional capacity, preventing thus, disability. In recent years the role of adipokines in the pathogenesis of rheumatoid arthritis has been discussed but results are still conflicting. Although results from some studies have shown the implications of adipokines in the pathophysiology of autoimmune diseases, including rheumatoid arthritis, their role in the pathogenesis of disease progression is not clear. Thus, this review aimed to describe the association of key adipokines (leptin, resistin, visfatin and adiponectin) and rheumatoid arthritis, given the high prevalence of this disease and the important social impact caused by this chronic disabling disease.

Keywords: Adipokines, Rheumatoid arthritis, Cytokines

Background

Rheumatoid arthritis (RA) is a chronic multisystem disease whose causes are unknown [1]. This disease presents a variety of systemic manifestations being the persistent inflammatory synovitis the most typical feature, compromising peripheral joints in a symmetric distribution. Mateen et al. (2016) [2] highlights RA as a disease, which is characterized in the majority of patients by the presence of rheumatoid factor (RF) and anti–citrullinated protein antibody (ACPA). The authors reinforce that cytokines such as tumor necrosis factor (TNF)-α, interleukin (IL)-1 and IL-17 have an important role in the pathophysiology of RA since serum concentrations of these substances may indicate the severity of the disease.

The diagnosis of RA must be at earlier stages of disease and treatment should aim to relieve pain, maintain or improve functional capacity, preventing thus, disability, and improving patients quality of life [3].

Barbosa et al. (2012) [4] reported the important role of mediators synthesized in adipose tissue, named adipokines, in RA. Hutcheson (2015) [5] points out that knowledge about adiposity has changed and currently it appears as an important regulator of several key processes, including inflammation. Furthermore, adipokines have hormonal action supporting the regulation of appetite and glucose metabolism, and some of them such as leptin, resistin, adiponectin and visfatin have been associated to RA development. However the results are still conflicting [4, 5].

Thus, this review aimed to describe the association of key adipokines (leptin, resistin, visfatin and adiponectin) and RA, given the high prevalence of this disease and the important social impact caused by chronic disabling diseases of the articular system.

Methods

Study selection

This review is in accordance with the guidelines of the Preferred Reporting Items for Systematic Reviews and Meta-Analyses (PRISMA) [6]. The search string was restricted to humans, including clinical studies, controlled clinical trials, meta-analysis, multicentric, observational studies, and randomized controlled trials. Relevant articles that were not retrieved in the main search but were cited in the publications were carefully reviewed and included if they met the criteria. As the main objective was to verify the association of adipokines with rheumatoid arthritis, most of the studies analyzed refer to observational studies such as cross-sectional, case-control and cohort studies presenting quantitative information regarding plasma or serum adipokines concentrations. The on line databases U.S. National Library of Medicine PUBMED, Periódicos

---

* Correspondence: elis.fatel@uffs.edu.br; elis.fatel@hotmail.com
[1]Postgraduate Program, Health Sciences Center, State University of Londrina, Londrina, Paraná, Brazil
[5]Department of Nutrition, University of Fronteira Sul, Rodovia PR 182 Km 466, CEP 85770-000, Realeza, Paraná Postal Code 253, Brazil
Full list of author information is available at the end of the article

Capes, Science Direct, and Scientific Electronic Library Online (SciELO) were searched for English, Spanish or Portuguese-language articles. The crossing of "rheumatoid arthritis" with the following descriptors separately was used to accomplish this review: "adipokines", "leptin", "resistin", "visfatin", and "adiponectin". No exclusion criteria were established in view of the small number of articles regarding this current issue. The study selection process is described in Fig. 1.

Data extraction

The information sources were the results described in the articles selected. The following data were extracted from articles included in this review: authors, year of publication, study design, number of participants, disease characteristics, control groups and results regarding associations between each adipokine and markers of disease activity.

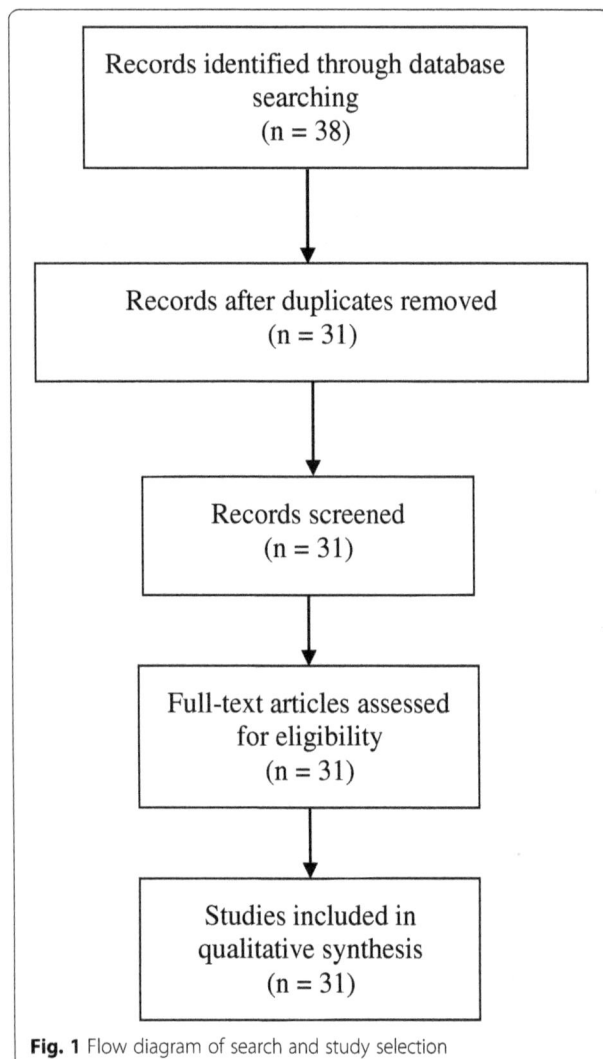

Fig. 1 Flow diagram of search and study selection

Results and discussion

Adipokines

Adipose tissue is a multifunctional organ responsible for lipid storage, thermogenesis, structural components and support of many organs such as joints, gastrointestinal tract and skin and nowadays also described as secretory and endocrine functions [7]. It is noteworthy in this context its role as an endocrine organ by synthesizing and secreting adipokines, which play an important role in the pathophysiology of insulin resistance, inflammation and atherogenesis [8, 9].

Leptin

Leptin is an adipokine produced in white adipose tissue. Discovered in 1994 [10], it is an *Ob* gene product [11], cloned and sequenced in mice and considered the adipokine responsible for the regulation of energy metabolism and homeostasis, as well as neuroendocrine functions [12]. It also assists the immunity and inflammation control through its receptor [13]. Thus, leptin is responsible for the regulation of various biological processes, being involved in the pathophysiology of many diseases. Leptin is considered a proinflammatory adipokine since it stimulates production of cytokines such as TNF-α, IL-6 and reactive oxygen species, and induces the production of CC chemokines by macrophages and alters the T helper (Th)1 / Th2 profile [13].

Paz-Filho et al. (2012) [14] described molecular mechanisms and pro-inflammatory systemic effects of leptin. It acts through its Ob receptor triggering inflammatory responses together with infectious and inflammatory stimuli of cytokines such as IL-1, lipopolysaccharide (LPS), and TNF-α, which may, in turn, increase levels of leptin. The interaction between leptin and inflammation are bidirectional, but all pro inflammatory since cytokines increases the synthesis and release of leptin, which in turn perpetuates the cycle of inflammation.

Leptin showed a significant effect on increasing the expression of Th1 cytokines. Experimental studies on mice demonstrated that these animals showed less severe stages of induced RA with lower levels of IL-1B and TNF-α in the synovial fluid and reduction in T-cell proliferative response induced by antigen [14]. However, clinical studies revealed paradoxical results about the effects of endogenous leptin in protecting joints in severe forms of erosive RA in humans [15].

In the last two decades, several studies have described the action of leptin in RA [16], leading researchers near to assume the hypothesis that this hormone has a key role in rheumatic diseases. [17] Thus, leptin levels may be a risk factor for the pathogenesis of RA [18].

Olama et al. (2012) [15] evaluated the ratio of synovial and serum leptin in patients with RA and found that the local utilization of leptin at the joint cavity has a protector role against the destructive course of RA. Rho et al. (2010) [19] also examined the hypothesis that the adipokines could influence insulin resistance and coronary atherosclerosis in patients with RA. Leptin was positively associated with insulin resistance assessed by Homeostasis Model Assessment - Insulin Resistance (HOMA-IR), even after adjusting for age, race, sex, body mass index (BMI), traditional cardiovascular risk factors and inflammation mediators. Targońska-Stepniak et al. (2010) [20] assessed leptin levels in patients with RA and demonstrated positive correlation between leptin levels and Disease Activity Score (DAS)-28. Yoshino et al. (2011) [21] found leptin levels significantly higher in RA patients compared to controls, and this adipokine correlated positively with C-Reactive Protein (CRP) levels, suggesting that leptin can act as a proinflammatory in this disease. On the other hand, Kontunen et al. (2011) [22] showed that leptin levels were increased only in patients with RA and concomitant diagnosis of metabolic syndrome (MetS).

Kang et al. (2013) [23] demonstrated that TNF-α was positively associated to leptin and the latter was associated with various metabolic risk factors, including insulin resistance. Bustos Rivera-Bahena et al. (2015) [24] evidenced that circulating levels of leptin correlate positively with clinical activity of RA, regardless of BMI. However, Xibille-Friedmann et al. (2015) [25] concluded that in a short term basal levels of leptin may predict disease activity independent of BMI. However, when submitted to treatment, this only occurred in patients with normal body weight.

Tian et al. (2014) [26] reported a review in which 23 studies were analyzed. The following results were obtained: 13 studies showed increased leptin levels; 8 studies did not demonstrate any significant difference and 2 had reduced leptin levels when compared to control subjects. Therefore, most of the studies have found higher levels of leptin in patients with RA, showing a possible role in the regulation of joint damage, and suggested that more studies are needed to understand the mechanisms of action of this adipokine. A meta-analysis conducted by Lee e Bae (2016) [27] confirmed these data showing that circulating levels of leptin were significantly higher in patients with RA with a positive correlation between this hormone and RA activity.

Despite the evidence demonstrated, some studies do not corroborate these associations. Allam e Radwan (2012) [28] and Abdalla et al. (2014) [29] found that although serum leptin level was significantly higher in RA patients than in control group, there was no correlation with clinical and laboratory markers of disease activity. Mirfeizi et al. (2014) [30] also stated that leptin has no effect on the process of joint damage in RA patients. Oner et al. (2015) [31] did not find any correlation between disease activity and serum leptin levels, indicating that this adipokine is not a good biomarker to monitor inflammation in RA.

Thus, leptin seems to have a role in the pathophysiology of RA and comorbidities associated, such as obesity and metabolic syndrome. Leptin is considered a pro inflammatory adipokine by the great majority of authors who suggest a predominantly deleterious action on the joint. Only one survey showed that increased levels of leptin can act as a protective factor against the destructive course of RA.

Table 1 summarizes the main findings of leptin in RA patients.

Resistin

Isolated in rodents, resistin was first described in 2001. It is a protein rich in cysteine, compounded by 108 amino acids, called RELMs (resistin-like molecules) also known as FIZZ 332 [32]. In humans, it is originated mainly from circulating monocytes and macrophages [33].

It was initially correlated to the pathogenesis of insulin resistance in obesity and some cardiovascular diseases (CVD) but now is also considered an important link between obesity and inflammation [34]. Resistin has been found in areas of inflammation and seems to be mediated by IL-6 and TNF α [35].

Due to its implication in inflammation processes, the involvement of resistin in the pathogenesis of RA has been investigated. Kassem et al. (2010) [36] studied if there is a role of resistin in the pathogenesis of RA by investigating possible correlations between resistin concentration in serum and synovial fluid with disease activity and radiographic joint damage. The authors' results supported the hypothesis that resistin is involved in the pathogenesis of RA and suggested serum resistin as a good marker of prognosis of the disease in RA patients. Yoshino et al. (2011) [21] compared serum resistin levels from RA patients and healthy control subjects. The authors found that the level of resistin in serum did not differ between patients and controls, but observed that serum resistin were positively associated with CRP levels in RA patients, suggesting a pro inflammatory action of this cytokine.

Kontunen et al. (2011) [22] reported that high levels of resistin are associated with RA, regardless of the presence of MetS. Fadda et al. (2013) [37] compared resistin levels in serum and synovial fluid of patients with RA and osteoarthritis and found higher levels in patients with RA. This result indicates a possible role of resistin in the pathogenesis of inflammatory rheumatic diseases. The high levels of this adipokine in the synovial fluid could suggest a

Table 1 Studies investigating the association of leptin and rheumatoid arthritis in humans

Authors	Study design	Subjects	Results/outcomes
Rho et al. (2010) [19]	Cross-sectional study evaluating correlation between HOMA-IR and serum adipokine levels.	169 RA patients	Positive correlation between serum leptin and insulin resistance.
Targońska-Stepniak et al. (2010) [20]	Cross-sectional study evaluating correlation between disease activity and serum adipokine levels.	80 RA patients	Positive correlation between serum leptin and DAS28.
Yoshino et al. (2011) [21]	Case-control study evaluating correlation between inflammation markers and serum adipokine levels.	141 RA patients 146 controls without RA	Positive correlation between serum leptin and CRP.
Kontunen et al. (2011) [22]	Cross-sectional study evaluating correlation between serum adipokines levels and markers of inflammation and MetS.	54 RA patients, 20 with MetS	Increased levels of serum leptin observed only in patients with MetS.
Olama et al. (2012) [15]	Case-control study evaluating differences between serum leptin and synovial/serum leptin ratio.	40 RA patients 30 controls without RA	Inverse correlation between leptin concentration and protection of joints in severe RA.
Allam e Radwan (2012) [28]	Case-control study evaluating correlation between serum leptin levels and disease activity.	37 RA patients 34 controls without RA	No correlation between leptin levels and disease activity.
Kang et al. (2013) [23]	Cross-sectional study evaluating correlation between adipokine levels, inflammation markers, insulin resistance and atherosclerosis.	192 RA patients	Positive correlation between serum leptin and TNF-α and metabolic risk, including insulin resistance
Mirfeizi et al. (2014) [30]	Cross-sectional study evaluating correlation between adipokine levels and radiographic joint damage.	54 RA patients (29 with erosion and 25 without erosion)	No differences in serum leptin between the two groups.
Abdalla et al. (2014) [29]	Case-control study evaluating correlation between serum leptin levels and clinical manifestations of disease activity.	60 RA patients 30 healthy controls	No correlation between leptin levels and clinical and laboratorial markers of disease activity.
Bustos Rivera-Bahena et al. (2015) [24]	Cross-sectional study evaluating correlation between adipokine levels and disease activity.	121 RA patients	Positive correlation between serum leptin and disease activity.
Xibille-Friedmann et al. (2015) [25]	Cohort study evaluating if baseline levels of adipokines may predict disease activity or response to treatment.	127 RA patients after 6 months of follow up; 91 after 1 year of follow up; 52 after 2 years of follow up	Positive correlation between serum leptin and prevention of disease activity progression.
Oner et al. (2015) [31]	Case-control study evaluating correlation between serum leptin levels and disease activity.	106 RA patients 52 healthy controls 37 osteoarthritis patients	No correlation between serum leptin and disease activity.
Lee e Bae (2016) [27]	Meta-analysis evaluating correlation between serum leptin levels and disease activity.	13 studies: 648 RA patients 426 controls without RA	Leptin levels significantly higher in RA patients and weak positive correlation between leptin levels and disease activity.

RA = rheumatoid arthritis; HOMA-IR = homeostatic model assessment-insulin resistance; DAS28 = Disease Activity Score-28; CRP = C-reactive protein; TNF-α = tumor necrosis factor-α; Metabolic Syndrome = MetS

bad prognosis for progression of RA, but the authors point out that more studies are needed to confirm if resistin is a good marker to evaluate the progression of this disease. Kang et al. (2013) [23] reinforced this hypothesis. The authors found an association between resistin levels and inflammatory markers in patients with RA. Recently, Bustos Rivera-Bahena et al. (2015) [24] demonstrated that resistin levels correlated positively with clinical manifestations of disease activity in patients with RA, albeit of patient body mass index. Huang et al. (2015) [38] in a meta-analysis concluded that serum resistin levels were significantly higher in RA patients compared to control group.

However, some authors did not show significant associations between serum resistin and HOMA-IR, nor differences between serum and synovial fluid resistin levels between RA patients and controls [19]. Al-Kady et al. (2010) [39] after studying the levels of resistin in of RA patients found no significant differences in resistin levels between RA patients and controls. Hammad et al. (2014) [40] also found no correlation between serum levels of resistin with clinical or laboratory markers in RA patients.

Thus, there is an important role of adipokines in the pathogenesis of obesity, CVD and inflammatory processes. The pro inflammatory action of resistin was observed in most studies of patients with RA, which suggest that this adipokines is a good marker to assess the progression of this disease.

Table 2 summarizes the main findings of resistin in RA patients.

Visfatin

Also known as PBEF (pre-B-cell colony-enhancing factor) or Nicotinamide Phosphoribosyltransferase (Nampt) [41], visfatin is a protein with molecular weight of 52 kDa, first described by Samal et al. (1994) [42]. It is primarily found in liver, bone marrow and muscle tissue, but also produced by adipose tissue and secreted by macrophage [43]. Its production is influenced by TNF-α, IL-6, Toll-like receptor (TLR) and chemokines [44]. Stofkova (2010) [45] reports that visfatin may contribute to inflammation processes, triggering production of cytokines and activation of nuclear factor kappa beta (NF-κβ). Thus, some studies have suggested some relation between this adipokine and the pathogenesis of type 2 diabetes and obesity [46] and increased cardiovascular risk [47].

Other studies have demonstrated a correlation between serum and synovial fluid levels of visfatin and the pathogenesis of RA [13, 41, 48, 49]. This adipokine can act as a regulator of inflammation and the destruction process of joints [35] and induce stimulation of great quantities of chemokines [50], thus possibly contributing to the inflammatory state of RA. However, its association to disease activity is not yet fully known [51].

Alkady et al. (2011) [52] showed that visfatin levels correlated with disease activity and may be involved in the progression of RA. Khalifa et al. (2013) [53] suggested that visfatin has a role in the pathogenesis of RA, and it may be considered as a marker of the disease and the radiographic bone lesion score. Therefore, it can be a potential therapeutic target for RA. El-Hini et al. (2013) [54] demonstrated positive and significant correlation between visfatin and insulin resistance and also with serum cholesterol, low density lipoprotein cholesterol (LDL-c) and triglycerides.

Table 2 Studies investigating the association of resistin and rheumatoid arthritis in humans

Authors	Study design	Subjects	Results/outcomes
Kassem et al. (2010) [36]	Case-control study evaluating correlation between serum and synovial resistin and inflammation markers, disease activity and radiographic joint damage.	30 RA patients 15 healthy controls	Significant correlation between serum resistin levels and CRP, ESR, rheumatoid factor and disease activity. Also considered a good prognostic marker of RA.
Rho et al. (2010) [19]	Cross-sectional study evaluating correlation between HOMA-IR and serum adipokine levels.	169 RA patients	No significant correlation between serum resistin and insulin resistance.
Al-Kady et al. (2010) [39]	Case-control study evaluating correlation between serum and synovial liquid adipokines and disease activity.	70 RA patients 30 controls	No differences between groups in serum resistin, but it was observed synovial liquid resistin levels significantly higher in patients with active disease.
Yoshino et al. (2011) [21]	Case-control study evaluating correlation between inflammation markers and serum adipokines levels.	141 RA patients 146 controls	No differences in serum resistin between groups, but in RA patients it was positively associated with CRP levels.
Kontunen et al. (2011) [22]	Cross-sectional study evaluating correlation between serum adipokine levels and markers of inflammation and MetS in RA.	54 RA patients, 20 with MetS	Increased levels of resistin were associated with RA irrespective of the presence of MetS.
Fadda et al. (2013) [37]	Case-control study comparing serum and synovial liquid resistin in patients with RA and osteoarthritis.	25 RA patients 25 osteoarthritis patients	Significant correlation between synovial liquid resistin and rheumatoid factor and ACPA, indicating a bad prognosis of disease.
Kang et al. (2013) [23]	Cross-sectional study evaluating correlation between adipokines levels, inflammation markers, insulin resistance and atherosclerosis.	192 RA patients	Significant correlation between serum resistin and inflammation markers ESR and CRP and disease duration.
Hammad et al. (2014) [40]	Case-control study comparing serum resistin in RA patients and a control group and its association to disease activity.	30 RA patients 30 controls	No correlation between serum resistin levels and clinical and laboratorial markers of disease activity.
Bustos Rivera-Bahena et al. (2015) [24]	Cross-sectional study evaluating correlation between adipokines levels and disease activity.	121 RA patients	Positive correlation between resistin levels and disease activity.
Huang et al. (2015) [38]	Meta-analysis evaluating correlation between serum resistin levels and RA.	8 studies with RA: 620 RA patients 460 controls	Serum resistin levels were significantly higher in patients with RA.

RA = rheumatoid arthritis; CRP = C-reactive protein; TNF-α = tumor necrosis factor-α; ESR = erythrocyte sedimentation rate; ACPA = anti-citrullinated protein antibody; HOMA-IR = homeostatic model assessment-insulin resistance; Metabolic Syndrome = MetS

Additionally, the disease activity score was positively correlated with visfatin.

Sglunda et al. (2014) [55] observed that visfatin levels in serum were significantly higher in RA patients compared to healthy individuals and suggested that reduction in visfatin concentrations could reduce disease activity in patients at early stage of RA. They also found positive association between this adipokine and elevated levels of total cholesterol, but not with the atherogenic index. Mirfeizi et al. (2014) [30] found that serum levels of visfatin in RA patients with radiographic joint damage were significantly higher than in patients without joint damage.

Nonetheless, Rho et al. (2010) [19] did not evidence relationship between visfatin and insulin resistance nor coronary atherosclerosis in patients with RA and Meyer et al. (2013) [56] did not show any correlation between serum levels of visfatin and radiographic progression of the disease.

Table 3 summarizes the main findings of visfatin in RA patients.

Adponectin

Adiponectin is an anti-inflammatory adipokine compounded by 244 amino acids and is produced and secreted mainly by adipocytes. [57, 58] Studies suggest that monomeric form of adiponectin appears to occur only in adipocytes, but there are three forms of adiponectin circulating in the body: trimmers (low molecular weight, LMW), hexamers (middle molecular weight, MMW) and multimers (high molecular weight, HMW) are the plasma circulating forms of adiponectin [58]. The receptors are AdipoR1and AdipoR2, respectively present at skeletal muscles and liver [59].

Several studies have demonstrated the role of this important anti-inflammatory cytokine in obesity, diabetes mellitus type 2, atherosclerosis and metabolic syndrome, being the highest levels a protective factor for these diseases [35, 60–62].

Paradoxically, in the pathogenesis of rheumatoid arthritis adiponectin seems to have proinflammatory effects in the joints, because its ability to stimulate the secretion of inflammatory mediators [63] and may also be associated to disease activity [52]. Scotece et al. (2012) [64] described the major effects of increased synovial and circulating levels of adiponectin in RA. They concluded that adiponectin in synovial fibroblasts induced prostaglandin (PG)E2, IL-6, IL-8, matrix metalloproteinase (MMP)-1 and MMP-13; in human chondrocytes induced nitric oxide (NO), IL-6, MMP-3, MMP-9, monocyte chemoattractant protein (MCP)-1 and IL-8 and promoted inflammation by increasing TNF-α, IL-6 and IL-8.

Krysiak et al. (2012) [65] suggested that these different actions can be explained by different mechanisms: LMW adiponectin has anti-inflammatory activities, while the HMW adiponectin has proinflammatory activities. However, Frommer et al. (2012) [66] showed a proinflammatory and destructive role of all isoforms

Table 3 Studies investigating the association of visfatin and rheumatoid arthritis in humans

Authors	Study design	Subjects	Results/outcomes
Rho et al. (2010) [19]	Cross-sectional study evaluating correlation between HOMA-IR and serum adipokine levels.	169 RA patients	No correlation between visfatin levels and IR
Alkady et al. (2011) [52]	Case-control study evaluating correlation between serum and synovial liquid adipokines and disease activity.	70 RA patients 30 controls	Positive correlation between serum visfatin levels and disease activity.
Khalifa et al. (2013) [53]	Case-control study evaluating correlation between serum visfatin and inflammation markers.	60 RA patients 20 controls	Positive correlation between visfatin levels and IL-6, CRP, ERS, TNF-α and DAS-28 in RA.
El-Hini et al. (2013) [54]	Case-control study evaluating metabolic disorder and its association with clinical characteristics of RA patients.	40 RA patients 40 controls	Positive correlations between serum visfatin levels and IR, cholesterol, triglycerides and LDL-C.
Meyer et al. (2013) [56]	Cohort study evaluating serum adipokine levels and radiographic progression of RA.	632 RA patients at early stage of disease and 159 with unspecific arthritis	No correlation between visfatin levels and progression of RA.
Sglunda et al. (2014) [55]	Prospective study evaluating visfatin level and its relationship with disease activity and serum lipids.	40 patients with early, treatment-naïve RA 30 controls	Correlation between visfatin levels and disease activity and reduced levels after treatment.
Mirfeizi et al. (2014) [30]	Cross-sectional study evaluating correlation between serum adipokines levels and radiographic joint damage.	54 RA patients (29 with erosion and 25 without erosion)	The levels of visfatin were higher in patients with radiographic joint damage and dependent on the duration of the disease.

RA = rheumatoid arthritis; IR = insulin resistance; MetS = metabolic syndrome; IL-6 = interleukin-6; CRP = C-reactive protein; ESR = erythrocyte sedimentation rate; DAS28 = Disease Activity Score-28; TNF-α = tumor necrosis factor α; LDL-C = low-density lipoprotein cholesterol

of adiponectin in patients with RA, suggesting a much more harmful than beneficial action of adiponectin in chronic inflammatory diseases. Several studies evidenced association of adiponectin in radiographic progression of RA [67, 68]. Thus, serum adiponectin levels could be a good biomarker to evaluate the early stages of disease progression [56]. However, this association was not mediated by the selective effect of HMW adiponectin. [69] Recently, Skalska and Kontny (2016) [18] observed that HMW and MMW adiponectins potentially stimulated the secretion of rheumatoid ASC (adipose-derived stem cells) in patients with RA, but did not exert a strong impact on ASC towards RA-FLS (fibroblast-like synoviocytes) and peripheral blood mononuclear cells.

Furthermore, Rho et al. (2010) [19] did not find any association between adiponectin levels and insulin resistance or coronary artery calcium score. Yoshino et al. (2011) [21] also observed higher levels of adiponectin in serum of RA patients, but it was negatively associated with CRP levels. Bustos Rivera-Bahena et al. (2015) [24] did not evidenced association between adiponectin and disease activity and Chennareddy et al. (2016) [70] reported that despite serum levels of adiponectin are higher in RA patients than in controls there was no correlation with disease activity, duration, BMI and waist-to-hip ratio.

Despite the protective effect of adiponectin in the pathogenesis of obesity, diabetes mellitus, atherosclerosis, and metabolic syndrome, it is unclear whether this effect is reproduced in RA. Several studies emphasize that adiponectin appears to play a pro inflammatory role in the pathogenesis of RA, particularly in the joints, by stimulating the secretion of inflammatory mediators. In this scenario, it highlights the importance of developing new research elucidating the real role of adipokines in the pathogenesis of RA.

Table 4 summarizes the main findings of adipnectin in RA patients.

Conclusion

In recent years, it has been studied the importance of adipokines in the pathogenesis of RA, however the results are still conflicting and the exactly role of adipose tissue in RA is not yet fully understood. Despite studies have been demonstrating the implications of adipokines in the pathophysiology of autoimmune diseases, including RA, it is not yet clear their role in the progression of disease. It is noteworthy the complex pathophysiology of this disease, thus requiring better knowledge about the mechanisms of action of these adipokines in RA as well as the changes that drugs can promote in the circulating levels of these adipokines in these patients.

Table 4 Studies investigating the association of adiponectin and rheumatoid arthritis in humans

Authors	Study design	Subjects	Results/outcomes
Rho et al. (2010) [19]	Cross-sectional study evaluating correlation between HOMA-IR and serum adipokine levels.	169 RA patients	No correlation between adiponectin and insulin resistance.
Alkady et al. (2011) [52]	Case-control study evaluating correlation between serum and synovial liquid adipokines and disease activity.	70 RA patients 30 controls	Positive correlation between serum and synovial adiponectin levels and disease activity.
Yoshino et al. (2011) [21]	Case-control study evaluating correlation between inflammation markers and serum adipokine levels.	141 RA patients 146 controls	No correlation between serum adiponectin levels and CRP.
Giles et al. (2011) [67]	Prospective study evaluating association of serum adipokine levels with progression of radiographic joint damage in patients with rheumatoid arthritis.	152 RA patients	Positive correlation between serum adiponectin levels and erosive joint destruction.
Klein-Wieringa et al. (2011) [68]	Cohort study evaluating baseline adipokine levels to predict radiographic progression of RA over a period of 4 years.	253 RA patients	Positive correlation between serum levels of adiponectin and radiographic progression of 4 RA.
Meyer et al. (2013) [56]	Cohort study evaluating serum adipokines levels and radiographic progression of RA.	632 RA patients at early stage of disease and 159 with unspecific arthritis	Positive association between serum adiponectin levels and radiographic progression of RA at early stage.
Bustos Rivera-Bahena et al. (2015) [24]	Cross-sectional study evaluating correlation between adipokines levels and disease activity.	121 RA patients	No correlation between serum adiponectin and clinical activity of RA, but negative correlation with TNFα and positive correlation with IL-1β.
Chennareddy et al. (2016) [70]	Cross-sectional study evaluating the serum concentrations of adiponectin and its impact on disease activity and radiographic joint damage.	43 RA patients 25 controls	Increased levels of serum adiponectin in RA, but no correlation with erosive and non-erosive disease, disease duration, BMI, waist-hip ratio and disease activity.

RA = rheumatoid arthritis; IR = insulin resistance; CRP = C-reactive protein; BMI = body mass index

Abbreviations

ACPA: Anti–citrullinated protein antibody; ASC: Adipose-derived stem cells; BMI: Body mass index; CRP: C-reactive protein; CVD: Cardiovascular diseases; DAS: Disease Activity Score; FLS: Fibroblast-like synoviocytes; HMW: High molecular weight; HOMA-IR: Homeostasis Model Assessment - Insulin Resistance; IL: Interleukin; LDL-c: Low density lipoprotein cholesterol; LMW: Low molecular weight; LPS: Lipopolysaccharide; MCP: Monocyte chemoattractant protein; MetS: Metabolic syndrome; MMP: Matrix metalloproteinase; MMW: Middle molecular weight; Nampt: Nicotinamide phosphoribosyltransferase; NF-κβ: Nuclear factor kappa beta; NO: Nitric oxide; PBEF: Pre-B-cell colony-enhancing factor; PG: Prostaglandina; PRISMA: Preferred Reporting Items for Systematic Reviews and Meta-Analyses; RA: Rheumatoid arthritis; RELM: Resistin-like molecules; RF: Rheumatoid factor; SciELO: Scientific Electronic Library Online; Th: T helper; TLR: Toll-like receptor; TNF: Tumor necrosis factor

Funding

The authors declare that they had no funding for this study.

Authors' contributions

ECSF and FTR made substantial contributions to acquisition and interpretation of data, and writing the manuscript. ANCS and ID contributed to conception of the study, and revising it critically. All authors read and approved the final manuscript.

Competing interests

The authors declare that they have no competing interests.

Author details

[1]Postgraduate Program, Health Sciences Center, State University of Londrina, Londrina, Paraná, Brazil. [2]Postgraduate Program, Experimental Pathology, State University of Londrina, Londrina, Paraná, Brazil. [3]Department of Pathology, Clinical Analysis and Toxicology, University Londrina, Londrina, Paraná, Brazil. [4]Department of Internal Medicine, University of Londrina, Londrina, Paraná, Brazil. [5]Department of Nutrition, University of Fronteira Sul, Rodovia PR 182 Km 466, CEP 85770-000, Realeza, Paraná Postal Code 253, Brazil.

References

1. Lipsky PE. Artrite Reumatoide. In: Medicina interna de Harrison. 14th ed. Rio de Janeiro: Amgh Editora; 1998. p. 1996–7.
2. Mateen S, Zafar A, Moin S, Khan AQ, Zubair S. Understanding the role of cytokines in the pathogenesis of rheumatoid arthritis. Clin Chim Acta. 2016; 455:161–71.
3. American College of Rheumatology Subcommittee on Rheumatoid Arthritis Guidelines. Guidelines for the management of rheumatoid arthritis: 2002 update. Arthritis Rheum. 2002;46(2):328–46. http://www.ncbi.nlm.nih.gov/pubmed/11840435
4. Barbosa VDS, Rêgo J, Antônio N. Possível papel das adipocinas no lúpus eritematoso sitêmico e na artrite reumatoide. Rev Bras Reumatol. 2012;52(2): 278–87.
5. Hutcheson J. Adipokines influence the inflammatory balance in autoimmunity. Cytokine. 2015;75(2):272–9.
6. Shamseer L, Moher D, Clarke M, Ghersi D, Liberati A, Petticrew M, et al. Preferred reporting items for systematic review and meta-analysis protocols (PRISMA-P) 2015: elaboration and explanation. BMJ. 2015;349 http://www.bmj.com/content/349/bmj.g7647
7. Neumann E, Frommer KW, Vasile M, Müller-Ladner U. Adipocytokines as driving forces in rheumatoid arthritis and related inflammatory diseases? Arthritis Rheum. 2011;63(5):1159–69.
8. Freitas Lima LC, Braga VA, do Socorro de França Silva M, Cruz JC, Sousa Santos SH, de Oliveira Monteiro MM, et al. Adipokines, diabetes and atherosclerosis: an inflammatory association. Front Physiol. 2015;6:1–15.
9. Dichi I, Simão ANC. Metabolic syndrome: new targets for an old problem. Expert Opin Ther Targets. 2012;16(2):147–50. http://www.tandfonline.com/doi/full/10.1517/14728222.2012.648924
10. Zhang Y, Proenca R, Maffei M, Barone M, Leopold L, Friedman JM. Positional cloning of the mouse obese gene and its human homologue. Nature. 1994;372(6505):425–32. http://www.ncbi.nlm.nih.gov/pubmed/7984236
11. Guimarães DED, Sardinha FL DC, Mizurini D DM, Das GT Do CM. Adipocitocinas: uma nova visão do tecido adiposo. Rev Nutr. 2007;20(5): 549–59. http://www.scielo.br/scielo.php?script=sci_arttext&pid=S1415-52732007000500010&lng=pt&nrm=iso&tlng=pt
12. Mantzoros CS, Magkos F, Brinkoetter M, Sienkiewicz E, Dardeno TA, Kim S, et al. Leptin in human physiology and pathophysiology. AJP Endocrinol Metab. 2011;301:567–84.
13. Del Prete A, Salvi V, Sozzani S. Adipokines as potential biomarkers in rheumatoid arthritis. Mediat Inflamm. 2014;2014:1–12.
14. Paz-Filho G, Mastronardi C, Franco CB, Wang KB, Wong M-L, Licinio J. Leptin: molecular mechanisms, systemic pro-inflammatory effects, and clinical implications. Arq Bras Endocrinol Metabol. 2012;56(9):597–607. http://www.ncbi.nlm.nih.gov/pubmed/23329181
15. Olama SM, Senna MK, Elarman M. Synovial/serum leptin ratio in rheumatoid arthritis: the association with activity and erosion. Rheumatol Int. 2012;32(3): 683–90. http://www.ncbi.nlm.nih.gov/pubmed/21140264
16. Toussirot É, Michel F, Binda D, Dumoulin G. The role of leptin in the pathophysiology of rheumatoid arthritis. Life Sci. 2015;140:29–36. http://linkinghub.elsevier.com/retrieve/pii/S002432051500257X
17. Scotece M, Conde J, López V, Lago F, Pino J, Gómez-Reino JJ, et al. Adiponectin and leptin: new targets in inflammation. Basic Clin Pharmacol Toxicol. 2014;114(1):97–102.
18. Skalska U, Kontny E. Adiponectin isoforms and Leptin impact on rheumatoid adipose Mesenchymal stem cells function. Stem Cells Int. 2016;2016:1–7.
19. Rho YH, Chung CP, Solus JF, Raggi P, Oeser A, Gebretsadik T, et al. Adipocytokines, insulin resistance, and coronary atherosclerosis in rheumatoid arthritis. Arthritis Rheum. 2010;62(5):1259–64.
20. Targońska-Stepniak B, Dryglewska M, Majdan M. Adiponectin and leptin serum concentrations in patients with rheumatoid arthritis. Rheumatol Int. 2010;30:731–7.
21. Yoshino T, Kusunoki N, Tanaka N, Kaneko K, Kusunoki Y, Endo H, et al. Elevated serum levels of resistin, leptin, and adiponectin are associated with C-reactive protein and also other clinical conditions in rheumatoid arthritis. Intern Med. 2011;50(4):269–75. https://www.ncbi.nlm.nih.gov/pubmed/21325757
22. Kontunen P, Vuolteenaho K, Nieminen R, Lehtimäki L, Kautiainen H, Kesäniemi Y, et al. Resistin is linked to inflammation, and leptin to metabolic syndrome, in women with inflammatory arthritis. Scand J Rheumatol. 2011; 40(4):256–62. http://www.ncbi.nlm.nih.gov/pubmed/21453187
23. Kang Y, Park H-J, Kang M-I, Lee H-S, Lee S-W, Lee S-K, et al. Adipokines, inflammation, insulin resistance, and carotid atherosclerosis in patients with rheumatoid arthritis. Arthritis Res Ther. 2013;15(6):1–7. http://www.ncbi.nlm.nih.gov/pubmed/24245495
24. Bustos Rivera-Bahena C, Xibillé-Friedmann DX, González-Christen J, Carrillo-Vázquez SM, Montiel-Hernández JL. Peripheral blood Leptin and Resistin levels as clinical activity biomarkers in Mexican rheumatoid arthritis patients. Reumatol Clin. 2016;12(6):323–6.
25. Xibille-Friedmann DX, Ortiz-Panozo E, Bustos Rivera-Bahena C, Sandoval-Rios M, Hernandez-Gongora SE, Dominguez-Hernandez L, et al. Leptin and adiponectin as predictors of disease activity in rheumatoid arthritis. Clin Exp Rheumatol. 2015;33(4):471–7.
26. Tian G, Liang J-N, Wang Z-Y, Zhou D. Emerging role of leptin in rheumatoid arthritis. Clin Exp Immunol. 2014;177(3):557–70. http://www.pubmedcentral.nih.gov/articlerender.fcgi?artid=4137840&tool=pmcentrez&rendertype=abstract
27. Lee YH, Bae S-C. Circulating leptin level in rheumatoid arthritis and its correlation with disease activity: a meta-analysis. Z Rheumatol. 2016;75(10): 1021–7.
28. Allam A, Radwan A. The relationship of serum leptin levels with disease activity in Egyptian patients with rheumatoid arthritis. Egypt Rheumatol. 2012;34(4):185–90.
29. Abdalla M, Effat D, Sheta M, Hamed WE. Serum Leptin levels in rheumatoid arthritis and relationship with disease activity. Egypt Rheumatol. 2014;36(1):1–5.

30. Mirfeizi Z, Noubakht Z, Rezaie AE, Jokar MH, Sarabi ZS. Plasma levels of leptin and visfatin in rheumatoid arthritis patients; is there any relationship with joint damage? Iran J Basic Med Sci. 2014;17(9):662–6. http://www.ncbi.nlm.nih.gov/pubmed/25691942

31. Oner SY, Volkan O, Oner C, Mengi A, Direskeneli H, Tasan DA. Serum leptin levels do not correlate with disease activity in rheumatoid arthritis. Acta Reumatol Port. 2015;40(1):50–4.

32. Steppan CM, Bailey ST, Bhat S, Brown EJ, Banerjee RR, Wright CM, et al. The hormone resistin links obesity to diabetes. Nature. 2001;409(6818):307–12. http://www.ncbi.nlm.nih.gov/pubmed/11201732

33. Lee JH, Chan JL, Yiannakouris N, Kontogianni M, Estrada E, Seip R, et al. Circulating resistin levels are not associated with obesity or insulin resistance in humans and are not regulated by fasting or leptin administration: cross-sectional and interventional studies in normal, insulin-resistant, and diabetic subjects. J Clin Endocrinol Metab. 2003;88(10):4848–56. http://www.ncbi.nlm.nih.gov/pubmed/14557464

34. Codoñer-Franch P, Alonso-Iglesias E. Resistin: insulin resistance to malignancy. Clin Chim Acta. 2015;438:46–54.

35. Abella V, Scotece M, Conde J, López V, Lazzaro V, Pino J, et al. Review article Adipokines. Metabolic Syndrome and Rheumatic Diseases J Immunol Researc. 2014;2014:1–15.

36. Kassem E, Mahmoud L, Salah W. Study of Resistin and YKL-40 in rheumatoid arthritis. J Am Sci. 2010;6(10):1004–12.

37. Fadda SMH, Gamal SM, Elsaid NY, Mohy AM. Resistin in inflammatory and degenerative rheumatologic diseases: relationship between resistin and rheumatoid arthritis disease progression. Z Rheumatol. 2013;72(6):594–600.

38. Huang Q, Tao S-S, Zhang Y-J, Zhang C, Li L-J, Zhao W, et al. Serum resistin levels in patients with rheumatoid arthritis and systemic lupus erythematosus: a meta-analysis. Clin Rheumatol. 2015:1713–20. http://link.springer.com/10.1007/s10067-015-2955-5

39. Al-kady EA, Ahmed HM, Tag L, Adel M, Al-Kady EA. Adipocytokines: Adiponectin, Resistin and Visfatin in serum and synovial fluid of rheumatoid arthritis patients and their relation to disease activity. Med J Cairo Univ. 2010;78(2):723–9.

40. Hammad MH, Nasef S, Musalam D, Ahmed MM, Osman I, Hammad MH. Resistin, an adipokine , its relation to inflammation in Systemic Lupus Erythematosus and Rheumatoid Arthritis. Middle East J Intern Med. 2014;7(3):3–9.

41. Bao JP, Chen WP, Wu LD. Visfatin: a potential therapeutic target for rheumatoid arthritis. J Int Med Res. 2009;37(6):1655–61. http://www.ncbi.nlm.nih.gov/entrez/query.fcgi?cmd=Retrieve&db=PubMed&dopt=Citation&list_uids=20146863

42. Samal B, Sun Y, Stearns G, Xie C, Suggs S, McNiece I. Cloning and characterization of the cDNA encoding a novel human pre-B-cell Colony-enhancing. Mol Cell Biol. 1994;14(2):1431–7.

43. Fukuhara A, Matsuda M, Nishizawa M, Segawa K, Tanaka M, Kishimoto K, et al. Visfatin: a protein secreted by visceral fat that mimics the effects of insulin. Science. 2005;307(5708):426–30. http://www.ncbi.nlm.nih.gov/pubmed/15604363

44. Kerekes G, Nurmohamed MT, González-Gay MA, Seres I, Paragh G, Kardos Z, et al. Rheumatoid arthritis and metabolic syndrome. Nat Rev Rheumatol. 2014;10(11):691–6. http://www.ncbi.nlm.nih.gov/pubmed/25090948

45. Stofkova A. Resistin and visfatin: regulators of insulin sensitivity, inflammation and immunity. Endocr Regul. 2010;44(1):25–36. http://www.ncbi.nlm.nih.gov/pubmed/20151765

46. Haider DG, Schindler K, Schaller G, Prager G, Wolzt M, Ludvik B. Increased plasma visfatin concentrations in morbidly obese subjects are reduced after gastric banding. J Clin Endocrinol Metab. 2006;91(4):1578–81. http://www.ncbi.nlm.nih.gov/pubmed/16449335

47. Romacho T, Sánchez-ferrer CF, Peiró C. Review article Visfatin / Nampt: an Adipokine with cardiovascular impact. Mediat Inflamm. 2013;2013:1–16.

48. Naguib A, Elsawy N, Aboul-enein F, Hossam N. The relation between serum visfatin levels and cardiovascular involvement in rheumatoid arthritis. Alexandria J Med. 2011;47(2):117–24. https://doi.org/10.1016/j.ajme.2011.07.005%5Cnhttp://linkinghub.elsevier.com/retrieve/pii/S2090506811000479

49. Gómez R, Suarez A, Villalvilla A, Herrero-Beaumont G, Largo R, Young DA. Visfatin: a new player in rheumatic diseases. Immunometabolism. 2013;1:10–5. http://www.degruyter.com/view/j/immun.2013.1.issue/immun-2013-0002/immun-2013-0002.xml

50. Meier FMP, Frommer KW, Peters MA, Brentano F, Lefèvre S, Schröder D, et al. Visfatin/pre-B-cell colony-enhancing factor (PBEF), a proinflammatory and cell motility-changing factor in rheumatoid arthritis. J Biol Chem.

2012;287(34):28378–85.

51. Kim KS, Choi HM, Ji HI, Song R, Yang HI, Lee SK, et al. Serum adipokine levels in rheumatoid arthritis patients and their contributions to the resistance to treatment. Mol Med Rep. 2014;9(1):255–60.

52. Alkady EAM, Ahmed HM, Tag L, Abdou MA. Adiponectin, Resistin und Visfatin in Serum und Gelenkflüssigkeit bei Patienten mit rheumatoider Arthritis. Z Rheumatol. 2011;70(7):602–8. http://link.springer.com/10.1007/s00393-011-0834-2

53. Khalifa IA, Abdelfattah A. Relation between serum visfatin and clinical severity in different stages of rheumatoid arthritis. Egypt Rheumatol Rehabil. 2013;40(1):1–8.

54. El-Hini SH, Mohamed FI, Hassan AA, Ali F, Mahmoud A, Ibraheem HM. Visfatin and adiponectin as novel markers for evaluation of metabolic disturbance in recently diagnosed rheumatoid arthritis patients. Rheumatol Int. 2013;33(9):2283–9.

55. Sglunda O, Mann H, Hulejová H, Kuklová M, Pecha O, Pleštilová L, et al. Decreased circulating visfatin is associated with improved disease activity in early rheumatoid arthritis: data from the PERAC cohort. PLoS One. 2014;9(7):1–5.

56. Meyer M, Sellam J, Fellahi S, Kotti S, Bastard J-P, Meyer O, et al. Serum level of adiponectin is a surrogate independent biomarker of radiographic disease progression in early rheumatoid arthritis: results from the ESPOIR cohort. Arthritis Res Ther. 2013;15(6):1–13.

57. Scherer PE, Williams S, Fogliano M, Baldini G, Lodish HF. A novel serum protein similar to C1q, produced exclusively in adipocytes. J Biol Chem. 1995;270(45):26746–9. http://www.ncbi.nlm.nih.gov/pubmed/7592907

58. Garaulet M, Hernández-Morante JJ, de Heredia FP, Tébar FJ. Adiponectin, the controversial hormone. Public Health Nutr. 2007;10(10A):1145–50. http://www.ncbi.nlm.nih.gov/pubmed/17903323

59. Yamauchi T, Nio Y, Maki T, Kobayashi M, Takazawa T, Iwabu M, et al. Targeted disruption of AdipoR1 and AdipoR2 causes abrogation of adiponectin binding and metabolic actions. Nat Med. 2007;13(3):332–9. http://www.ncbi.nlm.nih.gov/pubmed/17268472

60. Ohashi K, Ouchi N, Matsuzawa Y. Anti-inflammatory and anti-atherogenic properties of adiponectin. Biochimie. 2012;94(10):2137–42.

61. Fantuzzi G. Adiponectin in inflammatory and immune-mediated diseases. Cytokine. 2013;64(1):1–10. http://www.ncbi.nlm.nih.gov/pubmed/23850004

62. Simão TNC, Lozovoy MAB, Simão ANC, Oliveira SR, Venturini D, Morimoto HK, et al. Reduced-energy cranberry juice increases folic acid and adiponectin and reduces homocysteine and oxidative stress in patients with the metabolic syndrome. Br J Nutr. 2013;110(10):1885–94. http://www.journals.cambridge.org/abstract_S0007114513001207

63. Chen X, Lu J, Bao J, Guo J, Shi J, Wang Y. Adiponectin: a biomarker for rheumatoid arthritis? Cytokine Growth Factor Rev. 2013;24(1):83–9.

64. Scotece M, Conde J, Gómez R, López V, Pino J, González A, et al. Role of adipokines in atherosclerosis: interferences with cardiovascular complications in rheumatic diseases. Mediat Inflamm. 2012;2012:1–14.

65. Krysiak R, Handzlik-Orlik G, Okopien B. The role of adipokines in connective tissue diseases. Eur J Nutr. 2012;51(5):513–28.

66. Frommer KW, Schäffler A, Büchler C, Steinmeyer J, Rickert M, Rehart S, et al. Adiponectin isoforms: a potential therapeutic target in rheumatoid arthritis? Ann Rheum Dis. 2012;71(10):1724–32. http://www.ncbi.nlm.nih.gov/pubmed/22532632

67. Giles JT, van der Heijde DM, Bathon JM. Association of circulating adiponectin levels with progression of radiographic joint destruction in rheumatoid arthritis. Ann Rheum Dis [Internet]. 2011;70(9):1562–8. http://www.ncbi.nlm.nih.gov/pubmed/21571734

68. Klein-Wieringa IR, Van Der Linden MPM, Knevel R, Kwekkeboom JC, Van Beelen E, Huizinga TWJ, et al. Baseline serum adipokine levels predict radiographic progression in early rheumatoid arthritis. Arthritis Rheum. 2011;63(9):2567–74.

69. Klein-Wieringa IR, Andersen SN, Herb-Van Toorn L, Kwekkeboom JC, Van Der Helm-Van Mil AHM, Meulenbelt I, et al. Are baseline high molecular weight adiponectin levels associated with radiographic progression in rheumatoid arthritis and osteoarthritis? J Rheumatol. 2014;41(5):853–7.

70. Chennareddy S, Kishore Babu KV, Kommireddy S, Varaprasad R, Rajasekhar L. Serum adiponectin and its impact on disease activity and radiographic joint damage in early rheumatoid arthritis – a cross-sectional study. Indian J Rheumatol. 2016;11(2):82–5.

20

Favorable rituximab response in patients with refractory idiopathic inflammatory myopathies

Fernando Henrique Carlos de Souza[1], Renata Miossi[1], Júlio Cesar Bertacini de Moraes[1], Eloisa Bonfá[2] and Samuel Katsuyuki Shinjo[2*]

Abstract

Background: Interpretation of rituximab efficacy for refractory idiopathic inflammatory myopathies (IIM) is hampered by the absence of a uniform definition of refractory myositis and clinical response. Therefore, rigorous criteria of refractoriness, together with a homogenous definition of clinical improvement, were used to evaluate rituximab one-year response.

Methods: A retrospective cohort study including 43 IIM (15 antisynthetase syndrome, 16 dermatomyositis, 12 polymyositis) was conducted. All patients had refractory disease (inadequate response to at least two immunosuppressives/immunomodulatories and no less than three months sequentially or concomitantly glucocorticoid tapering) criteria. Clinical/laboratory improvement at one-year was based on modified International Myositis Assessment & Clinical Studies Group (IMACS) core set measures. The patients received two infusions of rituximab (1 g each) at baseline, followed by repeated dose after 6 months. Baseline immunosuppressive therapy was maintained and glucocorticoid dose was tapered according to clinical/laboratory parameters.

Results: Five patients had side effects at the first rituximab application and were excluded. Therefore, 38 out of 43 patients completed the one-year follow up. Almost 75% of the patients attained clinical and laboratory response after one-year. A significant reduction in median glucocorticoid dose (18.8 vs. 6.3 mg/day) was achieved and 42% patients were able to discontinue prednisone. In contrast, young individuals and patients with dysphagia had a tendency to be non-responders to rituximab. No severe infections were observed.

Conclusion: This study provides convincing evidence that rituximab is an effective and safe therapy for refractory IIM.

Keywords: Antibodies, Dermatomyositis, Myositis, Polymyositis, Rituximab

Background

Idiopathic inflammatory myopathies (IIM) constitute a heterogeneous group of chronic systemic autoimmune diseases with a high rate of morbidity and disability [1–3]. Based on their clinical, laboratory, histopathological and progression features, IIM can be classified as polymyositis (PM), dermatomyositis (DM), antisynthetase syndrome (ASS), inclusion body myositis, and others [2, 3].

A number of studies have suggested rituximab efficacy for refractory IIM, with response rates ranging from 61 to 83% [4–11]. This high and wide range of response rate is partly explained by the lack of a standardized definition for refractoriness and/or use of heterogeneous response parameters. In fact, refractory myositis has several definitions including intolerance to or an inadequate response to glucocorticoids and at least one other immunosuppressive agent, but few studies provide a clear description of whether the maximum tolerated therapeutic dose was achieved [5–11].

With regard to rituximab response parameters, most reports are limited to serum level of creatine phosphokinase and muscle strength improvements [6–11]. However, creatine phosphokinase may be not the best parameter, particularly if the evaluation includes different types of myositis,

* Correspondence: samuel.shinjo@gmail.com
[2]Division of Rheumatology, Faculdade de Medicina FMUSP, Universidade de Sao Paulo, Sao Paulo, Brazil
Full list of author information is available at the end of the article

such as DM and ASS, in which other target organ involvement is more relevant than muscular involvement [2]. Of note, the disease activity core set measures validated by the International Myositis Assessment & Clinical Studies Group (IMACS) [12, 13] have not been previously used to evaluate refractory IIM response to therapy. These measures defined response as a > 20% improvement on three out of any 6 of the following core set measures: Health Assessment Questionnaire (HAQ); Manual Muscle Testing-8 (MMT-8); Physician Global Activity - Visual Analogue Scale (VAS); Patient Global Activity - VAS; serum muscle enzymes; Myositis Disease Activity Assessment Tool (MDAAT); with no more than two core set measures worsening by > 25%, which cannot include MMT.

Therefore, the aim of the present study was to evaluate the efficacy and predictors of clinical improvement of rituximab in a homogeneous population of refractory IIM cases, using a rigorous definition of refractory disease and modified IMACS core set measures to evaluate long-term response.

Methods
Study design
This retrospective single-center cohort study conducted from 2011 to 2016 included 43 consecutive adult patients with refractory IIM: 15 ASS (defined as myositis, arthritis, pulmonary disease, positive antisynthetase antibody, with or without mechanic's hands, fever and/or Raynaud's phenomenon) [14]; 16 DM and 12 PM according to the criteria of Bohan and Peter [15].

Patient data
Patients with clinically amyopathic DM, overlap myositis, neoplasia associated myositis, necrotizing myopathies, acute and/or chronic infections were excluded.

Data were included in an ongoing electronic database protocol. Demographic, clinical, laboratory and therapeutic data were obtained by electronic medical records, containing previously standardized and parameterized data. The following parameters were analyzed: current age, gender, ethnicity, time between diagnosis and symptom onset, disease duration, gastrointestinal (upper dysphagia), pulmonary (moderate dyspnea or computed tomography disclosing evidence of interstitial pneumopathy and/or "ground-glass" pneumopathy), joint (arthralgia and/or arthritis), previous and current drug treatment.

Refractory myositis was defined as an inadequate response to at least two immunosuppressant/immunomodulatory drugs (cyclophosphamide, azathioprine, methotrexate, cyclosporine, leflunomide, mycophenolate mofetil and/or intravenous human immunoglobulin, in their full-dose, for a minimum period of 3 months) given sequentially or concomitantly, hampering glucocorticoid tapering. Upper dysphagia and pulmonary involvement were considered as disease severity parameters. Severe infection was defined as requiring hospitalization and/or intravenous antibiotic therapy.

Rituximab schedule
Rituximab treatment consisted of two infusions (1 g each, 2 weeks apart) and this same scheme was repeated 6 months after the first dose for patients showing no response or stable disease. The 6-month second dose was contraindicated for patients with recrudescent disease, hypogammaglobulinemia, side effects at first rituximab infusion and recurrent or severe infections. After starting on rituximab only one immunosuppressant was maintained at full-dose, and glucocorticoid tapering was started 2 months after initial rituximab treatment.

Disease activity
At the one-year evaluation, clinical and laboratory improvements were defined as > 20% improvement in at least three of the following modified IMACS core set measures: MMT-8 [12], physician' and patient' VAS [13], HAQ [16] and serum levels of muscle enzymes; with no more than two previous core set measures worsening by > 25%, which cannot include MMT.

Serum levels of creatine phosphokinase (normal range: 24–173 U/L) and aldolase (1.0–7.5 U/L) were evaluated. The following autoantibodies were investigated in this study: antinuclear factor (Hep2) and also anti-Jo-1, anti-OJ, anti-EJ, anti-PL-7, anti-PL-12, anti-Mi-2 and anti-SS-A/Ro-52. For the myositis-specific and myositis-associated autoantibodies' assessment, a commercially available line blot test kit (Myositis Profile Euroline Blot test kit, Euroimmun, Lübeck, Germany) was used according to the manufacturer's protocol and to the previously published study [17]. Reaction positivity was also defined according to a previously study [17].

Statistical analysis
The Kolmogorov-Smirnov test was used to evaluate the distribution of each parameter. The demographic and clinical features are expressed as mean ± standard deviation (SD) for the continuous variables or frequency (%) for the categorical variables. The median (25th - 75th interquartile range) was calculated for the continuous variables that were not normally distributed. Comparisons between different clinical, laboratory and treatment parameters at baseline and 12 months after rituximab infusion were performed using Student's t-test or the Mann-Whitney U-test for continuous variables, whereas the Chi-squared test or Fisher's exact test was used to evaluate the categorical variables. The 95% confidence interval (95% CI) of percentage was calculated by a binomial distribution. Age at Rituximab application sensitivity and specificity for identifying therapy responder were

calculated, and a receiver operating characteristic (ROC) curve was constructed. $P < 0.05$ was considered significant. All of the analyses were performed using the SPSS 15.0 statistics software (Chicago, USA).

Results

Five of the initial 43 patients were later excluded due to moderate allergic reactions to the first rituximab infusion ($N = 4$) or lost to follow-up ($N = 1$). There were no cases of patients with recrudescent disease, hypogammaglobulinemia or severe infections. Therefore, 38 patients remained in the study for 1 year: 15 (39.5%) patients with DM, 10 (26.3%) with PM, and 13 (34.2%) with ASS (Table 1).

Among the 38 patients assessed, mean current age was 42.6 ± 10.9 years, 84.2% were female gender and 68.4% had white ethnicity. Median disease time was 3.0 years, whereas median time between disease diagnosis and symptom onset was 4.5 months.

The antinuclear factor was present in 81.6% of patients with the following autoantibodies specificities: anti-Ro-52

Table 1 Demographic features, types of idiopathic inflammatory myopathies, autoantibody distribution and therapy of 38 patients immediately before rituximab application (Baseline)

Parameters	$N = 38$
Current age (years)	42.6 ± 10.9
Female gender	32 (84.2)
White ethnicity	26 (68.4)
Disease duration (years)	3.0 (2.0–6.5)
Duration time: diagnosis - symptom onset (months)	4.5 (3.9–9.0)
Idiopathic inflammatory myopathies	
Dermatomyositis	15 (39.5)
Polymyositis	10 (26.3)
Antisynthetase syndrome	13 (34.2)
Autoantibodies	
Antinuclear factor	31 (81.6)
Anti-Ro-52	16 (42.1)
Anti-Jo-1	13 (34.2)
Anti-Mi-2	4 (10.5)
Anti-OJ	0
Anti-EJ	0
Anti-PL-7	0
Anti-PL-12	0
Prednisone dose (mg/day)	18.8 (10.0–36.3)
Methylprednisolone + intravenous human immunoglobulin pulse therapy	23 (60.5)

Results expressed as mean ± standard deviation, median (25th - 75th interquartile range) or frequency (%)

(42.1%), anti Jo-1 (34.2%), anti-Mi-2 (10.5%), and no cases of anti-OJ, anti-EJ, anti-PL-7 or anti-PL-12 autoantibodies.

All 38 patients were in concomitant use of at least two immunosuppressive / immunomodulatory drugs, in their full-dose, for a minimum period of 3 months, hampering glucocorticoid tapering. Due to disease severity, 34 (89.5%) patients had also received methylprednisolone pulse therapy 1 g/day, for three consecutive days, and/or intravenous human immunoglobulin (1 g/kg/day, for 2 days, for two consecutive days). Moreover, immediately before the first dose of rituximab, 23 (60.5%) of 38 patients received again this same scheme (methylprednisolone and intravenous human immunoglobulin pulse therapies). At the time of rituximab application, median dose of prednisone was 18.8 mg/day.

Comparison of therapies at study entry vs. 12 months after rituximab application revealed a reduction in median glucocorticoid dose (18.8 vs. 6.3 mg/day; $P < 0.001$) (Table 2) and complete discontinuation of prednisone in 16 (42.1%) of the 38 patients.

Twenty-nine (72.5%) of the 38 patients achieved overall progress according to the modified core set of IMACS after 12 months of rituximab treatment.

With regard to adverse events in the 38 patients at one-year follow-up, none had severe infection, two (5.3%) patients had mild allergic reactions and one (2.6%) patient was diagnosed with non-Hodgkin's lymphoma (Table 2).

Further analysis of responders vs. non-responders at baseline identified younger age ($P = 0.008$) and higher frequency of dysphagia ($P = 0.038$) in non-responders (Table 3). The area under the ROC curve was 0.669 and age at 32 had 72% sensitivity and 67% specificity.

Female gender, ethnicity, disease duration and time between diagnosis and symptom onset were comparable between responder and non-responder groups. There was also no differences in myositis type (DM, PM or ASS), joint and pulmonary clinical symptoms, initial serum level of muscle enzymes, autoantibodies, or pre-treatment with methylprednisolone and intravenous human immunoglobulin pulse therapies ($P > 0.05$).

Discussion

In the present one-year study, long-term rituximab efficacy in refractory patients with IIM was demonstrated.

Rigorous criteria of refractoriness and also the modified IMACS disease activity response parameters were adopted in this research. Notably, due to disease severity, more than half of the patients also needed to receive methylprednisolone associated with intravenous human immunoglobulin pulse therapy to induce disease remission. In contrast, a less strict criterion of refractoriness was observed in previous studies and data on severe symptoms such as dysphagia were not reported hampering comparison with the present

Table 2 Evaluation at baseline, 6 and 12 months of 38 patients with idiopathic inflammatory myopathies after rituximab therapy

	Baseline	6 months	12 months	Δ% (12 months vs. Baseline)
Prednisone dose (mg/day)	18.8 (10.0–36.3)	8.8 (2.5–15.0)	6.3 (0.0–16.3)	–
MMT-8 (0–80)	68.5 (56.8–72.5)	72.0 (67.0–78.0)	74.0 (70.0–78.0)	+ 11.3
HAQ (0.00–3.00)	1.00 (0.50–1.51)	0.63 (0.25–1.00)	0.50 (0.03–1.16)	−53.0
Patient's VAS (0–10 cm)	5.0 (3.0–7.0)	3.0 (1.0–5.0)	2.0 (0.0–4.0)	− 57.0
Physician's VAS (0–10 cm)	5.0 (3.8–7.0)	3.0 (1.0–4.3)	2.0 (1.0–4.0)	−60.0
Creatine phosphokinase (U/L)	429 (123–971)	224 (83–527)	254 (83–551)	−8.6
Aldolase (U/L)	5.5 (4.0–10.6)	3.9 (3.2–6.9)	3.6 (3.2–7.0)	−29.0
Severe infections	–	0	0	–
Adverse events	–	0	2 (5.3)	–
Neoplasia	–	0	1 (2.6)	–

Results expressed as percentage (%), or median (25th - 75th). *VAS* Visual Analogue Scale, *MMT* Manual Muscle Testing, *HAQ* Healthy Assessment Questionnaire, *Δ%* percentage variation

Table 3 Frequency of rituximab response according to myosis type, clinical involvement, autoantibody profile and treatment

	Responders (N = 29)	Non-responders (N = 9)	P
Age at disease diagnosis (years)	39.6 ± 12.2	28.3 ± 9.0	0.008
Age at Rituximab application (years)	44.7 ± 11.0	35.8 ± 8.1	0.017
Female gender	24 (82.7)	8 (88.9)	1.000
White ethnicity	19 (65.5)	7 (77.8)	0.689
Disease duration (years)	3.0 (1.5–5.5)	3.0 (2.0–10.0)	0.919
Duration: diagnosis - symptoms (months)	5.0 (3.0–8.0)	4.0 (2.5–12.0)	0.589
Myositis			
Dermatomyositis	14 (48.3)	1 (11.2)	0.061
Polymyositis	6 (20.7)	4 (44.4)	0.205
Antisynthetase syndrome	9 (31.0)	4 (44.4)	0.389
Clinical and laboratory features			
Dysphagia	18 (62.1)	9 (100.0)	0.038
Articular	11 (37.9)	5 (55.6)	0.450
Pulmonary	11 (37.9)	3 (33.3)	1.000
Creatine phosphokinase (U/L)	5798 (2796–13,630)	9000 (4484–12,472)	0.457
Aldolase (U/L)	36.1 (18.7–42.3)	28.2 (20.6–40.6)	0.664
Autoantibodies			
Anti-Ro-52	11 (37.9)	5 (55.6)	0.450
Anti-Jo-1	9 (31.0)	4 (44.4)	0.689
Anti-Mi-2	4 (13.8)	0	–
Anti-OJ	0	0	–
Anti-EJ	0	0	–
Anti-PL-7	0	0	–
Anti-PL-12	0	0	–
Antinuclear factor	23 (73.9)	8 (88.9)	1.000
Pre-RTX infusion protocol			
Methylprednisolone + intravenous human immunoglobulin pulse therapy	16 (55.2)	7 (77.8)	0.273

Results expressed as mean ± standard deviation, median (25th - 75th) or percentage (%)
RTX Rituximab

analysis [4–11]. In fact, among patients evaluated in the present study, more than two-thirds had dysphagia, a known serious problem in patients with IIM that can be associated with nutritional deficiency, aspiration pneumonia and poor prognosis [18].

The rituximab protocol was a more aggressive approach than others previously reported [4–11], and included pre-infusion of methylprednisolone and intravenous human immunoglobulin for the majority of the patients. In addition, the rituximab fixed dose retreatment protocol was chosen as opposed to on-demand retreatment [4–11], taking into account refractoriness.

The long-term IMACS modified response rate obtained with the present protocol was comparable to that reported for the RIM trial [5], a remarkable result taking into consideration the disease severity and refractoriness of the patients selected. Our data reveals that this outcome occurred for all patients at 6 months and the improvement persisted at 1 year. In this regard, a highly successful prednisone taper was obtained, with a significant early mean dose reduction at 6 months and a substantial number of patients (42%) able to completely discontinue prednisone at 12 months. Reinforcing these results, a parallel improvement in MMT-8, HAQ, physician and patient' VAS, as well as in muscle enzymes occurred at 12 months.

Autoantibodies, especially anti-Jo-1 and anti-Mi-2, proved predictors of clinical improvement in a cohort of rituximab-treated myositis' patients, whereas at lack of definable autoantibodies was a predictor of no improvement [5]. Although this association was not found in the present study, the majority of patients with anti-Jo-1 and all with anti-Mi-2 autoantibodies, responded to a rituximab.

During the follow-up, rituximab was well-tolerated with few adverse reactions. The most common side effects in literature are infections (mainly respiratory tract infections), of which 5% were severe, requiring hospitalization. Infusion reactions rarely occurred and these were often mild and easily controlled with glucocorticoid. Notably, there were no cases of severe infections requiring hospitalization in the present study. The intravenous human immunoglobulin pre-rituximab may be contributed for these data. However, sustained clinical and laboratory improvement may be due to rituximab, since there was no difference between responders and non-responders regarding previous use of intravenous human immunoglobulin.

As a limitation of the present study, a small sample was included, given the rarity of the IIM and the strict inclusion and exclusion criteria applied. Moreover, a sequential analysis of the dysphagia (i.e.: manometry) and pulmonary function were not performed. Finally, it should be emphasized that the concomitant use of methylprednisolone associated with intravenous human immunoglobulin for the majority of the patients might have affected the outcomes.

Conclusions

The present study provides convincing evidence that rituximab treatment is an effective and safe therapy for refractory IIM with a sustained 1 year response and significant tapering/discontinuation of glucocorticoid therapy. Moreover, young individuals and patients with dysphagia have a tendency to be more refractory to rituximab.

Abbreviations
ASS: Antisynthetase syndrome; CI: Confidence interval; DM: Dermatomyositis; HAQ: Health Assessment Questionnaire; IIM: Idiopathic inflammatory myopathies; IMACS: International Myositis Assessment & Clinical Studies Group; MDAAT: Myositis Disease Activity Assessment Tool; MMT: Manual muscle testing; PM: Polymyositis; ROC: Receiver operating characteristic; SD: Standard deviation; VAS: Visual analogue scale

Acknowledgments
Not applicable.

Funding
Federico Foundation to EB and SKS; Fundação Faculdade de Medicina to SKS.

Authors' contributions
All authors contributed to write and review the manuscript. All authors read and approved the final manuscript.

Competing interests
All authors declare that they have no competing interests.

Author details
[1]Division of Rheumatology, Hospital das Clinicas HCFMUSP, Faculdade de Medicina, Universidade de Sao Paulo, Sao Paulo, Brazil. [2]Division of Rheumatology, Faculdade de Medicina FMUSP, Universidade de Sao Paulo, Sao Paulo, Brazil.

References
1. Feldman BM, Rider LG, Reed AM, Pachman LM. Juvenile dermatomyositis and other idiopathic inflammatory myopathies of childhood. Lancet. 2008; 371:2201–12.
2. Dalakas MC. Polymyositis, dermatomyositis and inclusion-body myositis. N Engl J Med. 1991;325:1487–98.
3. Fasano S, Gordon P, Hajji R, Loyo E, Isenberg DA. Rituximab in the treatment of inflammatory myopathies: a review. Rheumatology (Oxford). 2017;56:26–36.
4. Oddis CV, Reed AM, Aggarwal R, Rider LG, Ascherman DP, Levesque MC, et al. Rituximab in the treatment of refractory adult and juvenile dermatomyositis and adult polymyositis: a randomized, placebo-phase trial. Arthritis Rheum. 2013;65:314–24.
5. Aggarwal R, Bandos A, Reed AM, Ascherman DP, Barohn RJ, Feldman BM, et al; RIM Study Group, Oddis CV. Predictors of clinical improvement in rituximab-treated refractory adult and juvenile dermatomyositis and adult polymyositis. Arthritis Rheum. 2014;66:740–9.
6. Marie I, Dominique S, Janvresse A, Levesque H, Menard JF. Rituximab therapy for refractory interstitial lung disease related to anti-synthetase syndrome. Respir Med. 2012;106:581–7.
7. Levie TD. Rituximab in the treatment of dermatomyositis: an open-label pilot study. Arthritis Rheum. 2005;52:601–7.
8. Noss EH, Hausner-Sypek DL, Weinblatt ME. Rituximab as therapy for refractory polymyositis and dermatomyositis. J Rheumatol. 2006;33:1021–6.

9. Brulhart L, Waldburger JM, Gabay C. Rituximab in the treatment of antisynthetase syndrome. Ann Rheum Dis. 2006;65:974–5.

10. Dinh HV, McCormack C, Hall S, Prince HM. Rituximab for the treatment of the skin manifestations of dermatomyositis: a report of 3 cases. J Am Acad Dermatol. 2007;56:148–53.

11. Frikha F, Rigolet A, Behin A, Fautrel B, Herson S, Benveniste O. Efficacy of rituximab in refractory and relapsing myositis with anti-Jo-1 antibodies: a report of two cases. Rheumatology. 2009;48:1166–8.

12. Rider LG, Koziol D, Giannini EH, Jain MS, Smith MR, Whitney-Mahoney K, et al. Validation of manual muscle testing and a subset of eight muscles for adult and juvenile idiopathic inflammatory myopathies. Arthritis Care Res (Hoboken). 2010;62:465–72.

13. Sultan SM, Allen E, Oddis CV, Kiely P, Cooper RG, Lundberg IE, et al. Reliability and validity of the myositis disease activity assessment tool. Arthritis Rheum. 2008;58:3593–9.

14. Mahler M, Miller FW, Fritzler MJ. Idiopathic inflammatory myopathies and the anti-synthetase syndrome: a comprehensive review. Autoimmun Rev. 2014;13:367–71.

15. Bohan A, Peter JB. Polymyositis and dermatomyositis (first of two parts). N Engl J Med. 1975;292:344–7.

16. Bruce B, Fries JF. The Stanford health assessment questionnaire: dimensions and practical applications. Health Qual Life Outcomes. 2003;1:20.

17. Cruellas MG, Viana V dos S, Levy-Neto M, Souza FH, Shinjo SK. Myositis-specific and myositis-associated autoantibody profiles and their clinical associations in a large series of patients with polymyositis and dermatomyositis. Clinics. 2013;68:909–14.

18. Daković Z, Vesić S, Tomović M, Vuković J. Oropharyngeal dysphagia as dominant and life-threatening symptom in dermatomyositis. Vojnosanit Pregl. 2009;66:671–4.

21

A systematic review of the effects of strength training in patients with fibromyalgia: clinical outcomes and design considerations

Alexandro Andrade[1,2]* ⓘ, Ricardo de Azevedo Klumb Steffens[1,2,3] ⓘ, Sofia Mendes Sieczkowska[1,2] ⓘ, Leonardo Alexandre Peyré Tartaruga[4,5] ⓘ and Guilherme Torres Vilarino[1,2] ⓘ

Abstract

Background: Fibromyalgia (FM) is characterized by chronic and generalized musculoskeletal pain. There is currently no cure for FM, but palliative treatments are available. One type of treatment is strength training (ST). However, there is a need for more information on optimal training protocols, intensity, and volume needed to improve symptoms. The aim of this study was to analyze the effects of ST in the treatment of FM through a systematic review of experimental research.

Methods: Medical Subject Headings search terms and electronic databases including Scientific Electronic Library Online, PubMed, Science Direct, Web of Science, and Physiotherapy Evidence Database were used to identify studies.

Results: The inclusion criteria were met by 22 eligible studies. Most of the studies were conducted in the United States (36%), Finland (23%), Brazil (18%), and Sweden (18%). The studies showed that ST reduces the number of tender points, fatigue, depression, and anxiety, and improves sleep quality and quality of life in patients with FM. The intervention period ranged from 3 to 21 weeks, with sessions performed 2 times a week in 81.81% of the studies, at initial intensities of 40% of 1-repetition maximum. The repetitions ranged from 4 to 20, with no specific protocol defined for ST in FM.

Conclusion: The main results included reduction in pain, fatigue, number of tender points, depression, and anxiety, with increased functional capacity and quality of life. Current evidence demonstrates that ST is beneficial and can be used to treat FM.

Trial registration: CRD42016048480.

Keywords: Fibromyalgia, Resistance training, Health, Exercises, Therapy, Rehabilitation

Background

Fibromyalgia (FM) is a chronic disease characterized by generalized skeletal muscle pain [1, 2], and other common symptoms include fatigue, sleep disorders, depression, and excessive anxiety [3–6]. The pathogenesis of FM is still not well understood [7], and FM is considered by some researchers to be a neurobiological disease caused by abnormal processing of pain [8]. Owing to the lack of markers that can identify the disease, the diagnosis is made through clinical examination, according to the guidelines of the American College of Rheumatology [1, 3].

As FM has no cure, treatments are palliative, and multidisciplinary approaches involving the use of medications, physical exercise (PE), and psychological treatments are recommended [4, 9–12]. PE has been advised in several studies and guidelines for the treatment of FM

* Correspondence: alexandro.andrade.phd@gmail.com
[1]Health and Sports Science Center, CEFID / Santa Catarina State University – UDESC, Florianópolis, SC, Brazil
[2]Laboratory of Sports and Exercise Psychology - LAPE, Florianópolis, SC, Brazil
Full list of author information is available at the end of the article

[13–16], and the inclusion of aerobic, resistance, and water exercises has been strongly recommended [5, 15–17]. The severity of FM symptoms can affect the level of physical fitness, and patients commonly perform little physical activity because of pain [18–20].

The relationship between PE and FM has been investigated, and strength training (ST) has been compared with other PE modalities. Studies have shown that ST has favorable results on pain, sleep, depression, and the number of tender points [17, 21]. However, studies on the effect of PE present poor quality evidence owing to small sample sizes and methodological problems [22, 23]. Recent studies have attempted to better understand the effects of ST in patients with FM [21, 24–26]. However, research has emphasized physical aspects with conflicting results [27, 28]. Despite recent research on the effects of ST in patients with FM, the duration, frequency, and intensity required to improve the symptoms remain unknown because the protocols differ among studies [29–31]. Thus, there is no consensus on the use of ST in clinical practice. The aim of this study was to analyze the effects of ST in the treatment of FM through a systematic review of experimental research.

Methods

The present study followed the PRISMA (Preferred Reporting Items for Systematic Reviews and Meta-Analyses) guidelines [32]. The PRISMA Statement is a protocol that guides the construction of systematic reviews in a transparent and consistent manner using a checklist of 27 items and a 4-phase flow diagram [33]. This systematic review was registered as CRD42016048480 in the International Prospective Register of Systematic Reviews (PROSPERO) [34]. A primary goal of PROSPERO is to make known the intention to conduct a systematic review, in order to reduce duplication and to facilitate transparency in the review process [35].

Eligibility criteria

In order to include the entire publication period, no time limit was set. The eligibility criteria were determined according to the PICOS (Population, Intervention, Comparison, Outcomes, Setting) strategy.

Population

Adults 18 years and older with a diagnosis of FM according to the 1990 criteria of the American College of Rheumatology (1).

Intervention

Any intervention with ST or resistance training for patients with FM was included. We excluded studies with combined interventions, such as those with ST combined with aerobic training.

Comparison

With any other type of group (such as sedentary controls and healthy controls) and with other types of intervention (such as aerobic exercise and flexibility exercise).

Outcomes

All possible effects of ST and the intervention protocols used in the studies in patients with FM.

Type of study

Randomized or non-randomized trials reporting clinical outcomes demonstrating the effects of ST. The frequency of ST and the extent to which ST was provided were the minimum necessary data for a research to be defined as an intervention study. Revised articles, dissertations, theses, and congress abstracts were excluded.

Information sources

The studies were identified through electronic databases, including PubMed, Science Direct, Web of Science, Physiotherapy Evidence Database, and Scientific Electronic Library Online. The last survey was conducted in December 2017.

Search strategy

The search terms were defined by the researchers using the Medical Subject Headings (Table 1), and the search strategy in the PubMed database is shown in Additional file 1.

Study identification

The searches and selection of articles were independently performed by 2 researchers; in case of disagreement, a third party was asked to make the final decision. An initial analysis was performed based on reading the title. From these selected articles, the abstracts were read and the articles included in the review were read in their entirety. A review of the references and citations of these articles was also carried out in order to identify other potentially relevant studies. From the selected studies, an analysis of the use of ST for the treatment of patients with FM was performed.

Data extraction

For the analysis and discussion of the results, the following data were extracted: author and study design; study participant number, age, sex, and treatment group; type of exercise, time of intervention, intensity, and adherence (based on either the number of attending patients at the beginning and end of the study or from data provided by the authors); and conclusions of the study.

Quality of study and risk of Bias

This systematic review evaluated the quality of the included studies and the risk of bias using the Cochrane

Table 1 Search terms used in databases

Terms	Descriptors
1. Disease	"Fibromyalgia"
2. Exercise	"Resistance Training" OR "Strength Training" OR "Strength Training Program*" OR "Training Resistance" OR "Strengthening Program"
Combination	#1 AND #2

Collaboration Risk of Bias tool [36], which includes criteria to identify bias in the selected studies that can interfere with the interpretation and conclusion. Bias risk assessment was performed by 2 researchers. The kappa concordance index [37] between the reviewers for each of the criteria was determined, and differences were resolved by consulting a third reviewer for a final opinion.

Results

Identification and selection of studies
The first stage of selection using the databases identified 211 studies, with 1 additional study manually inserted. Sixty-two duplicate studies were excluded and 48 abstracts were selected after reading the titles. At the abstract review stage, 17 studies were excluded, of which 9 used combined exercise, 7 were congress abstracts, and 1 did not evaluate patients with FM. In the fourth stage, the complete texts of 31 studies were read; 5 were excluded because of the intervention protocol, 1 was a short communication, and 1 was a congress article. Thus, 22 studies were selected for the analysis, as shown in Fig. 1.

Characteristics of included studies
Of the 22 studies included in the review, the oldest was published in 2001 [38] and the most recent was published in 2017 [24, 39, 40] (Table 2). Most of the studies were conducted in the United States (36%, $n = 8$), followed by Finland (23%, $n = 5$), Brazil (18%, $n = 4$), Sweden (18%, $n = 4$), and Turkey (5%, $n = 1$). Women aged 18–65 years comprised the total sample, and the main variables analyzed were pain, strength, muscular activity, functional capacity, fatigue, quality of life, and sleep [24, 25, 27, 29, 38, 39, 41–44]. Among the tests used in the evaluations, the Fibromyalgia Impact Questionnaire, which evaluates the impact of FM on quality of life, was used in most of the studies [25, 27–29, 31, 45–48]. To measure strength, the 1-repetition maximum (1RM) was the most used test [27–29, 31, 38, 49, 50] and studies that verified muscle activity used electromyography [38, 41, 51–53]. The visual analogue scale was used to evaluate pain in most of the studies [29, 41, 42, 45, 48, 53]. Concerning adherence, most of the studies did not provide this information. Therefore, adherence was calculated based on the patients' attendance,

and an average adherence percentage of 84% (range, 54–100%) was obtained. Five studies provided the average attendance rate, ranging from 71 to 100%.

Summary of evidence and practical implications
The analysis of the results revealed that ST reduced the symptoms of patients with FM, such as pain, fatigue, number of tender points, depression, and anxiety, with improved functional capacity and quality of life [24, 25, 27, 29, 38, 39, 41, 42] (Table 2), despite the different training protocols used.

When analyzing the training protocol, 81.81% of the studies submitted the patients to interventions twice a week, whereas only 13% (3 studies) submitted the patients to 3 sessions per week and 1 study verified the effect of a single session. Concerning the intervention time, the shorter studies lasted for 3 weeks whereas the longer studies lasted for 21 weeks. Most of the studies had an intervention time of 21 (22.72%), 12 (22.72%), 16 (18.18%), and 15 (18.18%) weeks. The studies used similar training protocols, starting with 40% of 1RM and progressing to 85%. During the training, exercises using machines and free weights worked the large and small muscle groups.

Pain was the most studied variable, showing a reduction after ST [27, 29, 30, 45, 53–55]. No study reported increased pain after or during the intervention period. Kayo et al. [48] found at the end of 16 weeks of intervention that only 41.4% of patients in the ST group were using pain medication, whereas in 80% of the patients in the control group regularly used pain medication. Other well-analyzed variables were strength, quality of life, heart rate variability (HRV), and depression. With regard to muscle strength, increases between 33 and 63% were observed after 21 and 16 weeks [41, 49]. In terms of the variability of heart rate, the effects of ST on patients with FM presented controversial results; however, the evidence shows little effect on this variable [49]. Studies analyzing quality of life and functionality showed that ST is effective in improving these variables [28, 29, 31, 41, 42, 45].

The most investigated psychological variable was depression. The studies of Jones et al. [45], Gavi et al. [29], and Assumpção et al. [40] showed that ST reduces depressive symptoms; however, the study of Ericsson et al. [25] did not find a significant difference after 15 weeks of intervention.

We also analyzed the results related to sleep quality. Andrade et al. [24] found that sleep disorders were reduced after ST and that sleep correlated with pain. The results of Ericsson et al. [25] also disclosed that ST yielded better results than relaxation sessions in improving sleep quality. In addition, another important result is that patients with FM presented similar responses to

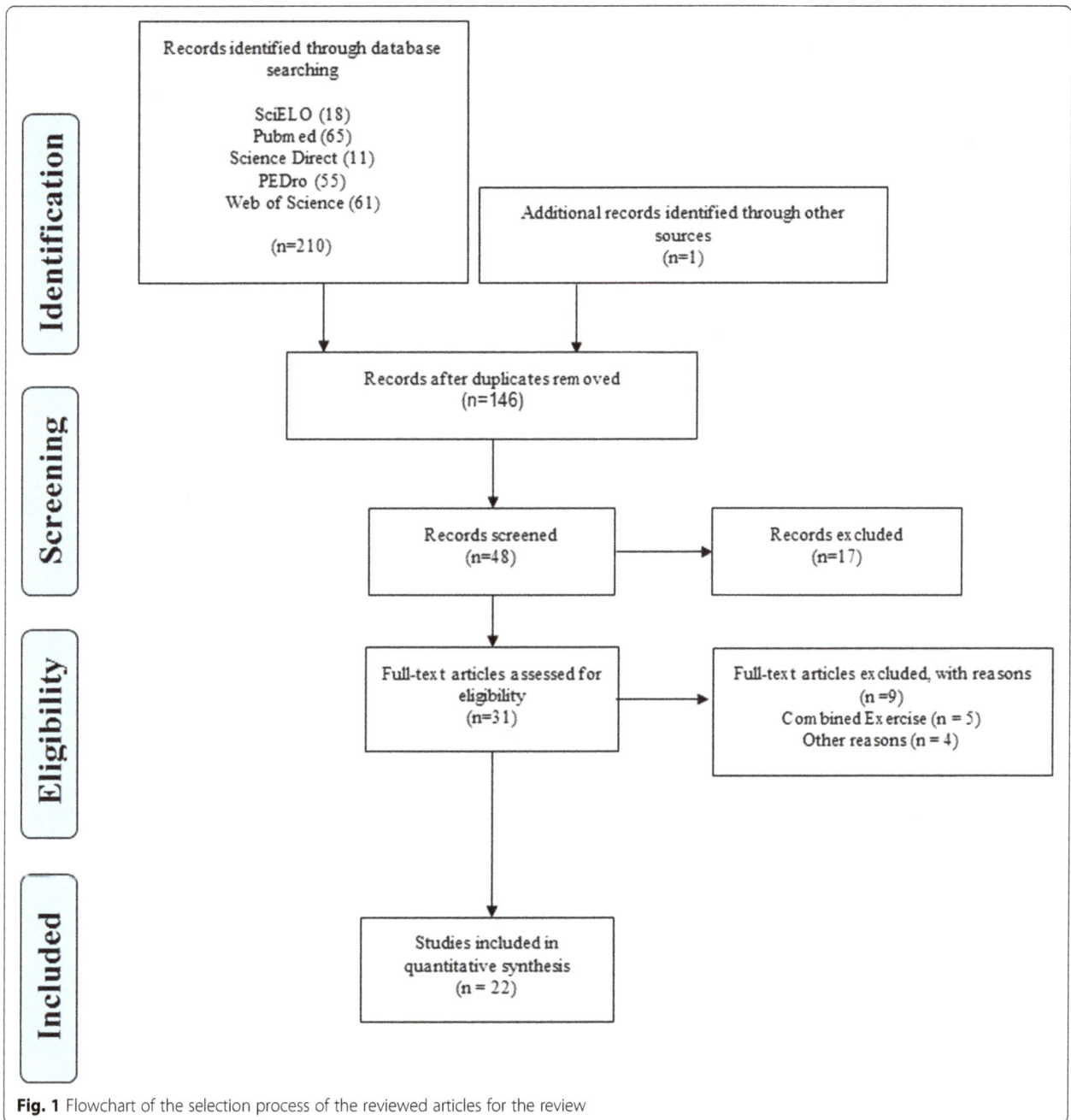

Fig. 1 Flowchart of the selection process of the reviewed articles for the review

those of healthy persons; thus, they recommended ST to assist in the treatment of patients.

The intervention protocols, results, and conclusions of each study are presented in Table 2.

Quality of studies and risk of Bias
The kappa concordance index between the two reviewers was 87.1% for all criteria. Of the 22 studies, 13 had low risk of adequate sequence generation bias; four were unclear regarding the risk of adequate sequence generation bias and six were not randomized. Only four studies had low risk of allocation concealment bias. Ten

studies had a high risk of blinded participant bias; only four had a low risk and eight were unclear. Twenty-one studies presented low risk of incomplete data bias. Similar findings were noted for selective results bias; only two studies were unclear. The descriptions of interventions (characteristics of exercises) were another source of bias, with only two studies having a high risk (Fig. 2).

Discussion
This systematic review aimed to analyze the efficacy of ST in the treatment of FM by examining the existing experimental research. The studies showed that the intervention

Table 2 Characteristics and results of experimental studies with strength training for patients with fibromyalgia syndrome

Study and Design	Sample	Intervention	Results	Conclusion
Hakkinen et al., (2001); RCT	21 women with FM (ST and CG) e 12 HC Age TF: 39 ± 6 years CG: 37 ± 5 years GS: 37 ± 6 years	Duration: 21 weeks; Weekly frequency: 2; Repetitions: Initially 15–20, from the 15th week; 5–10 Exercises: Supine, squats, extension and flexion of knees and trunk Adherence to ST: 100%	FM subjects increased their maximal and explosive strength and EMG activity to the same extent as the HC group. Moreover, the progressive strength training showed immediate benefits on subjectively perceived fatigue, depression, and neck pain of training patients with FM.	A similar maneuverability of the neuromuscular system occurs in women with FM and healthy women. ST is safe and can be used to decrease the impact of FM in the neuromuscular system
Hakkinen et al., (2002); RCT	21 women com FM, (ST and CG) and 12 HC Age TF: 39 ± 6 years CG: 37 ± 5 years GS: 37 ± 6 years	Duration: 21 weeks; Weekly frequency: 2; Series: 3–5 series per exercise; Intensity: 40–80% of 1RM; Repetitions: Initially 10–20, from the 14th week; 5–8. Exercises: leg press, extension and flexion of the knee, elbow and trunk, pulled high, adduction and abduction of the legs Adherence to ST: 100%	Maximal force increased by 18 ± 10% in the FM group, and by 22 ± 12% in the HC, while in the CG it remained unchanged. Maximum integrated EMG of the agonists (VL + VM/2) increased in HC by 22% and in the FM by 19%. Significant increases in the CSA of the QF were observed at 5 to 12/15 femur in FM and at 3 to 12/15 femur in HC, while in FM the CSA remained unchanged. A significant acute increase took place in the mean concentration of GH at pre-training in HC and in the FM, while at post-training the elevations after the loading remained elevated up to 15 min in HC and up to 30 min post-loading in the FM.	The time of neuromuscular and ST adaptations and the basal levels of anabolic hormones in women with FM are similar to healthy women
Jones et al., (2002); RCT	68 women (ST and FLEX); Age TF: 49.2 ± 6.36 years CG: 46.4 ± 8.56 years	Duration: 12 weeks; Weekly frequency: 2 Initially 1 series of 4–5, and progressively up to 12. Exercises: The main muscle groups were worked, but exercises were not specified. Adherence to ST:85%	No statistically significant differences between groups were found on independent t tests. Paired t tests revealed twice the number of significant improvements in the strengthening group compared to the stretching group. Effect size scores indicated that the magnitude of change was generally greater in the strengthening group than the stretching group.	The ST group decreased the total pain score, the number of tender points, increased leg strength, shoulder strength, improved quality of life and reduced depression. ST showed better results than FLEX.
Valkeinen et al., (2004); RCT	36 women (26 FM and 10 HC) Age ST: 60.2 ± 2.5 years CG: 59.1 ± 3.5 years HC: 64.2 ± 2.7 years	Duration: 21 weeks; Weekly frequency: 2; Initially 3 series of 15–20 progressively up to 4 series of 8–12 and up to 5 series of 5–10 . Exercises: The main muscle groups were worked, but exercises were not specified. Adherence to ST: 100%	The mean increases in maximal extension force during the training period in groups FM and in HC were 32 ± 33% and 24 ± 12% respectively and those of flexion were 13 ± 20% and 24 ± 17%. Explosive force of the extensors increased in both FM and in HC. The integrated EMGs of the vastus lateralis and medialis muscles increased in both FM and HC. Muscle forces and EMGs in group CG remained at the basal level. Walking speed, stair-climbing time and the HAQ index improved in group FM. The changes in the number of tender points and in perceived symptoms were in favors of the training group FM.	It improved the functional capacity and the strength in the extensor and flexor muscles of the knee in both groups submitted to the TF (FM and healthy). Patients with FM respond similarly to TF that healthy people of the same age.
Valkeinen et al., (2005); RCT	26 women (ST and CG); Age ST: 60 ± 2 years CG: 59 ± 4 years	Duration: 21 weeks; Weekly frequency: 2; Initially 3 series of 15–20; weeks 15 to 21 went to 5–10. Intensity: progressive increase of 40% to 80% of 1 RM Exercises: 6 to 7 for the main muscle groups Adherence to ST: not reported the	All patients were able to complete the training. In FM strength training led to increases of 36% and 33% in maximal isometric and concentric forces, respectively. The CSA increased by 5% and the EMG activity in isometric action by 47%	The ST increases strength, cross-sectional area and voluntary muscular activation in elderly women with FM. Patients with FM can be submitted to higher intensities without increasing symptoms

Table 2 Characteristics and results of experimental studies with strength training for patients with fibromyalgia syndrome *(Continued)*

Study and Design	Sample	Intervention	Results	Conclusion
		number of dropouts	and in concentric action by 57%. Basal serum hormone concentrations remained unaltered during strength training. The subjective perceived symptoms showed a minor decreasing tendency (ns). No statistically significant changes occurred in any of these parameters in CG.	
Kingsley et al., (2005); RCT	29 women (ST and CG); Age ST: 45 ± 9 years GC: 47 ± 4 years	Duration: 12 weeks; Weekly frequency: 2; 1 serie of 8–12 Intensity: 60 to 80% of 1RM Exercises: Supine, extension and flexion of knee and elbow, low row, shoulder and lumbar development Adherence to ST: 54%	The strength group significantly improved upper and lower body strength. And upper-body functionality measured by the Continuous-Scale Physical Functional Performance test improved significantly after training. Tender point sensitivity and fibromyalgia impact did not change.	At the end of study was a significant increase in muscle strength and improvement in functional capacity components in the ST group.
Valkeinen et al., (2006); Non RCT	23 women (13 ST and 10 CG) Age ST: 60 ± 2 years CG: 54 ± 3 years	Duration: 21 weeks; Weekly frequency: 2 Intensity: Started with 50% of 1RM and progressively up to 80%; Exercises: two Exercises for knee extensors and 4–5 Exercises for the rest of the body Adherence to ST: 100%	The ST led to large increases in maximal force and EMG activity of the muscles and contributed to the improvement in loading performance (average load/set) at week 21. The fatiguing loading sessions typically applied in strength training before and after the experimental period caused remarkable and comparable acute decreases in maximal force and increases in blood lactate concentration in both groups. Acute exercise-induced muscle pain increased similarly in both groups, and the pain level in women with FM was lowered after the 21-week training period.	An increase in maximal strength, blood lactate concentration and decrease in pain of the ST group was observed.
Bircan et al. (2008); RCT	26 women (ST and AE) Age ST: 46 ± 8,5 years AE: 48.3 ± 5.3 years	Duration: 8 weeks Weekly frequency: 3 Initially 1 serie of 4 repetitions and progressively up to 12 repetitions; Exercises were not specified, however, free weights were used and the patient's body weight Adherence to ST: 100%	There were significant improvements in both groups regarding pain, sleep, fatigue, tender point count, and fitness after treatment. HAD-depression scores improved significantly in both groups while no significant change occurred in HAD-anxiety scores. Bodily pain subscale of SF-36 and physical component summary improved significantly in the AE group, whereas seven subscales of SF-36, physical component summary, and mental component summary improved significantly in the ST group.	Aerobic exercise and strengthening exercise were similarly effective at improving symptoms, tender point count, fitness, psychological status, and quality of life in fibromyalgia patients.
Figueroa et al. 2008); RCT	19 women (10 FM and 9 HC) Age ST:50 ± 10 years HC: 49 ± 8 years	Duration: 16 weeks Weekly frequency: 2 1 serie of 8–12 repetitions; Intensity: Initially 50% 1RM and progressively up to 80%; Exercises: Supine, knee extension and flexion, Leg press, low row, shoulder development (performed on machine) Adherence to ST: 67%	RR interval, total power, log transformed (Ln) squared root of the standard deviation of RR interval (RMSSD), low-frequency power and BRS were lower, and HR and pulse pressure were higher in women with FM than in healthy controls. After ST, mean (SEM) total power increased, RMSSD increased and Ln of high-frequency power increased in women with FM. Upper and lower body muscle strength increased by 63% and 49%, and pain perception decreased by 39% in women with FM. There were no changes in BRS, HR and BP after ST.	The ST improves heart rate variability, parasympathetic activity, pain and the strength of women with FM with autonomic dysfunction.
Kingsley	18 women	Duration: acute effect	Variables were similar in both groups	The results showed lower muscle

Table 2 Characteristics and results of experimental studies with strength training for patients with fibromyalgia syndrome *(Continued)*

Study and Design	Sample	Intervention	Results	Conclusion
et al. (2009); Non RCT	(FM and HC) Age 48,0 years (21–59 years)	One session 30 min of ST, 1 serie of 12; Exercises: 10 exercises, were not specified. Adherence to ST: 100%	at rest. HFnu decreased in controls and increased in women with FM post. LFnu increased in controls and decreased in women with FM. The LFnu/HFnu ratio increased in controls with no change in women with FM, and BRS decreased in controls but not in women with FM.	strength in the FM group and after acute ST, women with FM responded differently from controls, demonstrated by lower sympathetic and higher vagal modulation without altering baroreceptor reflex sensitivity.
Panton et al. (2009); RCT	21 women (ST e ST-C); Age ST: 50 ± 7 years ST-C: 47 ± 12 years	Duration: 16 weeks; Weekly frequency: 2; 1 serie of 8–12 repetitions; Exercises: Supine, knee extension and flexion, Leg press, low row, shoulder development (performed on machine). Adherence: 82.8%	Both groups increased upper and lower body strength. There were similar improvements in FM impact in both groups. There were no group interactions for the functionality measures. Both groups improved in the strength domains; however, only ST-C significantly improved in the pre- to postfunctional domains of flexibility, balance and coordination, and endurance.	The ST improved FM impact on quality of life and strength. The practice of chiropractic in conjunction with TF assisted in adherence and functional capacity
Kingsley et al. (2010); Non RCT	29 women (9 FM and 20 HC) Age FM: 42 ± 5 years; HC: 45 ± 5 years	Duration: 12 weeks; Weekly frequency: 2; 3 series of 12 repetitions; Intensity: Initially 50% 1RM and progressively up to 85%; Exercises: Supine, extension and flexion of the knee, Leg press, low row (performed in machine) Adherence to ST: 88%	There was no group-by-time interaction for any variable. Number of active tender points, myalgic score, and FIQ score were decreased after ST in women with FM. Heart rate and natural log (Ln) high frequency (LnHF) were recovered, whereas Ln low frequency (LnLF) and LnLF/LnHF ratio were increased 20 min after acute leg resistance exercise. There were no significant effects of ST on HRV at rest or postexercise.	The ST increased strength in both groups and reduced pain and number of PT in patients with FM. The practice of ST does not change the resting HR, nor the variability of HR compared to healthy subjects.
Kingsley et al. (2011); Non RCT	23 women (9 FM and 14 HC); Age FM: 42 ± 5 years HC: 45 ± 5 years	Duration: 12 weeks; Weekly frequency: 2; 3 series of 12 repetitions; Intensity: Initially 50–60% 1RM Exercises: Supine, extension and flexion of the knee, Leg press, low row (performed in machine) Adherence to ST: 88%	Aortic and digital diastolic blood pressure (DBP) were significantly decreased and aortic and digital pulse pressures (PP) were significantly increased after acute exercise before ST. Acute resistance exercise had no effect on HR, wave reflection (augmentation index and reflection time), digital, or aortic systolic BP. ST improved muscle strength without affecting acute DBP and PP responses.	The results suggest that a leg-resistance exercise produces post-exercise diastolic hypotension and does not alter aortic systolic blood pressure and HR. In addition, vascular responses at rest and post-exercise are not altered after 12 weeks of ST in premenopausal women
Kayo et al. (2012); RCT	90 women with FM (30 ST, 30 AE and 30 CG) Age ST: 46.7 ± 6.3 years; AE: 47.7 ± 5.3 years; CG: 46.1 ± 6.4 years	Duration: 16 weeks; Weekly frequency: 3; 3 series of 10 repetitions; Exercises were not specified, however, free weights were used and the patient's body weight Adherence to ST: 73,5	All 3 groups showed improvement after the 16-week treatment compared to baseline. At the 28-week follow-up, pain reduction was similar for the AE and ST groups, but different from the control group. At the end of the treatment, 80% of subjects in the control group took pain medication, but only 46.7% in the AE and 41.4% in the ST groups. Mean FIQ total scores were lower for the AE and ST groups compared with the control group.	The ST was as effective as AE in reducing pain in relation to all study variables.
Hooten et al. (2012); RCT	72 FM (36 ST and 36 AE)	Duration: 3 weeks; Weekly frequency: 2; 1 serie of	Significant improvements in pain severity, peak Vo2, strength, and	The ST was effective in reducing pain in relation to all study

Table 2 Characteristics and results of experimental studies with strength training for patients with fibromyalgia syndrome *(Continued)*

Study and Design	Sample	Intervention	Results	Conclusion
	Age ST 47.3 ± 10.1 years AE 45.8 ± 11.5 years	10 repetitions; Exercises: Flexion and extension of the knee and arm Adherence to ST: 94,5%	pain thresholds were observed from baseline to week 3 in the intent-to-treat analysis; however, patients in the aerobic group experienced greater gains (in peak Vo2) compared to the strength group.	variables. ST practice reduced pain significantly, but there was no difference in relation to AE.
Gavi et al. (2014); RCT	76 FM (35 ST and 36 FLEX) Age ST: 44.34 ± 7.94 years FLEX: 48.65 ± 7.60 years	Duration: 16 weeks; Weekly frequency: 2; 1 serie of 10 repetitions; Intensity: 45% 1RM Exercises: Supine, extension and flexion of the knee, elbow and shoulder, Leg press, low paddling, fly, plantar flexion Adherence to ST: 87,5%	The ST group was more effective to strength gain for all muscles and pain control after 4 and 16 weeks. The FLEX group showed higher improvements in anxiety. Both groups showed improvements in the quality of life, and there was no significant difference observed between the groups. There was no change in the HRV of the ST and FLEX groups.	There was an increase in functionality, depression, quality of life in both groups, with no statistical difference between them. There was greater reduction of pain in the ST group.
Larsson et al. (2015); RCT	130 FM (67 ST, 63 RT) Age ST: 50.81 ± 9.05 years; RT: 52.10 ± 9.78 years	Duration: 15 weeks Weekly frequency: 2 Intensity: increased progressively Exercises: The main muscle groups were worked, but exercises were not specified. Adherence to ST: 71%	Significant improvements were found for isometric knee-extension force, health status, current pain intensity, 6MWT, isometric elbow flexion force, pain disability, and pain acceptance in the ST group when compared to the CG. Differed significantly in favor of the ST group at post-treatment examinations. No significant differences between ST group and the active CG were found regarding change in self-reported questionnaires from baseline to 13–18 months.	The ST was considered a viable exercise mode for women with FM, improving muscle strength, with a significant improvement in health-related quality of life and current pain intensity, when assessed immediately a fter the intervention.
Palstam et al. (2016); Non RCT	67 women com FM (67 ST) Age 51 ± 9.1 years	Duration: 15 weeks; Weekly frequency: 2; Intensity: Initially 40% 1RM and progressively up to 80%; Exercises: The main muscle groups were worked, but exercises were not specified. Adherence to ST: 71%	Reduced pain disability was explained by higher pain disability at baseline together with decreased fear avoidance beliefs about physical activity. The improvements in the disability domains of recreation and social activity were explained by decreased fear avoidance beliefs about physical activity together with higher baseline values of each disability domain respectively. The improvement in occupational disability was explained by higher baseline values of occupational disability.	The ST reduces pain, inability and fear of practicing Physical exercises and increased strength and level of physical activity.
Ericsson et al. (2016); RCT	105 women (56 ST and 49 RT) Range of age 22–64 years	Duration: 15 weeks; Weekly frequency: 2; Intensity: Initially 40% 1RM and progressively up to 80%; Exercises: The main muscle groups were worked, but exercises were not specified. Adherence to ST: 71%	A higher improvement was found at the post-treatment examination for change in the ST group; as compared to change in the active CG in the MFI-20 subscale of physical fatigue. Sleep efficiency was the strongest predictor of change in the MFI-20 subscale general fatigue. Participating in resistance exercise and working fewer hours per week were independent significant predictors of change in physical fatigue.	The ST group significantly reduced general, physical and mental fatigue and improved sleep efficiency in relation to the relaxation group; depression and anxiety did not decline after the intervention
Martinsen et al. (2017); Non RCT	54 women (31 ST and 23 HC) Age ST: 49 ± 6	Duration: 15 weeks Weekly frequency: 2 Exercises: exercises were not specified.	The FIQ ratings decreased following exercise in patients with FM, suggesting an improvement of FM symptoms. Furthermore, for the	The intervention had different effects on the speed of cognitive processing during SCWT in patients with FM and

Table 2 Characteristics and results of experimental studies with strength training for patients with fibromyalgia syndrome *(Continued)*

Study and Design	Sample	Intervention	Results	Conclusion
	HC: 47 ± 2	Adherence to ST: 65,5%	SF-36 PCS ratings we found a statistically significant effect of group and intervention, but no significant interaction between the factors, thus showing that exercise improved ratings of SF-36 PCS in both groups.	healthy controls. We found evidence of increased amygdala activation. In contrast, HC showed decreased RTs in incongruent and congruent stimuli. Exercise had no effect on distraction-induced analgesia or pressure pain thresholds in any of the groups but decreased the overall severity of FM symptoms.
Andrade, Vilarino e Bevilacqua (2017); Non RCT	52 FM (31 ST and 21 CG) Age ST: 54.42 ± 7.16 CG: 53.10 ± 8	Duration: 8 weeks Weekly frequency: 3 Exercises: knee extension, knee flexion, bench press, fly, adductors, low rowing, high pulley, elbow extension, lateral raise, arm curl, standing calf raise, and abdominal crunch. Adherence to ST: 81,5	After 8 weeks of intervention, significant differences were found between groups in subjective quality of sleep, sleep disturbance, daytime dysfunction, and total sleep score. The correlation analysis using Spearman's test indicated a positive relationship between the variables of pain intensity and sleep quality; when pain intensity increased in patients with fibromyalgia, sleep quality worsened.	A significant relationship was found between pain level and sleep disturbances in FM patients, and it was found that the higher the pain, the worse the sleep quality of these patients. The ST group reduced levels of sleep disturbance after 8 weeks of intervention.
Assumpção et al. (2017); RCT	53 FM (19 ST, 18 FLEX E 16 CG) Age ST: 45.7 ± 7.7 FLEX: 47.9 ± 5.3 CG: 46.9 ± 6.5	Duration: 12 weeks Weekly frequency: 2 Exercises: eight repetitions of strengthening exercises for the following muscles triceps sural, hip adductors and abductors, hip flexor, shoulder flexor and extensor, anterior and posterior deltoids, pectoralis major and rhomboids Adherence to ST: 89,5%	The ST group had the lowest depression score and; the control had the highest score of morning tiredness and stiffness, and the lowest score of vitality. In the clinical analyses, the stretching group had important improvement in quality of life for all SF-36 domains, and the strengthening group had important improvements in the impact on FM symptoms measured by the FIQ total score and in the quality of life for SF-36 domains of physical functioning, vitality, social function, role emotional and mental health.	The ST was more effective to reducing depression, while stretching exercises was better to improving quality of life, especially physical functioning and pain.

LEGEND: *FM* Fibromyalgia, *HC* Healthy Control, *RCT* Controlled and Randomized Study, *TP* Tender Points, *AE* Aerobic Group, *RT* Relaxation Therapy, *RM* 1 Maximum Repeat, *ST* Strength Training, *ST-C* Strength Training and chiropractic, *FLEX* Flexibility training, *HR* Heart Rate, *HRV* Heart Rate Variability, *CG* Control Group, *NMS* Neuro-muscular system, *SCWT* Test of colored words Stroop, *RTs* long reaction times, *FIQ* Fibromyalgia Impact Questionnaire, *SF-36* 36- Item Short Form Survey, *PCS* Physical Component, *MCS* Mental Components, *HAD* Hospital Anxiety and Depression Score, *6MWT* 6 min walking test, *PGIC* patient global impression of change, *VAS* Visual Analogue Scale, *MFI-20* Multidimensional Fatigue Inventory, *CSA* cross-sectional area, *QF* quadriceps femoris, *LF* low-frequency, *GH* growth hormone, *HAQ* Health Assessment Questionnaire, *EMG* Surface electromyographic, *Hfnu* normalized high-frequency, *Lfnu* normalized low-frequency, *RTs* reaction times

has favorable results, such as reducing physical and psychological symptoms. However, there are still gaps that need to be investigated.

Concerning the ST sessions, it was observed that there is no specific training protocol for patients with FM; thus, the researchers developed their own protocol. Jones et al. [45] submitted the patients to a series of four to five repetitions, progressively increasing the number of repetitions up to 12. This protocol was similar to that used by Bircan et al. [42], who instructed patients to perform a series of four repetitions and progressively increased the repetitions by up to 12. Kingsley et al. [28] and Figueroa et al. [49] also submitted the patients to a series in each exercise; however, from the beginning of the intervention, the patients were instructed to perform from 8 to 12 repetitions. As the first studies analyzed were published in 2001 and 2002, and at that time there was little knowledge about the development of the disease and the effects of ST on the patients, those first studies chose to use low load and series. On the basis of the results of the earlier studies, more studies were performed and chose to use more series with more repetitions from the beginning [24, 27, 44, 48]. Despite some differences in the protocols, the intensity of the exercises increased gradually. In some studies, the intensity reached 80% of 1RM at the end of the intervention [25, 27]. Another issue concerns weekly

Study	Sequence generation?	Allocation concealment?	Blinding of participants?	Incomplete outcome data	Selective outcome reporting?	Other sources of bias?
Hakkinen et al. (2001)	Low	Unclear	High	Low	Low	Low
Hakkinen et al. (2002)	Low	Unclear	Unclear	Low	Low	Low
Jones et al. (2002)	Low	Low	Low	Low	Low	Low
Valkeinen et al. (2004)	Unclear	Unclear	Unclear	Low	Low	Low
Valkeinen et al. (2005)	Unclear	Unclear	Unclear	Low	Low	Low
Kingsley et al. (2005)	Low	Unclear	Unclear	Low	Low	Low
Valkeinen et al. (2006)	Unclear	Unclear	Unclear	Low	Low	Low
Bircan et al. (2008)	Low	Unclear	High	Low	Low	Low
Figueroa et al. (2008)	Unclear	Unclear	Unclear	Low	Unclear	Low
Kingsley et al. (2009)	High	High	High	Unclear	Low	Low
Panton et al. (2009)	Low	Unclear	High	Low	Low	Low
Kingsley et al. (2010)	High	High	High	Low	Low	Low
Kingsley et al. (2011)	High	High	High	Low	Low	Low
Kayo et al. (2012)	Low	Low	Low	Low	Low	Low
Hooten et al. (2012)	Low	Low	High	Low	Unclear	Low
Gavi et al. (2014)	Low	Unclear	Low	Low	Low	Low
Larsson et al. (2015)	Low	Low	Low	Low	Low	High
Palstam et al. (2016)	High	High	High	Low	Low	Low
Ericsson et al. (2016)	Low	Unclear	High	Low	Low	Low
Martinsen et al. (2017)	Low	High	High	Low	Low	High
Andrade, Vilarino e Bevilacqua (2017)	High	High	Unclear	Low	Low	Low
Assumpção et al. (2017)	Low	Unclear	Unclear	Low	Low	Low

LEGEND: Low risk | High risk | Unclear risk

Fig. 2 Risk of bias in the studies analyzed

frequency, but this differed slightly between 2 and 3 weekly sessions. Despite the differences in the protocols, it was observed that, in general, the studies followed the recommendations of the American College of Sports Medicine for beginners in ST.

With regard to the main symptoms, there was a greater interest in pain, strength, quality of life, HRV, and depression. Pain is the main symptom of FM and is associated with other symptoms such as depression, sleep disorders, and poor quality of life [24, 56]; thus, finding treatments that improve these symptoms are of crucial clinical relevance for patients. The results of the present review demonstrate that the pain of patients with FM is significantly reduced by the ST intervention. Valkeinen et al. [53] evaluated 23 women with FM, of whom 13 were submitted to 2 ST sessions for 21 weeks and 10 were part of the control group. At the end of the 21 weeks of intervention, significant improvement in pain was observed. Other studies examined the effect of shorter periods of ST, and found that pain can be

reduced in a short time. Hooten et al. [30] analyzed the effect of 3-week ST on pain. Participants performed 2 weekly sessions, consisting of a series of 10 repetitions of knee and elbow flexion and extension exercises. At the end of the study, a significant reduction of pain was observed. This result is interesting for health professionals and for patients with FM, because it demonstrates that ST can help reduce symptoms in a few weeks and with few exercises.

Studies indicate that patients with FM have less strength and reduced functional capacity compared with healthy persons of the same age and without the disease [57]. The reduced muscle strength of patients with FM may be related to pain; because of pain, it is common for patients to avoid making physical efforts. However, studies that aimed to verify the responses of patients with FM after muscular effort showed positive results. In studies that applied ST, strength and hypertrophy were similar between patients with and those without the disease.

The first studies in this sense were those of Hakkinen et al. [38], Hakkinen et al. [51], Valkeinen et al. [41] and Valkeinen et al. [52]. The first 2 studies analyzed the effect of 21-week ST in patients with FM, and compared the results with those of healthy persons. From the results of these studies, it can be observed that there was an increase of force, activation, and hypertrophy in the ST group and in controls. Hakkinen et al. [51] verified an increase of 18% in the muscular strength of patients with FM, and of 22% in the control group, concluding that the neuromuscular adaptations derived from ST are similar between patients with FM and healthy persons. Reinforcing this result, Valkeinen et al. [41] observed a significant increase of the strength in the extension and flexion of the knee in patients with FM [33% and 20%, respectively], whereas in the control group the gains were 12% and 17%, respectively. Valkeinen et al. [52] that analyzed strength found that after 21 weeks of ST, patients with FM had a 36% increase in isometric force and 33% in concentric force. In addition, the authors verified a 5% increase in the cross-sectional area of the thigh and increased activation by 57%. After analyzing the results, the authors concluded that ST is safe for patients with FM and that the patients can undergo training with higher intensities.

Another variable that was investigated in the studies was the HRV. Some authors suggested that FM occurs because of dysregulation of the central nervous system [6, 8], causing an autonomic dysfunction that induces the appearance of some symptoms such as fatigue and anxiety. Figueroa et al. [49] verified the heart rate behavior of patients with FM who also had autonomic dysfunction. The researchers subjected the patients to 16 weeks of ST and verified improvements in HRV, parasympathetic activity, and pain reduction. Kingsley et al. [27] compared the effects of 12 weeks of ST on patients with FM and healthy women, in terms of various symptoms such as pain, number of tender points, impact of FM on quality of life, and HRV. The results showed an increase in strength in both groups, besides the reduction of pain and tender points in patients with FM; however, in terms of the behavior of HRV, no significant difference was observed between patients with FM and the healthy group. In contrast, in the study of Kingsley et al. [43] that aimed to verify the autonomic modulation of patients with FM after a ST session, the results demonstrated that patients with FM had a lower sympathetic response and greater vagal modulation, without altering the baroreflex sensitivity, a response different from that presented by the control group. Concerning a possible autonomic dysfunction in patients with FM, further studies need to be carried out in order to reach a conclusion.

Other symptoms investigated were quality of life, depression, and sleep disturbance. As quality of life is a variable that is directly related to other symptoms, the improvements observed in the other symptoms suggest that the quality of life could also be expected to increase. In the study of Gavi et al. [29], significant improvements in pain, functionality, quality of life, and depression were found after 16 weeks of ST. Similar results were found by Larsson et al. [54] and Palstam et al. [55]. In the first study, there was a reduction in pain and an increase in strength and quality of life. In the second study, in addition to the results seen in previous studies, the researchers noticed a reduction in the fear of performing exercises. With regard to sleep disturbance, some studies found a reduction after ST intervention [24, 25]. In addition, sleep quality correlated with pain, with patients having less pain experiencing less sleep disorders [24].

With the new possibility of using ST as an alternative treatment for patients with FM, some researchers began to compare the effects of ST with those of other physical exercise interventions. In the study of Bircan et al. [42], 13 women with FM were submitted to aerobic exercise and 13 were submitted to ST. The researchers found that both interventions have benefits for patients, including reduction of pain, fatigue, sleep disorders, and depression, and improvement of aerobic capacity. However, no significant improvements in anxiety were observed in either group. In the studies by Kayo et al. [48] and Hooten et al. [30], the effects of ST were also compared with those of aerobic exercise. It was noted that the 2 interventions presented similar results, particularly in reducing the pain of patients. In addition, other studies compared ST with relaxation or flexibility exercises. Assumpção et al. [40] verified the effects of ST and flexibility exercises after 12 weeks of intervention. The results demonstrated that ST is more effective in reducing depression, whereas flexibility exercises are better at improving the quality of life, especially physical function and pain. Gavi et al. [29] found similar results: ST and flexibility training were effective for reducing symptoms; however, the best results in terms of pain were found in the ST group. The study of Jones et al. [45] also compared ST and flexibility training, and verified that both interventions are effective; however, the most significant results were found in the ST group. Lorena et al. [58] performed a systematic review on the effects of stretching in patients with FM, and reported the importance of this intervention in improving the physical and mental aspects of patients. Nevertheless, they emphasized the need for studies with greater methodological rigor. The same can be emphasized in the present review: the positive effect of ST in patients with FM is visible, but it is necessary to carry out more studies with greater methodological rigor to address possible gaps.

Another interesting result is about adherence to treatments. It is known that patients with FM have difficulties adhering to the practice of physical exercise; however, few studies reported the adherence of patients to the interventions [59, 60]. In the present review, the mean adherence percentage was 84%, a result similar to that of the study by Sanz-Baños et al. [59] in patients undergoing aerobic exercises [adherence percentage 87.2%]. This result is a further indication that ST can be used as part of the treatment for patients with FM, because in addition to improving the symptoms, the patients show high adherence to the intervention.

Concerning the strengths and limitations of the study, we were able to verify through a broad literature review that ST improves the symptoms of patients with FM; however, some studies presented a high risk of bias and further studies are needed to consolidate the obtained results. In addition, future reviews including the gray literature are warranted in order to identify other studies on the subject.

Conclusion

In conclusion, ST had positive effects on physical and psychological symptoms, in terms of reducing pain, the number of tender points, and depression, and improving muscle strength, sleep quality, functional capacity, and quality of life. Intervention protocols should start at low intensity (40% of 1RM) and gradually increase the intensity. ST should be performed 2 or 3 times a week to exercise the main muscle groups. The current studies showed that ST is a safe and effective method of improving the major symptoms of FM and can be used to treat patients with this condition.

Abbreviations

1RM: One maximum repetition; FM: Fibromyalgia; HRV: Heart Rate Variability; PE: Physical Activity; ST: Strength Training

Acknowledgments

The authors thank FAPESC (Foundation for Research and Innovation of the State of Santa Catarina) for financial support through a research grant (Project No. 2442-2011/12), CAPES for a Master scholarship (grant No. 02/2017), and the State University of Santa Catarina for a UDESC study opportunity.

Funding

Foundation for Research and Innovation of the State of Santa Catarina grant (Project No. 2442–2011/12).

Authors' contributions

A.A., S.R.A.K, S.S.M, T.L.A.P drafted the manuscript. S.R.A.K, V.T.G., S.S.M., carried out the analysis. All authors discussed the results, commented on the manuscript and approved the final draft of the manuscript.

Competing interests

Alexandro Andrade, Ricardo de Azevedo Klumb Steffens, Sofia Mendes Sieczkowska, Leonardo Alexandre Peyré Tartaruga and Guilherme Torres Vilarino declare that they have no conflict of interest.

Author details

¹Health and Sports Science Center, CEFID / Santa Catarina State University – UDESC, Florianópolis, SC, Brazil. ²Laboratory of Sports and Exercise Psychology - LAPE, Florianópolis, SC, Brazil. ³Regional University of Blumenau - FURB, Blumenau, SC, Brazil. ⁴Human Movement Sciences and Pneumological Sciences, UFRGS- Federal University of Rio Grande do Sul, Porto Alegre, RS, Brazil. ⁵Research Laboratory of Exercise – LAPEX, Porto Alegre, RS, Brazil.

References

1. Wolfe F, Smythe HA, Yunus MB, Bennett RM, Bombardier C, Goldenberg DL, et al. The American College of Rheumatology 1990 criteria for the classification of fibromyalgia. Arthritis Rheum. 1990;33(2):160–72.
2. Wolfe F, Clauw DJ, Fitzcharles M-A, Goldenberg DL, Häuser W, Katz RL, et al. 2016 Revisions to the 2010/2011 fibromyalgia diagnostic criteria. Seminars in arthritis and rheumatism. 2016;46:319-29.
3. Wolfe F, Clauw DJ, Fitzcharles MA, Goldenberg DL, Katz RS, Mease P, et al. The American College of Rheumatology Preliminary Diagnostic Criteria for fibromyalgia and measurement of symptom severity. Arthritis Care Res. 2010;62(5):600–10 PubMed PMID: WOS:000280979600004.
4. Borchers AT, Gershwin ME. Fibromyalgia: a critical and comprehensive review. Clin Rev Allergy Immunol. 2015;49(2):100–51 PubMed PMID:WOS: 000362902500002.English.
5. McDowell CP, Cook DB, Herring MP. The effects of exercise training on anxiety in fibromyalgia patients: a meta-analysis. Med Sci Sports Exerc. 2017; 49(9):1868–76 PubMed PMID: 28419024.Epub 2017/04/19.eng.
6. Häuser W, Ablin J, Fitzcharles M-A, Littlejohn G, Luciano JV, Usui C, et al. Fibromyalgia. Nature reviews Disease primers. 2015;1:15022.
7. Andrade A, Vilarino GT, Sieczkowska SM, Coimbra DR, Steffens RAK, Vietta GG. Acute effects of physical exercises on the inflammatory markers of patients with fibromyalgia syndrome: a systematic review. J Neuroimmunol. 2018;316:40–9.
8. Sluka KA, Clauw DJ. Neurobiology of fibromyalgia and chronic widespread pain. Neuroscience. 2016;338:114–29 PubMed PMID:WOS:000386338200008.English.
9. Hauser W, Klose P, Langhorst J, Moradi B, Steinbach M, Schiltenwolf M, et al. Efficacy of different types of aerobic exercise in fibromyalgia syndrome: a systematic review and meta-analysis of randomised controlled trials. Arthritis Res Ther. 2010;12(3):R79 PubMed PMID: 20459730. PMCID: PMC2911859. Epub 2010/05/13.eng.
10. Arnold LM. Biology and therapy of fibromyalgia - New therapies in fibromyalgia. Arthritis Res Ther. 2006;8(4):20 PubMed PMID: WOS: 000240985200002.English.
11. Hauser W, Bernardy K, Arnold B, Offenbacher M, Schiltenwolf M. Efficacy of multicomponent treatment in fibromyalgia syndrome: a meta-analysis of randomized controlled clinical trials. Arthritis Rheum. 2009;61(2):216–24 PubMed PMID: 19177530. Epub 2009/01/30.eng.
12. Poole JL, Siegel P. Effectiveness of occupational therapy interventions for adults with fibromyalgia: a systematic review. Am J Occup Ther. 2017;71(1): 7101180040p1–p10 PubMed PMID. 28027011. Epub 2016/12/28.eng.
13. Sanz-Baños Y, Pastor-Mira MÁ, Lledó A, López-Roig S, Peñacoba C, & Sánchez-Meca, J. Do women with fibromyalgia adhere to walking for exercise programs to improve their health? Systematic review and meta-analysis. Disabil Rehabil. 2018;40(21):2475-87.
14. Bidonde J, Busch AJ, Schachter CL, Overend TJ, Kim SY, Góes SM, et al. Aerobic exercise training for adults with fibromyalgia. Cochrane Libr. 2017.
15. Brosseau L, Wells GA, Tugwell P, Egan M, Wilson KG, Dubouloz CJ, et al. Ottawa Panel evidence-based clinical practice guidelines for aerobic fitness exercises in the management of fibromyalgia: part 1. Phys Ther. 2008;88(7): 857–71 PubMed PMID: 18497301. Epub 2008/05/24. eng.
16. Brosseau L, Wells GA, Tugwell P, Egan M, Wilson KG, Dubouloz CJ, et al. Ottawa panel evidence-based clinical practice guidelines for strengthening exercises in the management of fibromyalgia: part 2. Phys Ther. 2008;88(7): 873–86 PubMed PMID: WOS:000257473000008. English.
17. Busch AJ, Webber SC, Richards RS, Bidonde J, Schachter CL, Schafer LA, et al. Resistance exercise training for fibromyalgia. Cochrane Database Syst Rev. 2013;(12):113 PubMed PMID: WOS:000329188500042. English.
18. Segura-Jimenez V, Castro-Pinero J, Soriano-Maldonado A, Alvarez-Gallardo IC, Estevez-Lopez F, Delgado-Fernandez M, et al. The association of total and central body fat with pain, fatigue and the impact of fibromyalgia in women; role of physical fitness. Eur J Pain. 2016;20(5):811–21 PubMed PMID: WOS:000373997600014.
19. Musumeci G. Effects of exercise on physical limitations and fatigue in rheumatic diseases. World J Orthop. 2015;6(10):762–9 PubMed PMID: 26601057. PMCID: 4644863. eng.

20. Segura-Jimenez V, Alvarez-Gallardo IC, Carbonell-Baeza A, Aparicio VA, Ortega FB, Casimiro AJ, et al. Fibromyalgia has a larger impact on physical health than on psychological health, yet both are markedly affected: the al-Andalus project. Semin Arthritis Rheum. 2015;44(5):563–70 PubMed PMID: WOS:000352923200013. English.

21. Nelson NL. Muscle strengthening activities and fibromyalgia: a review of pain and strength outcomes. J Bodyw Mov Ther. 2015;19(2):370–6 PubMed PMID: 25892394. Epub 2015/04/22. eng.

22. Bidonde J, Jean Busch A, Bath B, Milosavljevic S. Exercise for adults with fibromyalgia: an umbrella systematic review with synthesis of best evidence. Curr Rheumatol Rev. 2014;10(1):45–79.

23. Jones KD. Recommendations for resistance training in patients with fibromyalgia. Arthritis Res Ther. 2015;17(1):258.

24. Andrade A, Vilarino GT, Bevilacqua GG. What is the effect of strength training on pain and sleep in patients with fibromyalgia? Am J Phys Med Rehabil. 2017.

25. Ericsson A, Palstam A, Larsson A, Lofgren M, Bileviciute-Ljungar I, Bjersing J, et al. Resistance exercise improves physical fatigue in women with fibromyalgia: a randomized controlled trial. Arthritis Res Ther. 2016;18:12 PubMed PMID: WOS:000381728500002. English.

26. Larsson A, Palstam A, Lofgren M, Ernberg M, Bjersing J, Bileviciute-Ljungar I, et al. Resistance exercise improves muscle strength, health status and pain intensity in fibromyalgia--a randomized controlled trial. Arthritis Res Ther. 2015;17:161 PubMed PMID: 26084281. PMCID: PMC4489359. Epub 2015/06/19. eng.

27. Kingsley JD, McMillan V, Figueroa A. The effects of 12 weeks of resistance exercise training on disease severity and autonomic modulation at rest and after acute leg resistance exercise in women with fibromyalgia. Arch Phys Med Rehabil. 2010;91(10):1551–7 PubMed PMID: WOS:000282720300010. English.

28. Kingsley JD, Panton LB, Toole T, Sirithienthad P, Mathis R, McMillan V. The effects of a 12-week strength-training program on strength and functionality in women with fibromyalgia. Arch Phys Med Rehabil. 2005; 86(9):1713–21 PubMed PMID: WOS:000231747300001.

29. Gavi M, Vassalo DV, Amaral FT, DCF M, Gava PL, Dantas EM, et al. Strengthening exercises improve symptoms and quality of life but do not change autonomic modulation in fibromyalgia: a randomized clinical trial. PLoS One. 2014;9(3):–8 PubMed PMID: WOS:000333352800023. English.

30. Hooten WM, Qu WC, Townsend CO, Judd JW. Effects of strength vs aerobic exercise on pain severity in adults with fibromyalgia: A randomized equivalence trial. Pain. 2012;153(4):915–923. PubMed PMID: WOS: 000301877300027. English.

31. Panton LB, Figueroa A, Kingsley JD, Hornbuckle L, Wilson J, St John N, et al. Effects of resistance training and chiropractic treatment in women with fibromyalgia. J Altern Complement Med. 2009;15(3):321–8 PubMed PMID: 19249999. Epub 2009/03/03. eng.

32. Moher D, Shamseer L, Clarke M, Ghersi D, Liberati A, Petticrew M, et al. Preferred reporting items for systematic review and meta-analysis protocols (PRISMA-P) 2015 statement. Syst Rev. 2015;4(1):1.

33. Urrútia G, Bonfill X. La Declaración PRISMA: un paso adelante en la mejora de las publicaciones de la Revista Española de Salud Pública. Rev Española Salud Públ. 2013;87(2):99–102.

34. Booth A, Clarke M, Dooley G, Ghersi D, Moher D, Petticrew M, et al. The nuts and bolts of PROSPERO: an international prospective register of systematic reviews. Syst Rev. 2012;1(1):2.

35. Moher D, Booth A, Stewart L. How to reduce unnecessary duplication: use PROSPERO. Bjog-an International Journal of Obstetrics and Gynaecology. 2014;121(7):784–6 PubMed PMID: WOS:000336445300032.

36. Higgins JP, Altman DG, Gotzsche PC, Juni P, Moher D, Oxman AD, et al. The Cochrane Collaboration's tool for assessing risk of bias in randomised trials. BMJ (Clinical research ed). 2011;343:d5928. PubMed PMID: 22008217. PMCID: PMC3196245. Epub 2011/10/20. eng.

37. Cohen J. A coefficient of agreement for nominal scales. Educ Psychol Meas. 1960;20(1):37–46.

38. Hakkinen A, Hakkinen K, Hannonen P, Alen M. Strength training induced adaptations in neuromuscular function of premenopausal women with fibromyalgia: comparison with healthy women. Ann Rheum Dis. 2001;60(1): 21–6 PubMed PMID: WOS:000166008100005. English.

39. Martinsen S, Flodin P, Berrebi J, Lofgren M, Bileviciute-Ljungar I, Mannerkorpi K, et al. The role of long-term physical exercise on performance and brain activation during the Stroop colour word task in fibromyalgia patients. Clin Physiol Funct Imaging. 2017; PubMed PMID: 28627125. Epub 2017/06/20. eng.

40. Assumpção A ML, Yuan SL, Santos AS, Sauer J, Mango P, Marques AP. Muscle stretching exercises and resistance training in fibromyalgia: which is better? A three-arm randomized controlled trial. - PubMed - NCBI. 2017.

41. Valkeinen H, Alen M, Hannonen P, Hakkinen A, Airaksinen O, Hakkinen K. Changes in knee extension and flexion force, EMG and functional capacity during strength training in older females with fibromyalgia and healthy controls. Rheumatology. 2004;43(2):225–8 PubMed PMID: WOS: 000188850000018. English.

42. Bircan C, Karasel SA, Akgun B, El O, Alper S. Effects of muscle strengthening versus aerobic exercise program in fibromyalgia. Rheumatol Int. 2008;28(6): 527–32 PubMed PMID: WOS:000254206100004. English.

43. Kingsley JD, Panton LB, McMillan V, Figueroa A. Cardiovascular autonomic modulation after acute resistance exercise in women with fibromyalgia. Arch Phys Med Rehabil. 2009;90(9):1628–34 PubMed PMID: WOS:000269938100023.

44. Kingsley JD, McMillan V, Figueroa A. Resistance exercise training does not affect post-exercise hypotension and wave reflection in women with fibromyalgia. Appl Physiol Nutr Metab. 2011;36:254–63 PubMed PMID: WOS:000209142901618.

45. Jones KD, Burckhardt CS, Clark SR, Bennett RM, Potempa KM. A Randomized controlled trial of muscle strengthening versus flexibility training in fibromyalgia. J Rheumatol. 2002;29(5):1041–8 PubMed PMID: WOS: 000175430100030. English.

46. Rooks DS, Silverman CB, Kantrowitz FG. The effects of progressive strength training and aerobic exercise on muscle strength and cardiovascular fitness in women with fibromyalgia: a pilot study. Arthritis Rheum-Arthritis Care Res. 2002;47(1):22–8 PubMed PMID: WOS:000173803700005. English.

47. Rooks DS, Gautam S, Romeling M, Cross ML, Stratigakis D, Evans B, et al. Group exercise, education, and. combination self-management in women with fibromyalgia - A randomized trial. Arch Intern Med. 2007;167(20):2192–200 PubMed PMID: WOS:000250806200005. English.

48. Kayo AH, Peccin MS, Sanches CM, Trevisani VF. Effectiveness of physical activity in reducing pain in patients with fibromyalgia: a blinded randomized clinical trial. Rheumatol Int. 2012;32(8):2285–92 PubMed PMID: 21594719. Epub 2011/05/20.eng.

49. Figueroa A, Kingsley JD, McMillan V, Panton LB. Resistance exercise training improves heart rate variability in women with fibromyalgia. Clin Physiol Funct Imaging. 2008;28(1):49–54 PubMed PMID: WOS:000251629100008.

50. Kingsley JD, McMillan V, Figueroa A. Resistance Exercise Training Does Not Affect Post-exercise Hypotension And Wave Reflection In Women With Fibromyalgia. J Gen Intern Med. 2012;27:458 PubMed PMID: WOS:000209142901618.

51. Hakkinen K, Pakarinen A, Hannonen P, Hakkinen A, Airaksinen O, Valkeinen H, et al. Effects of strength training on muscle strength, cross-sectional area, maximal electromyographic activity, and serum hormones in premenopausal women with fibromyalgia. Journal of Rheumatology. 2002; 29(6):1287–95 PubMed PMID: WOS:000176033500028.

52. Valkeinen H, Hakkinen K, Pakarinen A, Hannonen P, Hakkinen A, Airaksinen O, et al. Muscle hypertrophy, strength development, and serum hormones during strength training in elderly women with fibromyalgia. Scand J Rheumatol. 2005;34(4):309–14 PubMed PMID: WOS:000231312100009.

53. Valkeinen H, Hakkinen A, Hannonen P, Hakkinen K, Alen M. Acute heavy-resistance exercise-induced pain and neuromuscular fatigue in elderly women with fibromyalgia and in healthy controls - effects of strength training. Arthritis Rheum. 2006;54(4):1334–9 PubMed PMID: WOS: 000236830800035. English.

54. Larsson A, Palstam A, Lofgren M, Ernberg M, Bjersing J, Bileviciute-Ljungar I, et al. Resistance exercise improves muscle strength, health status and pain intensity in fibromyalgia-a randomized controlled trial. Arthritis Research & Therapy. 2015;17:15 PubMed PMID: WOS:000357248900001. English.

55. Palstam A, Larsson A, Lofgren M, Ernberg M, Bjersing J, Bileviciute-Ljungar I, et al. Decrease of fear avoidance beliefs following person-centered

progressive resistance exercise contributes to reduced pain disability in women with fibromyalgia: secondary exploratory analyses from a randomized controlled trial. Arthritis Research & Therapy. 2016;18 PubMed PMID: WOS:000376372300006.

56. Andrade A, Vilarino GT, Sieczkowska SM, Coimbra DR, Bevilacqua GG, Steffens RAK. The relationship between sleep quality and fibromyalgia symptoms. J Health Psychol. 2018. https://doi.org/10.1177/1359105317751615.

57. Larsson A, Palstam A, Bjersing J, Löfgren M, Ernberg M, Kosek E, et al. Controlled, cross-sectional, multi-center study of physical capacity and associated factors in women with fibromyalgia. BMC Musculoskelet Disord. 2018;19(1):121.

58. Lorena SB, Lima Mdo C, Ranzolin A, Duarte AL. Effects of muscle stretching exercises in the treatment of fibromyalgia: a systematic review. Rev Bras Reumatol 2015;55(2):167–173. PubMed PMID: 25440706. Epub 2014/12/03. eng.

59. Sanz-Banos Y, Pastor-Mira MA, Lledo A, Lopez-Roig S, Penacoba C, Sanchez-Meca J. Do women with fibromyalgia adhere to walking for exercise programs to improve their health? Systematic review and meta-analysis. Disabil Rehabil. 2017;07:1–13 PubMed PMID: 28687050. Epub 2017/07/09. eng.

60. Thomas EN, Blotman F. Aerobic exercise in fibromyalgia: a practical review. Rheumatol Int. 2010;30(9):1143–50 PubMed PMID: 20340025. Epub 2010/03/27. eng.

22

Juvenile dermatomyositis: is periodontal disease associated with dyslipidemia?

Kátia T. Kozu[1*], Clovis A. Silva[1,2], Nadia E. Aikawa[2], Rosa M. R. Pereira[2], Adriana M. Sallum[1], Cynthia Savioli[3], Eduardo Borba[2] and Lucia M. Campos[1]

Abstract

Background: Association between periodontal disease and dyslipidemia was recently reported in healthy adults. However, a systematic evaluation of concomitant periodontal diseases and lipid profile was not carried out in juvenile dermatomyositis (JDM).

A cross-section study was performed in 25 JDM patients and 25 healthy controls, assessing demographic data, periodontal evaluation, fasting lipoproteins and anti-lipoprotein lipase antibodies. Disease parameters, laboratorial tests and treatment were also evaluated in JDM patients.

Results: The mean current age was similar in patients and controls (11.5 ± 3.75 vs. 11.2 ± 2.58 years,$p = 0.703$). Regarding lipid profile, the median triglycerides [80(31–340) vs. 61(19–182)mg/dL,$p = 0.011$] and VLDL[16(6–68) vs. 13(4–36)mg/dL,$p = 0.020$] were significantly higher in JDM patients versus controls. Gingival vasculopathy pattern was significantly higher in the former group (60% vs. 0%,$p = 0.0001$), as well as the median of gingival bleeding index (GBI) [24.1(4.2–69.4) vs. 11.1(0–66.6)%,$p = 0.001$] and probing pocket depth (PPD) [1.7(0.6–2.4) vs.1.4(0–2.12) mm,$p = 0.006$]. Comparison between JDM patients with and without dyslipidemia revealed that the median of dental plaque index (PI) [100(26.7–100) vs. 59(25–100)%,$p = 0.022$], PPD[1.9(0.6–2.4) vs. 1.4(1.2–1.8)mm,$p = 0.024$] and clinical attachment level (CAL) [1.31(0.7–1.7) vs. 0.8(0.6–1.7)mm,$p = 0.005$] were significantly higher in patients with dyslipidemia. Further analysis between JDM patients with and without gingivitis revealed that the median of current age [12.4 (8.3–18.4) vs. 9.2 (5.5–17.5) years, $p = 0.034$] and disease duration [7.09 ± 3.07 vs. 3.95 ± 2.1 years, $p = 0.008$] were significantly higher in the former group.

Conclusion: Our study showed that gingival inflammation seems to be related to dyslipidemia in JDM patients, suggesting underlying mechanisms for both complications.

Keywords: Juvenile dermatomyositis, Dyslipidemia, Periodontal disease, Gingivitis

Background

Juvenile dermatomyositis (JDM) is a multisystemic disease of unknown etiology characterized by chronic inflammation of striated muscles and skin [1, 2]. The survival rate, outcome and health related quality of life of JDM populations has been improving in the last years and some aspects, such as periodontal diseases [3, 4] and dyslipidemia [5–9] are particularly relevant for these patients.

Periodontal disease comprises gingivitis and periodontitis. It is defined as an immune inflammatory periodontal disorder characterized by chronic localized infections associated with inflammation [3]. Periodontitis is a progressive phenomenon, beginning with gingivitis, followed by the destruction of the periodontal ligaments and bone reabsorption and ending in dental attachment loss [4]. Gengivitis and/or periodontitis have been seldom studied in pediatric autoimmune diseases, like juvenile idiopathic arthritis and juvenile systemic lupus erythematosus [10–15] Recently the association between periodontal disease and dyslipidemia was reported in healthy adults [16].

Data of gingivitis and periodontal diseases are scarce in JDM patients. Of note, the association between gingival vasculopathy pattern, characterized by gingival erythema, capillary dilation and bush-loop formation and disease

---
* Correspondence: katia.kozu@hc.fm.usp.br; katia_kozu@hotmail.com
[1]Pediatric Rheumatology Unit, Hospital das Clinicas HCFMUSP, Faculdade de Medicina, Universidade de Sao Paulo, Rua Joel Jorge de Melo, 600 apto 121, Vila Mariana, São Paulo, SP 04128-081, Brazil
Full list of author information is available at the end of the article

activity was previously suggested [4, 17]. Moreover, dyslipidemia has been rarely reported in JDM patients [5–9], and was observed in 36% of JDM patients, characterized by low high-density lipoprotein (HDL) and high triglycerides (TG) levels [9].

However, to our knowledge, a systematic evaluation of concomitant periodontal diseases and lipid profile assessment was not carried out in JDM population.

Therefore, the aims of this study were to assess periodontal involvement and lipid profile in JDM patients and healthy controls, and to evaluate the possible associations between periodontal disease and dyslipidemia in this chronic inflammatory myopathy.

Materials and methods

JDM patients and controls

A cross-section study was performed from January 2009 to January 2011, and involved 52 JDM patients who were followed at the Pediatric Rheumatology Unit of our University Hospital. All of them fulfilled Bohan and Peter criteria for JDM diagnosis [18]. Exclusion criteria were: diabetes mellitus (fasting glycemia > 126 mg/dL); renal insufficiency (creatinine clearance < 70 ml/min/1.73m^2); proteinuria > 0.3 g/24 h; liver and thyroid dysfunction; neoplasia; infection in the last 15 days; hospitalization in the last month; previous/current smoking and alcohol use; current pregnancy; hormonal therapy; presence of orthodontic appliances and the use of lipid-lowering, anticonvulsant and antihypertensive drugs (thiazide, diuretics or betablockers). Twenty-seven JDM patients were excluded due to refusal to participate in this study ($n = 20$), presence of orthodontic appliances ($n = 4$) and incomplete evaluation ($n = 3$). Therefore, the final group was comprised by 25 JDM patients.

The healthy control group included 25 children and adolescents recruited from the families of JDM patients (either cousins or siblings) in order to minimize differences in some interfering aspects such as nutrition, constitutional and genetic factors. This study was approved by the Local Ethics Committee of our University Hospital and an age-appropriate written informed consent was obtained from all participants and their legal guardians.

Methods

Demographic, anthropometric data and body composition

Current age and gender were recorded for all subjects. For JDM patients, age at disease onset, and disease duration were also studied. Anthropometric data of patients and controls included blood pressure, weight in kilograms, height in meters, and body mass index (BMI) defined by the formula weight/height^2 (kg/m^2). For measurement of body composition, fat and lean mass and fat percentage were evaluated by dual-energy x-ray absorptiometry

(DXA) using the densitometer Hologic QDR 4500 with pediatric software (Discovery model; Hologic Inc. Bedford, MA, USA). A questionnaire of life style/life habits was applied to all JDM patients and healthy controls to assess information regarding breastfeeding, weekly physical activity in hours, and familial history of coronary disease and dyslipidemia [9].

Clinical evaluation and treatment

All JDM patients were examined by the same pediatric rheumatologist to assess the following disease parameters scores: Disease Activity Score (DAS) [19], Childhood Myositis Assessment Scale (CMAS) [20], Manual Muscle Testing (MMT) [20], Myositis Disease Activity Assessment Analogue Scale (MYOACT) [21] and Myositis Intention to Treat Activity Index (MYTAX) [21]. Functional ability score was assessed according to the validated Brazilian version of Childhood Health Assessment Questionnaire (CHAQ) [22].

Current use and cumulative dose of prednisone, hydroxychloroquine, immunosuppressive drugs (methotrexate, cyclosporine, azathioprine and cyclophosphamide) were also determined.

Periodontal assessment

Periodontal assessment was performed in all subjects by three standardized epidemiological parameters: gingival index (GI), dental plaque index (PI) [23] and gingival bleeding index (GBI) [24]. Clinical dental attachment was evaluated by three other indices: probing pocket depth (PPD), cementoenamel junction (CEJ) and clinical attachment level (CAL), at six sites per tooth [25]. The number of decayed, missing and filled teeth (DMF-T) was also counted [26]. PI was used to evaluate the level of oral hygiene, which was calculated according to the number of dental surfaces stained by a dental plaque disclosing agent, multiplied by 100 and divided by the total number of surfaces [23]. GBI was used to evaluate gingival inflammation, and was expressed as the number of bleeding surfaces after probing with a periodontal probe, which was then multiplied by 100 and divided by the total number of surfaces [24]. PPD was determined as the distance from the bottom of the pocket to the gingival margin (normal range < 3 mm). CEJ was measured as the distance from the gingival margin to the cementoenamel junction, identifying hyperplasia or recession. CAL was calculated as the sum of PPD and CEJ (normal range < 3 mm) [25]. Gingivitis was defined as inflammation of the gingiva in the absence of clinical attachment loss [27] with GBI > 25% [28]. Gingival vasculopathy pattern was defined according to the presence of concomitant gingival erythema, capillary dilation and bush-loop formation pattern, as previously described [3].

Laboratory analysis

Biochemical analyses were performed for JDM patients and controls on serum samples obtained after 12-h over-night fasting at the study entry.

Lipid profile

Total cholesterol (TC) and triglycerides (TG) were measured enzymatically on a Technicom RA 1000 System analyser (Boehringer Mannheim, Argentina and Merck, Alemanha) [29, 30]. High-density lipoprotein (HDL) cholesterol was obtained by colorimetric method (Roche Diagnostics) after precipitation of very low-density lipoprotein (VLDL) cholesterol and low-density lipoprotein (LDL) cholesterol by phosphotungstic acid and magnesium chloride [31]. Levels of VLDL were estimated using the formula of TG levels divided by 5 (TG/5), since all samples had a TG level < 400 mg/dL [32]; and LDL cholesterol levels were estimated using the following equation: TC - (HDL + VLDL) [32]. Normal values were defined according to national norms for metabolic data for children and adolescents as follow: TC ≤ 170 mg/dL, HDL ≥ 45 mg/dL, LDL ≤ 130 mg/dL, and TG ≤ 130 mg/

Table 1 Demographic and anthropometric data, body composition, laboratorial findings and periodontal evaluation in juvenile dermatomyositis (JDM) patients and healthy controls

Variables	JDM patients ($n=25$)	Controls ($n=25$)	p
Demographic data			
Current age, years	11.5 ± 3.75	11.2 ± 2.58	0.703
Female gender	14 (56)	13 (52)	0.500
Anthropometric data			
BMI, kg/m^2	19.1 (12.7–30)	17.1 (14.4–27.5)	0.954
Systolic blood pressure, mmHg	90 (80–118)	90 (80–110)	0.099
Dyastolic blood pressure, mmHg	60 (50–85)	60 (45–70)	0.211
Body composition			
Fat percentage	27.5 (10.9–45.4)	22.5 (10.2–42.3)	0.230
Fat mass, kg	10.7 (2.9–27.1)	6.7 (2.8–30.5)	0.274
Lean mass, kg	24.8 ± 6.4	25.4 ± 7.6	0.599
Lipid profile			
Dyslipidemia	17 (68)	10 (40)	0.087
Total cholesterol	151 (102–227)	151 (121–207)	0.941
≥ 170 mg/dL	8 (32)	4 (16)	0.320
HDL, mg/dL	44 (0–72)	50 (30–65)	0.117
≤ 45 mg/dL	10 (40)	7 (28)	0.550
LDL, mg/dL	87 (56–148)	91 (54–140)	0.675
≥ 130 mg/dL	1(4)	2(8)	1.000
VLDL, mg/dL	16 (6–68)	13 (4–36)	0.020
Triglycerides, mg/dL	80 (31–340)	61 (19–182)	0.011
≥ 130 mg/dL	5 (20)	1 (4)	0.189
Anti-LPL antibody	1 (4)	0	1.000
Periodontal assessment			
Gingival vasculopathy pattern	15 (60)	0 (0)	0.0001
DMF-T	2 (0–5)	2 (0–3)	0.862
PI, %	90.6 (25–100)	71.5 (19.8–100)	0.051
GBI, %	24.1 (4.2–69.4)	11.1 (0–66.6)	0.001
PPD, mm	1.7 (0.6–2.4)	1.4 (0–2.12)	0.006
CEJ, mm	−0.1 (−0.8–0)	−0.1 (−0.9–0)	0.570
CAL, mm	1.25 (0.7–1.7)	1 (0.6–1.7)	0.071

Values expressed in mean ± SD, median (range) and n (%); BMI (body mass index), HDL (high density lipoprotein), LDL (low density lipoprotein), VLDL (very low density), anti-LPL (anti-lipoprotein lipase antibody), DMF-T (decayed, missing and filled tooth index), PI (plaque index), GBI (gingival bleeding index), PPD (probing pocket depth), CEJ (cementoenamel juntion), CAL (clinical attachment level)

dL [33]. Dyslipidemia was defined when subjects presented lipid abnormalities in at least one of these lipid parameters [33].

Anti-lipoprotein lipase (LPL) antibodies

Anti-LPL IgG isotype antibodies were measured by double-enzyme-linked immunosorbent assay (ELISA). Costar polystyrene plates were coated overnight with commercially available LPL from bovine milk (5 µg/ml; Sigma, St Louis, MO) and then blocked with 15% adult bovine serum in Tris buffered saline (ABS-T) for one hour at room temperature. The test was performed with serum samples diluted at 1:100 in ABS-T incubated for one hour at room temperature. Anti-LPL IgG isotype antibodies were determined by alkaline phosphatase conjugated goat anti-human IgG (Sigma). The reaction was developed by means of p-nitrophenylphosphate and optical density (OD) was read at 405 nm with a labsystems Multiskan MS (Labsystems, Helsinki, Finland). Positive results were defined as OD values ≥3 standard deviation (SD) above the mean OD values of the 25 healthy control serum samples (cut-off value 0.36). To ensure consistency between assays, serial dilutions of known positive serum samples were included in each study [34].

Inflammatory profile and muscle enzymes

The following tests were performed in JDM patients only. Erythrocyte sedimentation rate (ESR) was evaluated using the Westergren method and C-reactive protein (CRP) by nephelometry. Skeletal muscle enzymes included creatinine kinase (CK) and aldolase measured by kinetic automated method, and lactate dehydrogenase

(LDH), aspartate aminotransferase (AST) and alanine aminotransferase (ALT) by kinetic method.

Statistical analysis

Data were presented in median (range) or mean (± SD) for continuous variables according to abnormal or normal distribution, respectively. Data were presented in number (percentage) for categorical variables. For continuous variables data were compared using Mann-Whitney test or t test to evaluate differences between JDM patients and controls, JDM patients with and without gingivitis, and also JDM patients with and without dyslipidemia according to demographic, anthropometric, laboratorial, treatments and dental parameters. For categorical variables, differences were assessed by Fisher exact test. P-values < 0.05 were considered as significant.

Results

JDM patients vs. healthy controls

Demographic, anthropometric data, body composition, laboratorial exams and periodontal evaluation in JDM patients and healthy controls are shown in Table 1. The mean of current age was similar in JDM patients and healthy controls (11.5 ± 3.75 vs. 11.2 ± 2.58 years, $p = 0.703$). Although trend of a higher frequency of dyslipidemia was observed in JDM patients compared to controls [68% vs. 40%, $p = 0.087$] it was not statistically significant. The median TG [80 (31–340) vs. 61 (19–182) mg/dL, $p = 0.011$] and VLDL [16 (6–68) vs. 13 (4–36) mg/dL, $p = 0.020$] were significantly higher in JDM patients versus controls. The frequency of gingival vasculopathy pattern was significantly higher in the former group (60% vs. 0%, $p = 0.0001$), as well as

Table 2 Demographic data and periodontal assessment in juvenile dermatomyositis (JDM) patients with and without dyslipidemia

Variables	JDM with dyslipidemia ($n = 17$)	JDM without dyslipidemia ($n = 8$)	p
Demographic data			
Current age, years	12.2 (5.5–18.4)	8.5 (7.2–17.8)	0.103
Age at disease presentation, years	6.56 ± 2.73	4.83 ± 2.46	0.159
Disease duration, years	5.49 ± 3.45	5.2 ± 1.55	0.840
Female gender	9 (52)	5 (62)	1.000
Periodontal assessment			
Gingival vasculopathy pattern	11 (64)	4 (50)	0.667
Gingivitis (GBI > 25%)	10 (59)	2 (25)	0.202
DMF-T	2 (0–12)	1 (0–6)	0.102
PI, %	100 (26.7–100)	59 (25–100)	0.022
GBI, %	29.7 (4.2–69.4)	19.6 (13–50)	0.923
PPD, mm	1.9 (0.6–2.4)	1.4 (1.2–1.8)	0.024
CEJ, mm	−0.12 (−0.8–0)	−0.1 (−0.5–0.04)	0.923
CAL, mm	1.31 (0.7–1.7)	0.8 (0.6–1.7)	0.005

Values expressed in mean ± SD, median (range) and n (%); *GBI* (gingival bleeding index), *DMF-T* (decayed, missing, filled teeth index), *PI* (plaque index), *PPD* (probing pocket depth), *CEJ* (cementoenamel juntion), *CAL* (clinical attachment level)

Table 3 Demographic and anthropometric data, body composition, laboratorial findings, juvenile dermatomyositis (JDM) scores and treatment in JDM patients with and without gingivitis

Variables	JDM with gingivitis (GBI > 25%, n = 12)	JDM without gingivitis (GBI ≤ 25%, n = 12)	p
Demographic data			
Current age, years	12.4 (8.3–18.4)	9.2 (5.5–17.5)	0.034
Age at disease presentation, years	4.8 (3.7–7.4)	5.2 (4.1–9.5)	0.580
Disease duration, years	7.09 ± 3.07	3.95 ± 2.1	0.008
Female gender	9 (75)	5 (41)	0.182
Anthropometric data			
BMI, kg/m^2	19.6 (14.5–30)	19.2 (15.3–25)	0.954
Body composition			
Fat percentual	28.2 (11.1–45.4)	26 (10.9–42)	0.789
Fat mass, kg	10.8 (5.0–27.1)	8.2 (2.9–20.2)	1.000
Lean mass, kg	26.4 (15.4–43.8)	27.2 (20–44.5)	0.423
Lipid profile			
Total cholesterol	151 (115–206)	151 (102–227)	0.913
≥ 170 mg/dL	5 (41)	3 (25)	0.666
HDL, mg/dL	43 (0–65)	49 (17–72)	0.328
≤ 45 mg/dL	9 (75)	4 (33)	0.099
LDL, mg/dL	92 (76–148)	77.5 (56–129)	0.265
≥ 130 mg/dL	1 (9)	0	1.000
VLDL, mg/dL	16 (9–42)	14.5 (9–68)	0.957
Triglycerides, mg/dL	82 (31–168)	72.5 (46 340)	0.935
≥130 mg/dL	1 (8)	3 (33)	0.316
Anti-LPL antibody	0	1 (8)	1.000
Muscle enzymes			
AST, U/L	28 (13–122)	29.5 (15–82)	0.703
ALT, U/L	36 (22–123)	34 (29–79)	0.744
CK, U/L	84 (33–478)	125 (62–179)	0.399
LDH, U/L	184 (107–1234)	216.5 (153–562)	0.355
Aldolase, U/L	5.7 (3.4–10.8)	6.35 (4.6–14.6)	0.231
Inflammatory profile			
ESR, mm/1SThour	20 (2–40)	19 (7–54)	0.624
CRP, mg/dL	0.59 (0.16–5.5)	1.61 (0.15–26)	0.242
JDM scores			
CMAS, 0–52	52 (10–52)	52 (17–52)	0.848
MMT, 0–80	80 (42–80)	80 (38–80)	0.742
DAS, 0–18	4 (0–12)	3 (0–18)	0.807
Cutaneous DAS, 0–9	1 (0–8)	1 (0–9)	0.663
Muscle DAS	2 (0–9)	2 (0–9)	0.853
MYOACT, 0–1	0.05 (0–0.16)	0.02 (0–0.3)	0.724
MITAX, 0–1	0.01 (0–0.23)	0 (0–0.28)	0.462
CHAQ	0 (0–1.75)	0.625 (0–2.5)	0.164
Treatment			
Prednisone			
Current use	1 (8)	8 (66)	0.303

Table 3 Demographic and anthropometric data, body composition, laboratorial findings, juvenile dermatomyositis (JDM) scores and treatment in JDM patients with and without gingivitis *(Continued)*

Variables	JDM with gingivitis (GBI > 25%, n = 12)	JDM without gingivitis (GBI ≤ 25%, n = 12)	p
Cumulative dose, g	13.6 (4.9–51.5)	15.1 (3.9–31.2)	0.531
Methotrexate			
Current use	3 (25)	8 (66)	0.277
Cumulative dose, g	2.2 (0.3–16.9)	1.9 (0.37–4.98)	0.79
Cyclosporine			
Current use	0	3 (25)	0.230
Cumulative dose, g	0 (0–3.6)	0	0.805

Values expressed in mean ± SD, median (range) and n (%), *GBI* (gingival bleeding index), *BMI* (body mass index), *HDL* (high density lipoprotein), *LDL* (low density lipoprotein), *VLDL* (very low density), *anti-LPL* (anti-lipoprotein lipase antibody), *AST* (aspartate aminotransferase), *ALT* (alanine aminotransferase), *CK* (creatine kinase), *LDH* (lactate dehydrogenase), *ESR* (erythrocyte sedimentation rate), *CRP* (C-reactive protein), *CMAS* (Childhood Myositis Assessment Scale), *MMT* (Manual Muscle Testing), *DAS* (Disease Activity Score), *MYOACT* (Myositis Disease Activity Assessment Analogue Scale), *MYTAX* (Myositis Intention To Treat Activity Index), *CHAQ* (childhood assessment questionnaire)

the median of GBI [24.1 (4.2–69.4) vs. 11.1 (0–66.6)%, $p = 0.001$] and PPD [1.7 (0.6–2.4) vs. 1.4 (0–2.12) mm, $p = 0.006$] (Table 1).

No differences were observed in breastfeeding duration [4 (0–7) vs. 3 (0–12) months, $p = 0.548$], weekly physical activity [4 (0–14) vs. 5 (5–30), hours, $p = 0.182$] and familial history of coronary disease (32% vs. 52%, $p = 0.251$) between JDM patients and healthy controls.

Periodontal assessment and dyslipidemia in JDM patients
Further analysis between JDM patients with and without dyslipidemia revealed that the median of PI [100 (26.7–100) vs. 59 (25–100)%, $p = 0.022$], PPD [1.9 (0.6–2.4) vs. 1.4 (1.2–1.8) mm, $p = 0.024$] and CAL [1.31 (0.7–1.7) vs. 0.8 (0.6–1.7) mm, $p = 0.005$] were significantly higher in JDM patients with dyslipidemia compared to those without this complication (Table 2).

Gingivitis (GBI > 25%) was observed in 12/24 (50%) of JDM patients and 9/12 (75%) had concomitantly gingivitis with gingival vasculopathy pattern that extends over the upper and/or lower teeth. Further analysis between JDM patients with and without gingivitis revealed that the median of current age [12.4 (8.3–18.4) vs. 9.2 (5.5–17.5) years, $p = 0.034$] and disease duration [7.09 ± 3.07 vs. 3.95 ± 2.1 years, $p = 0.008$] were significantly higher in the former group. No differences were observed in BMI, body composition, anti-LPL antibodies, muscle enzymes, inflammatory parameters, JDM scores and treatments in both groups (Table 3). None of the patients were classified as presenting lipodystrophy (data not shown).

Discussion
According to our study, gingival inflammation seems to be related to dyslipidemia in JDM patients, suggesting common underlying mechanisms for both complications.

The great advantage of the study was to assess a concomitant evaluation of periodontal and lipid parameters in JDM patients and healthy controls. Tobacco use, alcohol intake, diabetes mellitus and some medications may be related to periodontal disorders and therefore they were considered as exclusion criteria [13]. Moreover, the control group included only JDM siblings or relatives, to minimize risk factors associated with periodontal diseases and dyslipidemia, particularly tooth brushing habits, nutrition and genetic factors. However, the major limitations of the present study were a relative small sample, due to the restricted inclusion and exclusion criteria, and a cross-sectional study design.

We confirmed previous evidences of altered lipid profile in JDM populations [5–9]. Dyslipidemia occurred in approximately 70% of our JDM patients, with high levels of VLDL and triglycerides. The presence of anti-LPL antibodies, a specific autoantibody associated with hypertriglyceridemia in systemic lupus erythematosus patients [34], was not a possible explanation for the lipoprotein abnormalities seen in our JDM patients.

The gingival inflammation, that used to be considered a process restricted to oral cavity, can now be considered as responsible for systemic inflammation and associated to disease activity in children [4] and adult patients [35]. It is believed that in predisposed individuals, a metastatic inflammation can occur, that is, a systemic inflammatory reaction to the presence of microorganisms (aerobic and anaerobic bacteria) in the chronically inflamed gingiva and periodontal ligaments. Thus, in the presence of gingivitis or periodontitis, inflammatory cytokines such as IL1 and IL6 are produced and exert local and systemic action, leading to an increase in circulating immune complexes. Therefore, periodontal abnormalities could act as a trigger for local and systemic inflammatory process, which in turn predisposes to metabolic changes, explaining the association between the expressive plaque indexes found in our patients with JDM with dyslipidemia [16, 36].

In addition, three-quarter of our JDM patients with gingivitis (gingival bleeding index > 25%) had a concomitant clinical gingival vasculopathy pattern that extends over the upper and/or lower teeth, indicating a diffuse oral involvement. Of note, gingival alterations were not associated with treatment particularly with glucocorticoid and cyclosporine. This latter immunosuppressive drug is a well-known cause of gingival enlargement [37]. Moreover, gingival alterations could not be attributed to disease activity, since it was similar in JDM patients with and without gingivitis, with both groups presenting inactive disease or mild to moderate disease activity.

It was observed, however, that the group of patients with JDM and gingival alterations was composed by older individuals with longer disease duration. This fact suggests that the persistence of a chronic inflammatory process related to JDM disease could be responsible for the greater periodontal involvement and reinforces that periodontitis is a progressive phenomenon, beginning with gingivitis, followed by the destruction of the periodontal ligaments and bone reabsorption and ending in dental attachment loss [4]. In fact, although initial aspects of periodontitis, such as increased PCS and PCI, were associated with patients with JDM and dyslipidemia, none of the patients studied was classified as having periodontitis (PCI > 3 mm), which is rarely observed in pediatric age group [15]. Future prospective studies should be necessary to clarify this point.

The worst oral hygiene observed in the group of JDM patients with abnormal lipid profile alert to the risk of bacterial plaque accumulation inducing local inflammatory process, a condition that could contribute to aggravate periodontal and systemic inflammation, leading to lipid changes and increased risk of coronary artery diseases. Therefore, it is necessary to encourage patients and family members to maintain an adequate oral health [4, 36].

Conclusions

Gingival inflammation and attachment loss observed in the studied sample were associated with dyslipidemia and dental changes were more evident the longer was the disease duration.

Gingivitis and poor oral hygiene are important concerns in JDM dyslipidemic patients, especially after long-term disease. These findings indicate the importance of oral health prevention and treatment for these patients, aiming to reduce their early cardiovascular risk.

Acknowledgements

We thank Prof. Dr. Jose Siqueira Tadeu and Dr. Priscila Ribas Guardieiro for their suggestions and comments, and Dr. Ulysses Doria Filho for statistical analysis.

Funding

This study was supported by grants from Fundação de Amparo à Pesquisa do Estado de São Paulo (FAPESP 2008/58238-4 to CAS), Conselho Nacional de Desenvolvimento Científico e Tecnológico (CNPq 303422/2015-7 to CAS

and 301805/2013-0 to RMRP), Federico Foundation (to CAS and RMRP) and by Núcleo de Apoio à Pesquisa "Saúde da Criança e do Adolescente" of Universidade de São Paulo (NAP-CriAd) to CAS.

Authors' contributions

All authors contributed equally to this paper. All authors read and approved the final manuscript.

Competing interests

The authors declared that they have no competing interests.

Author details

[1]Pediatric Rheumatology Unit, Hospital das Clinicas HCFMUSP, Faculdade de Medicina, Universidade de Sao Paulo, Rua Joel Jorge de Melo, 600 apto 121, Vila Mariana, São Paulo, SP 04128-081, Brazil. [2]Division of Rheumatology, Hospital das Clinicas HCFMUSP, Faculdade de Medicina, Universidade de Sao Paulo, São Paulo, SP, Brazil. [3]Division of Dentistry, Hospital das Clinicas HCFMUSP, Faculdade de Medicina, Universidade de Sao Paulo, São Paulo, SP, Brazil.

References

1. Sato JO, Sallum AM, Ferriani VP, Marini R, Sacchetti SB, Okuda EM, et al. A Brazilian registry of juvenile dermatomyositis: onset features and classification of 189 cases. Clin Exp Rheumatol. 2009;27:1031-8.
2. Aikawa NE, Jesus AA, Liphaus BL, Silva CA, Carneiro-Sampaio M, Viana VS, et al. Organ-specific autoantibodies and autoimmune diseases in juvenile systemic lupus erythematosus and juvenile dermatomyositis patients. Clin Exp Rheumatol. 2012;30:126-31.
3. Savioli C, Silva CA, Fabri GM, Kozu K, Campos LM, Bonfá E, et al. Gingival capillary changes and oral motor weakness in juvenile dermatomyositis. Rheumatology (Oxford). 2010;49:1962-70.
4. Fabri GM, Savioli C, Siqueira JT, Campos LM, Bonfá E, Silva CA. Periodontal disease in pediatric rheumatic diseases. Rev Bras Reumatol. 2014;54:311-7.
5. Huemer C, Kitson H, Malleson PN, Sanderson S, Huemer M, Cabral DA, et al. Lipodystrophy in patients with juvenile dermatomyositis – evaluation of clinical and metabolic abnormalities. J Rheumatol. 2001;28:610-5.
6. Verma S, Singh S, Bhalla AK, Khullar M. Study of subcutaneous fat in children with juvenile dermatomyositis. Arthritis Rheum. 2006;55:564-8.
7. Bingham A, Mamyrova G, Rother KI, Oral E, Cochran E, Premkumar A, et al. Predictors of acquired lipodystrophy in juvenile-onset dermatomyositis and a gradient of. Medicine (Baltimore). 2008;87:70-86.
8. Coyle K, Rother KI, Weise M, Ahmed A, Miller FW, Rider LG. Metabolic abnormalities and cardiovascular risk factors in children with myositis. J Pediatr. 2009;155:882-7.
9. Kozu KT, Silva CA, Bonfá E, Sallum AM, Pereira RM, Viana VS, et al. Dyslipidaemia in juvenile dermatomyositis: the role of disease activity. Clin Exp Rheumatol. 2013;31:638-44.
10. Savioli C, Silva CA, Siqueira JT. Características morfológicas e funcionais do sistema estomatognático em pacientes portadores de artrite reumatóide juvenil. J Bras Ortodon Ortop Facial. 2000;25:70-8.
11. Savioli C, Silva CA, Ching LH, Campos LM, Prado EF, Siqueira JT. Dental and facial characteristics of patients with juvenile idiopathic arthritis. Rev Hosp Clin Fac Med Sao Paulo. 2004;59(3):93-8.
12. Fernandes EG, Savioli C, Siqueira JT, Silva CA. Oral health and the masticatory system in juvenile systemic lupus erythematosus. Lupus. 2007;16:713-9.
13. Pugliese C, van der Vinne RT, Campos LM, Guardieiro PR, Saviolli C, Bonfá E, et al. Juvenile idiopathic arthritis activity and function ability: deleterious effects in periodontal disease? Clin Rheumatol. 2016;35:81-91.
14. Figueredo CM, Areas A, Sztajnbok FR, Miceli V, Miranda LA, Gustafsson A. Higher elastase activity associated with lower IL-18 in GCF from juvenile systemic lupus patients. Oral Health Prev Dent. 2008;6:75-81.
15. Sete MR, Figueredo CM, Sztajnbok F. Periodontitis and systemic lupus erythematosus. Rev Bras Reumatol. 2016;56:165-70.
16. Jaramillo A, Lafaurie GI, Millán LV, Ardila CM, Duque A, Novoa C, et al. Association between periodontal disease and plasma levels of cholesterol and triglycerides. Colomb Med (Cali). 2013;44:80-6.

17. Rider LG, Atkinson JC. Images and clinical medicine: gingival and periungual vasculopathy of juvenile dermatomyositis. N Engl J Med. 2009;360:e21.

18. Bohan A, Peter JB. Polymyositis and dermatomyositis. N Engl J Med. 1975; 292:344–7.

19. Bode RK, Klein-Gitelman MS, Miller ML, Lechman TS, Pachman LM. Disease activity score for children with juvenile dermatomyositis: reliability and validity evidence. Arthritis Rheum. 2003;49:7–15.

20. Lovell DJ, Lindsley CB, Rennebohm RM, Ballinger SH, Bowyer SL, Giannini EH, et al. Development of validated disease activity and damage indices for the juvenile idiopathic inflammatory myopathies. II. The childhood myositis assessment scale (CMAS): a quantitative tool for the evaluation of muscle function. The juvenile dermatomyositis disease activity collaborative study group. Arthritis Rheum. 1999;42:2213–9.

21. Sultan SM, Allen E, Oddis CV, Kiely P, Cooper RG, Lundberg IE, et al. Reliability and validity of the myositis disease activity assessment tool. ArthritisRheum. 2008;58:3593–9.

22. Machado CS, Ruperto N, Silva CH, Ferriani VP, Roscoe I, Campos LM, et al. Paediatric Rheumatology International Trials Organisation. The Brazilian version of the childhood health assessment questionnaire (CHAQ) and the child health questionnaire (CHQ). Clin Exp Rheumatol. 2001;23:25–9.

23. Ainamo J, Bay I. Problems and proposals for recording gingivitis and plaque. Int Dent J. 1975;25:229–35.

24. O'Leary TJ. The periodontal screening examination. J Periodontol. 1967;38: 617–24.

25. Armitage GC. American Academy of periodontology. Periodontol record Ann Periodontol. 1999;4:1–6.

26. World Health Organization. Oral health surveys: basic methods. 4th ed. Geneva: World Health Organization; 1997.

27. Parameter on plaque-induced gingivitis. American Academy of Periodontology. J Periodontol. 2000;71:851–2.

28. Modéer T, Blomberg CC, Wondimu B, Julihn A, Marcus C. Association between obesity, flow rate of whole saliva, and dental caries in adolescents. Obesity. 2010;18:2367–73.

29. Fossati P, Prencipe L. Serum triglycerides determined colorimetrically with an enzyme that produces hydrogen peroxide. Clin Chem. 1982;28:2077–780.

30. Siedel J, Hägele EO, Ziegenhorn J, Wahlefeld AW. Reagent for the enzymatic determination of serum total cholesterol with improved lipolytic efficiency. Clin Chem. 1983;29:1075–80.

31. Warnick GR, Cheung MC, Albers JJ. Comparison of current methods for high – density lipoprotein cholesterol quantification. Clin Chem. 1979;25:596–604.

32. Friedewald WT, Levy RI, Fredrickson DS. Estimation of the concentration of low -density lipoprotein cholesterol in plasma, without use of the preparative ultracentrifuge. Clin Chem. 1972;18:499–502.

33. Xavier HT, Izar MC, Faria Neto JR, Assad MH, Rocha VZ, Sposito AC, et al. V Brazilian guidelines on dyslipidemias and prevention of atherosclerosis. Arq Bras Cardiol. 2013;101:1–20.

34. De Carvalho JF, Borba EF, Viana VS, Bueno C, Leon EP, Bonfá E. Anti-lipoprotein lipase antibodies: a new player in the complex atherosclerotic process in systematic lupus erythematosus? Arthritis Rheum. 2004;50:3610–5.

35. Venkataraman A, Almas K. Rheumatoid arthritis and periodontal disease. N Y State Dent J. 2015;81:30–6.

36. Noguchi E, Kato R, Ohno K, Mitsui A, Obama T, Hirano T, et al. The apolipoprotein B concentration in gingival crevicular fluid increases in patients with diabetes mellitus. Clin Biochem. 2014;47:67–71.

37. Shiboski CH, Krishnan S, Besten PD, Golinveaux M, Kawada P, Tornabene A, et al. Gingival enlargement in pediatric organ transplant recipients in relation to tacrolimus-based immunosuppressive regimens. Pediatr Dent. 2009;31:38–46.

23

The effects of cultural background on patient-perceived impact of psoriatic arthritis - a qualitative study conducted in Brazil and France

Penélope Esther Palominos[1,2*] (iD), Laure Gossec[3], Sarah Kreis[3], César Luis Hinckel[4], Rafael Mendonça da Silva Chakr[1,2,4], Ana Laura Didonet Moro[1], Willemina Campbell[5], Maarten de Wit[6], Niti Goel[7], Charles Lubianca Kohem[1,4] and Ricardo Machado Xavier[1,2,4]

Abstract

Background: In psoriatic arthritis (PsA) almost all qualitative studies have been performed in European populations. This work aimed to evaluate the impact of PsA in Brazilian and French subjects, as well as to explore cultural differences in the experience of disease and to recognize domains important for patients living with PsA outside Europe.

Methods: A qualitative study was conducted in two university hospitals in Brazil and France; outpatients fulfilling Classification Criteria for PsA participated in individual interviews regarding the impact of PsA; interviews were conducted in the local language. The sample size was defined by saturation; interviews were recorded and transcribed and content analysis was performed.

Results: Fifteen patients were interviewed in Brazil and 13 in France. Mean disease duration was 16.5 ± 12.5 years (range: 8 months to 47 years) and 14.4 ± 8.4 years (range 12 months to 29 years) for Brazilian and French subjects, respectively. A broad impact was perceived: 67 codes emerged from the interviews and were grouped in 41 categories. Although 2/3 of categories were common to both nationalities, some important health domains from the perspective of PsA patients from a non-European background were brought to light including sexual dysfunction, emotional impact of psoriasis and impact of prejudice on social and professional life.

Conclusions: This study highlights the importance of assessing the impact of PsA on a national level, emphasizing the common cross-cultural aspects but also revealing domains of interest for patients with PsA living outside Europe which merit further study.

Keywords: Psoriatic arthritis, Quality of life, Qualitative research, Disease burden

Background

Psoriatic arthritis (PsA) is a chronic rheumatic disease leading to altered quality of life, pain and functional disability, but also professional and emotional burden [1–5]. Perceptions of the impact of PsA differ between patients and physicians, with patients usually indicating a greater life impact compared to health professionals and describing aspects of impact which physicians may not acknowledge [6]. In this regard, qualitative studies are useful to obtain patients' opinions about the impact of disease.

Using qualitative methods to support the recognition of the most affected domains of health according to European patients, a questionnaire to evaluate patient-perceived impact of disease, the PsA Impact of Disease Questionnaire (PsAID) was recently developed [7].

* Correspondence: penelopepalominos@gmail.com
[1]Serviço de Reumatologia, Hospital de Clínicas de Porto Alegre, Ramiro Barcelos Street 2350, Porto Alegre Zip code 90035903, Brazil
[2]Programa de Pós Graduação em Ciências Médicas, Universidade Federal do Rio Grande do Sul (UFRGS), Ramiro Barcelos 2400, Porto Alegre Zip code 90035903, Brazil
Full list of author information is available at the end of the article

Qualitative methodology was also employed to verify if the questionnaires currently available to assess PsA include concepts important to patients [8].

A recent systematic literature review (SLR) analyzed the effects of PsA reported by patients in 13 qualitative studies and categorized them by a standardized reference system, the International Classification of Functioning, Disability and Health (ICF). The ICF component most represented was activities and participation (42.6%) rather than body structures (10.3%) or body functions (29.4%), indicating that the social impact of disease is very important for people living with PsA [9].

The impact of PsA from the patients' perspective has been well studied in European patients and to date, published qualitative studies in PsA have included patients mostly from Eastern and Western European countries [7, 8, 10–16]. Data on PsA impact are scarce for patients from countries outside of Europe.

In rheumatoid arthritis (RA) and systemic lupus erythematosus (SLE), it has been demonstrated, that even in the same country, distinct ethnic groups present different perceptions about the rheumatic disease and therapy [17–19]. In addition, RA patients from different nationalities have different priorities when attending a rheumatologic visit [20]. We can hypothesize that patients with PsA living in different countries would also present different perceptions on the impact of PsA.

Quantitative studies have indicated Brazilian patients with PsA have an impaired quality of life and suboptimal control of disease activity but qualitative studies aiming to obtain the patient-perceived impact of PsA in Brazil are lacking [21, 22]. Given the differences between Europe and the ethnic (diverse ethnicity), cultural, religious (diverse religious groups but mainly Catholic) and economic background of Brazil, it is of interest to explore potential similarities and differences in patient perceptions of disease. Indeed, since most patients prefer to be involved in decisions concerning PsA and its treatment, a better understanding on the impact of disease from the patients' perspective can lead physicians to optimize assessment of PsA and to facilitate shared decision-making [23].

The main objective of the present work was to evaluate the impact of PsA in Brazilian and French patients using a qualitative methodology. We also aimed to explore cultural differences in the experience of disease in Brazil and France and to recognize domains important to patients living with PsA outside the European background.

Methods

A qualitative study with individual interviews was conducted in two public academic tertiary hospitals: Hospital de Clínicas de Porto Alegre, in Porto Alegre, Brazil and Pitié-Salpêtrière Hospital, in Paris, France. The sample comprised outpatients fulfilling the Classification Criteria for PsA (CASPAR) able and willing to participate in a 1 h interview in the local language (Portuguese or French) [24]. In each country, the selection of participants aimed to ensure a broad spectrum of demographic aspects and different degrees of disease severity and manifestations through purposeful sampling.

Patients with a concomitant rheumatic disease other than PsA and patients not fluent in the local language were excluded [15].

The sample size was defined by saturation, i.e., the point when two consecutive interviews did not reveal additional concepts and the researcher obtained enough information about the subject [25]. New participants were interviewed until saturation was reached in each country.

Quantitative data collection

Demographic characteristics and data about PsA were collected by the patient and the interviewer (using the medical file when necessary) before the interview: age, gender, professional status, educational level, ethnicity, current medication, extent of skin disease, presence of joint deformities, functional assessment measured by the Health Assessment Questionnaire (HAQ), and patient assessment of pain, skin and global disease on a 0–100 mm visual analogue scale [26]. These data were not used as outcome measures but allowed the description of the patient sample.

Qualitative interview

Questions used in the interview were developed by the authors, with input from patient research partners of the Group for Research and Assessment of Psoriasis and Psoriatic Arthritis (GRAPPA) [27]. The semi-structured interview had three main questions: the first one was an open question which directly identified domains of health affected in PsA, "What is the impact of PsA on your life?". The additional questions encouraged patients to describe domains not routinely assessed by their health professionals and domains in which they expected improvement with therapy: "Is there any aspect of PsA that is important to you but is not often evaluated by doctors?", and "What do you expect from an effective treatment for PsA?". In addition, patients were encouraged to express themselves through prompt questions like: "Can you give us an example?", "What is your opinion about that?", "What do you do in these occasions?", "Could you talk more about that?"

Data analysis

In Brazil, the interviews were conducted in Portuguese by the first author (PEP) and recorded using Audacity version

2.1.2. In France, the interviews were conducted by two investigators (SK and LG) and recorded by audiotape.

Interviews were transcribed and analyzed in the original language using the qualitative content analysis method [28].

First, two researchers independently read the transcripts to gain a contextualized impression of the interview. Then, codes were assigned to each sentence of the interview by each researcher independently, a process called coding. A code is a word or short phrase that captures and summarizes what the patient says in a particular part of the interview. In the sentences "I can't dress myself, tie my shoelaces and buttons due to psoriatic arthritis" and "Now I can't walk outdoors on flat ground and climb up steps", for example, the codes "dressing" and "walking" could be used, respectively, to summarize the sentences.

The codes were created directly from data, without any preconceived ideas or theories. After coding the interview independently, the two researchers met to refine the codes: findings were shared, discussed and agreed by the two coders.

Then, codes were clustered together according to similarity and regularity creating categories. Category is a group of codes which share the same characteristics. In the previous example, the codes "dressing" and "walking" could be included inside the category "functional disability".

Codes and categories were then reviewed by a third researcher and disagreements were solved by consensus among the three investigators.

Interviews from Brazil were coded in Portuguese Language by PEP and RMSC and codes and categories reviewed by CLK. All three researchers were native Portuguese speakers. Interviews from France were coded in French Language by PEP and ALNM. Both researchers were fluent in the French Language but since they were not native French speakers, codes and categories were reviewed by LG, a native French researcher.

Categories were classified in three groups: those that were common to Brazil and France, those referred only by Brazilian participants and those referred only by French participants. The final interpretation of data was done by the first author (PEP – Brazilian researcher) and the second author (LG – French researcher) and reported in a descriptive manner using the English Language. This language was chosen since it was a common language to the six co-authors involved in the coding process and to the three patient research partners from GRAPPA who contributed to the project. The final reporting of results was finally read and agreed by all the six coders and patient research partners.

Results

Twenty-eight PsA patients were interviewed: 15 in Brazil and 13 in France. The individual demographic data and disease characteristics of participants are described in Table 1. A comparison between the French and Brazilian samples is shown in Table 2. The samples from Brazil and France had participants with a wide range of disease duration, including patients with early PsA to those with more than 20 years of diagnosis. Brazilian patients had higher disease activity, a higher proportion of participants with current or previous use of biological therapy and a lower educational level compared to the French sample (Table 2).

The analysis of the 28 transcripts found 67 different codes, grouped in 41 categories. Twenty-seven out of 41 categories (66%) were common to Brazilian and French participants (Table 3).

The physical impact of PsA

Eleven categories represented the physical impact of PsA (27% of the total 41 categories) and 6 of these (55%) were common to Brazilian and French participants (Table 3).

Pain was viewed as a disabling, intense and unremitting symptom by both nationalities, with participants usually describing an inflammatory rhythm associated with PsA pain: "the pain is worse in the morning, and everything is difficult, getting on and off the bus... Then, after work and movement, you feel better but I have pain all the time, you end up learning to live with it" (Male, 38 years old, Brazilian).

Functional disability, with impairment in motion, hygiene/ dressing and use of hands was widely cited in both samples. Patients expressed that PsA affected their ability to walk, run, go up and down stairs, get in and out of the car and use public transportation: "It is really difficult to walk, to sit down and get up off a chair is hard, to go to the bathroom is hard, to get up from the bed is hard, to go down stairs to go to the subway is exhausting" (Female, 37 years old, French).

Other activities such as washing oneself, tying shoelaces, putting on and taking off clothes, showering, and lowering/raising the toilet seat were also limited due to PsA. The involvement of hands was viewed as an obstacle to daily living activities such as picking up and carrying objects, opening and closing water taps, opening cans, cutting meat, cooking, handling cutlery, sweeping, washing clothes and peeling fruits and vegetables. "Before the treatment I could not hold the fork and knife anymore. I was invited to dinner by people who were not very close to me and it really makes me sad to say that I didn't eat because I couldn't cut my meat!" (Female, 67 years old, French). "The situation had reached a point where I could not take off my clothes, take a shower, put on a coat or a jacket, tie my shoes, it was unbearable" (Male, 19 years old, French). The code "loss of independence" due to functional disability emerged in both samples.

Table 1 Individual characteristics of the 28 PsA patients included in the study

Nationality	Higher education/ post secondary school	Disease duration since diagnosis (in years)	Disease duration since beginning of symptoms (in years)	Occupation	Patient global VAS	Patient skin VAS	Patient Pain VAS	HAQ	Current or previous biological therapy	Current BSA affected by psoriasis ≥10%	Joint deformity
BR	No	7	14	Retired due to disability	83	46	68	2.500	Yes	No	No
BR	No	11	13	Manager	79	48	76	1.625	Yes	No	No
BR	No	12	30	Retired due to disability	74	43	62	0.500	Yes	Yes	Yes
BR	No	10	14	Retired	41	6	24	0.750	No	No	Yes
BR	No	19	19	Retired	55	12	70	2.250	No	No	No
BR	No	3	16	Locksmith	58	46	78	1.750	No	Yes	No
BR	No	5	5	Retired	80	13	77	2.875	No	No	Yes
BR	No	27	27	Retired due to disability	70	50	63	1.625	No	No	Yes
BR	No	0.2	0.9	Housework	65	84	60	1.500	No	No	No
BR	No	0.1	0.7	Housework	92	81	78	2.125	No	No	No
BR	No	0.08	1	Tourism worker	20	27	10	1.125	No	No	No
BR	No	19	20	Retired due to disability	7	0	82	0.125	No	No	Yes
BR	No	20	24	Housework	26	2	3	1.750	Yes	No	Yes
BR	No	33	47	Retired due to disability	57	11	11	0.500	Yes	Yes	Yes
BR	No	6	16	Housework	86	47	56	1.625	No	No	Yes
FR	No	10	11	Photographer	4	58	87	1.875	No	No	Yes
FR	Yes	1	1	Retired	19	11	3	0.000	No	No	No
FR	Yes	0.25	3	Building worker	60	25	2	1.625	No	No	No
FR	No	8	9	Manager	12	30	60	1.000	Yes	No	No
FR	No	10	20	Manager	42	0	29	0.250	No	No	No
FR	No	19	20	Retired	66	10	37	0.375	No	No	No
FR	No	5	7	Student	35	0	43	0.375	Yes	No	No
FR	No	11	14	Salesman	65	0	36	0.250	No	No	No
FR	No	14	22	Retired	45	27	66	0.500	No	No	Yes
FR	Yes	1	17	Architect	54	25	35	0.750	No	No	No
FR	Yes	20	20	Engineer	0	24	54	0.375	No	No	Yes
FR	Yes	15	29	Engineer	43	0	0	0.000	No	No	No
FR	No	15	16	Retired	86	0	40	1.625	Yes	No	Yes

BR Brazil, FR France, VAS Visual analogue scale, HAQ Health assessment questionnaire, BSA Body surface area

Table 2 Comparison of demographic characteristics and disease activity of patients interviewed in Brazil and France

	Brazil (N = 15)	France (N = 13)
Age (in years), Mean ± SD, range	51 ± 11, 28–70	54 ± 17, 19–81
Female sex N (%)	8 (53.3)	6 (46.1)
Mean PsA duration since diagnosis (in years) ± SD, range	11.4 ± 10.0, 10 months to 33 years	9.5 ± 6.7, 3 months to 20 years
Mean PsA duration since beginning of symptoms (in years) ± SD, range	16.5 ± 12.5, 8 months to 47 years	14.4 ± 8.4, 1 to 29 years
Educational level: patients with higher education (university level) N (%)	0 (0.0)	5 (38.5)
Currently exerting professional activity N (%)	7 (46.6)	4 (30.8)
Current or previous use of biological therapy N (%)	5 (33.3)	3 (23.0)
Current BSA involved by psoriasis > 10% N (%)	3 (20.0)	0 (0.0)
Patients with joint deformities N (%)	8 (53.3)	4 (30.7)
Patient global VAS (0-100 mm) Mean ± SD, range	54 ± 27, 7–92	40 ± 26, 0–86
Patient skin VAS (0-100 mm) Mean ± SD, range	34 ± 26, 0–84	16 ± 17, 0–58
Patient pain VAS (0-100 mm) Mean ± SD, range	55 ± 27, 3–82	37 ± 25, 0–87
Disability measures by HAQ		
Mild (HAQ 0–1) N (%)	4 (26.7)	10 (76.9)
Moderate (HAQ > 1–2) N (%)	7 (46.4)	3 (23.0)
Severe (HAQ > 2–3) N (%)	4 (26.7)	0 (0.0)

SD Standard deviation, *N* Number, *PsA* Psoriatic arthritis, *BSA* Body surface area, *VAS* Visual analogue scale, *HAQ* Health assessment questionnaire

Table 3 Impact of PsA: comparison of categories found in Brazil and France

	Brazil	Common Categories	France
Physical Impact	Weight gain/loss Joint swelling Joint deformities Sexual dysfunction	Pain Fatigue Functional disability Sleep disorders Psoriasis Joint stiffness	Uveitis
Emotional Impact	Embarrassment/Shame	Anxiety Frustration Fear Lack of interest Depressed mood Low self esteem Irritability	Poor concentration
Professional Impact	Discrimination at work	Inability to perform job-related activities Absenteeism/job losses PsA symptoms impaired by occupational activity Financial impact Low productivity Inability to work full-time Necessity to delegate tasks and/or ask for other people's help	Difficulties to create a long term career plan Necessity to change position in company Necessity to change occupational activity Difficulties to get a job PsA impairing career advancement
Social Impact	Discrimination in social life	Patient perception of harming relatives Incomprehension of disability by relatives Limited activities with younger relatives Limitation to children's care Limitation to leisure activities Limitation to sports Sports impairing PsA symptoms	

Besides pain and functional disability, other categories were common to Brazilian and French patients: "fatigue", "joint stiffness", "sleep disorders" and "psoriasis/ skin impact". Fatigue seemed very important to patients and they usually described the fatigue of PsA as being more intense than "normal" fatigue, e.g., the tiredness which occur in healthy subjects after exercise or an intense day of work.

Since 20% of the Brazilian patients had more than 10% percent of body surface area covered by psoriasis, it appears this influenced the identification of more codes representing the characteristics of skin lesions (e.g., itching, burning, bleeding, scaling, fissures) and the consequences of psoriasis (e.g. psoriasis impairing sleep, discrimination due to skin lesions) in this sample.

Other categories of physical impact were described: Brazilian participants referenced "joint swelling", "joint deformities", "sexual dysfunction" and "weight gain/loss" while "uveitis" was cited by French patients.

The category "sexual dysfunction" was classified inside the domain "physical impact" because, in the opinion of participants, the effects of psoriasis on physical appearance was responsible for the decreased libido and decline in sexual activity, although the code "decreased libido" could also be viewed as an emotional impact of disease.

The increase in body weight was perceived by Brazilian patients as a consequence of restricted physical activity due to PsA and the use of corticosteroids, while lack of appetite and weight loss were perceived as consequences of medicines used to treat PsA.

The emotional impact of PsA

Nine categories of emotional impact were found in this study (22% of the total 41 categories) and 7 (78%) of those categories representing emotional impact were common to Brazilian and French participants.

Besides common categories as "anxiety", "low self-esteem", "frustration", "irritability", "fear", "lack of interest" and "depressed mood", the category "embarrassment/ shame" emerged in the Brazilian sample. The emotional impact of skin disease and the reporting of situations in which prejudice was experienced were repeatedly cited by Brazilians: "If you are waiting in a line, the person behind or the person in front of you looks at you, and takes a step to the side not to be too close. I think the prejudice is visible" (Male, 42 years old, Brazilian). "... in the crowded bus, the people were squeezed together standing, but no one sat next to me ... when I missed a medical visit, doctors said I could not miss it, but no one knew what I was feeling going there, taking the bus, suffering because of the prejudice, I got to the point that I took money from other things to buy gas and go to the clinic by car" (Female, 64 years old, Brazilian).

It was interesting that while the category "low self-esteem" for the Brazilian sample was mainly related to the prejudice and psoriasis, the same category in French subjects was more associated with functional disability: "I could not drive anymore, it was difficult to move around; it affects your self-esteem and the emotional side" (Male, 75 years old, French). "I felt different from others around me. This disease affects your self-esteem. I am 30 years married and my husband is a very good person to me. We lived many months without an intimate relationship due to the skin lesions" (Female, 54 years old, Brazilian).

Patients from both nationalities considered that the loss of independence due to pain and disability were contributing factors to depressed mood. Furthermore, the Brazilian patients perceived their depressed mood being driven primarily by the negative thoughts that other people had about them due to psoriasis.

The professional impact of PsA

Thirteen categories revealed the professional impact of PsA and represented 32% of the total number of categories in this study. Seven out of 13 (54%) were common to both nationalities (Table 3): "inability to perform job-related activities", "absenteeism/job loss", "PsA symptoms impaired by occupational activity", "financial impact", "low productivity", "inability to work full-time" and "necessity to delegate tasks and/or ask for other people's help".

Activities which involved the use of hands, heavy load lifting, immobility over long periods of time, major physical efforts and the obligatory wearing of high heels on the job were some examples of tasks impaired by PsA: "Some things I used to do, I can't do anymore; I went on rooftops using a ladder. But when you are using a ladder and fixing the roof, you must stand 10-15 minutes in the same position and I feel tired" (Male, 42 years old, Brazilian). "One year ago, the pain was so present and so permanent that I had to reject proposals. I could not accept more work because I was not able to work several hours in a day. My projects were put on hold because I could not work a whole day on the keyboard due to the pain in my hands" (Male, 33 years old, French).

Participants reported adapting their occupational activity, delegating tasks, slowing down the rhythm of work, adapting objects and tasks and even changing their occupation: "I used to work alone doing iron gates and grids but now I don't have strength in my wrists and I have to ask for other peoples' help. This is something that makes me sad because it's my business" (Male, 42 years old, Brazilian).

The social impact of PsA

Eight categories of social impact were found (20% of the total 41 categories) and 7 of these (87%) were common to Brazilian and French participants (Table 3).

Regarding family life, patients from both countries referenced having limited their leisure activities with children and grandchildren because they were not able to play and practice sports with them. The ability to take care of infants and newborns was perceived as impaired and participants reported they were afraid of dropping the babies and not being able to prevent accidents.

Participants reported that their relatives were not able to understand disability and pain caused by PsA: "It is difficult for other people to accept that you are sick. I try to look normal in the workplace; for three-quarters of the day it is as if nothing was wrong. When I get home, I am exhausted. And so, my husband doesn't accept it. He says: I don't understand, during the day you seem well and then, without any reason, when you're home you're tired and weak" (Female, 48 years old, French). "... in your social or family life it is not always simple because when you have pain you are not in the mood to do things, and not everyone understands it." (Male, 19 years old, French).

Brazilian and French patients reported limited participation in physical activities and sports, e.g., walking, football, running, volleyball, water aerobics, ski, biking, rowing and tennis. Pain, joint stiffness, functional disability and depressed mood were domains limiting leisure activities in both nationalities. Patients reported avoiding the beach and swimming pool due to psoriasis and refusing long trips due to pain and stiffness caused by extended periods of immobility. Dancing, going to parties, playing musical instruments, cooking, visiting friends and family, going out to dinner, swimming, diving and travelling by bus were some examples of leisure activities impaired by functional disability. Besides avoiding some activities, patients referenced that some leisure activities had to be adapted, e.g. replacing a beach trip by a city trip, visiting only one place instead of multiple places in the same day, slowing down the pace of activities.

Discussion

This study brings new and important information on patient-perceived impact of PsA and for the first time addresses cross-cultural similarities and differences in this regard. This qualitative study confirmed the broad impact perceived by PsA patients both in Brazil and in France: 41 categories emerged from the interviews, covering physical, emotional, professional and social domains. There were both similarities and differences between perceptions in Brazil and in France: 2/3 of categories were common to both nationalities in spite of cultural and economic differences between the countries, as well as variances between the public health systems. However, some important health domains from the perspective of PsA patients from a non-European background were revealed including sexual dysfunction, emotional impact of psoriasis and impact of prejudice on social and professional life.

This study has strengths and weaknesses: the Brazilian sample of this study was recruited in the most southern state of Brazil, a region characterized by European colonization with a predominance of Caucasian inhabitants. Since Brazil is a large country with a multicultural population, we can hypothesize that the impact of PsA could be different if patients from other regions were interviewed. In France, the sample was ethnically representative but in both countries, the recruitment of Black and Asian patients was difficult because they are minorities among the population of patients attending the tertiary health centers which recruited participants to the study. Education levels were high, mainly in the sample from France, which is often the case in qualitative studies [29]. The characteristics of the sample may limit generalizability.

However, patient sampling did strive for a wide spread of patient characteristics. And rather than to obtain generalizability, this methodology intends to create new hypotheses that should be consequently tested in quantitative studies. The sample size was small but saturation was reached which strengthens our results. Content analyses were performed in an undirected way thus leading to both known aspects of impact, and some new aspects. Although this study is limited by the small sample size, rigorous data interpretation methods were applied and comparisons were performed with the literature. Thus, this qualitative study allowed a first exploration of patients' experiences of impact of PsA in South America, and we believe some important insights have been gained.

The present study found a wide diversity of health domains affected by PsA, thus confirming previous studies but including information on individuals from a different cultural background [30–32]. The impact of PsA is not only physical (the aspect most easily recognized by health professionals) but it is also psychological and social. Most domains perceived as important for the patients interviewed in our work were also highlighted in other studies and are covered by questionnaires assessing impact and quality of life in PsA [4, 7, 8, 32]. Fatigue, functional disability, social participation and emotional impact, for example, are assessed by the PsAID, the Psoriatic Arthritis Quality of Life (PsA-QoL) and the Nottingham Health Profile (NHP) [7, 11, 33]. Sleep disorders are also assessed by the PsAID and the NHP instruments [7, 32]. Thus this study confirms the global impact of PsA may be cross-culturally true and current questionnaires such as the PsAID may hold well as valid across cultures, but still need to be validated through quantitative studies.

Despite the substantial overlap of experiences of Brazilian and French PsA patients, there were important differences that legitimately require further research. Some aspects appeared more important for patients from Brazil than for patients from France. This includes sexual dysfunction, emotional impact of psoriasis (mainly embarrassment/shame due to skin lesions) and impact of prejudice on social and professional life.

A systematic review of articles reporting sexual dysfunction in PsA found that the severity of skin findings, the psychological effects of the condition, concerns of the sexual partner and side effects of medical treatments were associated with sexual disorders in PsA. This work emphasized that this type of symptomatology is frequently neglected in medical practice and also highlighted the lack of studies about the subject in Brazilian patients [34].

In the present work, the impact of prejudice due to skin lesions seemed more marked in Brazilians; categories such as, "discrimination at work", "discrimination in social life" and "embarrassment/shame" emerged only in the Brazilian sample. It is very probable, that in our work, the impact of prejudice due to skin disease was more intense in participants from Brazil because they had more severe psoriasis compared to subjects recruited in France. South of Brazil and Île-de-France, the two regions where patients were recruited, have similar climate, with four well defined seasons (contrasting with the North and Northeast regions of Brazil where high temperatures predominate throughout the year). The patients were recruited in both countries over a 2-year period, meaning that interviews were conducted in both countries during all seasons. It seems less probable that the climate, sun exposure or clothing could be the responsible for the difference in the perceived impact of psoriasis referred by patients in Brazil and France.

The hypothesis that the impact of prejudice is higher in Brazil due to the lower educational level of the population in this country or due to cultural differences among countries is unsupported: a recent study with 1005 healthy French subjects showed that more than 60% of them recognized a lack of information about psoriasis and 50% of respondents showed discriminatory behavior toward psoriasis patients reflected by reluctance to maintain friendship ties/a relationship of friendliness (7.6%), to have lunch or dinner with a person with visible manifestations (17.9%), to give a kiss on the cheek in greeting (29.7%), to shake hands (28.8%) and to have sexual relations/intercourse (44.1%) [35]. In that work, educational level was not associated with an increased prevalence of misconceptions and/or perceived discriminatory behaviors [35]. The impact of prejudice has also been previously recognized in another qualitative study which recruited European patients with PsA [36].

Conclusion

In conclusion, this study highlights the importance of assessing the impact of PsA on a national level, emphasizing the common cross-cultural impact of PsA but also exploring domains of interest for the Brazilian population which merit further studies.

Abbreviations

CASPAR: Classification Criteria for Psoriatic Arthritis; GRAPPA: Group for Research and Assessment of Psoriasis and Psoriatic Arthritis; HAQ: Health Assessment Questionnaire; ICF: International Classification of Functioning, Disability and Health; NHP: Nottingham Health Profile; PsA: Psoriatic arthritis; PsAID: Psoriatic Arthritis Impact of Disease Questionnaire; PsAQoL: Psoriatic Arthritis Quality of Life; RA: Rheumatoid arthritis; SLE: Systemic lupus erythematosus; SLR: Systematic literature review

Acknowledgements

We thanks Professor Odirlei André Monticielo from Universidade Federal do Rio Grande do Sul, Porto Alegre, Brazil and Professor Cláudia Diniz Lopes Marques from Universidade Federal de Pernambuco, Recife, Brazil for their suggestions to the manuscript.

Funding

The first author Penélope Palominos conducted the work with own resources. Professor Xavier received a research grant from National Council for Scientific and Technological Development (CNPq).

Authors' contributions

PEP, LG, WC, MdeW, NG, CLK, RMSC and RMX contributed to the conception and design of study. PEP, LG, SK, CLH, RMSC, ALDM, CLK contributed to acquisition of data. PEP, LG, RMX, WC, MdeW, NG, ALDM, CLH and SK contributed to analysis and interpretations of data. PEP and LG drafted the manuscript and all authors revised the manuscript critically for intellectual content. All authors read and approved the final manuscript.

Competing interests

Niti Goel is an employee of Quintiles IMS but declares no conflict of interest regarding this manuscript. The other authors have disclosed no conflict of interest.

Author details

[1]Serviço de Reumatologia, Hospital de Clínicas de Porto Alegre, Ramiro Barcelos Street 2350, Porto Alegre Zip code 90035903, Brazil. [2]Programa de Pós Graduação em Ciências Médicas, Universidade Federal do Rio Grande do Sul (UFRGS), Ramiro Barcelos 2400, Porto Alegre Zip code 90035903, Brazil. [3]Institut Pierre Louis d'Epidémiologie et de Santé Publique. Pitié-Salpetrière Hospital, AP-HP, Rheumatology Department, Sorbonne Universités, UPMC Univ Paris 6, GRC-08, 83 Boulevard de l'Hôpital, 75013 Paris, France. [4]Faculdade de Medicina, Departamento de Medicina Interna, Universidade Federal do Rio Grande do Sul (UFRGS), Ramiro Barcelos 2400, Porto Alegre Zip code 90035903, Brazil. [5]Patient Research Partner, Group for Research and Assessment of Psoriasis and Psoriatic Arthritis (GRAPPA), University Health Network, Toronto Western Hospital, 399 Street Toronto, Bathurst, ON M5T 2S8, Canada. [6]Department of Medical Humanities, Patient Research Partner, VU University Medical Centre, de Boelenlaan 1089a, 1081 HV Amsterdam, Netherlands. [7]Patient Research Partner; Advisory Services, Quintiles; Division of Rheumatology, Duke University School of Medicine, Durham, North Carolina 27705, USA.

References

1. Tezel N, Yilmaz Tasdelen O, Bodur H, Gul U, Kulcu Cakmak S, Oguz ID, et al. Is the health-related quality of life and functional status of patients with psoriatic arthritis worse than that of patients with psoriasis alone? Int J Rheum Dis. 2015;18:63–9.

2. Sokoll KB, Helliwell PS. Comparison of disability and quality of life in rheumatoid and psoriatic arthritis. J Rheumatol. 2001;28:1842–6.

3. Husted JA, Gladman DD, Farewell VT, Cook RJ. Health-related quality of life of patients with psoriatic arthritis: a comparison with patients with rheumatoid arthritis. Arthritis Rheum. 2001;45:151–8.

4. Kavanaugh A, Helliwell P, Ritchlin CT. Psoriatic arthritis and burden of disease: patient perspectives from the population-based multinational assessment of psoriasis and psoriatic arthritis (MAPP) survey. Rheumatol Ter. 2016;3:91–102.

5. Hagberg KW, Li L, Peng M, Shah K, Paris M, Jick S. Incidence rates of suicidal behaviors and treated depression in patients with and without psoriatic arthritis using the Clinical Practice Research Datalink. Mod Rheumatol. 2016;26:774–9.

6. Desthieux C, Granger B, Balanescu AR, Balint P, Braun J, Canete J, et al. Determinants of patient-physician discordance in global assessment in psoriatic arthritis: a multicenter European study. Arthritis Care Res (Hoboken). 2016. https://doi.org/10.1002/acr.23172 [Epub ahead of print].

7. Gossec L, de Wit M, Kiltz U, Braun J, Kalyoncu U, Scrivo R, et al. A patient-derived and patient-reported outcome measure for assessing psoriatic arthritis: elaboration and preliminary validation of the Psoriatic Arthritis Impact of Disease (PsAID) questionnaire, a 13-country EULAR initiative. Ann Rheum Dis. 2014;73:1012–9.

8. Stam TA, Nell V, Mathis M, Coenen M, Aletaha D, Cieza A. Concepts important to patients with psoriatic arthritis are not adequately covered by standard measures of functioning. Arthritis Care Res. 2007;57:487–94.

9. Gudu T, Kiltz U, de Wit M, Kvien TK, Gossec L. Mapping the Effect of Psoriatic Arthritis Using the International Classification of Functioning, Disability and Health. J Rheumatol. 2017;44:193–200.

10. Torre-Alonso JC, Gratacós J, Rey-Rey JS, Valdazo de Diego JP, Urriticoechea-Arana A, Daudén E, et al. Development and validation of a new instrument to measure health-related quality of life in patients with psoriatic arthritis: the VITACORA-19. J Rheumatol. 2014;41:2008–17.

11. Billing E, McKenna SP, Staun M, Lindqvist U. Adaptation of the Psoriatic Arthritis Quality of Life (PsAQoL) instrument for Sweden. Scand J Rheumatol. 2010;39:223–8.

12. McKenna SP, Doward LC, Whalley D, Tennant A, Emery P, Veale DJ. Development of the PsAQoL: a quality of life instrument specific to psoriatic arthritis. Ann Rheum Dis. 2004;63:162–9.

13. Wink F, Arends S, McKenna SP, Houtman PM, Brouwer E, Spoorenberg A. Validity and reliability of the Dutch adaptation of the psoriatic arthritis quality of life (PsAQoL) questionnaire. PLoS One. 2013;8:e55912.

14. Chisholm A, Pearce CJ, Chinoy H, Warren RB, Bundy C. Distress, misperceptions, poor coping and suicidal ideation in psoriatic arthritis: a qualitative study. Rheumatology (Oxford). 2016; [Epub ahead of print].

15. Stam T, Hieblinger R, Boström C, Mihai C, Birrell F, Thorstensson C, et al. Similar problem in the activities of daily living but different experience: a qualitative analysis in six rheumatic conditions and eight European countries. Musculoskelet Care. 2014;12:22–33.

16. Moverley AR, Vinall-Collier KA, Helliwell PS. It's not just the joints, it's the whole thing: qualitative analysis of patients's experience of flare in psoriatic arthritis. Rheumatology (Oxford). 2015;54:1448–53.

17. Kumar K, Gordon C, Barry R, Shaw K, Horne R, Raza K. 'It's like taking poison to kill poison but I have to get better': a qualitative study of beliefs about medicines in rheumatoid arthritis and systemic lupus erythematosus patients of south Asian origin. Lupus. 2011;20:837–44.

18. Sanderson T, Calnan M, Kumar K. The moral experience of illness and its impact on normalisation: examples from narratives with Punjabi women living with rheumatoid arthritis in the UK. Sociol Heal Illn. 2015;37(8):1218–35.

19. Kumar K, Gordon C, Toescu V, Buckley CD, Horne R, Nightingale PG, et al. Beliefs about medicines in patients with rheumatoid arthritis and systemic lupus erythematosus: a comparison between patients of South Asian and White British origin. Rheumatology (Oxford). 2008;47:690–7.

20. Wen H, Ralph Schumacher H, Li X, Gu J, Ma L, Wei H, et al. Comparison of expectations of physicians and patients with rheumatoid arthritis for rheumatology clinic visits: a pilot, multicenter, international study. Int J Rheum Dis. 2012;15:380–9.

21. Ribeiro SL, Albuquerque EN, Bortoluzzo AB, Gonçalves CR, da Silva JA, Ximenes AC, et al. Quality of life in spondyloarthritis: analysis of a large Brazilian cohort. Rev Bras Reumatol. 2016;56:22–7.

22. da Costa IP, Bortoluzzo AB, Gonçalves CR, da Silva JA, Ximenes AC, Bértolo MB, et al. Evaluation of performance of BASDAI (Bath ankylosing spondylitis disease activity index) in Brazilian cohort of 1,492 patients with spondyloarthritis: data from the Brazilian registry of Spondyloarthritides (RBE). Rev Bras Reumatol. 2015;55:48–54.

23. Nota I, Drossaert CH, Taal E, Vonkeman HE, van de Laar MA. Patient participation in decisions about disease modifying anti-rheumatic drugs: a cross-sectional survey. BMC Musculoskelet Disord. 2014;15:333.

24. Taylor W, Gladman D, Helliwell P, Marchesoni A, Mease P, Mielants H. Classification criteria for psoriatic arthritis: development of new criteria from a large international study. Arthritis Rheum. 2006;54:2665–73.

25. Depoy E, Gitlin LN. Introduction to research. St. Louis: Mosby; 1998.

26. Bruce B, Fries JF. The Stanford health assessment questionnaire (HAQ): a review of its history, issues, progress, and documentation. J Rheumatol. 2003;30:167–78.

27. Szentpetery A, Johnson MAN, Ritchlin CT. GRAPPA Trainees Symposium 2013: A Report from the GRAPPA 2013 Annual Meeting. J Rheumatol. 2014;41:1200–5.

28. Crabtree B, Miller W. Doing qualitative research. London: SAGE; 1999. p. 406.

29. Hewlett S, Nicklin J, Bode C, Carmona L, Dures E, Engelbrecht M, et al. Translating patient reported outcome measures: methodological issues explored using cognitive interviewing with three rheumatoid arthritis measures in six European languages. Rheumatology (Oxford). 2016;55:1009–16.

30. Kalyoncu U, Ogdie A, Campbell W, Bingham CO 3rd, de Wit M, Gladman DD, et al. Systematic literature review of domains assessed in psoriatic arthritis to inform the update of the psoriatic arthritis core domain set. RMD Open. 2016;2:e000217.

31. Palominos PE, Gaujoux-Viala C, Fautrel B, Dougados M, Gossec L. Clinical outcomes in psoriatic arthritis: A systematic literature review. Arthritis Care Res (Hoboken). 2012;64:397–406.

32. Orbai AM, de Wit M, Mease P, Shea JA, Gossec L, Leung YY, et al. International patient and physician consensus on a psoriatic arthritis core outcome set for clinical trials. Ann Rheum Dis. 2016. https://doi.org/10.1136/annrheumdis-2016-210242 [Epub ahead of print].

33. Hunt SM, McKenna SP, MEwen J, Backtt EM, Williams J, Papp E. A quantitative approach to perceived health status: a validation study. J Epidemiol Community Health. 1980;34:281–6.

34. Kurizky PS, Mota LM. Sexual dysfunction in patients with psoriasis and psoriatic arthritis - a systematic review. Rev Bras Reumatol. 2012;52:943–8.

35. Halioua B, Sid-Mohand D, Roussel ME, Maury-le-Breton A, de Fontaubert A, Stalder JF. Extent of misconceptions, negative prejudices and discriminatory behaviour to psoriasis patients in France. J Eur Acad Dermatol Venereol. 2016;30:650–4.

36. Uttjek M, Nygren L, Stenberg B, Dufåker M. Marked by visibility of psoriasis in everyday life. Qual Health Res. 2007;17:364–72.

24

Cardiac and vascular complications of Behçet disease in the Tunisian context: clinical characteristics and predictive factors

Melek Kechida[1*], Sana Salah[2], Rim Kahloun[3], Rim Klii[1], Sonia Hammami[1] and Ines Khochtali[1]

Abstract

Background: Cardiac and vascular involvement in Behçet disease (BD), also referred as vasculo BD, is frequent. We aimed to describe clinical characteristics, predictive factors and management of vasculo BD in the Tunisian context.

Methods: We retrospectively studied 213 records of all BD patients followed between January 2004 and May 2016 in the Internal Medicine Department and who fulfilled the ISGBD criteria. We described first clinical features of BD with cardiac and vascular involvement then predictive factors were studied in univariate then multivariate analysis.

Results: Among the 213 patients, 64 (30%) were diagnosed as having vasculo BD. The mean age at diagnosis was 31.5 years. About 81.25% of them were males and 18.75% females. Vascular involvement associated or not with cardiac involvement was found in 64 patients (30%). Deep venous thromboses are most common (62.5%) compared with superficial ones (23.4%), pulmonary arterial thrombosis (14.1%) or aneurysms (9.4%). Cardiac involvement is ranging from pericarditis (1.6%) to intra cardiac thrombosis (3.1%) and myocardial infarction (1.6%). Predictive factors associated with cardiac and vascular involvement in BD are male gender (OR = 3.043, 95% CI = 1.436–6.447, $p = 0.004$), erythema nodosum (OR = 4.134, 95% CI = 1.541–11.091, $p = 0.005$) and neurologic involvement (OR = 2.46, 95% CI = 1.02–5.89, $p = 0.043$).

Conclusion: Cardiac and vascular involvement in BD is frequent in the Tunisian context with a broad spectrum of manifestations ranging from vascular involvement to cardiac one. Male gender, patients with erythema nodosum or neurologic involvement are prone to develop cardiac or vascular features of BD needing therefore a close monitoring.

Keywords: Behcet syndrome, Cardiovascular system, Risk factors

Background

Behçet disease (BD) is a systemic vasculitis of unknown origin with a remitting and relapsing course. It is prevalent along the "silk road" extending from Japan to the Middle Eastern and the Mediterranean countries [1]. BD usually affects patients around the third or fourth decade of life [1]. Sex distribution is roughly equal with some particularities all over the world. In fact, BD would be more prevalent in males in some Middle Eastern and the Mediterranean countries and less frequent in females in Japan and Korea [1].

BD is mainly characterized by recurrent oral and genital aphthosis associated with other cutaneous and ocular manifestations. It may also involve, in a lesser extent, the gastro intestinal tract, joints and the central nervous system. These clinical signs seem to vary in prevalence according to the ethnic groups and geographical regions.

Cardiac and vascular involvement, also referred as vasculo BD, is frequent. It can reach 46% of patients according to the literature [2] affecting all sizes of arteries and veins as well as all the cardiac layers and accounting for the major cause of mortality.

As clinical signs are varying according to the ethnic groups and the geographical regions, and as data regarding prevalence and management of vasculo BD in the North African countries are lacking, we aimed in this

---

* Correspondence: kechida_mel_lek@hotmail.com
[1]Internal Medicine and Endocrinology Department, Fattouma Bourguiba University Hospital, 1st June Avenue, 5000 Monastir, Tunisia
Full list of author information is available at the end of the article

work to describe clinical characteristics, predictive factors and management of cardiac and vascular involvement in BD in the Tunisian context.

Methods

We retrospectively studied records of Behçet Disease patients followed in Internal Medicine Department of Fattouma Bourguiba University Hospital between January 2004 and May 2016. All patients fulfilled the International Study Group for Behçet Disease criteria [2].

Patients with cardiac involvement are defined as having pericarditis and/or myocarditis and/or intra cardiac thrombosis and/or myocardial infarction associated or not to vascular involvement. Patients with vascular involvement are those having deep venous thrombosis and/or superficial venous thrombosis and/or pulmonary embolism and/or arterial aneurysm without cardiac involvement.

Cardiac and vascular involvement diagnosis was based on clinical examination and imaging techniques including Computed Tomography Angiography, Magnetic Resonance Angiography and Doppler ultrasound. Screening for cardiac and vascular involvement was performed in symptomatic patients only.

We described first clinical features of BD with cardiac and vascular involvement then a comparative study was performed between patients with (group 1) and without cardiac and/or vascular involvement (group2). Predictive factors of cardiac and/or vascular involvement were studied in univariate then multivariate analysis.

The t test was used to analyze the continuous variables. The chi-square test was used to analyze the categorical variables. Multivariate analysis of variables significantly associated with cardiac and vascular involvement in univariate analysis was performed using binary logistic regression. Results are expressed as odds ratios (OR) with accompanying 95% confidence interval (95% CI). A p value < 0.05 was considered significant and if needed Fisher's exact test was used. Only relevant predictive factors highly associated with cardiac and vascular involvement were analyzed according to the goodness of fit of Hosmer-Lemeshow test. All data were assessed on computer using a SPSS 21.0 software package.

Results

Out of 213 BD patients studied, 145 (68.1%) were males and 68 (31.9%) were females. Sex ratio M/F was 2.13. Mean age at diagnosis was 30.6 years. Oral ulcers were found in 210 patients (98.6%) at presentation occurring then in all patients during follow-up. Cutaneous manifestations were present in 190 patients (89.2%). Pathergy test done in 174 patients was positive in 108 of cases (62.06%). Clinical characteristics of the patients are reported in Table 1. HLA 51 done in 113 patients (53.05%) was positive in 18 patients (15.92%).

Among the 213 patients, 64 (30%) were diagnosed as having vasculo BD. The mean age at diagnosis was 31.5 years. About 81.25% of them were males and 18.75% were females.

Vascular involvement was found in 59 patients (27.7%), isolated cardiac involvement in 2 patients (0.9%) and the association of cardiac and vascular involvement was found in 3 patients (1.4%).

Eight patients (12.5%) had cardiac or vascular involvement as a first manifestation of the disease. Deep venous thrombosis were reported in 40 patients (62.5%). Venous thrombosis occurred in more than one site in 3 cases (7.5%).

Superficial venous thrombosis affected 15 patients (23.4%). Arterial involvement was found in 16 patients (25.1%) with pulmonary embolism in 9 patients (14.1%), pulmonary aneurysm in 6 patients (9.4%) and aorta aneurysm in 1 case (1.6%). Cardiac involvement was found in 5 patients (7.9%).

Cardiac and vascular involvement is detailed in Table 2.

Management of cardiac or vascular involvement in BD consisted in colchicine in all patients, corticotherapy in 22 patients (46%) and immunosuppressors in 17 patients (26.6%) which were Cyclophasphamide or Azathioprine. Oral anticoagulation was associated in 44 patients (72.1%). Arterial Embolisation was performed in 2 patients (3.3%).

Table 1 clinical features of patients with Beçet Disease syndrome

Clinical features	Results
Sex	
- Male (n) (%)	145 (68.1)
- Female (n) (%)	68 (31.9)
Age at diagnosis (years)	30.6
Family history of BD (n) (%)	27 (13.8)
Oral ulcers (n) (%)	210 (98.6)
Genital ulceration (n) (%)	178 (83.6)
Pseudofolliculitis (n) (%)	169 (79.3)
Erythema nodosum (n) (%)	21 (9.99)
Positive pathergy reaction (n) (%)	108(62.06)
Joint involvement (n) (%)	94(44.3)
Ophthalmic involvement (n) (%)	67 (31.6)
Neurological manifestations (n) (%)	26 (12.3)
Cardiovascular complications (n) (%)	64 (30)
Gastrointestinal involvement (n) (%)	1(0.5)
Orchitis (n) (%)	12 (5.6)

Table 2 cardiovascular features in Behçet Disease patients

Cardiovascular features	Patients (n)(%)
Vascular involvement (n) (%)	73 (34.27)
Deep venous thrombosis (n) (%)	40 (62.5)
- Upper limb (n) (%)	8(12.5)
- Lower limb (n) (%)	16(25)
- Bilateral lower limb (n) (%)	3 (4.7)
- Inferior vena cava (n) (%)	8(12.5)
- More than one site (n) (%)	3(4.7)
- Budd Chiari syndrome (n) (%)	1(1.55)
- Mesenteric vein (n) (%)	1(1.55)
Superficial venous thrombosis (n) (%)	15 (23.4)
Pulmonary embolism (n) (%)	9 (14.1)
Pulmonary arterial aneurysm (n) (%)	6 (9.4)
Ascending aorta aneurysm (n) (%)	1 (1.6)
Cardiac involvement (n) (%)	5 (2.4)
- Pericarditis (n) (%)	1 (1.6)
-Myocarditis (n) (%)	1 (1.6)
- Intra cardiac thrombosis (n) (%)	2 (3.1)
- Myocardial infarction (n) (%)	1 (1.6)

Table 3 Comparison of clinical features in Behçet Disease patients with and without vascular involvement

	Patients with cardiovascular involvement (group1) ($n = 64$)	Patients without cardiovascular involvement (group 2) ($n = 149$)	P value
Sex			
- Males (n) (%)	52(81.3)	93(62.4)	**0.007***
- Females (n) (%)	12(18.8)	56(37.6)	
Age (years)	31.5	30.21	0.43
Familiar history of BD (n) (%)	5 (8.9)	22(15.8)	0.2
Oral aphthosis (n) (%)	63(98.4)	147(98.7)	0.9
Genital ulcerations (n) (%)	53(82.8)	125(83.9)	0.84
Pseudofolliculitis (n) (%)	54(84.4)	115(77.2)	0.23
Erythema nodosum (n) (%)	11(17.2)	10(6.7)	**0.019***
Ophthalmic involvement (n) (%)	20(31.3)	47(31.5)	0.96
Neurological involvement (n) (%)	12(18.8)	14(9.4)	0.056
Orchitis (n) (%)	7(10.9)	5(3.4)	**0.047*** (exact Fisher test)

*$p < 0.05$

Comparative study between patients with (group 1) and without cardiac or vascular involvement (group 2) revealed significant prevalence of males in group 1 (81.3% vs 62.4%) ($p = 0.007$), and increased frequency of patients with erythema nodosum (17.2% vs 6.7%) ($p = 0.019$) and with orchitis (10.9% vs 3.4%) ($p = 0.047$) (Exact Fisher test) (Table 3).

Multivariable analysis performed on this model showed that predictive factors for cardiac or vascular involvement were male gender (OR = 3.043, 95% CI = 1.436–6.447, $p = 0.004$), erythema nodosum (OR = 4.134, 95% CI = 1.541–11.091, $p = 0.005$) and neurologic involvement (OR = 2.46, 95% CI = 1.02–5.89, $p = 0.043$) (Table 4).

Discussion

Cardiac and vascular involvement in BD is rarely reported in African countries. To the best of our knowledge, this study is the first to focus on cardiac and vascular spectrum in BD patients in a Tunisian cohort.

Cardiac and vascular involvement is frequent in our cohort, diagnosed in 30% of our patients. It is estimated to range from 7 to 46%, [3] according to the published data, and to affect about 27% in the Tunisian multicenter study of 519 patients [4]. Predictive factors of cardiac and vascular involvement found in our cohort were male gender (OR = 3.043, 95% CI = 1.436–6.447, $p = 0.004$), erythema nodosum (OR = 4.134, 95% CI = 1.541–11.091, $p = 0.005$) and neurologic involvement (OR = 2.46, 95%

CI = 1.02–5.89, $p = 0.043$). All studies dealing with cardiac or vascular involvement in BD are unanimous on the fact that the frequency of these complications is higher in males [4–7]. Some authors found that eye involvement, genital ulcers and arthritis were less frequent in vasculo-BD patients [8], which was not the case in our study.

Cardiac or vascular complications revealed the disease in 12.5% of cases in our patients. In the study of Fei et al. [6], 27.5% of patients presented with vascular involvement as the initial manifestation.

There is a broad spectrum of cardiac and vascular involvement in BD patients and we found that vascular manifestations are more frequent than cardiac ones.

Table 4 Predictive factors independently associated with cardiovascular involvement in patients with BD in multivariate analysis

Variable	Odds ratio	95% CI	p value
Male gender	3.043	1.436–6.447	0.004*
Erythema nodosum	4.134	1.541–11.091	0.005*
Neurological involvement	2.462	1.028–5.893	0.043*

CI confidence interval; *$p < 0.05$

Cardiac involvement is accounting for 1 to 6% [5] and occurred in 2.4% of patients in our study. The main types of cardiac features are pericarditis, valvular insufficiency, intra cardiac thrombosis and myocardial infarction. Pericardial involvement has been reported as the most common manifestation in some series [3, 9]. Clinical presentation may be acute pericarditis, recurrent pericarditis, constrictive pericarditis, hemorrhagic pericarditis tamponade or even asymptomatic pericardial effusion [3, 5]. But unlike literature findings, pericarditis was not the first most frequent cardiac feature in our cohort (1.6%), it was intra cardiac thrombosis (3.1% of cases). This probably could be explained by the asymptomatic character of pericarditis which can be missed as echocardiography was not systematically done for all the patients. Intra cardiac thrombosis is generally considered one of the serious cardiac complications which may cause pulmonary embolism [3] like in one of our patients or cerebral emboli by passing through the patent foramen ovale. The right ventricle is usually involved, which was the case of all our patients [3]. But it has been demonstrated that the left ventricle can also be involved [10, 11].

Myocardial infarction diagnosed in one of our patients was caused by coronary aneurysm. Coronary lesions are usually proximal [5] and some of them may be asymptomatic [3]. Sinus Valsalva aneurysms may occur alone or with other sinus aneurysms and may lead to acute or chronic aortic failure [3].

We reported a rare case of myocarditis revealing BD which was diagnosed in a patient with fever and chest pain confirmed with MRI findings. Few data is found in this field, Geri et al. [5] reported only one case in a series of 52 European patients and two cases were reported in a Japanese autopsy series [12].

Vascular system involvement emerged in approximately 1.8 to 51.6% of BD patients affecting all sizes of arteries and veins and accounting for the major cause of mortality [6]. It was estimated at 34.27% in our study.

Vascular lesions mainly consist in venous and arterial thrombosis and various types of arterial aneurysms. Venous lesions were more common in our cohort reaching 85.9% in agreement of literature findings which demonstrated that venous lesions were more frequently affected than arterial lesions [6]. Venous involvement can affect lower extremities as well as upper limb. Others including inferior vena cava, Budd-Chiari syndrome (hepatic vein thrombosis) and mesenteric vein thrombosis are rarely seen [13].

Arterial involvement is less common than venous one [3]. It consists in thrombosis or aneurysms. Pulmonary embolism, although found in 14.1% in our study, is thought to be rare in the literature given that the thrombi in the inflamed veins of the lower extremities are strongly adherent. [6, 14]. Aneurysms are considered to be the most severe complications given the high risk of rupture [6]. They mainly affect pulmonary arteries (9.4% in our cohort) but can be located in systemic circulation. We described the first case of ascending aortic aneurysm associated with deep vein thrombosis revealing BD. Few articles reported cases of Hughes Stovin Syndrome revealing BD. It's a rare entity defined as thrombophlebitis associated with pulmonary aneurysms [15]. Few cases were reported with associated aneurysm of the systemic circulation such bronchial, external carotid, iliac artery aneurysm and left hepatic artery [16] but no association with ascending aorta aneurysm was reported.

Treatment of BD is still based on a low level of evidence [3, 17]. All of our patients were treated with colchicine associated to steroids and immunosuppressors in 46 and 26.6% of cases, respectively. Corticosteroids and immunosuppressive agents like Cyclophasphamide are usually used for the management of cardiac lesions or if there is evidence of severe vascular manifestations. Thrombotic complications too may require immunosuppressors given that vascular inflammation plays a major role in thrombus formation. However treatment of arterial aneurysms remains challenging. Anticoagulant treatment should be administered cautiously with a close control in association to steroids and immunosuppressors given the risk of bleeding.

Surgical treatment may be problematic leading to pseudo aneurysms. Therefore surgical treatment should not be applied in the active phase of the disease [6].

The major limitation of our work is that it is a retrospective study especially faced to the incompleteness in data collection. It would be interesting to prospectively monitor how BD patients with predictive risk factors will evolve and how many will develop cardiac or vascular features.

Conclusion

Cardiac and vascular involvement in BD is frequent in the Tunisian context having sometimes threatening complications. It can occur during follow up or reveal the disease as the initial manifestation. Vascular manifestations are the most frequent affecting both veins and arteries. Deep venous thromboses are most common. Cardiac involvement can affect all layers ranging from pericarditis to intra cardiac thrombosis and myocardial infarction. We found that male gender is more prone to developing such complications in addition to patients presenting with erythema nodosum or neurologic involvement, needing therefore close monitoring.

Management of cardiac and vascular involvement in Behçet disease is still lacking standardization as treatment is still based on a low level of evidence. Cardiologists should always be aware of such disease as they could be the first physicians to deal with the cardiac and vascular complications.

Authors' contributions
MK: wrote the manuscript and done the bibliography research. SS: corrected the statistics. R. Kahloun: corrected the language and the final form of the manuscript. R. Klii, SH, and IK: participates with data. All authors read and approved the final manuscript.

Competing interests
The authors declare that they have no competing interests.

Author details
[1]Internal Medicine and Endocrinology Department, Fattouma Bourguiba University Hospital, 1st June Avenue, 5000 Monastir, Tunisia. [2]Physical Medicine and Rehabilitaion Department, Fattouma Bourguiba University Hospital, Monastir, Tunisia. [3]Ophtalmology Department, Fattouma Bourguiba University Hospital, Monastir, Tunisia.

References
1. Alpsoy E. Behcet's disease: a comprehensive review with a focus on epidemiology, etiology and clinical features, and management of mucocutaneous lesions. J Dermatol. 2016;43:620–32.
2. International Study Group for Behçet's disease. Criteria for diagnosis of Behçet's disease. Lancet. 1990;335:1078–80.
3. Demirelli S, Degirmenci H, Inci S, Arisoy A. Cardiac manifestations in Behçet's disease. Intractable Rare Dis Res. 2015;4(2):70–75.
4. B'chir Hamzaoui S, Harmel A, Bouslama K, Abdallah M, Ennafaa M, M'rad S, le groupe tunisien d'étude Sur la maladie de Behçet, et al. Behçet's disease in Tunisia. Clinical study of 519 cases. La Revue de médecine interne. 2006; 27:742–50.
5. Geri G, Wechsler B, Thi Huong du L, Isnard R, Piette JC, Amoura Z, et al. Spectrum of cardiac lesions in Behçet disease. A series of 52 patients and review of the literature. Medicine. 2012;91:25–34.
6. Fei Y, Li X, Lin S, Song X, Wu Q, Zhu Y, et al. Major vascular involvement in Behçet's disease: a retrospective study of 796 patients. Clin Rheumatol. 2013;32:845–52.
7. Bang D, Lee JH, Lee ES, Lee S, Choi JS, Kim YK, et al. Epidemiologic and clinical survey of Behcet's disease in Korea: the first multicenter study. J Korean Med Sci. 2001;16(5):615–8.
8. Sakane T, Takeno M, Suzuki N, Inaba G. Behçet's disease. Engl J Med. 1999; 341(17):1284–91.
9. Bono W, Filali-Ansary N, Mohattane A, Tazi-Mezalek Z, Adnaoui M, Aouni M, et al. Cardiac and pulmonary artery manifestations during Behcet's disease. Rev Med Interne. 2000;21:905–7.
10. Fekih M, Fennira S, Ghodbane L, Zaouali RM. Intracardiac thrombosis: unusual complication of Behcet's disease. Tunis Med. 2004;82:785–90.
11. Darie C, Knezinsky M, Demolombe-Rague S, Pinède L, Périnetti M, Ninet JF, et al. Cardiac pseudotumor revealing Behcet's disease. Rev Med Interne. 2005;26:420–4.
12. Lakhanpal S, Tani K, Lie JT, Katoh K, Ishigatsubo Y, Ohokubo T. Pathologic features of Behcet's syndrome: a review of Japanese autopsy registry data. Hum Pathol. 1985;16:790–5.
13. Ma WG, Zheng J, Zhu JM, Liu YM, Li M, Sun LZ. Aortic regurgitation caused by Behcet's disease: surgical experience during an 11-year period. J Card Surg. 2012;27:39–44.
14. Tohmé A, Aoun N, El-Rassi B, Ghayad E. Vascular manifestations of Behcet's disease. Eighteen cases among 140 patients. Joint Bone Spine. 2003;70:384–9.
15. Jambeih R, Salem G, Huard DR, Jones KR, Awab A. Hughes Stovin syndrome presenting with hematuria. Am J Med Sci. 2015;(5):425–6.
16. Balci NC, Semelka RC, Noone TC, Worawattanakul S. Multiple pulmonary aneurysms secondary to Hughes-Stovin syndrome: demonstration by MR angiography. J Magn Reson Imaging. 1998;(6):1323–5.
17. Hatemi G, Silman A, Bang D, Bodaghi B, Chamberlain AM, Gul A, et al. EULAR recommendations for the management of Behcet disease. Ann Rheum Dis. 2008;67:1656–62.

25

Comparison between treatment naive juvenile and adult dermatomyositis muscle biopsies: difference of inflammatory cells phenotyping

Samuel Katsuyuki Shinjo[1*], Adriana Maluf Elias Sallum[2], Sueli Mieko Oba-Shinjo[3], Marilda Guimarães Silva[1], Clovis Artur Silva[2] and Suely Kazue Nagahashi Marie[3]

Abstract

Background: Different inflammatory cells (i.e., CD4, CD8, CD20 and CD68) are involved in pathogenesis of DM muscle. In this context, the aim of this study was to assess and compare these inflammatory cell phenotyping in muscle samples of treatment naive juvenile and adult patients with dermatomyositis.

Methods: This is a cross-sectional study, in which 28 untreated juvenile and 28 adult untreated dermatomyositis patients were included. Immunohistochemical analysis was performed on serial frozen muscle sections. Inflammatory cell phenotyping was analyzed quantitatively in endomysium, perimysium, and perivascular (endomysium and perimysium) area.

Results: Mean age at disease onset was 7.3 and 42.0 years in juvenile and adult dermatomyositis, respectively. Both groups had comparable time duration from symptom's onset to biopsy performance. CD4 and CD8 positive cells distributions were similar in both groups in all analyzed area, except for more predominance of CD4 in perimysium at juvenile muscle biopsies. The CD20 and CD68 positive cells were predominantly observed in adult muscle biopsy sections, when compared to juvenile samples, except for similar distribution of CD20 in perivascular endomysium, and CD68 in perimysium.

Conclusions: These data show that the differences between juvenile and adult dermatomyositis may be restricted not only to patients' age, but also to different inflammatory cell distribution, particularly, in new-onset disease. Further studies are necessary to confirm the present study data and to analyze meaning of the different inflammatory cell phenotyping distribution finding in these both diseases.

Keywords: Dermatomyositis, Immunohistochemistry, Juvenile dermatomyositis, Myositis, Muscle biopsy

Introduction

Dermatomyositis (DM) is a rare systemic autoimmune myositis with characteristic cutaneous manifestations, such as heliotrope rash and Gottron's papules [1–7]. The annual incidence of DM is 5–10 cases per million, with the adult DM primarily affecting patients between 45 and 55 years old, whereas the juvenile DM affects individuals between 5 and 10 years of age [3, 4].

Muscle biopsy is one of the important diagnostic procedures in DM. The classical findings of muscle biopsies for DM evident are presence of mononuclear, inflammatory cell exudate arranged in a perivascular and perifascicular distribution with degenerating and regenerating muscle fibers and perifascicular atrophy [3–8]. Furthermore, the major histocompatibility complex expression and inflammatory cell phenotyping have been extensively described in both juvenile and adult DM muscle biopsies [3–9]. Until recently, these two parameters have not been simultaneously assessed and compared in both juvenile and adult DM. In that point, a recent study has

* Correspondence: samuel.shinjo@gmail.com
[1]Disciplina de Reumatologia, Faculdade de Medicina FMUSP, Universidade de Sao Paulo, Sao Paulo, Brazil
Full list of author information is available at the end of the article

shown at the first time that there is different major histocompatibility complex expression in simultaneously analysed juvenile and adult myositis [9]. However, the inflammatory cell phenotyping had not yet been studied.

Therefore, the aim of the present study was to compare the inflammatory cell phenotyping in the naive juvenile and adult DM muscle samples.

Subject and methods

Twenty-eight juvenile and 28 adult DM consecutive patients fulfilling Bohan and Peter's criteria [1, 2] were included in this cross-sectional study. The study was approved by the local Research Ethics Committee (Number 0335/11).

The patients were followed between 1990 and 2010 in the Pediatric Rheumatology Unit and the Inflammatory Myopathies Unit of our tertiary center.

All demographic, clinical, laboratory parameters were based on the previous study [9]. Demographics and clinical manifestations at disease onset (cutaneous involvement: heliotrope rash and Gottron's papules; articular involvement: arthralgia and/or arthritis; pulmonary involvement: pulmonary alterations in computer tomography and with symptoms like dyspnea; muscular strength of the limbs (degree 0: absence of muscle contraction, degree I: signs of mild contractility, degree II: normal amplitude movements but that do not overcome the action of gravity, degree III: normal amplitude movements against the action of gravity; degree IV: integral mobility against the action of gravity and some degree of resistance, degree V: complete mobility against severe resistance and against the action of gravity) [10]; and laboratory data were obtained through a systematic review of patients records.

The laboratory data corresponds to information collected at disease onset. Creatine phosphokinase (normal range: 24–173 U/L) and aldolase (normal range: 1.0–7.5 U/L) were determined by the automated kinetic method.

Sequential frozen 5 μm-thickness sections were stained for haematoxylin-eosine (HE), and then by immunohistochemistry. Monoclonal antibodies (CD4 and CD8: EnVision-AP technique, CD20 and CD68: LSB+ system) were used in immunohistochemical analysis. Frozen sections were fixed for 10 min in acetone at 4 °C. Endogenous peroxidase was blocked with H_2O_2 1% in absolute methanol three times for 10 min. After a rinse in phosphate-buffered-saline (PBS 0.01 M, pH 7.4) for 5 min, the specimens were incubated in fetal serum in a wet chamber for 1 h at 37 °C. Primary antibodies diluted in PBS and bovine serum albumin 1% were applied in a wet chamber at 37 °C, overnight. Slides were then washed in PBS, the prepared secondary mouse biotinylated (StreptABComplex/HRP) was applied for 30 min at 37 °C, and rinsed in PBS. Subsequently, the prepared

StreptABComplex/HRP complex was applied and incubated for 30 min at 37 °C. After rinsing in PBS, reactions were visualized after incubation with a chromogenic substrate (3.3′-diaminobenzidine tetrahydrochloride) solution for peroxidase. After a final rinse, haematoxylin counterstaining was performed. Slides were mounted and cover-slipped with an aqueous based mounting medium. The preparations of all muscle specimens were done at the same time as a batch. Human tonsil was used as a positive control. Inflammatory cell phenotyping (CD4, CD8, CD20, CD68) was analyzed quantitatively in endomysium, perimysium, pericapillar (endomysium and perimysium) areas in 10 distinct fields (200x magnification). Each muscle biopsy specimen was coded and analyzed by two independent investigators (SKS and AMES), blinded to diagnosis and clinical status. When any discrepancy was noted, the case was reviewed concomitantly.

Statistical analysis. The Kolmogorov-Smirnov test was used to evaluate the distribution of each parameter. The data were expressed as mean ± standard deviation or median (25th - 75th interquartile range). Comparisons between juvenile and adult DM patient parameters were made using Student's t-test or the Mann-Whitney test. All of the analyses were performed using the SPSS 15.0 statistics software (Chicago, Illinois, EUA). $P < 0.05$ was considered to indicate statistical significance.

Results

The demographic, clinical, laboratory parameters of adult and juvenile DM are shown in the Table 1. Mean age at onset of disease was 7.3 ± 3.4 and 42.0 ± 15.9 years-old in juvenile and adult DM, respectively, whereas median disease time within muscle biopsy was similar in both groups: 4.0 (2.0–16.5) vs. 7.0 (3.3–12.0) months, $P = 0.274$. There was no difference between both groups in relation to clinical and laboratory data, except for higher hampered muscle strength (upper limbs) in juvenile DM group.

Concerning immunohistochemical analysis, CD4 and CD8 positive inflammatory cells distributions in muscle biopsies were comparable between juvenile and adult DM, except for a higher number of CD4 positive cells in perimysium area in juvenile DM, when compared to adult DM (Fig. 1). Cells expressing CD20 were predominantly present in adult DM muscle biopsies (endomysium, perimysium, pericapillar perimysium) in relation to juvenile DM, whereas the distribution of CD20 positive cells was similar in pericapillar endomysium in both groups. Additionally, inflammatory cells which express CD68 were also predominant in adult DM muscle biopsies (endomysium, pericapillar endomysium and perimysium), except in perimysium, where CD68 positive cells distribution was similar in both groups.

Table 1 Demographic, clinical and laboratory features of adult and juvenile dermatomyositis

Features	Adult DM (N = 28)	Juvenile DM (N = 28)	P value
Age at disease onset (years)	42.0 ± 15.9	7.3 ± 3.4	
Disease duration (months)	7.0 [3.3–12.0]	4.0 [2.0–16.5]	0.274
Gender: female	24 (85.7)	20 (71.4)	0.329
Cutaneous involvement			
Heliotrope rash	26 (92.9)	21 (75.0)	0.243
Gottron's papules	28 (100.0)	22 (78.6)	0.481
Muscle strength			
Upper limbs (Degree: 0-V)	IV [IV-IV]	III [III-IV]	< 0.001
Lower limbs (Degree: 0-V)	III [III-IV]	III [III-IV]	0.652
Articular involvement	11 (39.3)	8 (28.6)	0.577
Pulmonary involvement	7 (25.0)	3 (10.7)	0.295
Laboratory alterations			
Creatine phosphokinase (U/L)	640 [144–8069]	556 [155–1659]	0.407
Aldolase (U/L)	14 [8–60]	16 [14–24]	0.783

Data expressed as mean ± standard deviation, median [interquartile 25th - 75th] or percentage (%)
DM dermatomyositis

Moreover, all inflammatory cells distributions (CD4, CD8, CD20 and CD68) did not correlate to any demographics, to clinical data and to laboratory features (P > 0.05).

Discussion

Similarly to major histocompatibility complex expression in juvenile and adult DM [9], the present study showed that there is different inflammatory cell phenotyping distribution in juvenile and adult DM muscle biopsy samples.

DM is an autoimmune systemic myopathy characterized by the presence of cellular infiltrates in muscle biopsies, autoantibodies in the peripheral blood and association with major histocompatibility complex overexpression [3, 5, 11, 12]. In this context, the presence and activation of CD4+ and CD8+ T cells as well as B cells in muscle tissues promote the humoral mediated pathogenesis in DM [11, 12]. However, corroborating with literature data, there were few inflammatory cell infiltrations in muscle biopsies, because an early histological and primarily feature in DM is a complement-mediated microangiopathy leading to capillary drop-out, necrosis of muscle fibers [11], even in the absence of inflammation [6, 13].

In the present study, even with few inflammatory cell infiltrations in muscle biopsies, a different inflammatory cell phenotype aspect was observed. There was a higher CD4+ T-cell distribution on perimysium area in juvenile DM biopsy, in contrast to a more evident CD20+ and CD68+ cells in muscle tissue areas of adult DM.

The predominance of CD4+ T lymphocyte infiltrations had also observed in juvenile DM muscle biopsies [14]. These cells are important to active CD20+ and autoantibody production in DM. On the other hand, CD20+ and CD68+ cells were more predominant in adult DM muscle biopsies. The relevance of CD20+ in DM is supported by the favorable clinical response to rituximab, a B cell blocking immunobiologic [15–17].

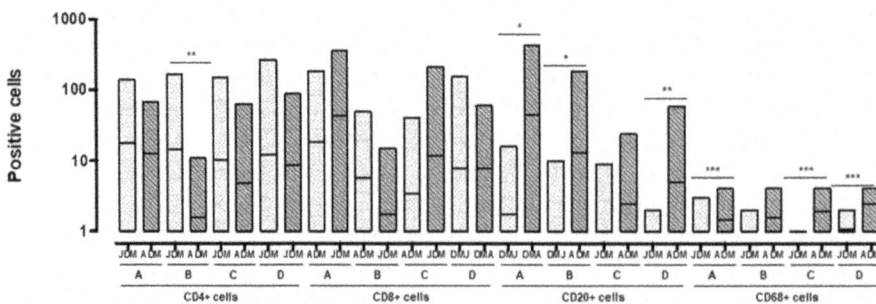

Fig. 1 Absolute number of inflammatory cell infiltrations in 10 different areas of muscle biopsies from untreated adult and juvenile dermatomyositis patients at 200x magnification. Bars represent the lower and higher values and the mean of the group. ADM: adult dermatomyositis; JDM: juvenile dermatomyositis; muscle areas: **a**, endomysium; **b**, perimysium; **c**, pericapillar endomysium; **d**, pericapillar perimysium *P < 0.05; **P = 0.001; ***P < 0.001

Additionally, in a recent report, it was demonstrated that Th2 T cells are increased in juvenile DM compared to adult DM muscle, indicating different immune cells regulation [18]. CD4 T-cells, and also B lymphocytes and macrophage cells may also play a major role [19, 20] in a immunological-mediated mechanism underlying an important pathologic aspect of this disease.

Overall, all these different immunohistochemical aspects can partially explain why patients with DM show different disease prognosis, clinical manifestations and/ or response to conventional treatment.

Further multicentric and international studies will be necessary to confirm the present study data and to analyse the meaning of the different inflammatory cell phenotyping distribution finding in both diseases.

Conclusions

Our data show that the differences between juvenile and adult DM could be restricted not only to age of onset, but also possibly to histological muscle biopsies with different inflammatory cell distribution, particularly, in new-onset disease.

Abbreviations
DM: Dermatomyositis; HE: Haematoxylin-eosine; PBS: Phosphate-buffered-saline

Acknowledgments
Not applicable.

Funding
Federico Foundation, Fundação Faculdade de Medicina, Fundação de Amparo à Pesquisa do Estado de São Paulo (FAPESP) #2014/09079–1 to SKS.

Authors' contributions
All authors contributed to write and review the manuscript.

Competing interests
The authors declare that they have no competing interests.

Author details
[1]Disciplina de Reumatologia, Faculdade de Medicina FMUSP, Universidade de Sao Paulo, Sao Paulo, Brazil. [2]Instituto da Criança, Hospital das Clinicas HCMFUSP, Faculdade de Medicina, Universidade de Sao Paulo, Sao Paulo, Brazil. [3]Laboratório de Biologia Molecular e Celular, Faculdade de Medicina, Universidade de Sao Paulo, Sao Paulo, Brazil.

References
1. Bohan A, Peter JB. Polymyositis and dermatomyositis (first of two parts). N Engl J Med. 1975;292:344–7.
2. Bohan A, Peter JB. Polymyositis and dermatomyositis (second of two parts). N Engl J Med. 1975;292:403–7.
3. Dalakas MC. Inflammatory muscle diseases. N Engl J Med. 2015;373:393–4.
4. Drake LA, Dinehart SM, Farmer ER, Goltz RW, Graham GF, Hordinsky MK, et al. Guidelines of care for dermatomyositis. American Academy of Dermatology. J Am Acad Dermatol. 1996;34:824–9.
5. Dalakas MC, Sivakumar K. The immunopathologic and inflammatory differences between dermatomyositis, polymyositis and sporadic inclusion body myositis. Curr Opin Neurol. 1996;9:235–9.
6. Emslie-Smith AM, Engel AG. Microvascular changes in early and advanced dermatomyositis: a quantitative study. Ann Neurol. 1990;27:343–56.
7. Engel AG, Arahata K. Mononuclear cells in myopathies: quantitation of functionally distinct subsets, recognition of antigen-specific cell-mediated cytotoxicity in some diseases, and implications for the pathogenesis of the different inflammatory myopathies. Hum Pathol. 1986;17:704–21.
8. Lorenzoni PJ, Scola RH, Kay CS, Prevedello PG, Espindola G, Weneck LC. Idiopathic inflammatory myopathies in childhood: a brief review of 27 cases. Pediatr Neurol. 2011;45:17–22.
9. Shinjo SK, Sallum AME, Silva CA, Marie SKN. Skeletal muscle major histocompatibility complex class I and II expression differences in adult and juvenile dermatomyositis. Clinics. 2012;67:885–90.
10. Medical Research Council. Aids to the examination of the peripheral nervous system. War memorandum (revised 2nd edition). London: HMSO, 1943.
11. Dalakas MC. An update on inflammatory and autoimnmune myopathies. Neuropathol Appl Neurobiol. 2011;37:226–42.
12. Haq SA, Tournadre A. Idiopathic inflammatory myopathies: from immunopathogenesis to new therapeutic targets. Int J Rheum Dis. 2015;18:818–25.
13. Engel AG, Hohlfeld R, Banker BQ. The polymyositis and dermatomyositis syndrome. In: Engel AG, Franzini-Armstrong C, editors. Myology. New York: McGraw-Hill; 2006. p. 1135.83.
14. Papa V, Romanin B, Bergamaschi R, Cordelli DM, Costa R, De Giorgi LB, et al. Juvenile dermatomyositis: a report of three cases. Ultrastruct Pathol. 2016; 40:83–5.
15. Krystufkova O, Vallerskog T, Helmers SB, Mann H, Putová I, Belácek J, et al. Increased serum levels of B cell activating factor (BAFF) in subsets of patients with idiopathic inflammatory myopathies. Ann Rheum Dis. 2009;68(6):836–43.
16. Oddis CV, Reed AM, Aggarwa R, Rider LG, Ascherman DP, Levesque MC, et al. Rituximabe in the treatment of refractory adult and juvenile dermatomyositis an adult polymyositis: a randomized, placebo-phase trial. Arthritis Rheum. 2013;65:314–24.
17. Couderc M, Gottenberg JE, Mariette X, Hachulla E, Sibilia J, Fain O, et al. Efficacy and safety of rituximab in the treatment of refractory inflammatory myopathies in adults: results from the AIR registry. Rheumatology. 2011;50:2283–9.
18. López De Padilla CM, Crowson CS, Hein MS, Pendegraft RS, Strausbauch MA, Niewold TB, et al. Gene expression profiling in blood and affected muscle tissues reveals differential activation pathways in patients with new-onset juvenile and adult dermatomyositis. J Rheumatol. 2017;44:117–24.
19. Arahata K, Engel AG. Monoclonal antibody analysis of mononuclear cells in myopathies: I: quantitation of subsets according to diagnosis and sites of accumulation and demonstration and counts of muscle fibers invaded by T cells. Ann Neurol. 1984;16:193–208.
20. Engel AK. Monoclonal antibody analysis of mononuclear cells in myopathies. III: Immunoelectron microscopy aspects of cell-mediated muscle fiber injury. Ann Neurol. 1986;19:119–25.

26

Quadriceps muscle weakness influences the gait pattern in women with knee osteoarthritis

Deborah Hebling Spinoso[1,5*], Natane Ceccatto Bellei[2], Nise Ribeiro Marques[3] and Marcelo Tavella Navega[4]

Abstract

Background: Osteoarthritis is the most prevalent rheumatic disease in the population and is characterized by limitation of main functional activities of daily living, as the gait. Muscle strength is a variable that may be related to performance in daily tasks.Therefore, we to analyze the gait pattern in individuals with knee osteoarthritis (KOA) and to determine associations of gait variables with the level of muscle strength of knee extensors.

Methods: Sixty-seven female volunteers divided into 2 groups, a KOA group (KOAG, $n = 36$, 66.69 ± 7.69 years) and control ($n = 31$, 63.68 ± 6.97 years), participated in the study. The volunteers walked on a 10-m platform at their usual gait speed, using 2 pressure sensors positioned at the base of the hallux and calcaneus. The mean step time, support and double support times, swing time and gait speed were calculated. The evaluation of the quadriceps isometric torque was performed in an extensor chair, with hip and knee flexion at 90°. The procedure consisted of three maximal contractions of knee extension. Peak torque was determined by the highest torque value obtained after the onset of muscle contraction. For statistical analysis, one-way ANOVA and Pearson's correlation were used, with $p < 0.05$.

Results: The KOAG had a 54.76% longer support time, a 13% longer step time ($p < 0.001$), a 30% decrease in swing time ($p < 0.001$) and a 10.7% decrease in gait speed ($p = 0.001$) compared with controls. The quadriceps isometric torque was 34% ($p = 0.001$) lower in the KOAG. There was a correlation between kinematic variables and quadriceps torque.

Conclusion: Weakness of the quadriceps muscle in women with KOA influences gait pattern, resulting in reduced speed associated with a shorter swing time and longer support time.

Keywords: Kinematics, Torque, Falls

Background

Osteoarthritis (OA) is the most prevalent rheumatic disease in the population, characterized by progressive degeneration of cartilage and periarticular tissue, which results in changes in joint mechanics and may result in functional disability [1]. OA has a high incidence in the population; at least 30% of men and women over 65 years old have some radiographic alterations, and one-third of them are symptomatic [2]. In addition, in the age group of over 75 years old, the incidence increases to 85% because the older the population, the greater the number of individuals affected by the disease [3].

It is estimated that 4% of the Brazilian population has OA in at least one joint [4]. In 37% of these cases, the knee is the main affected region because in occupational and leisure activities, it is exposed to maximal compressive loads that can exceed three times that produced by the individual's body weight during walking. This stress favors high injury rates and cartilage degeneration, contributing to a greater incidence of OA in this joint [4].

Approximately 25% of individuals with knee osteoarthritis (KOA) cannot perform the main activities of daily living due to pain, muscle weakness, reduced balance,

* Correspondence: deborahebling@yahoo.com.br
[1]Department of Physical Education, São Paulo State University, UNESP, Rio Claro, SP, Brazil
[5]Departamento de Fisioterapia e Terapia Ocupacional, Universidade Estadual Paulista, Avenida Hygino Muzzi Filho, 737, CEP, Marília, SP 17525-000, Brazil
Full list of author information is available at the end of the article

proprioception deficits, reduced joint range of motion and joint instability [5, 6]. Among the possible limitations caused by KOA, gait difficulty has great clinical relevance because it is the most performed daily life activity and ensures functional independence [7].

The gait is a complex task and requires a perfect harmony of the sensory, motor and cognitive systems to produce a stable, efficient and safe gait pattern [8]. Biomechanical gait pattern changes, such as reduction of gait speed, step length and width, increase of the double support phase time, shorter swing phase time and reduction of heel contact with the ground, among other parameters, can be observed through kinematic gait analysis [8]. These gait pattern changes are often reported in the elderly, and the causes are multifactorial, but the main factor related to gait performance is decreased muscular strength of the lower limbs [9].

In individuals with KOA, the reduction of the knee extensor strength has been noted as the main symptom of the disease because there is a reduction of approximately 50–60% of quadriceps maximum torque in relation to the young population, possibly resulting from atrophy by disuse, secondary to joint pain and arthrogenic muscle inhibition [10–12]. This loss of strength is more significant than that presented by the healthy population in the same age group that reaches 30 to 40% of maximum capacity [12]. The quadriceps weakness observed in this population can decrease the shock absorption capacity during walking, leading to accentuated symptoms and, consequently, gait pattern alteration as a strategy to minimize pain and maintain functionality [9, 13].

Previous studies have noted that the quadriceps is one of the main muscle groups responsible for increasing gait speed and has an important role in maintaining functional mobility. Weakness of this muscle group may be responsible for increased metabolic expenditure during functional activities, which limits the intensity and duration of these tasks [14, 15]. Therefore, reduced ability to generate quadriceps strength, characteristic in patients with KOA, can negatively affect gait pattern, with a greater probability of becoming dependent on daily tasks, which leads to a decrease in quality of life and an increase in public expenditures to care services for this population [12, 13].

In this sense, gait analysis in patients with KOA can help identify changes in the gait pattern caused by the disease and, consequently, can help guide treatment and prevention programs for functionality loss in this population. The aim of the present study was to analyze the gait patterns of healthy individuals with KOA and to test for associations of gait variables with the strength level of the knee extensor muscles. We hypothesize that individuals with KOA will show decreased gait speed and swing time and longer step time in relation to controls and that these modifications are associated with lower knee extensor muscle strength in this population.

Methods
Subjects
Seventy-one female subjects, divided into a knee osteoarthritis group (KOAG) and a control group (CG), participated in this study. For the KOAG ($n = 38$, 66.4 ± 7.6 years), the individuals presented radiological diagnosis of tibiofemoral OA, confirmed according to the criteria of the American College of Rheumatology, and with grades II-III, based on the radiological grading scale of osteoarthritis described by Kellgren-Lawrence and WOMAC [16] pain scores greater than 21. For the CG ($n = 31$, 64.5 ± 7.1 years), the subjects had no history of changes related to chronic-degenerative diseases in the lower limbs. The sample size was determined by the G*Power program and was based on data obtained from pilot studies (effect = 0.85, power = 0.95, error $\alpha = 0.05$, sample $N = 15$).

The eligibility criteria for this study were as follows: age between 50 and 75 years, able to walk without gait devices and no other rheumatic diseases in the lower limbs, patellofemoral osteoarthritis, total or partial knee and/or hip arthroplasty, lesions in the lower limbs in the 6 months preceding the study or other diseases that made it impossible to perform the tests.

The present study was approved by the local ethics committee (n. 9032/2015), and obtained written informed consent from the patients for publication of data and images.

Evaluation procedures
The procedures for data collection were performed on 2 days, with an interval of two to 7 days between the collection days [17]. On the first day, anamnesis was performed to characterize the sample according to the anthropometric data and applying the WOMAC questionnaires to the KOAG. Subsequently, subjects were familiarized with isometric knee torque evaluation. On the second day, the isometric muscle strength of the knee and the gait were evaluated.

Gait evaluation
The gait evaluation was performed on a 14-m-long and 2-m-wide catwalk, with the first 2 m and the last 2 m of the catwalk being disregarded for data analysis to avoid possible influences from the gait acceleration and deceleration process [18, 19].

After being familiarized with the gait test, the volunteers were instructed, through verbal stimulation, to walk on the catwalk at the speed they performed their

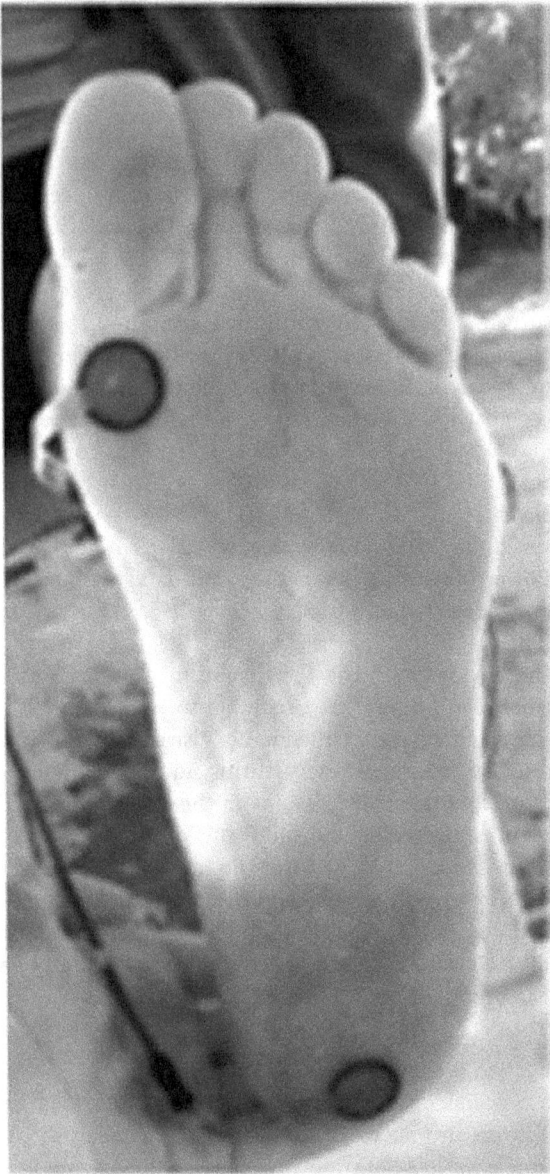

Fig. 1 Positioning of pressure sensors for gait analysis

between the familiarization and the beginning of the data collection procedures to avoid fatiguing the evaluated muscle group.

The evaluation protocol consisted of 3 maximal voluntary isometric contractions for the movement of the knee joint extension for a period of 5 s, with a 30-s interval between each contraction [23]. The volunteers were seated in the chair extensor with hip and knee at 90° flexion (0° of full extension). The trunk and the contralateral lower limb were stabilized by belts. A loading cell (Noraxon®) was coupled to the extensor chair lever for acquiring joint torque data. Figure 2 shows the positioning of the volunteer. The volunteers were instructed and encouraged to perform the movement as strongly and as quickly as possible.

The calculation of knee extensor torque was calculated from the following equation:

$$Knee\ extensor\ torque = Force\ (N)\ x\ Distance \times sen\ 90^o$$

Data analysis
Cardoso, B.C et al. [24]for gait data analysis, 40 steps and a 4th-order Butterworth filter with a cutoff frequency of 6 Hz were used. The mean step time (i.e., the

daily activities [20, 21]. Five attempts to evaluate the gait were performed.

FootSwitch (Noraxon®) pressure sensors positioned bilaterally on the calcaneus and at the hallux base were used to determine gait phases, as shown in Fig. 1.

Evaluation of knee extensor torque
The evaluation of knee extensor torque was performed on the affected lower limb for KOAG and on the dominant lower limb for the CG. Before the beginning of the evaluation protocol, a familiarization with the equipment, consisting of 2 submaximal contractions and 2 maximal contractions of the muscle group to be evaluated, was performed [22]. There was a 5-min interval

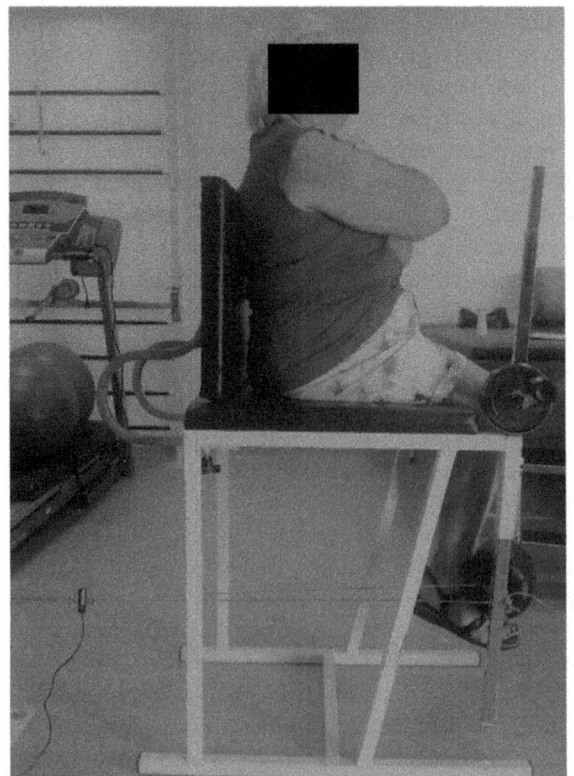

Fig. 2 Positioning of the volunteer for evaluation of muscle torque

time between the touch of the right calcaneus until the same limb touched the ground again), support time (i.e., the time between the touch of the right calcaneus and the touch of the hallux of the same limb), swing time (i.e., the time between removal of the right hallux and the next touch of the calcaneus of the same limb), double support time and gait speed were calculated.

Muscle torque data were processed in routines developed in the Matlab environment (Mathworks®) using a 4th-order Butterworth filter with cutoff frequency of 15 Hz [25]. Torque data were normalized for the volunteers' body mass. Peak torque was determined from the highest torque value obtained after the onset of muscle contraction.

Statistical analysis

For statistical analysis, the program PASW statistics 18.0® (SPSS) was used. After verifying the normality of the data, one-way ANOVA for comparisons between the groups and Pearson's correlation were applied, considering $p < 0.05$.

Results

Table 1 presents the characteristics of the study participants. There were no differences between groups for anthropometric characteristics. Regarding the limb affected by the disease, 32 volunteers presented diagnosis in the dominant limb and 6 in the non-dominant limb.

The one-way ANOVA showed a significant difference between the groups, with the KOAG presenting a 54.76% ($p < 0.001$) greater support time and a greater step time ($p < 0.001$). In addition, the swing time and the gait speed were 30% ($p < 0.001$) and 10.7% ($p = 0.001$) lower, respectively, than those of the control volunteers. The double support time in the KOAG was 33% greater than the CG ($p = 0.02$), as shown in Table 2.

Regarding the muscle torque of knee extensors, the KOAG presented a 34% ($p = 0.001$) reduction in peak torque compared with healthy individuals.

Table 1 Sample characterization

	KOAG ($n = 38$)	CG ($n = 33$)	P
Age (years)	66.49 ± 7.64	64.52 ± 7.12	0.36
Body weight (kg)	76.51 ± 14.77	67.42 ± 11.39	0.22
Height (m)	1.56 ± 0.06	1.55 ± 0.05	0.88
BMI (kg/m²)	31.01 ± 4.86	27.94 ± 4.58	0.96
WOMAC questionnaire			
Pain intensity (0–20)	8.87 ± 2.93	0.33 ± 0.56	< 0.001*
Stiffness (0–8)	3.08 ± 1.61	0	< 0.001*
Physical fitness (0–68)	30.70 ± 6.06	5.70 ± 2.33	< 0.001*
Total (0–96)	42.66 ± 8.61	6.04 ± 2.36	< 0.001*

Mean values ± standard deviation, *KOAG* knee osteoarthritis group, *CG* control group, *kg* kilograms, *m* meters

Table 2 Comparison of gait kinematic variables and quadriceps strength in subjects with KOA and healthy subjects

	KOA	Healthy subjects	P
Speed (m/s)	1.00 ± 0.13	1.12 ± 0.15	0.001
Support time (s)	0.65 ± 0.20	0.42 ± 0.10	< 0.001
Swing time (s)	0.42 ± 0.13	0.60 ± 0.13	< 0.001
Step time (s)	1.13 ± 0.12	1.00 ± 0.10	< 0.001
Knee extensor torque (Nm/kg)	0.96 ± 0.35	1.44 ± 0.42	0.001

Mean values ± standard deviations, *m* meters, *s* seconds, *Nm/kg* Newton meters per kilogram

There were correlations between the knee extensor torque and the support time ($r = -0.552$, $p = 0.03$), step time ($r = -0.492$, $p = 0.017$) and gait speed ($r = 0.442$, $p = 0.04$), as shown in Table 3.

Discussion

The results of this study corroborate the initial hypotheses that individuals with KOA show impairments in all gait kinematic parameters compared with healthy volunteers, and these biomechanical changes are correlated with knee extensor weakness.

Changes in the movement patterns during gait occur with advancing age and are well established in the literature. However, in individuals with KOA, these changes are more pronounced and have a negative impact on the independence level in performing daily tasks [9]. Muscle pain and weakness are the main symptoms of the disease associated with changes in the spatial-temporal gait parameters that aim to minimize pain and protect the knee joint [9]. In the present study, women in the KOAG had a 34% decrease in knee extensor strength compared with the control. According to Park et al. [12], the muscle strength deficit in KOA affects all lower limbs and is more pronounced in the knee extensors, being 40% lower in relation to individuals of the same age group without KOA. Strength levels also showed a negative correlation with support/step time, indicating that muscle weakness results in gait temporal changes that lead to reduced gait speed. These findings corroborate studies by Resende et al. (2011) and Feber et al. (2016), who observed that gait pattern changes are associated with knee pain symptoms and weakness of the anterior thigh muscles [10, 11, 26].

Table 3 Correlation between knee extensor torque and gait variables

	Support time	Step time	Swing time	Gait speed
Torque				
R²	−0.552	−0.492	−0.318	0.442
P	0.003	0.017	0.08	0.04

According to Ploutz-Snyder et al. [27] and Manini et al. (2010), individuals with knee extensor torque values below 1.5 Nm/kg are classified as having mobility limitations and difficulty in performing daily tasks due to less capacity to generate force in the quadriceps [27, 28]. In the present study, the volunteers with KOA showed extensor torque values that were 36% below the threshold proposed by those authors, and the CG presented values that were 4% below proposed values, which indicates greater functionality impairment of these individuals observed through the score obtained in the WOMAC questionnaire.

The muscles around the knee produce movement but also provide stability and control the load imposed on the joint; therefore, these muscles are related to the development and progression of KOA [12, 29, 30]. According to Kean et al. [31], maximal knee joint loads during gait occur because of muscle weakness, especially of knee extensors, which compromise the lower limb deceleration function before contact with the ground to reduce impact. Therefore, the strategy adopted by KOA patients is to reduce gait speed.

According to Kaufman et al. [32], patients with KOA tend to walk at slower speeds and with greater joint stiffness to avoid high external joint movements on the joint, i.e., the gait speed reduction is a strategy to decrease the vertical component of the soil reaction force imposed on the knee joint, reducing the functional demand in this joint. The lower usual gait speed observed in the KOAG can be considered a compensatory response to reduce joint stress during movement.

The literature establishes an ideal value for gait speed of 1.2–1.4 m/s to perform daily tasks, including street crossing [33]. The women with KOA who participated in the present study had an average speed below the threshold value for what is considered safe, corroborating the findings of Tas et al. [34] and Gill et al. [35], which point to this speed reduction in KOA as a risk factor for future falls, functional decline and mortality in this population.

Modifications in the gait kinematic pattern may also justify the speed reduction observed in the KOAG. The decrease in the swing time observed in the KOAG (30% lower) is in agreement with Bennell et al. (2013), who mentioned that the shorter swing time is due to weakness of the knee extensor muscles, which are not able to provide dynamic stability during the total weight placed over the limb at that gait phase. However, the increases in support time, step time and double support may be related to the possibility of generating a greater load distribution in the healthy limb. However, this compensatory response may contribute to joint wear and tear in the long term. According to Resende et al. (2011), if

individuals with KOA stayed in the support phase longer, it is possible that the prolonged effect of a minor overload would be close to the short effect of an intense joint stress, i.e., the protective neuromuscular response may cause pain and joint damage. Thus, when the strategy of the movement changes due to pain or reduced capacity to stabilize a segment, joint overloads and early fatigue occur [13].

The limitations of this study are related to the approach involving only the knee extensor muscles, as this muscular group is the most affected by the disease. However, it is known that muscular weakness affects the entire lower limb, and studies by Bennell et al. (2010) and Amiri et al. [29] emphasize the importance of the hip abductor muscles and plantar flexors, respectively, in the gait pattern of individuals with KOA as a strategy to compensate for the deficit of quadriceps strength. Therefore, future studies should include other muscle groups of the lower limb to better understand the biomechanical gait changes in KOA.

Conclusion

There is a potential relationship between gait kinematic variables and knee extensor strength, and the weakness of the quadriceps muscle influences the gait pattern in individuals with KOA. This relationship results in the reduction of gait speed, associated with greater support/step time and shorter swing time. Given that KOA has no cure and changes in gait are progressive and increase as the degenerative disease progresses, this study aims to contribute to directing physiotherapeutic interventions in KOA treatment by identifying the relationships between knee extensor strength and gait kinematic variables. Thus, physiotherapy can develop strategies focused on lower limb strength training, with a greater emphasis on the quadriceps muscle, which is more compromised in this population, and on activities that aim at gait training, seeking a better distribution of body weight in both limbs and improvements of range of motion and muscle recruitment, thereby improving the performance of the individual during daily tasks and contributing to slow down the progression of OA.

Acknowledgements
The authors appreciate the participation of all the volunteers of this research and financial support FAPESP.

Funding
The São Paulo Research Foundation (FAPESP) for financial support.

Authors' contributions
Data Collection: D.H. Spinoso and N.C. Bellei. Data Analysis: D.H. Spinoso, N.C.Bellei, N.R. Marques. Manuscript Writing: D.H. Spinoso, N.R. Marques, and M.T. Navega. The authors further declare that this manuscript was approved for publication in the Brazilian Journal of Rheumatology.

Competing interests

The authors declare that none had any conflict of interest which could bias the results of this study and the material in this manuscript has not been and will not be submitted for publication elsewhere.

Author details

[1]Department of Physical Education, São Paulo State University, UNESP, Rio Claro, SP, Brazil. [2]Department of Physiotherapy and Occupational Therapy, São Paulo State University, UNESP, Marília, SP, Brazil. [3]Department of Health Sciences, University of the Sacred Heart, USC, Bauru, SP, Brazil. [4]Lecturer in Musculoskeletal Physiotherapy Department of Physiotherapy and Occupational Therapy, São Paulo State University, UNESP, Marília, SP, Brazil. [5]Departamento de Fisioterapia e Terapia Ocupacional, Universidade Estadual Paulista, Avenida Hygino Muzzi Filho, 737, CEP, Marília, SP 17525-000, Brazil.

References

1. Lim J, Tchai E, Jang SN. Effectiveness of aquatic exercise for obese patients with knee osteoarthritis: a randomized controlled trial. Am Acad Phys Med Rehabil. 2010;2(8):723–31.

2. Fernandes WC, Machado A, Borella C, Carpes F. Influência da velocidade da marcha sobre a pressão plantar em sujeitos com osteoartrite unilateral de joelho. Rev Bras Reumatol. 2014;54(6):441–5.

3. Neto EMF, Queluz TT, Freire BF. Atividade física e sua associação com qualidade de vida em pacientes com osteoartrite. Rev Bras Reumatol. 2011; 51(6):539–49.

4. Senna ER, De Barros AL, Silva EO, Costa IF, Pereira LV, Ciconelli RM, et al. Prevalence of rheumatic diseases in Brazil: a study using the COPCORD approach. J Rheumatol. 2004;31(3):594–7.

5. Jorge RT, Souza MC, Chiari A, Jones A, Fernandes AD, Junior IL, et al. Progressive resistance exercise in women with osteoarthritis of the knee: a randomized controlled trial. Clin Rheabil. 2014;29(3):234–43.

6. Edmonds DW, Mcconnell J, Ebert JR, Ackland TR, Donnelly CJ. Biomechanical, neuromuscular and knee pain effects following therapeutic knee taping among patients with knee osteoarthritis during walking gait. Clin Biomech. 2016;39:28–43.

7. Alkjaer T, Raffalt PC, Dalsgaard H, Simonsen EB, Petersen NC, Bliddal H, et al. Gait variability and motor control in people with knee osteoarthritis. Gait Posture. 2015;42:479–84.

8. Jahn K, Zwergal A, Schniepp R. Gait disturbances in old age. Deutsches Arteblatt International. 2010;107(17):306–16.

9. Clermont CA, Barden JM. Accelerometer-based determination of gait variability in older adults with knee osteoarthritis. Gait Posture. 2016;50:126–30.

10. Callahan DM, Tourville TW, Slauterbeck JR, Ades PA, Stevens-lapsley J, Beynnon BD, et al. Reduced rate of knee extensor torque development in older adults with knee osteoarthritis is associated with intrinsic muscle contractile deficits. Exp Gerontol. 2015;72:16–21.

11. Davison MJ, Maly MR, Keir PJ, Hapuhennedige SM, Kron AT, Adachi JD, et al. Lean muscle volume of the thigh has a stronger relationship with muscle power than muscle strength in women with knee osteoarthritis. Clin Biomech. 2017;41:92–7.

12. Park SK, Kobsar D, Ferber R. Relationship between lower limb muscle strength, self-reported pain and function, and frontal plane gait kinematics in knee osteoarthritis. Clin Biomech. 2016;38:68–74.

13. Kierkegaard S, Jorgensen PB, Dalgas U, Soballe K, Mechlenburg I. Pelvic movement strategies and leg extension power in patients with end-stage medial compartment knee osteoarthritis: a cross-sectional study. Arch Orthop Trauma Sur. 2015;135(9):1217–26.

14. Abreu SSE, Caldas CP. Velocidade de marcha, equilíbrio e idade: um estudo correlacional entre idosas praticantes e idosas não praticantes de um programa de exercícios terapêuticos. Rev Bras Fisioter. 2008;12(4):324–30.

15. Marques NR, LaRoche DP, Hallal CZ, Crozara LF, Morcelli MH, Karuka AH, Navega MT, Gonçalves M. Association between energy cost of walking, muscle activation, and biomechanical parameters in older female fallers and non-fallers. Clin Biomech. 2013;28(3):330–6.

16. Murray AM, Thomas AC, Armstrong CW, Pietrosimone BG, Tevald MA. The associations between quadriceps muscle strength, power, and knee joint mechanics in knee osteoarthritis: a cross-sectional study. Clin Biomech. 2015;30:1140–5.

17. LaRoche DP, Millett ED, Kralian RJ. Low strength is related to diminished ground reaction forces and walking performance in older women. Gait Posture. 2011;33(4):668–72.

18. Doi T, Yamaguchi R, Asai T, Komatsu M, Makiura D, Shimamura M, Hirata S, Ando H, Kurosaka M. The effects of shoe fit on gait in community-dwelling older adults. Gait Posture. 2010;32(2):274–8.

19. Hollman JH, Kovask FM, Kubit JJ, Linbo RA. Age-related differences in spatiotemporal markers of gait stability during dual task walking. Gait Posture. 2007;26(1):113–7.

20. Bertucco M, Cesari P. Dimensional analysis and ground reaction forces for stair climbing: effects of age and task difficulty. Gait Posture. 2009;29(2):326–31.

21. Perry CJ, Kiriella JB, Hawkins KM, Shanahan CJ, Moore AE, Gage WH. The effects of anterior load carriage on lower limb gait parameters during obstacle clearance. Gait Posture. 2010;32(1):57–61.

22. Costa RA, Oliveira LM, Watanabe SH, Jones A, Natour J. Isokinetic assessment of the hip muscles in patients with osteoarthritis of the knee. Clinics. 2010;65(12):1253–9.

23. Hartmann A, Knols R, Murer K, Bruin ED. Reproducibility of an isokinetic strength-testing protocol of the knee and ankle in older adults. Gerontology. 2009;55(3):259–68.

24. Cardoso, B.C.; Pimentel, N.L.; Bellei, N.C.; Nishiomoto, D.N.; Navega, M.T.; Spinoso, D.H. Efeito da bandagem elástica na ativação muscular do quadríceps e torque isométrico dos extensores de joelho em indivíduos com osteoartrite de joelho. Revista Brasileira de Educação Física e Esporte, jan/mar, 2017.

25. Crozara LF, Morcelli MH, Marques NR, Hallal CZ, Spinoso DH, Neto AA, et al. Motor readiness and joint torque production in lower limbs of older women fallers and non-fallers. J Electromyogr Kinesiol. 2013;23(5):1131–8.

26. Ferber R, Kobsar D, Park S. Relationship between lower limb muscle strength, self-reported pain and function, and frontal plane gait kinematics in knee osteoarthritis. Clin Biomech. 2016;38:68–74.

27. Ploutz-Snyder LL, Manini T, Ploutz-Snyder RJ, Wolf DA. Functionally relevant thresholds of quadriceps Femoris strength. J Gerontol. 2002;57(4):144–52.

28. Manini TM, Newman AB, Fielding R, Blair SN, Perri MG, Anton SD, et al. Effects of exercise on mobility in obese and nonobese older adults. Obesity (Silver Spring). 2011;18(6):1168–75.

29. Amiri P, Hubley-Kozey CL, Landry SC, Stanish WD, Astephen-Wilson JL. Obesity is associated with prolonged activity of the quadriceps and gastrocnemii during gait. J Electromyogr Kinesiol. 2015;25(6):951–8.

30. Hodges PW, Van Den HW, WRigley TV, Hinman RS, Bowles KA, Cicuttini F, et al. Increased duration of co-contraction of medial knee muscles is associated with greater progression of knee osteoarthritis. Man Ther. 2016;21:151–8.

31. Kean CO, Hinman RS, Wrigley TV, Lim BW, Bennell KL. Impact loading following quadriceps strength training in individuals with medial knee osteoarthritis and varus alignment. Clin Biomech. 2017;42:20–4.

32. Kaufman KR, Hughes C, Morrey BF, Morrey M, An K. Gait characteristics of patients with knee osteoarthritis. J Biomech. 2001;34(7):907–15.

33. Lui B, Hu X, Zhang Q, Fan Y, Li J, Zou R, Zhang M, et al. Usual walking speed and all-cause mortality risk in older people: A systematic review and meta-analysis. Gait Posture. 2016;44:172–7.

34. Tas S, Güneri S, Baki A, Yildirim T, Kaymak B, Erden Z. Effects of severity of osteoarthritis on the temporospatial gait parameters in patients with knee osteoarthritis. Acta Orthop Traumatol Turc. 2014;48(6):635–41.

35. Gill SV, Hicks GE, Zhang Y, Niu J, Apovian CM, White DK. The association of waist circumference with walking difficulty among adults with or at risk of knee osteoarthritis: the osteoarthritis initiative. Osteoarthritis Cartilage. 2017; 25(1):60–6.

27

Ultrasound and its clinical use in rheumatoid arthritis: where do we stand?

Aline Defaveri do Prado[1,2]*, Henrique Luiz Staub[2], Melissa Cláudia Bisi[2], Inês Guimarães da Silveira[2], José Alexandre Mendonça[3], Joaquim Polido-Pereira[4,5] and João Eurico Fonseca[4,5]

Abstract

High-resolution musculoskeletal ultrasound (MSUS) has been increasingly employed in daily rheumatological practice and in clinical research. In rheumatoid arthritis (RA), MSUS can be now considered a complement to physical examination. This method evaluates synovitis through gray-scale and power Doppler and it is also able to identify bone erosions. The utilization of MSUS as a marker of RA activity has received attention in recent literature. Current data account for good correlation of MSUS with classical measures of clinical activity; in some instances, MSUS appears to perform even better. Diagnosis of subclinical synovitis by MSUS might help the physician in RA management. With some variation, interobserver MSUS agreement seems excellent for erosion and good for synovitis. However, lack of MSUS score standardization is still an unmet need. In this review, we describe several MSUS scores, as well as their correlation with clinical RA activity and response to therapy. Finally, we look at the relationship of MSUS with synovial tissue inflammation and discuss future perspectives for a better interpretation and integration of this imaging method into clinical practice.

Keywords: Musculoskeletal ultrasound, Gray-scale, Power Doppler, Cytokines, Rheumatoid arthritis

Background

Rheumatoid arthritis (RA) is a chronic inflammatory immune mediated disorder where synovial proliferation, pannus formation and bone erosions are histological hallmarks [1]. Proinflammatory cytokines play a major role in development of disease and clinical progression. Anti-cytokine therapy has brought a major impact in RA management [2].

Clinical assessment of RA patients includes history, physical examination, scores of disease activity and questionnaires addressing quality of life. As far as imaging is concerned, conventional radiograms and magnetic resonance imaging (MRI) are well-recognized support methods for clinical assessment and response to therapy. They have intrinsic problems, nevertheless. Radiograms cannot evaluate joint inflammation and show low sensitivity for damage; MRI, although sensitive, is expensive and not widely available [1, 2].

In recent years, high-resolution musculoskeletal ultrasound (MSUS) has been increasingly used in rheumatological practice worldwide [3]. While MSUS gray-scale (GS) usually identifies synovial proliferation, power Doppler (pD) may recognize active inflammation and neoangiogenesis. Both parameters seem worthy of utilization in the follow-up of RA patients [4]. In addition, MSUS is also reliable for the detection of bone erosions [5] as well as for the detection of subclinical synovitis and prediction of disease relapse and structural progression [6].

Although unequivocally useful in RA, MSUS has intrinsic reproducibility issues that may be optimized through standardized training and recommendations. In 2010, a multinational group of 25 Rheumatologists from the American Continent participated in a consensus-based questionnaire and established the first recommendations and guidelines for MSUS course training in the Americas [7]. Besides, EULAR consensual advice for use of imaging techniques (MSUS included) in the management of RA has been recently proposed [8].

* Correspondence: adprado@gmail.com
[1]Rheumatology Unit, Nossa Senhora da Conceição Hospital, Porto Alegre, RS, Brazil
[2]Rheumatology Department, Sao Lucas Hospital, Faculty of Medicine of Pontifical Catholic University of Rio Grande do Sul (PUCRS), Av. Ipiranga, 6690/220, Porto Alegre 90610-000, Brazil
Full list of author information is available at the end of the article

In this paper, we review the correlation of MSUS findings with synovial tissue inflammation in RA patients and its implications for a better clinical utilization of this imaging technique. Also, we discuss MSUS clinical application as compared to classical activity parameters. Lastly, we update MSUS techniques and interobserver reliability in RA.

Ultrasound parameters and synovial tissue

Comparison of MSUS findings with features of synovial tissue allows characterizing how far this technique can capture the inflammatory activity that is actually ongoing inside joints.

Andersen et al. studied the correlation between histological synovitis and GS and pD in RA patients and found fairly good correlations between pD and histological features of inflammation and proliferation, namely synovium expression of CD3, CD68, Ki67 and von Willebrand factor (r between 0,44 and 0,57). There were areas of histological inflammation where no pD could be identified [9]. Other authors showed that 5 RA patients in DAS remission who had GS but negative pD had low likelihood of relapse after TNF inhibitor tapering and histologically had low infiltrates of macrophages (CD68+), T (CD3+) a B (CD20+) cells [10].

In a study of 14 RA patients in remission who were submitted to surgery, 15 synovial samples were collected. GS changes were found in 80% patients, pD detected in 60% of the individuals and MRI synovitis in 86%. Histologically, 4 samples had severe inflammation, 6 moderate, 3 mild and 2 minimal [11].

In another study in 20 patients with knee arthritis, pD showed better correlation with histological synovitis than contrast-enhanced MRI [12]. In the setting of rheumatoid synovium, the thickness of synovial lining and the number of vessels are increased, although it is not clear whether the angiogenesis is a cause or a consequence of the inflammatory process [13, 14].

Koski et al. found that in RA synovium there was a good correlation between the number of vessels and the inflammatory state (synovium inflammatory infiltrate), but not with pD. They concluded that chronic histological synovitis was not always related with a positive pD [15] In fact, in another study by the same authors, pD was not always translating synovial inflammation and could be related with other pathologic processes, such as fibrosis [16]. Waltheret al found a correlation between the number of vessels and pD, but did not report on the inflammatory state [17].

In healthy synovial joints, the presence of pD signal associated with serum levels of vascular endothelial growth factor (VEGF), but not with other growth factors or cytokines. This could support a role of VEGF in neo-angiogenesis in RA [18]. In a survey of 55 RA patients in clinical remission, pD correlated with VEGF levels and other angiogenesis markers [19]. On the contrary, a correlation between pD and serum vascular endothelium growth factor could not be established in RA patients according to a 2004 study [20].

Contrast-enhanced Doppler ultrasound may be superior to pD in translating a dynamic process such as synovitis in RA, in which perfusion may be determinant, but little is known about the correlation of these findings with histological features in the synovium RA. This method has proved to be superior to pD in defining active synovitis, using arthroscopy, but not MRI, as the gold standard [21–24].

Worthy of note, synovial production of IL-6 was found to associate with synovitis as detected by MRI and pD [25]. This in accordance with our own results, depicting that IL-6, but not other cytokines, correlated positively with DAS28, swollen joint count, 10-joint pD score and GS/pD of both wrists. In multiple linear regression, the association of IL-6 with 10-joint pD score was maintained even after adjustment for DAS28. There was no correlation of IL-6 with tender joint count, 10-joint GS score, or bone erosion [26].

Interestingly, Ball et al. described association of serum IL-6 with arthritis on physical examination and pD score in patients with systemic lupus erythematosus [27]. Overall, these findings [26, 27] may result from a prominent synovial production of IL-6. In fact, IL-6 stimulates angiogenesis [28], and this could eventually explain the association of IL-6 concentrations with a positive pD in RA. A recent report accounted for association of serum IL-6 with MSUS parameters of synovitis in patients with early RA; of importance, serial measurements of IL-6 were linked to structural damage [29].

In patients with established RA, a correlation of serum IL-17 with synovial hypertrophy and pD in hand MSUS was documented [30]. Interestingly, the presence of Th-17 lymphocytes in synovial tissue was associated with a persistent pD signal, according to a 2010 study [31].

As seen, the study of the relationship of MSUS parameters with synovial tissue features is clearly a field open to research, which may add new pathogenic information and help to clarify MSUS usefulness in RA management.

Correlation of MSUS with physical examination, inflammatory markers and patient reported outcomes

For many years, Rheumatologists have been using the disease activity score of 28 joints (DAS28) and other composite scores as gold standard for assessment of RA activity; these tools have clearly brought great progress in treatment monitoring. Even though they are the most extensively validated methods for measuring disease activity to date [32], the precise way of objectively defining inflammation is still lacking. MSUS can be worthwhile in this context, since it is more sensitive than physical examination for detection of arthritis according to a number of studies [33–37].

In patients with joint inflammatory symptoms lasting less than 12 months, MSUS significantly increased the classification of patients as RA (31% pretest, 61% post-test) [38]. In individuals with established RA, synovial hypertrophy and pD scores of wrists and MCP correlated significantly with physician-recorded clinical outcomes and helped the rheumatologist in clinical decision [39].

Of great importance, preliminary data indicated that the MSUS methodology improved the accuracy of the 2010 ACR/EULAR criteria for identifying patients needing methotrexate treatment. $GS \geq 2$ and $pD \geq 1$ were good indicators of synovitis [40].

According to a study published in 2001, pD scan of MCP joints was a reliable method in assessment of synovitis of RA patients, considering MRI as standard [41]. In a systematic review and metanalyis of 21 studies, MSUS was more effective than conventional radiograms for detection of bone erosions; efficacy was comparable to MRI and reproducibility was good [42]. In another systematic review, MSUS added value to clinical findings for the diagnosis of RA when studying at least MCP, wrist and MTP joints; to evaluate remission, scanning of at least wrist and MCP joints of the dominant side was advocated. In both circumstances, pD was a more reliable instrument as compared to GS [43].

Recent data suggested that both MSUS and clinical examination were relevant to appraise risk of subsequent structural damage in RA patients [44]. Subclinical joint inflammation detected by imaging techniques as MSUS probably accounts for the paradoxical structural deterioration seen in RA patients allegedly in clinical remission [45]. Of note, Peluso et al. demonstrated that remission as confirmed by pD was much more prevalent in patients with early than long-standing RA [46].

We have previously reported that pD, GS and bone erosion on MSUS were associated with swollen joint count, but not with joint tenderness [47]. Concordance of physical examinationand MSUS assessment seems poor (not more than 50% between the most affected joint and pD signal), and RA structural progression has been more associated with swollen joint count than with pain [48–50].

Correlations studies of MSUS with disease activity are a matter of debate. In a study employing pD score of 22 joints and GS score of 28 joints, a defined correlation of MSUS parameters with classical measures of RA activity (acute phase proteins, DAS28) was found. Differently, correlation of MSUS scores with health assessment questionnaires were weak to moderate [51].

In a 2014 study, concordance level of standard activity measures with MSUS was evaluated. For such, a pD score of hands, radiocarpal and MTP joints was utilized. Discrepancies between pD and DAS28 occurred in 29% of cases, promoting changes in therapeutic decision, in other words, supporting DMARD escalation in patients with continuing subclinical synovitis and preventing escalation in symptomatic patients without ultrasonographic synovitis [52]. Likewise, Gartner et al. demonstrated pD signal in up to 20% of patients in remission according to DAS28 [53].

Recently, it has been shown that the 7-joint GS/pD Backhaus score showed performance comparable to clinical and laboratory data in RA patients under various therapies. Higher score predicted bone erosions after one year. Of interest, Backhaus method was sensitive enough to demonstrate decline in bone erosions in patients who switched biological agents [54]. In patients in remission, a link of GS/pD positivity with risk of clinical flare and structural progression was demonstrated by metanalysis in 2014 [55].

A 2012 study revealed that the presence of pD signal was an accurate predictor of flare in RA patients in remission [56]. Synovitis detected by pD may predict biologic therapy tapering failure in RA patients in sustained remission, according to a very recent report [57]. Adding of pD was able to identify RA patients in DAS28 remission, with subclinically active disease. The same authors reported that the combination of clinical and pD parameters recognized patients in remission who could undergo anti-TNF dose tapering [58].

It has been observed that subclinical synovitis is long-lasting in RA patients in clinical remission [59]. In a study dated from 2012, pD, but not low-field MRI, predicted relapse and radiographic progression in RA patients with low levels of disease activity [60]. In early RA patients on conventional therapy, pD-positive synovial hypertrophy identified ongoing inflammation, even during remission and also predicted a short-term relapse [61].

In an observational study of 307 RA patients, Zufferey et al. demonstrated that many subjects in clinical remission according to classical parameters (DAS28 and ACR/EULAR criteria) showed residual synovitis on GS and pD scan [62]. Yoshimi et al. documented synovitis by pD in patients in clinical inactivity and suggested that the pD parameter is essential to confirm "true remission" of RA [63].

Recently, a group of authors originally approached the correlation of MSUS with clinical scores in RA patients with and without fibromyalgia. While GS scores correlated with classical parameters in both groups, the pD analysis was more precise by correlating with clinical scores only in patients without fibromyalgia [64].

In 68 RA patients evaluated with a six-joint pD method (two MCP, wrists, knees), the global MSUS score correlated moderately with the DAS28; in this survey, pD positivity was a sensitive-to-change method for monitoring the short-term response to anti-TNF agents [65]. In a cross-sectional study of 97 RA patients, an inactive disease status defined by a 12-joint pD score (but not clinical parameters) associated, interestingly, with decrease in complement levels in patients treated with biologics [66].

In 2015, the ARTIC trial addressed the question if MSUS could correlate with DAS28 defined RA remission criteria. In 238 patients with early RA randomized to perform or not GS/pD MSUS in addition to DAS28, both strategies (MSUS included or not) were effective to estimate remission after two years of therapy [67].

In summary, there has been plenty of recent literature looking at the role of MSUS either as a complement to physical examination or as a measure of disease activity. It seems the discrepancies between US findings and clinical findings on articular examination are more important in long standing RA and/or fibromyalgia associated RA patients, where metrics are less reliable (due to difficulties in physical examinations and on pain exacerbation). It remains an open question if MSUS would work as additional or preferential criteria for assessing RA activity. MSUS looks a promising instrument for monitoring RA disease activity, but a greater body of evidence still is required.

Intra and interobserver agreement

Another critical aspect when using MSUS in the evaluation of RA is reproductibility. Inter-reader analysis of the clinical assessment of joint inflammation can itself show some discrepancy [68, 69]. Intra and interobserver discrepancies in both acquisition of image and image interpretation have been a matter of concern.

A study dated from 2007 reported that the interobserver agreement of a 3-dimensional pD scan was better (> 0.80) than a 2-dimensional quantitative pD method [70]. In healthy subjects, MSUS of MCP joints using an 18 MHz transducer yielded an excellent interobserver kappa (0.83) for erosions [71]. A fair to good concordance (kappa 0.36–0.76) of a semiquantitative MCP score for cartilage damage was described in RA patients in 2010 [72].

Subclinical joint changes in asymptomatic feet of RA patients were recently assessed. Concordance between MSUS and radiograms was low (kappa 0.08–0.40). Inter-reader agreement was excellent for bone erosion (kappa = 1), good for quantitative synovitis (0.64) and moderate (0.47) for pD signal [73].In 2011, the interobserver reliability of a synovitis MSUS resulted in moderate concordance (kappa 0.50) for quantification of synovitis in the radiocarpal joint [74].

Szkudlarek et al showed in thirty RA patients with active disease that MSUS agreement was good for erosions (kappa 0.78) and pD (0.72), and excellent for synovitis (0.81) evaluatingfive joints (second and third MCP, second PIP, first and second MTP) that were scanned by two experienced sonographers. [75]

The Swiss Sonography in Arthritis and Rheumatism (SONAR) group had previously developed a consistent MSUS method for assessing RA activity utilizing B-mode and pD scores [76]. The same group evaluated synovitis and erosion in six differentMSUS machines. Overall, agreement was not more than moderate. Considering only high-quality machines, kappa concordance was better for synovitis (0.64) than erosion (0.41) [77].

Yet in 2005, the EULAR promoted the "Train the trainers" course aiming to evaluate MSUS interobserver reliability in RA. Clinically dominant joint regions (shoulder, knee, ankle/toe, wrist/finger) were examined. Concordance was particularly high for bone lesions, bursitis, and tendon tears (kappa = 1). As a whole, interobserver concordance, sensitivities, and specificities were comparable with MRI [78].

The reliability of the Backhaus 7-joint score was evaluated in 2012 and the best interobserver concordance was obtained for bone erosions in second MTP (plantar side), with kappa of 1. Agreement for pD in palmar side of wrist was good (0.79). Intraobserver reliability of the method was moderate to substantial [79].

In our own experience, we have been employing a 10-joint score exclusively of hand/wrist joints (dorsal aspects of wrists and second and third MCP, and volar aspect of second and third PIP joints of both hands). After evaluating 1380 joints of 60 RA patients, kappa agreement for synovitis ranged from fair to good (0.30–0.70); for cartilage changes, also from fair to good (0.28–0.63; for pD signal, from moderate to absolute agreement (0.53–1); and for erosions, from good to excellent (0.70–0.97) [80].

In 2014, the LUMINA European study assessed the reliability of grading MSUS videoclips with hand pathology in RA by employing non-sophisticated internet tools. Intra-reader concordance for GS/pD synovitis was moderate to good (0.52/0.62), while the interobserver agreement for global synovitis (synovitis and tenosynovitis) was not more than moderate (0.45) [81].

Also recently, a short collegiate consensus attempted to improve MSUS interobserver reliability. Concordance was good for B mode synovitis (0.75) and excellent for pD (0.88). Kappa values were excelllent for small hand joints, but poor to fair in wrists, elbows, ankles and MTP. Admittedly, the consensus meeting was useful to improve agreement in synovits scores of still images. Moreover, the consensus strongly emphasized the need for standards of image acquisition and interpretation [82].

The several studies [68–82] evaluating reliability of MSUS scores have revealed some variation. As a whole, MSUS seems very reliable for bone erosions (kappa ranging from good to excellent); in turn, the grade of agreement for synovitis, although generally moderate to good, has shown more fluctuation. Standardized training seems essential to improve all these outcomes.

Ultrasound scores

A high-resolution machine with a linear high-frequency probe (7.5–18 MHz) should be utilized for evaluation of small joints. In the most widely used scoring systems, semiquantitative GS, generated in the B-mode, synovial proliferation is classified as: zero (absent); 1) mild (slight hipoechoic or anechoic image in articular capsule); 2) moderate (presence of elevation of articular capsule); 3) severe or marked (important distension of articular capsule). The semiquantitative scale of pD signal stratifies inflammatory activity and angiogenesis as follows: zero (absent); 1) mild (one pD signal); 2) moderate (two or more pD signal, meaning < 50% of intraarticular flow); 3) severe or marked (> 50% of intraarticular flow) [83]. In addition, Carotti et al. reported that the resistive index (RI), using spectral Doppler, quantified inflammation in microvessels of finger joints and wrists and discriminated RA synovitis (higher values) from normal subjects [84]. Bone erosions, in turn, are defined according to the OMERACT criteria and are classified as present or absent [85]. Figure 1 illustrates MSUS findings in normal and RA hand joints.

There has been no agreement regarding which joints and tendons should be systematically examined in MSUS of RA patients. A number of different methods and scores have been advocated, without wide concordance to date. As a whole, it was proposed to include dorsal and volar exam of the hands in daily practice and clinical trials [33], but volar examination might not be consensual.

Historically, MSUS scores were firstly proposed in 2005 by two groups of authors [83, 86]. Scheel et al. described different MCP and PIP scores for GS and pD [86]. In 2006, Loeuille et al. reported a 7-joint GS/pD score including wrist, MCP and MTP of dominant side [87]. One year later, an 8-joint system evaluating GS/pD of MCP and MTP of dominant side was proposed by Hensch et al. [88]. In 2008, Iagnocco et al. designed a 10-joint method including MCP, PIP, wrist and knee including tenosynovitis, bursitis and erosion in addition to GS/pD [89]. Also in 2008, a 12-joint simplified MSUS including elbow, wrist, MCP, knee and ankle was reported by Naredo [90].

The 7-joint MSUS score proposed by Backaus et al. in 2009 has been the most largely utilized in recent

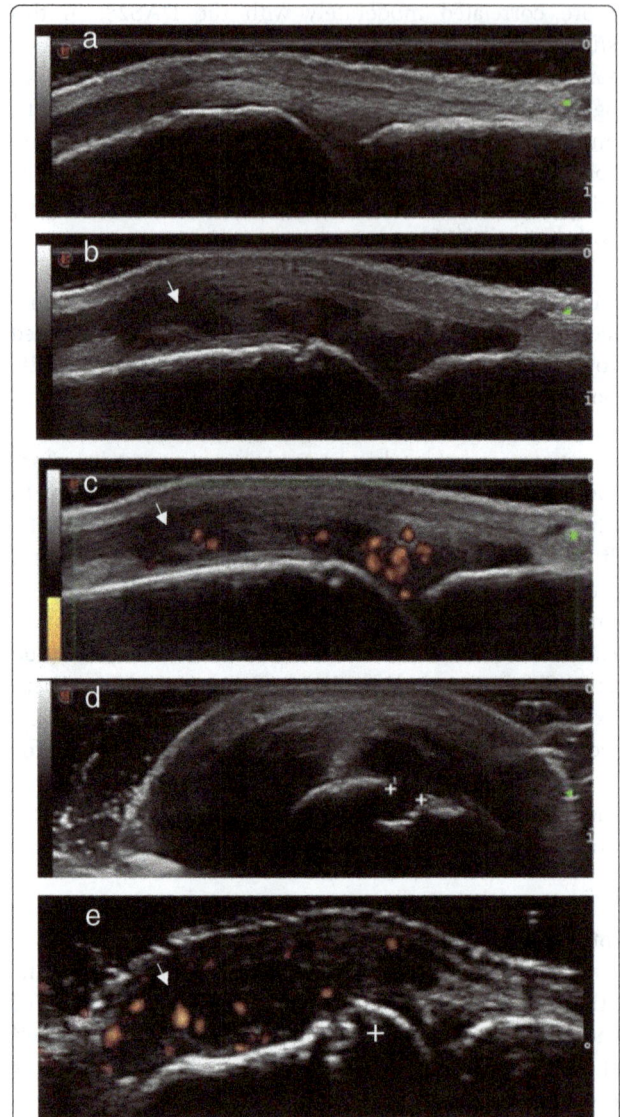

Fig. 1 Imagens of a normal MCP joint and an abnormal MCP joint of a RA patient. **a** Normal musculoskeletal ultrasound (MSUS) of third metacarpophalangeal (MCP) joint, longitudinal dorsal aspect; **b** Synovial proliferation grade 3 on second MCP, longitudinal dorsal aspect (arrow in hypoechoic area); **c** Synovial proliferation (arrow) and power Doppler (pD) captation grade 2 on second MCP, longitudinal dorsal aspect; **d** Interruption of cortical bone (erosion) on second MCP, radial aspect, longitudinal scan (plus sign); **e** MSUS of a patient with long-standing rheumatoid arthritis. Findings of second MCP (longitudinal dorsal aspect) include synovial proliferation grade 3 (arrow), pDcaptation grade 2 and bone erosion (plus sign)

literature and includes five hand and two foot joints of the clinically dominant side: wrist, second and third MCP and proximal interphalangeal (PIP), and second and fifth metatarsophalangeal (MTP) joints. This score also evaluated tenosynovitis and erosive changes [91].

In 2010, Hammer et al. proposed a 78-joint GS/pD score [92]. In 2012, a 6-joint MSUS score of wrists,

MCP and knees utilized synovial effusion in conjunction with the synovial proliferation and pD parameters. This score was practical, trustworthy and sensitive-to-change for evaluating synovial inflammation in RA [93].

Of note, a semi-quantitative 10-joint score of synovial thickness and pD which included only MCP joints was proved a reliable endpoint in a clinical trial [94]. A modified 7-joint score adding dorsal and palmar recesses of the wrists, as well as of small joints of hands and feet, was described in 2014. In a survey of 32 patients with early RA (832 joints examined), GS and pD were sensitive to detect synovitis [95]. A total pD score of 8-joint (bilateral wrist, knee, and the second and third MCP joints), reported in 2015, was found to be a simple and effective tool for monitoring RA activity [96].

Also very recently, a 12-joint score evaluating synovial hypertrophy by B-mode technology and synovitis by pD signal was described. The wrist–hand–ankle–MTP assessments were able to predict unstable remission in RA patients presumably inactive on methotrexate therapy [97].

With such heterogeneity in the previously mentioned scores, it is important to verify if scores with low number of joints correlate well with scores involving more joints, in order to find a set feasible for clinical daily practice. For instance, the 7-joint Backaus score significantly correlated with a 12-joint instrument for monitoring of response to infliximab in RA patients, according to a 2016 study [98].

A novel GS/pD score composed of a bilateral approach of six hand joints (first, second and third MCP joints, second and third PIP joints and radiocarpal joint), two feet joints (second and third MTP) and, in addition, one tendon (extensor carpi ulnaris), performed better than previous scores in a longitudinal analysis [99]. Using a data-driven approach, the same group of authors set out to validate a new MSUS score in a large survey of early or established RA. The set comprising GS/pD scores of seven joints/two tendons (first and second MCP, second MCP, third PIP, radiocarpal, elbow, first and second MTP, tibialis posterior tendon, extensor carpi ulnaris tendon) preserved most of the information when compared to a 9-joint score (which added fifth MCP and fifth MTP) [100].

A systematic review of 14 studies published in 2011 did not yield a consensus as to the minimal number of joints to be included in a global MSUS score [101]. Newer recommendations after critical analysis of the most recent MSUS scores are expected. Table 1 lists, in chronological order, the MSUS scores described so far.

Conclusion

MSUS is an useful instrument to complement the physical examination of RA patients. The method is quick and safe. The GS/pD scales are helpful to detect early synovitis and MSUS is also sensitive in the identification of bone erosions.

The method is of interest to identify subclinical disease activity in patients considered to be in clinical remission and might add relevant information regarding response to therapy. Whether targeted therapy to pD activity would provide superior outcomes compared with treating to clinical targets alone, it is still a matter of open discussion, which was recently highlighted by the Targeted Ultrasound Initiative group [102]. Proper clinical trials are warranted to clarify this point.

Table 1 Musculoskeletal ultrasound scores described in chronological order

Author/reference	Year	Joint characteristic/score elements
Naredo et al. [83]	2005	12-joint (wrists, MCP, PIP, knees); GS/pD
Scheel et al. [86]	2005	Three different MCP/PIP scores; GS/pD
Loeuille et al. [87]	2006	7-joint (wrists, MCP, MTP); GS/pD
Hensch et al. [88]	2007	8-joint (MCP, MTP); GS/pD
Iagnocco et al. [89]	2008	10-joint (MCP, PIP, wrist, knee); GS/pD, tenosynovitis, bursitis, erosion
Naredo et al. [90]	2008	12-joint (elbow, wrist, MCP, knee, ankle); GS/pD, tenosynovitis, bursitis
Backhaus et al. [91]	2009	7-joint (wrist, MCP, PIP, MTP); GS/pD, tenosynovitis, erosion
Hammer et al. [92]	2010	78-joint; GS/pD
Perricone et al. [93]	2012	6-joint (wrists, second MCP and knees); synovial effusion, GS/pD
Seymour et al. [94]	2012	10-joint (MCP); GS/pD
Mendonça et al. [95]	2014	7-joint (wrists, MCP, MTF); GS/pD
Yoshimi et al. [96]	2015	8-joint (wrists, knees, MCP); pD
Aga A et al. [99]	2015	6-joint (MCP, PIP,radiocarpal, MTP, extensor carpi ulnaris); GS/pD
Aga A et al. [100]	2015	7-joint/2 tendon (MCP, PIP, radiocarpal, elbow, MTP, tibialis posterior tendon, extensor carpi ulnaris tendon); GS/pD
Janta I et al. [97]	2016	12-joint (wrist, hand,ankle,MTP); B-mode, pD, tenosynovitis

GS gray scale, *pD* power Doppler, *MCP* metacarpophalangeal joint, *PIP* proximal interphalangeal joint, *MTP* metatarsophalangeal joint

Correlation of MSUS parameters with synovial tissue inflammatory activity and cytokines is also an area to be searched. Exploring this field may disclose new physiopathological features of synovitis and also better clarify the meaning of MSUS parameters.

Importantly, MSUS is practical, feasible and less expensive than MRI. Quality of MSUS devices is surely an item of major importance. Better training and competency of sonographers, allied to incorporation of modern ultrasound will certainly improve MSUS performance in the following years [103].

For the time being, a number of points regarding employment of MSUS in rheumatological daily practice demand elucidation. Validity and reproducibility of MSUS scores have still to be improved (interobserver concordance is yet variable – just like clinical assessment). Choice of equipment and selection of parameters to be utilized (pD alone, pD plus GS, bone erosions, cartilage changes, synovial effusion, tenosynovitis, spectral Doppler) are also pending issues.

Since a pD signal can be also seen in healthy joints [104], the adding of spectral Doppler and estimate of RI might provide useful information regarding the flow in synovial membrane (low RI are seen in inflamed joints) [105]. New data on reliability of RI as a measure of synovial flow and microvessel inflammation should be available shortly.

Above all, MSUS score standardization, considering the particularities of each affected joint or tendon, is surely a requirement. Solved these questions, MSUS will consolidate its role as a reliable instrument to complement physical examination, appraise disease activity and monitor response to therapy in RA management.

Key messages

1) MSUS can be nowadays considered a complement to physical exam in patients with rheumatoid arthritis (RA).
2) MSUS seems to correlate well with indexes of disease activity in RA patients. Subclinical synovitis seen on MSUS could help the physician in clinical decisions.
3) Standardization of MSUS techniques is necessary to consolidate the method in clinical practice.

Abbreviations
ACR: American College of Rheumatology; DAS: Disease Activity Score; DAS28: Disease Activity Score in 28 joints; EULAR: Europena League Against Rheumatism; GS: gray scale; IL-17: interleukin 17; IL-6: interleukin 6; MCP: metacarpophangeal joint; MRI: magnetic resonance imaging; MSUS: musculoskeletal ultrasound; MTP: metatarsophalangeal joint; OMERACT: Outcome Measures in Rheumatology; pD: power Doppler; RA: rheumatoid arthritis; TNF: tumor necrosis factor; VEGF: vascular endothelial growth factor

Authors' contributions
AP, HS, JPP, IGS, JAM, MCB and JEF carried out literature search and reviewed the articles. AP and HS wrote the manuscript. JPP, IGS, JAM, MCB and JEF reviewed the manuscript and made adjustments to the text and contributed to update the review. All authors read and approved the final manuscript.

Authors' information
JAM is currently the chief of the "Image in Rheumatology" Committee of the Brazilian Society of Rheumatology.
AP and IGS teach rheumatology fellows on the use of ultrasound in Rheumatology.

Competing interests
The authors declare that they have no competing interests.

Author details
[1]Rheumatology Unit, Nossa Senhora da Conceição Hospital, Porto Alegre, RS, Brazil. [2]Rheumatology Department, Sao Lucas Hospital, Faculty of Medicine of Pontifical Catholic University of Rio Grande do Sul (PUCRS), Av. Ipiranga, 6690/220, Porto Alegre 90610-000, Brazil. [3]Rheumatology Unit, Pontifical Catholic University of Campinas (PUCCAMP), Campinas, SP, Brazil. [4]Rheumatology Research Unit, Instituto de Medicina Molecular, Faculdade de Medicina, Universidade de Lisboa, Lisbon, Portugal. [5]Rheumatology Department, Hospital de Santa Maria, Lisbon Academic Medical Centre, Lisbon, Portugal.

References
1. Scott D, Wolfe F, Huizinga T. Rheumatoid arthritis. Lancet. 2010;376:1094–108.
2. McInnes I, Schett G. Cytokines in the pathogenesis of rheumatoid arthritis. Nat Rev Immunol. 2007;7:429–42.
3. Ohrndorf S, Backhaus M. Pro musculoskeletal ultrasonography in rheumatoid arthritis. Clin Exp Rheumatol. 2015;33:S50–3.
4. Filippucci E, Iagnocco A, Meenagh G. Ultrasound imaging for the rheumatologist. Clin Exp Rheumatol. 2006;24:1–5.
5. Zayat AS, Ellegaard K, Conaghan PG, Terslev L, EM a H, Freeston JE, et al. The specificity of ultrasound-detected bone erosions for rheumatoid arthritis. Ann Rheum Dis. 2015;74:897–903.
6. Iwamoto T, Ikeda K, Hosokawa J, Yamagata M, Tanaka S, Norimoto A, Sanayama Y, Nakagomi D, et al. Prediction of relapse after discontinuation of biologic agents by ultrasonographic assessment in patients with rheumatoid arthritis in clinical remission: high predictive values of total gray-scale and power Doppler scores that represent residual synovial. Arthritis Care Res. 2014;66:1576–81.
7. Pineda C, Reginato AM, Flores V, Aliste M, Alva M, Aragón-Laínez RA, et al. Pan-American league of associations for rheumatology (PANLAR) recommendations and guidelines for musculoskeletal ultrasound training in the Americas for rheumatologists. J Clin Rheumatol. 2010;16:113–8.
8. Colebatch A, Edwards C, Østergaard M, van der Heijde D, Balint P, D'Agostino M, et al. EULAR recommendations for the use of imaging of the joints in the clinical management of rheumatoid arthritis. Ann Rheum Dis. 2013;72:804–14.
9. Andersen M, Ellegaard K, Hebsgaard JB, Christensen R, Torp-Pedersen S, Kvist PH, et al. Ultrasound colour Doppler is associated with synovial pathology in biopsies from hand joints in rheumatoid arthritis patients: a cross-sectional study. Ann Rheum Dis. 2014;73:678–83.
10. Alivernini S, Peluso G, Fedele AL, Tolusso B, Gremese E, Ferraccioli G. Tapering and discontinuation of TNF-α blockers without disease relapse using ultrasonography as a tool to identify patients with rheumatoid arthritis in clinical and histological remission. Arthritis Res Ther. 2016;18:39.
11. Anandarajah A, Thiele R, Giampoli E, Monu J, Seo GS, Feng C, et al. Patients with rheumatoid arthritis in clinical remission manifest persistent joint inflammation on histology and imaging studies. J Rheumatol. 2014;41:2153–60.
12. Takase K, Ohno S, Takeno M, Hama M, Kirino Y, Ihata A, et al. Simultaneous evaluation of long-lasting knee synovitis in patients undergoing arthroplasty

by power Dopplerultrasonography and contrast-enhanced MRI in comparison with histopathology. Clin Exp Rheumatol. 2012;30:85–92.

13. Koski J. Doppler Imaging and Histology of the Synovium. J Rheumatol. 2012;39:452–3.

14. Paleolog EM. The vasculature in rheumatoid arthritis: cause or consequence? Int J Exp Pathol. 2009;90:249–61.

15. Koski JM, Saarakkala S, Helle M, Hakulinen U, Heikkinen JO, Hermunen H. Power Doppler ultrasonography and synovitis: correlating ultrasound imaging with histopathological findings and evaluating the performance of ultrasound equipments. Ann Rheum Dis. 2006;65:1590–5.

16. Koski JM, Saarakkala S, Helle M, Hakulinen U, Heikkinen JO, Hermunen H, et al. Assessing the intra- and inter-reader reliability of dynamic ultrasound images in power Doppler ultrasonography. Ann Rheum Dis. 2006;65:1658–60.

17. Walther M, Harms H, Krenn V, Radke S, Faehndrich TP, Gohlke F. Correlation of power Doppler sonography with vascularity of the synovial tissue of the knee joint in patients with osteoarthritis and rheumatoid arthritis. Arthritis Rheum. 2001;44:331–8.

18. Kitchen J, Kane D. Greyscale and power Doppler ultrasonographic evaluation of normal synovial joints: correlation with pro- and anti-inflammatory cytokines and angiogenic factors. Rheumatology (Oxford). 2015;54:458–62.

19. Ramirez J, Ruiz-Esquide V, Pomes I, Celis R, Cuervo A, Hernandez M, et al. Patients with rheumatoid arthritis in clinical remission and ultrasound-defined active synovitis exhibit higher disease activity and incresed serum levels of angiogenic biomarkers. Arthritis Res Ther. 2014;16:R5.

20. Strunk J, Heineman E, Neeck G, Schmidt KL, Lange U. A new approach to studying angiogenesis in rheumatoid arthritis by means of power Doppler ultrasonography and measurement of serum vascular endothelial growth factor. Rheumatology. 2004;43:1480–3.

21. Terslev L, Torp-Pedersen S, Bang N, Koenig MJ, Nielsen MB, Bliddal H. Doppler ultrasound findings in healthy wrists and finger joints before and after use of two different contrast agents. Ann Rheum Dis. 2005;64:824–7.

22. Klauser A, Frauscher F, Schirmer M, Halpern E, Pallwein L, Herold M, et al. The value of contrast-enhanced color Doppler ultrasound in the detection of vascularization of finger joints in patients with rheumatoid arthritis. Arthritis Rheum. 2002;46:647–53.

23. Fiocco U, Ferro F, Cozzi L, Vezzù M, Sfriso P, Checchetto C, et al. Contrast medium in power Doppler ultrasound for assessment of synovial vascularity: comparison with arthroscopy. J Rheumatol. 2003;30:2170–6.

24. Szkudlarek M, Court-Payen M, Strandberg C, Klarlund M, Klausen T, Østergaard M. Contrast-enhanced power Doppler ultrasonography of the metacarpophalangeal joints in rheumatoid arthritis. Eur Radiol. 2003;13:163–8.

25. Andersen M, Boesen M, Ellegaard K, Christensen R, Söderström K, Søe N, et al. Synovial explant inflammatory mediator production corresponds to rheumatoid arthritis imaging hallmarks: a cross-sectional study. Arthritis Res Ther. 2014;16:R107.

26. Do Prado AD, Bisi MC, Piovesan DM, Bredemeier M, Batista TS, Petersen L, et al. Ultrasound power Doppler synovitis is associated with plasma IL-6 in established rheumatoid arthritis. Cytokine. 2016;83:27–32.

27. Ball E, Gibson D, Rooney AB. Plasma IL-6 levels correlate with clinical and ultrasound measures of arthritis in patients with systemic lupus erythematosus. Lupus. 2014;23:46–56.

28. Brzustewicz E, Bryl E. The role of cytokines in the pathogenesis of rheumatoid arthritis. Practical and potential application of cytokines as biomarkers and targets of personalized therapy. Cytokine. 2015;76:527–36.

29. Baillet A, Gossec L, Paternotte L, Paternotte S, Etcheto A, Combe B, et al. Evaluation of serum Interleukin-6 level as a surrogate marker of synovial inflammation and as a factor of structural progression in early rheumatoid arthritis: results from a French National Multicenter Cohort. Arthritis Care Res (Hoboken). 2015;67:905–12.

30. Fazaa A, Ben Abdelghani K, Abdeladhim M, Laatar A, Ben Ahmed M, Zakraoui L. The level of interleukin-17 in serum is linked to synovial hypervascularization in rheumatoid arthritis. Jt Bone Spine. 2014;81:550–1.

31. Gullick N, Evans H, Church L, Javaraj D, Filer A. Linking power Doppler ultrasound to the presence of Th17 cells in the rheumatoid. PLoS One. 2010;5:e12516.

32. Van der Heijde D, van 't Hof M, van Riel P, Theunisse L, Lubberts E, van Leeuwen M, et al. Judging disease activity in clinical practice in rheumatoid arthritis: first step in the development of a disease activity score. Ann Rheum Dis. 1990;49:916–20.

33. Vlad V, Berghea F, Libianu S, Balanescu A, Bojinca V, Constantinescu C, Abobului M, Predeteanu D, Ionescu R. Ultrasound in rheumatoid arthritis: volar versus dorsal synovitis evaluation and scoring. BMC Musculoskelet Disord. 2011;12:124.

34. Szkudlarek M, Narvestad E, Klarlund M, Court-Payen M, Thomsen HS, Østergaard M. Ultrasonography of the metatarsophalangeal joints in rheumatoid arthritis: comparison with magnetic resonance imaging, conventional radiography, and clinical examination. Arthritis Rheum. 2004; 50:2103–12.

35. Salaffi F, Filippucci E, Carotti M, Naredo E, Meenagh G, Ciapetti A, et al. Inter-observer agreement of standard joint counts in early rheumatoid arthritis: a comparison with grey scale ultrasonography - a preliminary study. Rheumatology (Oxford). 2008;47:54–8.

36. Ogishima H, Tsuboi H, Umeda N, Horikoshi M, Kondo Y, Sugihara M. Analysis of subclinical synovitis detected by ultrasonography and low-field magnetic resonance imaging in patients with rheumatoid arthritis. Mod Rheumatol. 2014;24:60–8.

37. Mendonca J, Yazbek M, Laurindo I, Bertolo M. Wrist ultrasound analysis of patients with early rheumatoid arthritis. Braz J Med Biol Res. 2011;44:11–5.

38. Rezaei H, Torp-Pedersen S, af Klint E, Backheden M, Kisten Y, Gyori N, et al. Diagnostic utility of musculoskeletal ultrasound in patients with suspected arthritis - a probabilistic approach. Arthritis Res Ther. 2014;16:448–55.

39. Ceponis A, Onishi M, Bluestein H, Kalunian K, Townsend J, Kavanaugh A. Utility of the ultrasound examination of the hand and wrist joints in the management of established rheumatoid arthritis. Arthritis Care Res. 2014;66:236–44.

40. Nakagomi D, Ikeda K, Okubo A, Iwamoto T, Sanayama Y, Takahashi K, et al. Ultrasound can improve the accuracy of the 2010 American College of Rheumatology/European league against rheumatism classification criteria for rheumatoid arthritis to predict the requirement for methotrexate treatment. Arthritis Rheum. 2013;65:890–8.

41. Szkudlarek M, Court-Payen M, Strandberg C, Klarlund M, Klausen T, Ostergaard M. Power Doppler ultrasonography for assessment of synovitis in the metacarpophalangeal joints of patients with rheumatoid arthritis: a comparison with dynamic magnetic resonance imaging. Arthritis Rheum. 2001;44:2018–23.

42. Baillet A, Gaujoux-Viala C, Mouterde G, Pham T, Tebib J, Saraux A, Fautrel B, Cantagrel A, Le Loët X, Gaudin P. Comparison of the efficacy of sonography, magnetic resonance imaging and conventional radiography for the detection of bone erosions in rheumatoid arthritis patients: a systematic review and meta-analysis. Rheumatology (Oxford). 2011;50:1137–47.

43. Ten Cate DF, Luime JJ, Swen N, Gerards AH, De Jager MH, Basoski NM. Role of ultrasonography in diagnosing early rheumatoid arthritis and remission of rheumatoid arthritis - a systematic review of the literature. Arthritis Res Ther. 2013;15:R4.

44. Dougados M, DEvauchelle-Pensec V, Ferlet J, Jousse-Joulin S, D'Agostino M, Backhaus M. The ability of synovitis to predict structural damage in rheumatoid arthritis: a comparative study between clinical examination and ultrasound. Ann Rheum Dis. 2013;72:665–71.

45. Brown A, Conaghan P, Karim Z, Quinn M, Ikeda K, Peterfy C, et al. An explanation for the apparent dissociation between clinical remission and continued structural deterioration in rheumatoid arthritis. Arthritis Rheum. 2008;58:2958–67.

46. Peluso G, Michelutti A, Bosello S, Gremese E, Toluso B, Ferraccioli G. Clinical and ultrasonographic remission determines different changes of relapse in early and long standing rheumatoid arthritis. Ann Rheum Dis. 2011;70:172–5.

47. Do Prado AD, Bisi M, Piovesan D, Bredemeier M, Silveira I, Mendonça J, et al. Association of clinical examination with gray scale and power Doppler ultrassonography in established rheumatoid arthritis. J Clin Rheumatol. 2016; in press

48. Yoshimi R, Toyota Y, Tsuchida N, Sugiyama Y, Kunishita Y, Kishimoto D, et al. Considerable discrepancy between Patient's assessment and ultrasonography assessment on the most affected joint in rheumatoid arthritis [abstract]. Arthritis Rheumatol. 2015;67:S10.

49. Filer A, de Pablo P, Allen G, Nightingale P, Jordan A, Jobanputra P. Utility of ultrasound joint counts in the prediction of rheumatoid arthritis in patients with very early synovitis. Ann Rheum Dis. 2011;70:500–7.

50. Smolen J, Van Der Heijde D, St Clair E, Emery P, Bathon J, Keystone E, et al. Predictors of joint damage in patients with early rheumatoid arthritis treated with high-dose methotrexate with or without concomitant infliximab: results from the ASPIRE trial. Arthritis Rheum. 2006;54:702–10.

51. Damjanov N, Radunovic G, Prodanovic S, Vukovic V, Milic V, SimicPasalic K. Construct validity and reliability of ultrasound disease activity score in assessing joint inflammation in RA: comparison with DAS-28. Rheumatology (Oxford). 2012;51:120–8.

52. Dale J, Purves D, McConnachie A, McInnes I, Porter D. Tightening up? Impact of musculoskeletal ultrasound disease activity assessment on early rheumatoid arthritis patients treated using a treat to target strategy. Arthritis Care Res. 2014;66:19–26.

53. Gärtner M, Mandl P, Radner H, Supp G, Machold K, Aletaha D, et al. Sonographic joint assessment in rheumatoid arthritis: associations with clinical joint assessment during a state of remission. Arthritis Rheum. 2013; 65:2005–14.

54. Backhaus T, Ohrndorf S, Kellner H, Strunk J, Hartung W, Sattler H, et al. The US7 score is sensitive to change in a large cohort of patients with rheumatoid arthritis over 12 months of therapy. Ann Rheum Dis. 2013;72:1163–9.

55. Nguyen H, Ruyssen-Witrand A, Gandjbakhch F, Constantin A, Foltz V, Cantagrel A. Prevalence of ultrasound-detected residual synovitis and risk of relapse and structural progression in rheumatoid arthritis patients in clinical remission: a systematic review and meta-analysis. Rheumatology. 2014;53:2110–8.

56. Saleem B, Brown A, Quinn M, Karim Z, Hensor E, Conaghan P, et al. Can flare be predicted in DMARD treated RA patients in remission, and is it important? A cohort study. Ann Rheum Dis. 2012;71:1316–21.

57. Naredo E, Valor L, De la Torre I, Montoro M, Bello N, Martinez-Barrio J, et al. Predictive value of Doppler ultrasound-detected synovitis in relation to failed tapering of biologic therapy in patients with rheumatoid arthritis. Rheumatology. 2015;54:1408–14.

58. Marks J, Holroyd C, Dimitrov B, Armstrong R, Calogeras A, Cooper C, et al. Does combined clinical and ultrasound assessment allow selection of individuals with rheumatoid arthritis for susteined reduction of anti-tumor necrosis factor therapy? Arthritis Care Res. 2015;67:746–53.

59. Gärtner M, Alasti F, Supp G, Mandl P, Smolen J, Aletaha D. Persistence of subclinical sonographic joint activity in rheumatoid arthritis in sustained clinical remission. Ann Rheum Dis. 2015;74:2050–3.

60. Foltz V, Gandjbakhch F, Etchepare F, Rosenberg C, Tanguy M, Rozenberg S, et al. Power Doppler ultrasound, but not low-field magnetic resonance imaging, predicts relapse and radiographic disease progression in rheumatoid arthritis patients with low levels of disease activity. Arthritis Rheum. 2012;64:67–76.

61. Scirè C, Montecucco C, Codullo V, Epis O, Todoerti M, Caporali R. Ultrasonographic evaluation of joint involvement in early rheumatoid arthritis in clinical remission: power Doppler signal predicts short-term relapse. Rheumatol. 2009;48:1092–7.

62. Zufferey P, Möller B, Brulhart L, Tamborrini G, Scherer A, Finckh A, et al. Persistence of ultrasound synovitis in patients with rheumatoid arthritis fulfilling the DAS28 and/or the new ACR/EULAR RA remission definitions: results of an observational cohort study. Joint Bone Spine. 2014;81:426–32.

63. Yoshimi R, Hama M, Takase K, Ihata A, Kishimoto D, Terauchi K, et al. Ultrasonography is a potent tool for the prediction of progressive joint destruction during clinical remission of rheumatoid arthritis. Mod Rheumatol. 2013;23:456–65.

64. da Silva Chakr RM, Brenol JC, Behar M, Mendonça JA, Kohem CL, Monticielo OA, et al. Is ultrasound a better target than clinical disease activity scores in rheumatoid arthritis with fibromyalgia? A case-control study. PLoS One. 2015;10:e0118620.

65. Iagnocco A, Finucci A, Ceccarelli F, Perricone C, Iorgoveanu V, Valesini G. Power Doppler ultrasound monitoring of response to anti-tumour necrosis factor alpha treatment in patients with rheumatoid arthritis. Rheumatology (Oxford). 2015;54:1890–6.

66. Montoro Alvarez M, Chong OY, Janta I, González C, López-Longo J, Monteagudo I, Valor L, et al. Relation of Doppler ultrasound synovitis versus clinical synovitis with changes in native complement component levels in rheumatoid arthritis patients treated with biologic disease-modifying antirheumatic drugs. Clin Exp Rheumatol. 2015;33:141–5.

67. Haavardsholm E, Aga A, Olsen I, Hammer H, Uhlig T, Fremstad H, et al. Aiming for remission in rheumatoid arthritis: clinical and radiographic outcomes from a randomized controlled strategy trial investigating the added value of ultrasonography in a treat-to-target regimen [abstract]. Arthritis Rheumatol. 2015;67:S10.

68. Hart LE, Tugwell P, Buchanan WW, Norman GR, Grace EM, Southwell D. Grading of tenderness as a source of interrater error in the Ritchie articular index. J Rheumatol. 1985;12:716–7.

69. Thompson PW, Hart LE, Goldsmith CH, Spector TD, Bell MJ, Ramsden MF. Comparison of four articular indices for use in clinical trials in rheumatoid arthritis: patient, order and observer variation. J Rheumatol. 1991;18:661–5.

70. Strunk J, Strube K, Rumbaur C, Lange U, Müller-Ladner U. Interobserver agreement in two- and three-dimensional power Doppler sonographic assessment of synovial vascularity during anti-inflammatory treatment in patients with rheumatoid arthritis. Ultraschall Med. 2007;28:409–15.

71. Fodor D, Felea I, Popescu D, Motei A, Ene P, Serban O, Micu M. Ultrasonography of the metacarpophalangeal joints in healthy subjects using an 18 MHz transducer. Med Ultrason. 2015;17:185–91.

72. Filippucci E, da Luz KR, Di Geso L, Salaffi F, Tardella M, Carotti M, et al. Interobserver reliability of ultrasonography in the assessment of cartilage damage in rheumatoid arthritis. Ann Rheum Dis. 2010;69:1845–8.

73. Sant'Ana Petterle G, Natour J, Rodrigues da Luz K, Soares Machado F, dos Santos MF, da Rocha Correa Fernandes A, et al. Usefulness of US to show subclinical joint abnormalities in asymptomatic feet of RA patients compared to healthy controls. Clin Exp Rheumatol. 2013;31:904–12.

74. Luz KR, Furtado R, Mitraud SV, Porglhof J, Nunes C, Fernandes AR, Natour J. Interobserver reliability in ultrasound assessment of rheumatoid wrist joints. ActaReumatol Port. 2011;36:245–50.

75. Szkudlarek M, Court-Payen M, Jacobsen S, Klarlund M, Thomsen HS, Østergaard M. Interobserver agreement in ultrasonography of the finger and toe joints in rheumatoid arthritis. Arthritis Rheum. 2003;48:955–62.

76. Zufferey P, Brulhart L, Tamborrini G, Finckh A, Scherer A, Moller B, et al. Ultrasound evaluation of synovitis in RA: correlation with clinical disease activity and sensitivity to change in an observational cohort study. Jt Bone Spine. 2014;81:222–7.

77. Brulhart L, Ziswiler HR, Tamborrini G, Zufferey P, SONAR/SCQM programmes. The importance of sonographer experience and machine quality with regards to the role of musculoskeletal ultrasound in routine care of rheumatoid arthritis patients. Clin Exp Rheumatol. 2015;33:98–101.

78. Scheel AK, Schmidt WA, Hermann KG, Bruyn GA, D'Agostino MA, Grassi W, et al. Interobserver reliability of rheumatologists performing musculoskeletal ultrasonography: results from a EULAR "train the trainers" course. Ann Rheum Dis. 2005;64:1043–9.

79. Ohrndorf S, Fischer IU, Kellner H, Strunk J, Hartung W, Reiche B, et al. Reliability of the novel 7-joint ultrasound score: results from an inter- and intraobserver study performed by rheumatologists. Arthritis Care Res (Hoboken). 2012;64:1238–43.

80. Bisi M, do Prado A, Rabelo C, Brollo F, da Silveira I, JA M, et al. Articular ultrasonography: interobserver reliability in rheumatoid arthritis. Rev Bras Reumatol. 2014;54:250–4.

81. Vlad V, Berghea F, Iagnocco A, Micu M, Damjanov N, Skakic V, et al. Inter & intra-observer reliability of grading ultrasound videoclips with hand pathology in rheumatoid arthritis by using non- sophisticated internet tools (LUMINA study). Med Ultrason. 2014;16:32–6.

82. Cheung PP, Kong KO, Chew LC, Chia FL, Law WG, Lian TY, Tan YK, Cheng YK. Achieving consensus in ultrasonography synovitis scoring in rheumatoid arthritis. Int J Rheum Dis. 2014;17:776–81.

83. Naredo E, Bonilla G, Gamero F, Uson J, Carmona L, Laffon A. Assessment of inflammatory activity in rheumatoid arthritis: a comparative study of clinical evaluation with grey scale and power Doppler ultrassonography. Ann Rheum Dis. 2005;64:375–81.

84. Carotti M, Salaffi F, Morbiducci J, Ciapetti A, Bartolucci L, Gasparini S, et al. Colour Doppler ultrasonography evaluation of vascularization in the wrist and finger joints in rheumatoid arthritis patients and healthy subjects. Eur J Radiol. 2012;81:1834–8.

85. Wakefield R, Balint P, Szkudlarek M, Fillipucci E, Backhaus M, D'Agostino M. OMERACT 7 Special Interest Group. Musculoskeletal ultrasound including definitions for ultrasonographic pathology. J Rheumatol. 2005;32:2485–7.

86. Scheel AK, Hermann KG, Kahler E, et al. A novel ultrasonografic synovitis scoring system suitable for analyzing finger joint inflammation in rheumatoid arthritis. Arthritis Rheum. 2005;52:733–43.

87. Loeuille D, Sommier JP. ScUSI, an ultrasound inflammatory score, predicts sharp progression at 7 months in RA patients. Arthritis Rheum. 2006;54:S139.

88. Hensch A, Hermann KG. Impact of B mode, power Doppler and contrast enhanced ultrasonography in RA patients on anti-TNF alfa therapy. Arthritis Rheum. 2007;56:S280.

89. Iagnocco A, Filippucci E, Perella C, Ceccarelli F, Cassarà E, Alessandri C, et al. Clinical and ultrasonographic monitoring of response to adalimumabe treatment in rheumatoid arthritis. J Rheumatol. 2008;35:35–40.

Ultrasound and its clinical use in rheumatoid arthritis: where do we...

203

90. Naredo E, Rodríguez M, Campos C, Rodríguez-Heredia JM, Medina JA, Giner E, Martínez O, et al. Validity, reproducibility, and responsiveness of a twelve-joint simplified power dopplerultrasonographic assessment of joint inflammation in rheumatoid arthritis. Arthritis Rheum. 2008;59:515–22.

91. Backhaus M, Ohrndorf S, Kellner H, Strunk J, Backhaus T, Hartung W. Evaluation of a novel 7-joint ultrasound score in daily rheumatologic practise: a pilot project. Arthritis Rheum. 2009;61:1194–201.

92. Hammer HB, Sveinsson M, Kongtorp AK, Kvien TK. A 78-joints ultrasonographic assessment is associated with clinical assessments and is highly responsive to improvement in a longitudinal study of patients with rheumatoid arthritis starting adalimumab treatment. Ann Rheum Dis. 2010;69:1349–51.

93. Perricone C, Ceccarelli F, Modesti M, Vavala C, Di Franco M, Valesini G, Iagnocco A. The 6-joint ultrasonographic assessment: a valid, sensitive-to-change and feasible method for evaluating joint inflammation in RA. Rheumatology (Oxford). 2012;51:866–73.

94. Seymour M, Pétavy F, Chiesa F, Perry H, Lukey PT, Binks M, et al. Ultrasonographic measures of synovitis in an early phase clinical trial: a double-blind, randomized, placebo and comparator controlled phase IIa trial of GW274150 (a selective inducible nitric oxide synthase inhibitor in rheumatoid arthritis. Clin Exp Rheumatol. 2012;30:254-61.

95. Mendonça JA, Yazbek MA, Costallat BL, Gutiérrez M, Bértolo MB. The modified US7 score in the assessment of synovitis in early rheumatoid arthritis. Rev Bras Reumatol. 2014;54:287–94.

96. Yoshimi R, Ihata A, Kunishita Y, Kishimoto D, Kamiyama R, Minegishi K, et al. A novel 8-joint ultrasound score is useful in daily practice for rheumatoid arthritis. Mod Rheumatol. 2015;25:379–85.

97. Janta I, Valor L, De la Torre I, MartínezEstupiñán L, Nieto JC, Ovalles-Bonilla JG, et al. Ultrasound-detected activity in rheumatoid arthritis on methotrexate therapy: which joints and tendons should be assessed to predict unstable remission? Rheumatol Int. 2016;36:387–96.

98. Leng X, Xiao W, Xu Z, Zhu X, Liu Y, Zhao D, et al. Ultrasound7 versus ultrasound12 in monitoring the response to infliximab in patients with rheumatoid arthritis. Clin Rheumatol. 2016;35:587–95.

99. Aga A, Lie E, Olsen I, Hammer H, Uhlig T, van der Heijde D, et al. Development of an ultrasound joint inflammation score for rheumatoid arthritis through a data-driven approach. Arthritis Rheumatol. 2015;67:S10.

100. Aga AB, Hammer HB, Olsen IC, Uhlig T, Kvien TK, van der Heijde D, et al. First step in the development of an ultrasound joint inflammation score for rheumatoid arthritis using a data-driven approach. Ann Rheum Dis. 2016;75:1444–51.

101. Mandl P, Naredo E, Wakefield R, Conaghan P, D'Agostino M, OMERACT Ultrasound Task Force, et al. A systematic literature review analysis of ultrasound joint count and scoring systems to assess synovitis in rheumatoid arthritis according to the OMERACT filter. J Rheumatol. 2011;38:2055–62.

102. Wakefield RJ, D'Agostino MA, Naredo E, Buch MH, Iagnocco A, Terslev L, et al. After treat-to-target: can a targeted ultrasound initiative improve RA outcomes? Ann Rheum Dis. 2012;71:799–803.

103. Gutierrez M, Okano T, Reginato AM, Cazenave T, Ventura-Rios L, Bertolazzi C, Pineda C. Pan-American League Against Rheumatisms (PANLAR) Ultrasound Study Group. New Ultrasound Modalities in Rheumatology. J Clin Rheumatol. 2015;21:427–34.

104. Terslev L, Torp-Pedersen E, Qvistgaard E, von der Recke P, Bliddal H. Doppler ultrasound findings in healthy wrists and finger joints. Ann Rheum Dis. 2004;63:644–8.

105. Vlad V, Micu M, Porta F, Radunovic G, Nestorova R, Petranova T, et al. Ultrasound of the hand and wrist in rheumatology. Med Ultrason. 2012;14:42–8.

28

Characterization of scrotal involvement in children and adolescents with IgA vasculitis

Izabel M. Buscatti[1], Henrique M. Abrão[2], Katia Kozu[1], Victor L. S. Marques[1], Roberta C. Gomes[1], Adriana M. E. Sallum[1] and Clovis A. Silva[3]* ⓘ

Abstract

Objective: To characterize scrotal involvement in children and adolescents with IgA vasculitis.

Methods: A cross-sectional retrospective study included 296 IgA vasculitis (EULAR/PRINTO/PRES criteria) patients, 150/296 (51%) were males and assessed by demographic/clinical/laboratory and treatments. Scrotal involvement was defined by the presence of scrotal edema and/or pain/tenderness in physical examination and/or testicular Doppler ultrasound abnormalities.

Results: Scrotal involvement was observed in 28/150 (19%) IgA vasculitis patients. This complication was evidenced at IgA vasculitis diagnosis in 27/28 (96%). Acute recurrent scrotal involvement was observed in 2/150 (1%) and none had chronic subtype. Further analysis of patients with scrotal involvement at first episode ($n = 27$) compared to those without this complication ($n = 122$) revealed that the median age at diagnosis [4.0 (2.0–12) vs. 6 (1.3–13) years, $p = 0.249$] was similar in both groups. The frequency of elevated serum IgA was significantly lower in IgA vasculitis patients with scrotal involvement versus without this manifestation (18% vs. 57%, $p = 0.017$), whereas glucocorticoid (93% vs. 49%, $p < 0.0001$) and ranitidine use (63% vs. 30%, $p = 0.003$) were significantly higher in the former group.

Conclusions: The scrotal involvement occurred in almost one fifth of IgA vasculitis patients and was commonly evidenced as acute subtype at diagnosis. Scrotal signs/symptoms improved after a prompt use of glucocorticoid and was associated with low frequency of elevated IgA serum levels.

Keywords: IgA vasculitis, Henoch-Schönlein purpura, Scrotal vasculitis, Children, Glucocorticoid, Testicular ultrasound

Background

Immunoglobulin A (IgA) vasculitis previously known as Henoch-Schönlein purpura (HSP), is the most frequent systemic vasculitis of small vessels with IgA dominant immune complexes deposits [1–7]. The most common manifestations at diagnosis are cutaneous, articular, gastrointestinal and renal [1, 2, 4].

Scrotal involvement in children and adolescents with IgA vasculitis is generally acute, resulting in scrotal edema, pain and/or tenderness in physical examination [1, 3, 7–11]. Doppler testicular ultrasound may help to confirm the scrotal involvement and to exclude testicular torsion [7, 12].

In 2010, validated classification criteria for IgA vasculitis were established and proposed by European League Against Rheumatism (EULAR), Paediatric Rheumatology International Trials Organisation (PRINTO) and Paediatric Rheumatology European Society (PRES) [13]. Data of scrotal involvement in IgA vasculitis patients are limited due to the small representation of this complication in previous case reports or case series [1, 3, 5, 8–12] precluding an accurate analysis of associated factors and outcomes in patients with and without this complication, particularly using the EULAR/PRINTO/PRESS IgA vasculitis classification criteria [9].

Therefore, the objective of the present study was to characterize scrotal involvement in children and adolescents with IgA vasculitis, and to evaluate the possible association of demographic data, clinical manifestations,

* Correspondence: clovis.silva@hc.fm.usp.br
[3]Pediatric Rheumatology Unit, Children's Institute, Hospital das Clinicas HCFMUSP, Faculdade de Medicina, Universidade de Sao Paulo, SP, Av. Dr. Eneas Carvalho Aguiar, 647 - Cerqueira César, São Paulo, SP 05403-000, Brazil
Full list of author information is available at the end of the article

laboratorial abnormalities and treatments in patients with and without scrotal involvement.

Methods

Data from 322 children and adolescents with IgA vasculitis followed at the Pediatric Rheumatology Department of our University Hospital during a 32-year period (January 1983 to December 2015) were retrospectively evaluated. Twenty-six patients were excluded due to incomplete data in medical charts. All 296 patients fulfilled IgA vasculitis validated EULAR/PRINTO/PRES classification criteria [13]. Out of them, 150/296 (51%) IgA vasculitis patients were males and were assessed by demographic data, clinical manifestations, laboratory exams and treatments. The Ethics Committee of the University Hospital approved this study. Informed consent was obtained from all participants and their legal guardians.

Scrotal involvement was defined by the presence of scrotal edema and/or pain/tenderness in physical examination and/or testicular Doppler ultrasound abnormalities [3, 9]. Patients with only petechiae or purpuric rash on scrotum were excluded [9]. This manifestation was characterized by three subtypes: acute scrotal involvement, acute recurrent (new presence of scrotal signs/symptoms and/or testicular Doppler ultrasound abnormalities after total recovery) [1] and chronic (presence of scrotal signs/symptoms and/or testicular Doppler ultrasound abnormalities with more than 3 months duration) [14].

The demographic data included: age at diagnosis, disease duration and body mass index (BMI). BMI was defined as weight in kilograms divided by the square of the body height (m^2).

Recurrent purpura/petechiae was considered as new skin lesions after total recovery and persistent purpura/petechiae, as cutaneous lesions persisting for more than one month [1]. Arthritis was defined by joint swelling or joint pain with limitation on motion. Arthralgia was characterized by joint pain without joint edema or limitation on motion [13]. Recurrent arthritis was considered as new joint inflammation after total recovery [1].

Abdominal pain was determined as colicky and diffuse pain with acute onset. Severe abdominal pain was defined as the presence of at least one of them: abdominal angina, bowel intussusception and gastrointestinal bleeding. Recurrence was defined as new abdominal pain after complete resolution [1]. Abdominal Doppler ultrasound was performed to evaluate severe abdominal involvement [1].

Renal involvement was defined by proteinuria > 0.1 g/m^2/day and/or hematuria > 5 red blood cells/high power field or red blood cells casts in the urinary sediment. Nephrotic syndrome was characterized by edema, serum albumin < 2.5 g/L and proteinuria > 1 g/m^2/day [1]. High blood pressure was defined as systolic and/or diastolic blood pressures ≥95th percentile for gender, age and height on ≥3 occasions [15]. Acute kidney injury was determined by sudden increase in serum creatinine above 2 mg/dl [16] or by modified RIFLE (Risk, Injury, Failure, Loss of kidney function and End-stage kidney disease) criteria [17]. Chronic renal disease was defined as structural or functional abnormalities of the kidney for ≥3 months (with or without decreased glomerular filtration rate) or glomerular filtration rate < 60 ml/min/1.73 m^2 for ≥3 months [18]. Renal replacement therapies (hemodialysis, peritoneal dialysis and hemofiltration and renal transplantation) were also assessed. Renal biopsy was performed in all patients with severe nephritis and/or persistent renal alterations.

Neuropsychiatric involvement was defined as the presence of at least one neuropsychiatric manifestation, such as: headaches, seizures, hemiparesis, aphasia, cortical blindness and impaired consciousness [19].

Current treatment data were also recorded: prednisone/prednisolone, intravenous methylprednisolone, ranitidine, intravenous immunoglobulin (IVIG), azathioprine, cyclosporine, intravenous cyclophosphamide (IVCYC) and plasmapheresis.

IgA vasculitis patients were also divided in two groups: with scrotal involvement at first episode and without scrotal involvement.

Statistical analysis

Results were presented as median (range) or mean ± standard deviation for continuous variables and number (%) for categorical variables. Mann Whitney or t tests were used for comparing continuous variables to evaluate the differences between the two study groups (with scrotal involvement at first episode and without scrotal involvement). Fisher's exact test analyzed the differences for categorical variables. For all statistical tests the level of significance was defined as "p" value less than 0.05.

Results

Scrotal involvement (scrotal edema with pain/tenderness) was observed in 28/150 (19%) IgA vasculitis patients during disease course or follow up. Twenty-two of 150 patients (15%) had unilateral involvement and 6/150 (4%) had bilateral involvement. None of the patients had scrotal edema as the first sign/symptom of IgA vasculitis. This complication was evidenced at IgA vasculitis diagnosis in 27/28 (96%). During follow-up, only one of them was diagnosed after one year of disease onset.

Regarding characterization of scrotal involvement subtypes in IgA vasculitis patients: acute subtype was observed in 26/150 (17%), acute recurrent subtype in 2/150 (1%) and none of them had chronic subtype.

Thirteen patients underwent testicular Doppler ultrasound and the findings were described in Table 1. None of them had torsion, atrophy, tumor, necrosis and/or cysts on testicles. All of these 13 IgA vasculitis patients were followed-up, 11 of them remained without scrotal symptoms after total recovery and did not carry-out testicular Doppler ultrasound. Gastrointestinal involvement was observed in 7/13 (54%) IgA vasculitis with testicular abnormalities on ultrasound examination. Two of 13 patients had acute recurrent involvement and were submitted to the second testicular Doppler ultrasound after total recovery, in one month and one year respectively, showing epididymitis-orchitis in both.

Regarding treatment, a short course of prednisolone/prednisone (0.5–2.0 mg/kg/day) was administered in 25/27 (93%), with resolution of scrotal signs/symptoms.

Further analysis of IgA vasculitis patients with scrotal involvement at first episode ($n = 26$) compared to those without this complication ($n = 122$) revealed that the median age at diagnosis [4.0 (2.0–12) vs. 6 (1.3–13) years, $p = 0.249$] and purpura duration [18.5 (5–60) vs. 14 (1–120) days, $p = 0.101$] were similar in both groups. The frequency of elevated serum IgA was significantly lower in IgA vasculitis patients with scrotal involvement versus without this manifestation (18% vs. 57%, $p = 0.017$), whereas glucocorticoid (93% vs. 49%, $p < 0.0001$) and ranitidine use (63% vs. 30%, $p = 0.001$) were significantly higher in the former group (Table 2).

The frequencies of persistent purpura/petechiae, arthritis/arthralgia, abdominal pain, nephritis and neuropsychiatric involvements were also similar in IgA vasculitis patients with scrotal involvement at first episode compared to those without this complication ($p > 0.05$) (Table 2). No differences were evidenced of gastrointestinal involvement in IgA vasculitis patients with scrotal involvement confirmed by testicular Doppler ultrasound compared to those with scrotal involvement that did underwent testicular Doppler ultrasound [7/13 (54%) vs. 12/14 (86%), $p = 0.103$].

None of IgA vasculitis patients had chronic renal disease, underwent renal replacement therapies or died.

Discussion

This study characterized scrotal involvement in IgA vasculitis patients using EULAR/PRINTO/PRES classification criteria [13]. This complication occurred in almost one fifth of male with IgA vasculitis and was commonly evidenced as acute subtype at diagnosis. Acute recurrent involvement was rarely observed. Scrotal signs/symptoms improved after a prompt use of glucocorticoid and was associated with low frequency of elevated IgA serum levels.

The strength of this study was inclusion of IgA vasculitis patients fulfilled the validated classification criteria [13] and use of standardized database to minimize bias. The characterization of scrotal involvement subtypes was also relevant, allowing to differentiate disease severity. However, the main weakness observed herein was the retrospective design, with potential missing data. We also did not evaluate the IgA glycosylation test [20].

The prevalence of acute scrotal involvement in IgA vasculitis patients observed in the present study was similar to other previous reports, ranging from 2 to 32% [1, 8, 9, 21, 22]. Bilateral involvement was observed in 20% of IgA vasculitis patients with scrotal involvement, as observed in Korean patients. Acute scrotal involvement as the first signs/symptoms of disease was also rarely been described [9].

One relevant point reported herein was the evaluation of severity according to scrotal involvements subtypes. Indeed, acute recurrent involvement was rarely evidenced in IgA vasculitis and none of them had complications with chronic scrotal pain and/or edema. These findings suggest a predominant acute and mild/moderate scrotal involvement.

IgA vasculitis is a primary vasculitis characterized by leukocytoclastic vasculitis involving the capillaries (mainly in skin, gastrointestinal and kidneys), with high levels of serum IgA (up to 40%) and deposition of IgA immune complexes in these organs and systems [1, 23, 24]. Rare cases of IgA vasculitis patients also demonstrated deposition of IgA-containing immune complexes in the testicular vessels, supports the notion that testis is a target organ of this systemic vasculitis [25].

Interestingly, elevated serum IgA was lower in IgA vasculitis patients with scrotal involvement, and had similar frequencies of skin, articular, gastrointestinal and renal involvements [1]. These results may be related to different immunopathogenesis mechanisms in patients with autoimmune orchitis. Further studies will be necessary to clarify this point.

Table 1 Testicular Doppler ultrasound findings in 13 IgA vasculitis patients

Testicular Doppler ultrasound findings	$n = 13$
Unilateral scrotal edema with soft tissue thickening, epidydimal swelling with normal blood flow	3 (23)
Bilateral scrotal edema with soft tissue thickening, epidydimal swelling with normal blood flow	3 (23)
Unilateral epidydimal swelling, hydrocele and scrotal wall thickening	5 (39)
Bilateral epidydimal swelling, hydrocele and scrotal wall thickening	2 (15)

Results are presented as n (%), hydrocele - fluids accumulation around testicle

Table 2 Demographic data, clinical manifestations and treatments in patients with scrotal involvement at first episode compared to those without this condition in 149 IgA vasculitis patients

Variables at diagnosis, n (%)	With scrotal involvement (n = 27)	Without scrotal involvement (n = 122)
Demographic data		
Age at diagnosis, years	4.0 (2.0–12.0)	6.0 (1.3–13.0)
Body mass index, kg/m², n = 139	16.4 (13.2–20.3)	16 (12.5–32.7)
Clinical/laboratorial involvements		
Persistent purpura/petechiae, n = 146	6/27 (22)	25/119 (21)
Recurrent purpura/petechiae	7 (26)	20 (16)
Purpura/petechiae duration, days, n = 140	18.5 (5–60)	14 (1–120)
Arthritis/arthralgia	21 (78)	95 (77)
Recurrent arthritis/arthralgia	1 (4)	6 (5)
Arthritis/arthralgia duration, days, n = 100	4 (2–13)	6 (1–113)
Abdominal pain	20 (74)	73 (59)
Recurrent abdominal pain, n = 149	3/26 (12)	16/123 (13)
Severe abdominal pain, n = 92	7/20 (35)	26/72 (36)
Abdominal pain duration, days, n = 83	4.5 (1–40)	5 (1–60)
Gastrointestinal bleeding, n = 149	6/27 (22)	23/122 (19)
Bowel intussusception	0 (0)	1 (0.8)
Nephritis, n = 147	10/27 (37)	56/120 (47)
Arterial hypertension, n = 122	4/22 (18)	16/100 (16)
Nephrotic syndrome, n = 147	0/26 (0)	3/121 (3)
Acute kidney injury, n = 145	0/27 (0)	2/118 (2)
Leukocyturia, n = 146	0/27 (0)	14/119 (12)
Urinary casts, n = 146	2/27 (7)	13/119 (11)
Hematuria, n = 146	7/27 (26)	39/119 (33)
Proteinuria, n = 108	5/17 (29)	34/91 (37)
Neuropsychiatric involvement	0 (0)	1 (1)
Increased serum IgA, n = 76	2/11 (18)	37/65 (57)*
Treatments		
Prednisone	25 (93)	60 (49)*
Intravenous metilprednisolone	0 (0)	1 (1)
Prednisone dose, mg/kg/day, n = 72	2 (0.5–2)	1 (0.2–30)
Glucorticosteroid duration, days, n = 76	47.5 (7–140)	37.5 (1–240)
Ranitidine, n = 149	17/27 (63)	37/122 (30)*
Ranitidine duration, days, n = 57	35 (2–90)	60 (5–425)
Immunosuppressive agents	0 (0)	0 (0)
IVIG	1 (4)	1 (1)

Results are presented as median (minimum value - maximum value) or n (%), increased serum IgA (> 255 mg/dL), *IVIG* - intravenous immunoglobulin, *p value < 0.05 and the other comparisons between two groups were non-significant

IgA vasculitis patients with scrotal involvement had higher frequencies of glucocorticoid and ranitidine use, with resolution of scrotal signs/symptoms. There is clinical expertise guidance for glucocorticoid treatment in this condition [3, 7]. We suggest prompt therapy with prednisone/prednisolone (1-2 mg/kg/day) and then gradually withdrawal from two to four weeks. This management may have minimized the severity and chronicity of this manifestation.

The IgA vasculitis severity, particularly renal and gastrointestinal involvements, was similar between male and female patients [1, 22, 26]. A study from Turkey showed that renal involvement was higher in IgA vasculitis patients with scrotal involvement compared to those without this condition [22], suggesting a more severe and multisystemic disease in male patients.

Scrotal ultrasound was performed in more than 50% of IgA vasculitis of the present study. We suggest to evaluate this exam in all male patients with IgA vasculitis to accurately diagnose scrotal involvement, excluding testicular torsion. Our IgA vasculitis patients were pre-pubertal subjects without testicular complications. In spite of that, additional evaluation of gonadal hormones, sperm and anti-sperm antibodies analysis will be necessary to assess fertility [7].

Conclusion

Scrotal involvement occurred in almost 20% of IgA vasculitis patients and was frequently evidenced as acute subtypes at diagnosis. Scrotal signs/symptoms improved after prompt glucocorticoid use and was associated with low frequency of elevated IgA serum levels.

Acknowledgements
Our gratitude to Ulysses Doria-Filho for the statistical analysis.

Funding
This study was supported by grants from Conselho Nacional de Desenvolvimento Científico e Tecnológico (CNPq 303422/2015-7 to CAS), Fundação de Amparo à Pesquisa do Estado de São Paulo (FAPESP 2015/03756-4 to CAS), Federico Foundation (to CAS) and by Núcleo de Apoio à Pesquisa "Saúde da Criança e do Adolescente" da USP (NAP-CriAd) to CAS.

Authors' contributions
IMB, HMA, KK, VLSM, RCG, AMES, CAS analyzed and interpreted the patient data regarding scrotal involvement in Henoch Shönlein purpura. IMB and CAS were the major contributor in writing the manuscript. All authors read and approved the final manuscript.

Author details
[1]Pediatric Rheumatology Unit, Children's Institute, Hospital das Clinicas HCFMUSP, Faculdade de Medicina, Universidade de Sao Paulo, São Paulo, Brazil. [2]Universidade de Santo Amaro – UNISA, São Paulo, Brazil. [3]Pediatric Rheumatology Unit, Children's Institute, Hospital das Clinicas HCFMUSP, Faculdade de Medicina, Universidade de Sao Paulo, SP, Av. Dr. Eneas Carvalho Aguiar, 647 - Cerqueira César, São Paulo, SP 05403-000, Brazil.

References
1. de Almeida JL, Campos LM, Paim LB, Leone C, Koch VH, Silva CA. Renal involvement in Henoch-Schönlein purpura: a multivariate analysis of initial prognostic factors. J Pediatr. 2007;83:259–66.
2. Ozen S, Acar-Ozen NP. Recent advances in childhood vasculitis. Curr Opin Rheumatol. 2017;29:530–4.
3. Modi S, Mohan M, Jennings A. Acute scrotal swelling in Henoch-Schönlein purpura: case report and review of the literature. Urol Case Rep. 2016;6:9–11.
4. Júnior CR, Yamaguti R, Ribeiro AM, Melo BA, Campos LA, Silva CA. Hemorrhagic vesicle-bullous lesions in Henoch-Schönlein purpura and review of literature. Acta Reumatol Port. 2008;33:452–6.
5. Jauhola O, Ronkainen J, Koskimies O, Ala-Houhala M, Arikoski P, Hölttä T, et al. Clinical course of extrarenal symptoms in Henoch-Schönlein purpura: a 6-month prospective study. Arch Dis Child. 2010;95:871–6.
6. Suehiro RM, Soares BS, Eisencraft AP, Campos LM, Silva CA. Acute hemorrhagic edema of childhood. Turk J Pediatr. 2007;49:189–92.
7. Silva CA, Cocuzza M, Borba EF, Bonfá E. Cutting-edge issues in autoimmune orchitis. Clin Rev Allergy Immunol. 2012;42:256–63.
8. Chamberlain RS, Greenberg LW. Scrotal involvement in Henoch-Schönlein purpura: a case report and review of the literature. Pediatr Emerg Care. 1992;8:213–5.
9. Ha TS, Lee JS. Scrotal involvement in childhood Henoch-Schönlein purpura. Acta Paediatr. 2007;96:552–5.
10. Güneş M, Kaya C, Koca O, Keles MO, Karaman MI. Acute scrotum in Henoch-Schönlein purpura: fact or fiction? Turk J Pediatr. 2012;54:194–7.
11. Verim L, Cebeci F, Erdem MR, Somay A. Henoch-Schönlein purpura without systemic involvement beginning with acute scrotum and mimicking torsion of testis. Arch Ital Urol Androl. 2013;85:50–2.
12. Lim Y, Yi BH, Lee HK, Hong HS, Lee MH, Choi SY, et al. Henoch-Schonlein purpura: ultrasonography of scrotal and penile involvement. Ultrasonography. 2015;34:144–7.
13. Ozen S, Pistorio A, Iusan SM, Bakkaloglu A, Herlin T, Brik R, et al. EULAR/PRINTO/PRES criteria for Henoch-Schönlein purpura, childhood polyarteritis nodosa, childhood Wegener granulomatosis and childhood Takayasu arteritis: Ankara 2008. Part II: final classification criteria. Ann Rheum Dis. 2010;69:798–806.
14. Rottenstreich M, Glick Y, Gofrit ON. Chronic scrotal pain in young adults. BMC Res Notes. 2017;10:241.
15. National High Blood Pressure Education Program Working Group on High Blood Pressure in Children and Adolescents. The fourth report on the diagnosis, evaluation, and treatment of high blood pressure in children and adolescents. Pediatrics. 2004;114:555–76.
16. Chan JC, Williams DM, Roth KS. Kidney failure in infants and children. Pediatr Rev. 2002;23:47–60.
17. Akcan-Arikan A, Zappitelli M, Loftis LL, Washburn KK, Jefferson LS, Goldstein SL. Modified RIFLE criteria in critically ill children with acute kidney injury. Kidney Int. 2007;71:1028–35.
18. National Kidney Foundation. K/DOQI clinical practice guidelines for chronic kidney disease: evaluation, classification, and stratification. Am J Kidney Dis. 2002;39:S1–266.
19. Pacheva IH, Ivanov IS, Stefanova K, Chepisheva E, Chochkova L, Grozeva D, et al. Central nervous system involvement in Henoch-Schonlein Purpura in children and adolescents. Case Rep Pediatr. 2017;2017:5483543.
20. Kiryluk K, Moldoveanu Z, Sanders JT, Eison TM, Suzuki H, Julian BA, et al. Aberrant glycosylation of IgA1 is inherited in both pediatric IgA nephropathy and Henoch-Schönlein purpura nephritis. Kidney Int. 2011;80:79–87.
21. Ben-Sira L, Laor T. Severe scrotal pain in boys with Henoch-Schönlein purpura: incidence and sonography. Pediatr Radiol. 2000;30:125.
22. Tabel Y, Inanc FC, Dogan DG, Elmas AT. Clinical features of children with Henoch-Schonlein purpura: risk factors associated with renal involvement. Iran J Kidney Dis. 2012;6:269–74.
23. Kawasaki Y, Ono A, Ohara S, Suzuki Y, Suyama K, Suzuki J, et al. Henoch-Schönlein purpura nephritis in childhood: pathogenesis, prognostic factors and treatment. Fukushima J Med Sci. 2013;59:15–26.
24. Calvo-Río V, Loricera J, Mata C, Martín L, Ortiz-Sanjuán F, Alvarez L, et al. Henoch-Schönlein purpura in northern Spain: clinical spectrum of the disease in 417 patients from a single center. Medicine. 2014;93:106–13.
25. Zhao L, Zheng S, Ma X, Yan W. Henoch-Schönlein Purpura With Testicular Necrosis: Sonographic Findings at the Onset, During Treatment, and at Follow-up. Urology. 2017;107:223–5.
26. Buscatti IM, Casella BB, Aikawa NE, Watanabe A, Farhat SCL, Campos LMA, et al. Henoch-Schönlein purpura nephritis: initial risk factors and outcomes in a Latin American tertiary center. Clin Rheumatol. 2018;37:1319–24.

29

Assessment of gesture behavior and knowledge on low back pain among nurses

Hisa Costa Morimoto[1], Anamaria Jones[1] and Jamil Natour[1,2]*

Abstract

Background: Low back pain is particularly problematic among nursing professionals. Education is part of the rehabilitation process for low back pain and has been heavily studied. In parallel, gestural behaviors play an important role during the evaluation of the low back pain, especially while performing the activities of daily living. The aim of the present study was to evaluate gesture behavior and knowledge on LBP among nurses with and without LBP and correlate these factors with pain, physical functioning and quality of life.

Methods: An observational, controlled, cross-sectional study was carried out in 120 female nurses: 60 with LBP and 60 without LBP. The two groups were matched for age. The measures used for the evaluation were the Gesture Behavior Test, LBP Knowledge Questionnaire, Numerical Pain Scale for LBP, Roland Morris Disability Questionnaire and the Short Form-36 (SF-36) to assess quality of life.

Results: Mean age in both groups was 31 years. In the group with LBP, the mean Numerical Pain Scale score was 5.6 cm and the mean score on the Roland Morris questionnaire was 2.7. No statistically differences between groups were found regarding the scores of the LBP Knowledge Questionnaire or Gesture Behavior Test ($p = 0.531$ and $p = 0.292$, respectively). Statistically lower scores were found in the group with LBP for the following SF-36 domains: physical functioning ($p < 0.001$), physical role ($p = 0.015$), pain ($p = 0.001$), general health perceptions ($p = 0.015$), vitality ($p < 0.001$) and mental health ($p = 0.001$).

Conclusions: No differences were found when comparing nurses with or without LBP regarding gesture behavior or knowledge on LBP. Nurses with LBP showed a decrease in some domains of quality of life.

Keywords: Low back pain, Nurses, Behavior and patient's knowledge

Background

Low back pain is one of the most painful disorders, it is also a common cause of morbidity and is associated with significant social and economic impact worldwide. Epidemiological studies indicate that the prevalence of low back pain in the general population is between 60 and 80% [1, 2]. The literature reports that 90% of adults will experience back pain at least once in their lives [1, 3].

Low back pain is particularly problematic among nursing professionals in terms of absenteeism and litigation processes; it is also an important source of morbidity in this population. Its prevalence seems to be higher among nurses and nurses' aids than in the rest of the population, ranging between 56 and 90% respectively. Emotional stress, physical and psychosocial factors at work are crucial to the onset of low back pain [4–6].

Flexion, twisting, weight transfer and sudden movements were related to low back pain [7]. Similar findings were observed in another study, considering hoisting associated with spinal twisting, previous injury and excess of weight as risk factors for low back pain in nurses [8].

In 2008, researchers conducted a cross-sectional study of nurses with an average age of 26 years, in which they assessed the risk of developing low back pain due to occupational exposure in new nurses and students [9]. They concluded that over the course of one year in the profession, the risk of experiencing an increase in back pain was 90%, suggesting that the act of transferring patients in bed was detrimental and that preventive strategies should be aimed at this population.

Education is part of the rehabilitation process for low back pain and has been heavily studied. In parallel, gestural behaviors play an important role during the evaluation of the low back pain, especially while performing the activities of daily living (ADLs). Assessment

* Correspondence: jnatour@unifesp.br
[1]Rheumatology Division, Universidade Federal de São Paulo, São Paulo, Brazil
[2]Disciplina de Reumatologia, Rua Botucatu, 740, Sao Paulo, SP 04023-090, Brazil

instruments, such as the low back pain knowledge questionnaire (LKQ) and the gestural behavior test (GBT), were created and validated to expand the ways to evaluate the patient in a more specific manner [10, 11]. Because gestural behavior and knowledge of the disease are important variables in the management of low back pain, the aim of the present study was to evaluate the gestural and knowledge of low back pain in nurses with low back pain and compare with nurses without low back pain, as there are no studies in the literature for this purpose.

Methods

Sample

A hundred twenty nurses from the Hospital Sao Paulo - Universidade Federal de São Paulo / Escola Paulista de Medicina (UNIFESP / EPM) were included: 60 nurses with low back pain and 60 nurses who served as controls without back pain. The nurses in the control group were matched by age with the low back pain group. The study was approved by the Ethics and Research Committee of the University.

Sample size was calculated using GBT as the main parameter, with a standard deviation of 5 points.11 For the determination of a minimal difference of 3 points between groups among healthcare professionals, a 5% α error and a power of 90% were established. The calculation determinate a minimal sample of 60 nurses per group.

The low back pain group included nurses in activity, aged between 22 and 60 years, working in different hospital sectors (wards, emergency room and/or intensive care units) with a minimum workload of 6 h/day who experienced back pain on most days during the last three months, with a report of pain greater than 3 cm on a numerical pain scale (NPS) 0–10 cm. The control group included nurses with the same features but without back pain.

Nurses in situations of dispute, with prior surgery of the spine and/or a current pregnancy, were excluded from the study.

Outcomes

The participants completed an evaluation form with demographic (age, marital status, body mass index), clinical and professional information (disease duration and time since graduation), information's regarding smoking habits and life style and applied assessment tools to specify the level of low back pain. Almost all questionnaires were self-applied, only the GBT evaluation, was done by evaluator not blinded.

The assessment instruments used included the following:

- Gesture Behavior Test (GBT): this test evaluates the gestural behavior of patients with chronic non- specific low back pain. It consists of five functional tasks:

  ○ Task 1: getting out of bed after sleeping;
  ○ Task 2: sweep under the bed;
  ○ Task 3: lift and carry a garbage disposal;
  ○ Task 4: simulate tying shoelaces without help;
  ○ Task 5: organize objects with various weights on shelves of various heights.

Each task is characterized by an instruction, allowing several standardized scoring criteria. The score ranges from 0 to 32, with a higher score indicating a better gestural behavior [11].

- Low Back Pain Knowledge Questionnaire (LKQ): this instrument assesses knowledge about back pain. Composed of 16 questions, divided into the following categories: general aspects, concepts and treatment. The score ranges from 0 to 24 points, with a higher score denoting a better knowledge of low back pain [10].
- Numerical Pain Scale (NPS): this instrument subjectively assesses pain. The nurse quantifies the intensity of low back pain following a line of 0–10 cm, 0 being no pain and 10 being unbearable pain [12].
- Roland Morris Disability Questionnaire (RM): this instrument assesses the functional disability in patients with low back pain. It consists of 24 questions of self - response (yes or no), and the score ranges from zero (no disability) to 24 points (severe disability) [13].
- Short Form - 36 (SF-36): generic questionnaire that assesses quality of life, with 36 items about general health that fall into eight domains: physical functioning, role limitations due to physical health, bodily pain, general health, vitality, social health, emotional health and mental health. The score for each domain ranges from 0 to 100, and higher scores indicate a better quality of life [14].

Statistical analysis

The statistical program SPSS 19.0 was used. The level of significance was set to 0.05.

Descriptive statistics were presented by the frequency and percentage for categorical data and the mean with standard deviation for quantitative data. The Kolmogorov-Smirnov test was applied to assess the normality of the variables. To evaluate the homogeneity of the sample at baseline, chi-square tests, Student t-tests and Mann-Whitney tests were performed. The Spearman correlation test was used to assess the quantitative variables [15, 16].

Results

Table 1 summarizes the mean and standard deviation (SD) of the sociodemographic data, demonstrating the homogeneity of the sample for these parameters. The mean age of total sample was 31.6 years. The groups were similar in terms of age, body mass index (BMI),

Table 1 Sample characteristics

	LBP group N = 60	Control group N = 60	P intergrupo
Age (years)	31,7 ± 7,8	31,6 ± 7,5	0,979[b]
BMI (kg/m²)	24,6 ± 4,9	23,5 ± 3,2	0,518[b]
Marital status	–	–	0,727[a]
Single	39 (65%)	41 (68,3%)	–
Maried	19 (31,7%)	16 (26,7%)	–
Divorced	2 (3,3%)	3 (5,0%)	–
Time since graduation (years)	7,2 ± 6,9	6,6 ± 6,0	0,983[b]
Disease duration (years)	4,2 ± 2,6	–	–
NPS (cm)	5,6 ± 1,7	–	–
Roland Morris	2,7 ± 2,5	–	–

Data presented as mean ± standard deviation or percentage (%)
BMI body mass index, NPS numeric pain scale, p significance value in the comparison between groups
[a]chi-square test
[b]Mann-Whitney

marital status and training time. The mean duration of symptoms in the low back pain group was 4.2 years. Table 1 also shows the NPS and RM scores of the low back pain group.

According to the lifestyle evaluation of the nurses, the groups were homogeneous regarding inactivity ($p = 0.838$) and smoking ($p = 0.679$). The proportions are presented in Table 2.

With respect to the variables of GBT and LKQ, we found no significant differences between the groups ($p = 0.292$ and $p = 0.531$, respectively). The means and standard deviation scores are presented in Table 3.

In the quality of life assessment using the SF-36, there were significant differences between the groups in the following domains: physical functioning ($p = 0.001$), role limitations due to physical health ($p = 0.015$), pain ($p < 0.001$), general health ($p = 0.015$), vitality ($p < 0.001$) and mental health ($p = 0.001$). There were no significant differences between the groups in the areas of social and emotional health (Table 4).

In Table 5 shows the statistically significant correlations between the SF-36 domains, LKQ and GBT scores in the

Table 2 Ratio of sedentary and smoking among nurses

	LBP group N = 60	Control group N = 60	P intergrupo
Sedentary	–	–	0,838
Yes	44 (73,3%)	43 (71,7%)	–
No	16 (26,7%)	17 (28,3%)	–
Smoking	–	–	0,679
Yes	4 (6,7%)	2 (3,3%)	–
No	56 (93,3%)	58 (96,7%)	–

Data presented as n and percentage (%) using the Chi-square test
p significance value in the comparison between groups

Table 3 Scores of the Gestural Behavior Test (GBT) and Low Back Pain Knowledge Questionnaire (LKQ)

	LBP group N = 60	Control group N = 60	P intergrupo
GBT	17,7 ± 3,9	18,5 ± 4,3	0,292
LKQ	–	–	–
General aspects	8,2 ± 1,0	8,0 ± 0,8	0,217
Concept	3,1 ± 1,1	3,1 ± 0,9	0,867
Treatment	8,0 ± 1,8	8,0 ± 1,7	0,781
Total	19,2 ± 3,1	19,1 ± 2,5	0,531

Data presented as mean ± standard deviation using the Mann-Whitney test
GBT gestural behavior test, LKQ low back pain knowledge questionnaire, p significance value in the comparison between groups

control and low back pain groups. No correlations were found between the RM, LKQ and GBT questionnaires.

Discussion

LBP is the most prevalent and costly musculoskeletal disorder worldwide. Studies in nurses with low back pain have reported strong associations among work environment, lifestyle and postural factors [17].

The aim of this study was to evaluate the gestures and knowledge of disease in nurses because the literature indicates that these variables are relevant in the perpetuation and management of low back pain.

Our study evaluated only nurses and not nurses aids. It is known that in Brazil, these professionals have distinct and unique roles, commonly involving activities that require constant movement of the lumbar spine, such as caring for patients in bed and performing transfers. However, a regulation imposed by the Board of Nursing describes the full range of functions for nursing professionals, which includes being exposed to physical and biomechanical factors that can trigger back pain. Therefore, to avoid bias, we chose to only evaluate nurses because each group has a professional profile and distinct function. The study evaluated nurses' aids and nurses within a single group [18].

d'Ericco et al. in 2013, investigated the prevalence of back pain and the association with absenteeism in nurses and concluded that the prevalence was 58.2%, being 55.9% to chronic low back pain and 61.9% to acute low back pain. Relative to the nurses' aids, the prevalence was higher (67.5% among the nurses and 36.4% among the nurses' aids) [19].

Our sample included only women to ensure a homogeneous sample by gender, as male hospital nurses represent a minority. Some of the other studies previously in the literature also opted for a heterogeneous sample by gender [20–22].

The average age of the nurses assessed was 31.7 years. These data are similar to Yip and Jaromi et al. studies

Table 4 Evaluation of the SF-36 demonstrated as mean and standard deviation

	LBP group N = 60	Control group N = 60	P intergrupo
Physical functioning	82,1 ± 16,6	91,8 ± 9,1	< 0,001[a]
Role limitations due to physical health	72,5 ± 32,1	84,2 ± 26,4	0,015[a]
Bodily pain	56,4 ± 16,2	74,0 ± 21,8	< 0,001[a]
General health	74,7 ± 15,6	81,4 ± 14,6	0,015[a]
Vitality	52,1 ± 17,5	64,3 ± 16,0	< 0,001[a]
Social Health	74,8 ± 20,9	80,0 ± 18,7	0,179
Emotional health	72,8 ± 35,0	75,0 ± 30,5	0,970
Mental health	66,5 ± 16,7	75,5 ± 13,1	0,001[a]

Data presented as mean ± standard deviation using the Mann-Whitney test
p significance value in the comparison between groups
[a]Value statistically significant

and are consistent with the literature, which places the age group with the highest incidence of low back pain between 18 and 65 years [23, 24]. A study by Sikiru & Hanifa [22], showed that the prevalence of back pain increased with age. The group < 35 years showed a prevalence of 6.3%; the group 36–45 years showed a prevalence of 27%; and the group > 46 years showed a prevalence of 66.7%.

Other variables, such as physical inactivity and smoking, were also collected to characterize the sample. Physical inactivity and smoking, in association with other variables, have been reported as important factors for increasing the risk of low back pain [25]. In this study, 73% of the nurses were sedentary. In contrast, only 6% of the sample were smokers. In Vieira et al. [21] study, the nurses were less sedentary (55%) but included more smokers (35%). Yip found no significant correlation between inactivity and low back pain in nurses.

The GBT was the instrument chosen to assess the gestural behavior of the nurses. This test was initially created to evaluate the gestures of patients with chronic nonspecific low back pain who have participated in an educational program that typically consists of information on joint protection and energy conservation, as well as advice on spinal anatomy, conservative treatment, medication and disease management.

Importantly, the literature does not describe a specific test for evaluating the gestural behavior of nurses. The GBT does not evaluate gestures performed during the work activities of a nurse but rather those performed while simulating the activities of daily living. We believe that the behaviors that nurses adopt in their day-to-day will also adapt to their work environment.

Although this is a cross-sectional study and does not propose an educational intervention for nurses, it is interesting to evaluate the gestural behavior of this

Table 5 Correlations between of SF-36 domains, the Gestural Behavior Test (GBT) and Low Back Pain Knowledge Questionnaire (LKQ) scores in the control and low back pain groups

SF-36	LKQ -GA	LKQ -Concept	LKQ -Treatment	LKQ - Total	GBT
Control group					
Bodily Pain	NS	0.270 (0.037)	NS	NS	NS
Global health	NS	NS	NS	NS	0.290 (0.024)
Vitality	NS	NS	NS	NS	0.290 (0.049)
LBP group					
Physical functioning	NS	0.258 (0.047)	NS	NS	NS
Bodily pain	0.227 (0.032)	NS	NS	NS	NS
General health	NS	0.312 (0.015)	NS	NS	NS
Social Health	NS	0.269 (0.038)	NS	NS	NS
Emotional health	NS	NS	0.268 (0.038)	NS	NS
Mental health	NS	NS	NS	0.256 (0.048)	NS

Correlations presented were statistically significant (p < 0.05)
LKQ low back pain knowledge questionnaire, GA general aspects, LKQ low back pain knowledge questionnaire, LBP low back pain, NS non significant

population because the relationship between physical factors and low back pain has been heavily discussed in the literature, and to date, no other study has used this instrument.

Regarding the assessment of knowledge of the disease, the only specific questionnaire addressing low back pain in the literature is the LKQ. This is the first study to evaluate the knowledge of low back pain in nurses using the LKQ.

Sikiru & Hanifa evaluated the knowledge of joint protection of the spine in 300 nurses with low back pain using a no validated questionnaire formulated by the authors themselves [22]. They observed that 80 nurses (26.6%) exhibited knowledge about joint protection, whereas 220 (73.3%) had no knowledge on this topic. There was a significant correlation between the knowledge of joint protection of the spine with the incidence of low back pain. In this study, it would be appropriate to use the LKQ that include issues regarding joint protection and energy conservation.

Pain and disability are important variables in the characterization of low back pain. There are many instruments that assess pain and functional disability in low back pain. For pain assessment, the NPS was chosen because of its easy application and improved understanding, and the RM was used to assess functional disability due to its status as a questionnaire widely used in the literature. The nurses presented an average pain level of 5.6 cm (SD = 1.7) and showed no severe disability according to the RM questionnaire. In a study by Lin et al. in 2012, nurses were evaluated using the Visual Analogue Scale (VAS) 0–100 mm, and the average pain level was 41.6 mm [26]. With respect to functional disability, we cannot compare our data with those in the literature because we did not find any studies that evaluated low back pain in nurses and utilized the RM.

The quality of life, assessed using the SF-36, was worse in terms of functional capacity, role limitations due to physical health, bodily pain, general health, vitality and mental health in the low back pain group compared to the control group. Carugno et al. showed similar results to those of our study [27]. The authors used the mental health domain of SF-36 to evaluate 751 nurses and found that nurses with musculoskeletal disorders, including back pain, presented worse mental health. No studies that correlated the SF-36 with the instruments used in our study were found.

Regarding knowledge of disease and gestural behavior, we found no statistical differences between the groups. Regarding the GBT, the total average score in the two groups was 19 points, with a maximum score of 32 points. In a study by Furtado et al., the average score among all patients with low back pain was 16.3, whereas rehabilitation professionals without back pain had a mean score of 26 points. Despite the smaller scores within the general population, these results are similar to those of nurses, indicating a low level of knowledge in this area even among health professionals [11].

Regarding the assessment using the LKQ, the mean score for nurses was 19 points, in a total score of 24 points. Maciel et al. [10] showed that the mean total score of patients with chronic low back pain was 9 points, far below the results observed for our sample.

Based on these results, we believe that both nurses with low back pain and the control group have a good level of knowledge about the important aspects of low back pain but do not use this knowledge in their day-to-day lives, resulting in behaviors that include inappropriate gestures. This line of thought further strengthens the importance and necessity of adopting a behavioral approach during the treatment of chronic nonspecific low back pain that includes disease management, adherence to therapy and conservative treatment, thereby improving both mental and physical behaviors.

Although the nurses showed no difference between gestural behavior and knowledge of the disease, we found positive (weak and moderate) correlations between some SF-36 domains with GBT and LKQ. These data reflect that the two variables are directly related to the quality of life, mainly in the physical aspects and vice versa.

We found no correlation between pain and disability using the GBT and LKQ. Similarly, a study by Furtado et al. [11], found no correlation between pain and GBT. However, our data showed a correlation between RM and GBT. The authors believe that the disability caused by chronic low back pain leads the patient to adopt copping towards protecting and not overloading the spine. It is likely that our results did not agree with those of the study by Furtado et al. because nurses with LBP have only low disability, according to the assessment by RM.

This study has some limitations, among them the small sample, the lack of men in the sample and also the lack of blind evaluator.

We believe that no difference was found between the groups in GBT and LKQ, because the nurses in the low back pain group did not show an important disability. As shown in the results, according to the RM, the nurses were classified as having mild disability. A possible explanation for RM results may be the level of knowledge of the sample, because it is a health professional and because of the classification of low back pain. The study chose to evaluate nurses with chronic low back pain. Perhaps in the acute phase, the results would be different from those presented in the present study. It is important to note that GBT is not specific to assess the disease's impairment. We believe that RM is more sensitive to evaluate this variable.

As seen in the literature, there are few studies evaluating the variables evaluated in our study. Therefore, it is necessary that new controlled studies be carried out in order to deepen the use of these instruments and to corroborate the results of the present study; epidemiological studies with large samples to evaluate the prevalence of low back pain in nurses; and other studies with educational intervention.

Conclusion

Nurses with back pain do not show differences in behavior or in gestural knowledge about back pain when compared to nurses without low back pain. However, nurses with low back pain show less quality of life.

Authors' contributions

All authors contributed to conception and design of the study, analysis and interpretation of data, drafting the article and revising it critically for important intellectual content and final approval of the version to be submitted. HCM and AJ contributed with the data acquisition too.

Competing interests

The authors declare that they have no competing interests.

References

1. Deyo RA, Weinstein JN. Primary care - low back pain. N Engl J Med. 2001; 344(5):363–70.
2. Jaromi M, Nemeth A, Kranicz J, Laczko T, Betlehem J. Treatment and ergonomics training of work-related lower back pain and body posture problems for nurses. J Clin Nurs. 2012;21(11–12):1776–84.
3. Frymoyer JW, Pope MH, Constanza MC, Osen JC, Goggin JE, Wilder DJ. Epidemiologic studies of low back pain. Spine. 1980;5:419–23.
4. Maul I, Laubli T, Klipstein A, Krueger H. Course of low back pain among nurses: a longitudinal study across eight years. Occup Environ Med. 2003;60:497–503.
5. Smedley J, Trevelyan F, Inskip H, Bucle P, Cooper C, Coggon D. Impact of ergonomic intervention on back pain among nurses. Scand J Work Environ Health. 2003;29(2):117–23.
6. Eriksen W, Bruusgaard D, Knardahl S. Work factors as predictors of intense a disabling low back pain; a prospective study of nurses' aides. Occup Environ Med. 2004;61:398–404.
7. Punnet L, Fine LJ, Keyserling WM, Hersen GD, Chaffin DB. Back disorders and nonneutral trunk postures of automobile assembly workers. Scand J of Work, Environ Health. 1991;17(5):337–46.
8. Fuortes LJ, Shi Y, Zhang M, Zwerling C, Schootman M. Epidemiology of back injury in university hospital nurses from review of workers compensation records and a case-control survey. J Occup Med. 1994; 36:1022–6.
9. Mitchell T, O'Sullivan PB, Burnett AF, Straker I, Rudd C. Low back pain chacteristics from undergraduate student to working nurse in Australia: a cross-sectional survey. Int J Nurs Stud. 2008;45(11):1636–44.
10. Maciel SC, Jennings F, Jones A, Natour J. The development and validation of a low back pain knowledge questionnaire – LKQ. Clinics. 2009;64(12):1167–75.
11. Furtado R, Jones A, Furtado RNV, Jennings F, Natour J. Validation of the Brazilian portuguese version of the gesture behavior test for patients with non-specific chronic low back pain. Clinics. 2009;64(2):83–90.
12. Ferraz MB, Oliveira LM, Araujo PM, Atra E, Tugwell P. Crosscultural reability of physicalability dimension of the health assessment questionaire. J Rheumatol. 1990a;17(6):813–7.
13. Nusbaum L, Natour J, Ferraz MB, Goldenberg J. Translation, adaptation and validation of the Roland-Morris questionnaire – Brazil Roland-Morris. Braz J Med Biol Res. 2001;34(2):203–10.
14. Ciconelli RM, Ferraz MB, Santos W, Meinão I, Quaresma MR. Tradução para a língua portuguesa e validação do questionário genérico de avaliação de qualidade de vida SF-36 (Brasil SF-36). Rev Bras Reumatol. 1999;39(3):143–50.
15. Zar JH. Biostatistical analysis. Upper Saddle River: Prentice Hall; 1999.
16. Brunner E, Langer F. Nonparametric análisis of ordered categorical data in designs with longitudinal observations and small sample sizes. Biom J. 2000; 42(6):663–75.
17. Woolf AD, Pfleger B. Burden of major musculoskeletal conditions. Bull World Health Organ. 2003;81(9):646–56.
18. Hartvigsen J, Lauritzen S, Lings S, Lauritzen T. Intensive education combined with low tech ergonomic intervention does not prevent low back pain in nurses. Occup Environ Med. 2005;62:13–7.
19. d'Errico A, Viotti S, Baratti A, Mottura B, Barocelli AP, Tagna M, et al. Low back pain and associated presenteeism among hospital nursing staff. J Ocupp Health. 2013;55(4):276–83.
20. Yip VY. New low back pain in nurses: work activies, work stress and sedentary lifestyle. J Adv Nurs. 2004;46(4):430–40.
21. Vieira ER, Kumar S, Coury HJCG, Narayan Y. Low back problems and possible improvements in nursing jobs. J Adv Nurs. 2006;55(1):79–89.
22. Sikiru L, Hanifa S. Prevalence and risk factors of low back pain among nurses in a typical Nigerian hospital. Afr Health Sci. 2010;10(1):26–30.
23. Leclaire R, Esdaile JM, Suissa S, Rossignol M, Proulx R, Dupuis M. Back school in a first episode of compensated acute low back pain: a clinical trial to assess efficacy and prevent relapse. Arch Phys Med Rehabil. 1996;77(7):673–9.
24. Glomsrod B, Loon JH, Soukup MG, Bo K, Larsen S. (2001). Active back school. Prophylactic management for low back pain: three year follow-up of a randomized controlled trial. J Rehab Med. 2001;33:26–30.
25. Bejia I, Younes M, Jamila HB, Khalfallah T, Bem Salem K, Touzi M, et al. Prevalence and factors associated to low back pain among hospital staff. Joint Bone Spine. 2005;72(3):254–9.
26. Lin PH, Tsai YA, Chen WC, Huang SF. Prevalence, characteristics, and work-related risk factors of low back pain among hospital nurses in Taiwan: a cross-sectional survey. Int J Occup Med Environ Health. 2012;25(1):41–50.
27. Carugno M, Pesatori AC, Ferrario MM, Ferrari AL, Silva FJ, Martins AC, et al. Physical and psychosocial risk factors for musculoskeletal disorders in Brazilian and Italian nurses. Cad Saude Publica. 2012;28(9):1632–42.

30

Endothelial progenitor cells and vascular endothelial growth factor in patients with Takayasu's arteritis

Luiz Samuel Gomes Machado*⬛, Ana Cecilia Diniz Oliveira, Patricia Semedo-Kuriki, Alexandre Wagner Silva de Souza and Emilia Inoue Sato

Abstract

Background: Endothelial progenitor cells (EPCs) are responsible for endothelial damage repair. Takayasu's arteritis (TA) is a chronic inflammatory disease that affects large vessels. The aim of the study was to evaluate the number of EPCs and the levels of vascular endothelial growth factor (VEGF) and the relationship of these variables in patients with TA.

Methods: Thirty women with TA and 30 healthy controls were included. EPCs were assessed by flow cytometry and cell culture and VEGF quantification was performed by commercial ELISA kits.

Results: Ages of patients and controls were similar. The number of EPCs in patients and controls (median (interquartile range) were 0.0073% (0.0081%) vs. 0.0062% (0.0089%), $p = 0.779$ by flow cytometry and 27.0 (42.3) colony forming units (CFUs) vs. 27.0 (20.5) CFUs, $p = 0.473$ by cells culture, respectively. VEGF levels in patients and controls was 274.5 (395.5) pg/ml vs. 243.5 (255.3) pg/ml, $p = 0.460$. There was no difference in the number of EPCs and VEGF level between patients with active and inactive disease. There was a tendency of the number of angioblast-like EPCs in patients taking anti-TNFs to be higher; and in patients using methotrexate to be lower.

Conclusion: No significant difference was found in the quantification of EPCs and VEGF levels in TA patients compared to controls, and no difference was observed between patients with active and inactive disease.

Keywords: Endothelial cells, Vascular endothelial growth factor, Takayasu's arteritis

Background

Takayasu's arteritis (TA) is a chronic granulomatous vasculitis that affects mainly large vessels as aorta and its branches. TA patients also present premature atherosclerosis [1–4], as reported in other inflammatory rheumatic diseases [5, 6]. The pathogenesis of atherosclerosis in this arteritis is likely multifactorial and may be related to inflammatory process of vessels, chronic systemic inflammation and increased traditional cardiovascular risk factors [3, 7, 8]. In some diseases such as systemic lupus erythematosus (SLE) and rheumatoid arthritis (RA), premature atherosclerosis is explained in part by decreased levels of endothelial progenitor cells (EPCs) [9–11].

The EPCs are bone marrow-derived cells that contribute to the reendothelialization of injured vessels, as well as for neovascularization after ischemic injury [12]. These cells are rare [13] and are considered independent predictors of morbidity and mortality in patients with cardiovascular disease [14]. There are two main types of EPCs: angioblast-like EPCs, as assessed by flow cytometry and monocytic EPCs as measured by colony forming units (CFUs) in cell culture [13]. VEGF and stromal cell-derived factor-1 (SDF-1) are hypoxia-induced oxygen-sensitive cytokines [15] and play a key role in the mobilization of EPCs from the bone marrow, maturing these into mature endothelial cells and targeting to sites with ischemic tissue [16, 17].

Studies have shown traditional cardiovascular risk factors reduce the count of EPCs [18–21] while medication as statins [22] and angiotensin converting enzyme inhibitors [23],

* Correspondence: luizmachado67@gmail.com
Rheumatology Division, Escola Paulista de Medicina UNIFESP (Universidade Federal de São Paulo), Rua Doutor Diogo de Faria, 561, apt 12, Vila, Clementin São Paulo-SP CEP: 04037-000, Brazil

neoplastic diseases [24, 25] and aerobic activity [26] increase the count of EPCs.

In relation to rheumatic diseases, most studies have shown a smaller number of EPCs in patients than controls in RA [9, 27, 28], SLE [10, 11, 29–31], thromboangiitis obliterans [32], ANCA-associated vasculitis [33, 34], Kawasaki disease [35] and Behçet's disease [36]. On the contrary, most studies in patients with systemic sclerosis (SSc) showed a greater number of EPCs when compared to controls [37–42].

In 2014, Dogan et al. published the first study evaluating EPCs in TA patients in Turkey and found no significant difference between TA and controls. However, the number of EPCs measured by flow cytometry in patients with active disease was higher than healthy control. Similar results were found for VEGF level [43].

In analogy to other inflammatory rheumatic diseases, we hypothesized that EPCs could also be involved in the physio pathogenesis of TA. The aim of the study was to quantify both angioblast-like and monocytic EPCs and VEGF levels in Brazilian patients with TA, as well to assess the number of EPCs and VEGF levels in relation to disease activity, presence of hypertension and dyslipidemia, and the use of medications.

Methods

This was a cross-sectional study carried out at the Federal University of São Paulo/Hospital São Paulo. All participants signed the consent form approved by the Ethics Committee of the institution. Participants were 30 women with TA, aged between 18 and 50 years, who met the classification criteria for TA of the American College of Rheumatology [44]. The control group consisted of 30 female healthy volunteers matched for age. We excluded patients who were current smokers, individuals with diabetes, end-stage kidney disease, coronary disease, infection, malignancy, with another autoimmune rheumatic disease or who had used cyclophosphamide until three months before the study.

TA activity was assessed by criteria of the National Institute of Health (Kerr' criteria) 1994 [45]. Thirty-five mL of peripheral blood was collected from all participants for cells count, erythrocyte sedimentation rate (ESR), creatinine, glucose and serum cholesterol and triglycerides, as well as to quantify angioblast-like and monocytic EPCs and to measure VEGF levels.

Quantification of angioblast-like EPCs by flow cytometry

Angioblast-like EPCs was quantified from peripheral blood mononuclear cells (PBMCs) isolated through density gradient medium with Ficoll-Paque Plus (GE Healthcare, Uppsala, Sweden) and stored at – 80 °C for 2 to 6 weeks. After thawing, the cells were incubated with 7AAD (Southern Biotechnology Associates Inc., Alabama,

USA), anti-KDR-APC (R & D Systems, Inc., Minnesota, USA), anti-CD34-FITC (Southern Biotechnology Associates Inc.) and anti-CD133-PE (Miltenyi Biotec, California, USA) for 40 min. The quantification of EPCs was performed using a FACS Canto II cytometer (BD Becton Dickinson, California, USA). EPCs were defined as 7AAD-negative, CD34-positive, CD133-positive and KDR-positive lymphmononuclear cells [13]. The percentage of viable cells (7AAD-negative) were similar between patients and controls (50.1 (11.4)% vs 51,0 (14.1)%, respectively; $p = 0.684$).

Analyzes were performed using the Flow-Jo software program (Oregon, USA) acquiring on average, 450,000 events for each sample. The technique of fluorescence minus one (FMO) was used for the final analysis. The EPCs quantification was presented as a percentage of the absolute number of EPCs among viable lymphomononuclear cells.

Quantification of monocytic EPCs by cell culture

Monocytic EPCs was quantified according the literature [13]. PBMCs were incubated in 6-well plates coated with fibronectin (BD - Becton Dickinson) for 48 h at 37 °C. Each well contained 5×10^6 PBMCs suspended in 2 mL of Endocult medium (Stemcell Technologies, Washington, USA) supplemented with penicillin G streptomycin + amphotericin B (Invitrogen, California, USA). After incubation, the supernatant was aspirated, and a new cell count was performed and 1×10^6 cells were added in fibronectin-coated plates with 24 wells (BD - Becton Dickinson) suspended again in endothelial cell medium with antibiotic. Incubation was performed for another 72 h and stained with Giemsa 1% (EMD Chemicals Inc., New Jersey, USA). CFU counts were carried out though of inverted microscope (CK2, Olympus, New York, USA). CFUs were characterized by cell clusters surrounded by elongated and spiculated cells and the results are presenting as number of CFUs.

Confirmation of the endothelial lineage of CFUs

To confirm the endothelial lineage of CFUs, the same procedure for EPCs culture was conducted, with two incubations performed in 48 and 72 h, but in the last incubation fibronectin-coated plates with 24 wells were replaced by glass slides coated with fibronectin (BD BioCoat Fibronectin Coated Coverslips). After 72 hs incubation, coverslips were incubated with 12 µg/mL of 1,1′–dioctadecyl-3,3,3′,3-tetramethyl-indocarbocyanine perchlorate labeled acetylated low-density lipoprotein (Dil-Ac-LDL) (Invitrogen) for 4 h, fixed with methanol and incubated again with 10 µg/mL fluorescein isothiocyanate-conjugated *Ulex europaeus* agglutinin type I (FITC-UEA-I) (Sigma, Missouri, USA) [46]. Both are markers of endothelial lineage cells. Observation and image capture was performed by immunofluorescence-specific microscopy (Carl Zeiss, Oberkochen, Germany) and confirmed that the cells which constituted the UFCs were endothelial lineage cells.

Quantification of VEGF

VEGF dosage was performed by ELISA using a commercial kit (Human, VEGF Quantikine ELISA - R & D Systems) according to manufacturer's manual.

Statistical analysis

Statistical Package for the Sciences (SPSS) version 15.0 (Chicago, USA) was used for statistical analysis. All data were considered having non-normal distribution by Kolmogorov and Shapiro-Wilk tests. Then, data were shown as median and interquartile range. Mann-Whitney U test was used for comparisons regarding the quantification of EPCs and VEGF levels between groups of patients and controls as well as among subgroups of patients. Chi-square and Fisher's exact test were used for comparisons of categorical variables between subgroups of patients. Values of $P < 0.05$ were considered significant and values between 0.05 and 0.10 were considered as a trend toward significance.

Results

The mean age of the patients and controls were comparable (32.5 (15.3) vs. 30.0 (5.3) years; $p = 0.646$). The mean time of diagnosis was 8.3 ± 6.5 years. Twenty-three (76,7%) patients were hypertensive [47], 18 (60%) were dyslipidemic [48] and 8 (27%) were obese (47). As expected the frequency of these variables were higher than in controls (Table 1).

With respect to medication 16 patients were using statins (53.3%), all were using acetyl salicylic acid (100%) and 22 were on some antihypertensive medication (73.3%). In relation to the specific treatment of arteritis, 23 patients (76.7%) were using corticosteroids and 24 were using immunosuppressive drugs and five were using anti-TNF (Table 2). According to Kerr's criteria, nine patients were classified as having active disease (30%).

No significant differences were found when comparing the subgroups of patients with and without disease activity in relation to hypertension, dyslipidemia, and use of statin, antihypertensive drugs, different doses of corticosteroids and different immunosuppressive drugs (Table 2).

EPC count and VEGF dosage in patients and controls

Flow cytometry showed that the proportion of EPCs between lymphomononuclear-viable cells was 0.0073% (0.0081%) in patients and 0.0062% (0.0089%) in controls ($p = 0.779$). In cell culture the mean of colony-forming units of EPCs were 27.0 (42.3) in patients and 27.0 (20.5) CFUs in controls ($P = 0.473$).

There was no difference in VEGF levels between patients and controls (**274.5 (395.5) pg/ml vs. 243.5 (255.3) pg/ml, $p = 0.460$**).

EPCs and VEGF in patients with and without active disease

Quantification of EPCs in cell culture and by flow cytometry, as well as VEGF levels did not differ between patients with and without disease activity (Table 3).

Medications

Comparing the subgroup of patients with and without anti-TNFα, no difference was found in relation to the quantification of monocytic EPCs and VEGF dosage. However, there was a tendency for patients using anti-TNF-α to have a higher number of angioblast-like EPCs (Table 4).

The use of methotrexate did not affect the quantification of EPCs by cell culture or VEGF dosage. However, we observed a tendency of patients using this medication to have a lower number of EPCs assessed by flow cytometry (Table 5).

There was no difference in the number of angioblast-like and monocytic EPCs when comparing subgroups of patients with and without use of leflunomide, statins and different doses of prednisone (data not shown).

Table 1 Demographic and clinical characteristics of the Takayasu's arteritis patients and controls

Variables	Takayasu's arteritis patients (30)	Controls (30)	p
mean age (years)	(32.5 (15.3)	30.0 (5.3)	0.646
mean time of diagnosis (years)	8.3 ± 6.5	–	
Skin color	White:18 (60%) Not White:12 (40%)	White: 20 (66%) Not White: 10 (34%)	0,592
patients with disease activity	9	–	
obesity (BMI > 30)	8 (27%)	1 (3%)	0,01
Hypertension	23 (76%)	2 (6%)	0,001
dyslipidemia	18 (60%)	4 (13%)	0,001

BMI Body Mass Index

Table 2 Frequency of hypertension, dyslipidemia, and use of medication in patients with and without Takayasu's arteritis activity

Variables	Without activity N = 21 N (%)	With activity N = 9 N (%)	p
Hypertension	16 (76.2)	07 (77.8)	1.00
Dyslipidemia	12 (57.1)	06 (66.7)	0.704
Statins	11 (52.4)	05 (55.6)	1.00
ACE inhibitors	10 (47.6)	05 (55.6)	1.00
ARB	02 (9.5)	01 (11.1)	1.00
Beta-blockers	05 (23.8)	04 (44.4)	0.389
Calcium channel blockers	05 (23.8)	03 (33.3)	0.666
Acetyl salicylic acid	21 (100)	09 (100)	1.00
Prednisone	16 (76.2)	07 (77.8)	0.166
	Dose ≤5 mg: 06 (37.5)	Dose ≤5 mg: 0	
	Dose > 5 mg: 10 (62.5)	Dose > 5 mg: 07 (100)	
Immunosuppressive drugs	17 (80,9)	07 (77,7)	1,00
	Leflunomide: 06 (35)	Leflunomide: 05 (71,4)	0,225
	Methotrexate: 09 (53)	Methotrexate: 01(14,2)	0,204
	Azathioprine: 02 (12)	Azathioprine: 01 (14,2)	1,00
users of anti-TNF	03 (14,2)	02 (22,2)	0,622

ACE angiotensin-converting enzyme, ARB angiotensin receptor blocker
TNF tumor necrosis factor

Hypertension and dyslipidemia

There were no differences in the number of angioblast-like and monocytic EPCs, as well as the levels of VEGF when compared TA patients with and without hypertension and dyslipidemia (data not shown).

Discussion

Contrary to our expectation, and in opposition of the only one study in the literature [43], in the present study TA patients showed no significant difference compared to healthy women with respect to quantification of EPCs by flow cytometry, which evaluates angioblast-like EPCs or by cells culture with early growth, which evaluates monocytic EPCs. There was also no significant difference in relation to VEGF dosage between groups.

TA is a chronic inflammatory disease associated with elevated levels of several inflammatory cytokines [49, 50]. In our previous study TA patients with active disease showed increased TNF and IL-6 levels compared to inactive [51]. Many studies have evaluated EPCs in other rheumatic diseases. Holmen et al. (33) showed than the numbers of EPC colony-forming units are lower in patients with active granulomatosis with polyangiitis (GPA) as compared with those in remission and healthy individuals, probably caused by high levels of IL-8, epithelial neutrophil activating peptide-78 (ENA-78), macrophage inflammatory protein-1α (MIP-1α), and growth-related oncogene-α (GRO-α) found in supernatants from patients with active disease. Patients with RA also have a lower number of EPCs than healthy individuals [9, 27, 28], however in RA, different than SLE, the cytokine responsible for the reduction of these cells seems to be TNF-α [52, 53]. Since TA is

Table 3 EPCs and VEGF in Takayasu's arteritis patients with and without disease activity

Variables	With activity N = 09 Median (IQ)	Without activity N = 21 Median (IQ)	p
Monocytic EPCs (number of CFUs)	27.0 (40.0)	27.0 (43.0)	0.929
Angioblast-like EPCs (%)	0.0038 (0.0067)	0.0074 (0.0118)	0.326
VEGF (pg/ml)	279.0 (625.0)	272.0 (295.0)	0.657

IQ Interquartil Range
EPCs endothelial progenitor cells
VEGF vascular endothelial growth factor

Table 4 EPCs and VEGF in Takayasu's arteritis patients users and nonusers of anti-TNF

Variables	With anti-TNF N = 5 Median (IQ)	Without anti-TNF N = 25 Median (IQ)	p
Monocytic EPCs (number of CFUs)	49.0 (59.5)	27.0 (39.0)	0.706
Angioblast-like EPCs (%)	0.0108 (0.0068)	0.0038 (0.0079)	0.085
VEGF (pg/ml)	272.0 (478.0)	277.0 (453.0)	0.787

IQ Interquartil Range
EPCs endothelial progenitor cells
VEGF vascular endothelial growth factor

Table 5 EPCs and VEGF in Takayasu's arteritis patients users and nonusers of methotrexate

VARIABLES	With methotrexate N = 10 Median (IQ)	Without methotrexate N = 20 Median (IQ)	p
Monocytic EPCs - (number of CFUs)	27.5 (34.3)	27.0 (43.2)	0.746
Angioblast-like EPCs - (%)	0.0033 (0.0065)	0.0088 (0.0098)	0.061
VEGF (pg/ml)	217.5 (419.8)	293.0 (442.3)	0.286

IQ Interquartil Range
EPCs endothelial progenitor cells
VEGF vascular endothelial growth factor

a chronic inflammatory disease, where increased levels of TNF-α and other cytokines are also described [49, 50], we expected to find lower numbers of EPCs in this vasculitis.

The absence of the difference in the quantification of EPCs between TA patients and healthy controls can be explained, in part, by the balancing between intrinsic factors of Takayasu's arteritis, some of them that inhibit the formation of EPCs and others that stimulate their formation. Among the inhibiting factors, the most relevant are the chronic inflammatory nature of this disease [49, 50] and the high prevalence of hypertension and dyslipidemia. Regarding stimulatory factors, the most important is the chronic ischemic state observed in this arteritis [45]. Chronic ischemic states, such as those that occur in systemic sclerosis (SSc), promote the increase of EPCs [37–42]. Del Papa et al. [40, 41] reported a significant increase in VEGF, a cytokine-induced hypoxia, in SSc patients [15], which was associated with elevated levels of EPCs, thus showing the importance of hypoxia as a stimulator of EPCs. Although SSc and TA affect vessels with different caliber, ischemia/chronic hypoxia also can occur in TA, which could, in theory, contribute to the increase in EPCs. Usually TA patients with severe arterial stenosis/occlusion present collateral arteries formation that needs the presence of VEGF and EPCs.

The concomitant presence of inflammation and ischemia in TA may also explain the lack of difference in the levels of VEGF compared to controls. Inflammation, beyond reducing the number of EPCs, may be at least partially responsible by the reduction in VEGF serum levels, as observed in SLE patients [29]. Ischemia, in turn, can raise levels of this angiogenic cytokine, a situation found in systemic sclerosis [40, 41].

To assess the influence of inflammation on the quantification of EPCs, we analyzed subgroups of patients divided according to disease activity and no difference was observed between patients classified as active and inactive disease using Kerr's criteria. We know these criteria fail in the characterization of disease activity [44], but there is no criterion considered ideal. Therefore, the

formation of subgroups may not have been adequate, which may have affected the outcome.

The Dogan study [43] found no difference of EPC between TA patients and controls, however they found a higher EPC number measured by cytometry, in subgroup of active disease comparing to controls. They also found higher levels of VEGF in TA patients with active disease than controls. This study presented a different patient's profile. Their patients were older, and smoker, diabetes and coronary disease were not excluded, for other hand our patients had higher frequency of dyslipidemia and hypertension. However, all these conditions are associated with lower EPC number and cannot explain the difference between studies. Although sample size and the methods to EPC measuring were similar, some difference between our and their study could be due to the ethnic variability. They did not evaluated the monocytic EPC by culture, than we could not compare with our result.

As several TA patients had factors known to influence the quantification of EPCs, we made comparative analysis between patients with and without hypertension and dyslipidemia, and no difference was observed between these subgroups. This results are according with Dogan study, which also did not find differences between patients with and without cardiovascular risk factor. One possible explanation for these results is that the majority of hypertensive and dyslipidemic patients were using medications, such as statins and ACE inhibitors, and studies have shown that the use of these medications increases quantification of EPCs [22, 23].

There was a tendency of increased angioblast-like EPCs in the subgroup of TA patients using anti-TNFα therapy, suggesting the importance of inhibition of this cytokine to increase EPCs. In RA patients, Ablin et al. [53] reported increased number of EPCs, assessed by cell culture, after infliximab use. Furthermore, Grisar et al. [52] demonstrated in vitro that cultured EPCs in the presence of TNFα showed reduced formation of CFUs.

The subgroup of TA patients using methotrexate showed a trend to have fewer angioblast-like EPCs when compared to patients without this medication. Only one study assessed the effect of methotrexate in cultured EPCs, observing an increase in apoptosis of those cells. [27]. This may be a possible mechanism to explain our data.

The limitations of our study were: a) a small sample due to the rarity of the disease; b) the use of frozen cells for cell counts, reducing the number of lymphomononuclear-viable cells, however, there was no difference in the percentage of viable cells between patients and controls, and; c) the cross-sectional design to assess disease activity and effect of medication. Ideally, a prospective study would better evaluate the effect of these variables.

Conclusion

In conclusion, no significant difference was found in the quantification of EPCs and VEGF levels in TA patients compared to controls, and no difference was observed between patients with active and inactive disease.

Acknowledgements

To our study group of autoimmune rheumatic diseases - Frederico Augusto Gurgel Pinheiro MD, Olívia Barbosa MD, Henrique Ataíde Mariz MD and Edgard Torres dos Reis Neto MD and to Neusa Pereira Silva,PhD.

Funding

This work was supported by FAPESP (São Paulo Research Foundation) [grant number 2009/15987-0].

Authors' contributions

LSGM did a literature review, wrote the article and participated in flow cytometry and cell culture; ACDO did the clinical evaluation of patients; PSK developed the standardization of flow cytometry and cell culture; AWSS support in statistical analysis and bibliographic review; EIS idealized the project and did revision of the manuscript. All authors read and approved the final manuscript.

Competing interests

The authors declare that they have no competing interests.

References

1. Filer A, Nicholls D, Corston R, Carey P, Bacon P. Takayasu arteritis and atherosclerosis: illustrating the consequences of endothelial damage. J Rheumatol. 2001;28:2752-3.
2. Hotchi M. Pathological studies on Takayasu arteritis. Heart Vessel. 1992;7:11-7.
3. Seyahi E, Ugurlu S, Cumali R, Balci H, Seyahi N, Yurdakul S, et al. Atherosclerosis in Takayasu arteritis. Ann Rheum Dis. 2006;65:1202-7.
4. Sharma S, Sharma S, Taneja K, Gupta AK, Rajani M. Morphologic mural changes in the aorta revealed by CT in patients with nonspecific aortoarteritis (Takayasu's arteritis). Am J Roentgenol. 1996;167:1321-5.
5. Shoenfeld Y, Gerli R, Doria A, Matsuura E, Cerinic MM, Ronda N, et al. Accelerated atherosclerosis in autoimmune rheumatic diseases. Circulation. 2005;112:3337-47.
6. Haque S, Mirjafari H, Bruce IN. Atherosclerosis in rheumatoid arthritis and systemic lupus erythematosus. Curr Opin Lipidol. 2008;19:338-43.
7. Souza AWS, Mariz HA, Neto ETR, Arraes AED, Silva NP, Sato EI. Risk factors for cardiovascular disease and endothelin-1 levels in Takayasu arteritis patients. Clin Rheumatol. 2009;28:379-83.
8. Carvalho JF, Bonfá E, Bezerra MC, Pereira RMR. High frequency of lipoprotein risk levels for cardiovascular disease in Takayasu arteritis. Clin Rheumatol. 2009;28:801-5.
9. Grisar J, Aletaha D, Steiner CW, Kapral T, Steiner S, Seidinger D, et al. Depletion of endothelial progenitor cells in the peripheral blood of patients with rheumatoid arthritis. Circulation. 2005;111:204-11.
10. Lee PY, Li Y, Richards HB, Chan FS, Zhuang H, Narain S, et al. Type I interferon as a novel risk factor for endothelial progenitor cell depletion and endothelial dysfunction in systemic lupus erythematosus. Arthritis Rheum. 2007;56:3759-69.
11. Westerweel PE, Luijten RKMA, Hoefer IE, Koomans HA, Derksen RHWM, Verhaar MC. Haematopoietic and endothelial progenitor cells are deficient in quiescent systemic lupus erythematosus. Ann Rheum Dis. 2007;66:865 70.
12. Asahara T, Murohara T, Sullivan A, Silver M, van der Zee R, Li T, et al. Isolation of putative progenitor endothelial cells for angiogenesis. Science. 1997;275:964-7.
13. Distler JH, Allanore Y, Avouac J, Giacomelli R, Guiducci S, Moritz F, et al. EULAR Scleroderma Trials and Research group. EULAR scleroderma trials and research group statement and recommendations on endothelial precursor cells. Ann Rheum Dis. 2009;68(2):163-8.
14. Werner N, Kosiol S, Schiegl T, Ahlers P, Walenta K, Link A, et al. Circulating endothelial progenitor cells and cardiovascular outcomes. N Engl J Med. 2005;353:999-1007.
15. Distler JH, Wenger RH, GassmannM KM, Hirth A, Gay S, et al. Physiologic responses to hypoxia and implications for hypoxia-inducible factors in the pathogenesis of rheumatoid arthritis [review]. Arthritis Rheum. 2004;50:10-23.
16. Kalka C, Masuda H, Takahashi T, Gordon R, Tepper O, Gravereaux E, et al. Vascular endothelial growth factor gene transfer augments circulating endothelial progenitor cells in human subjects. Circ Res. 2000;86:1198-202.
17. Yamaguchi J, Kusano KF, Masuo O, Kawamoto A, Silver M, Murasawa S, et al. Stromal cell-derived factor-1 effects on ex vivo expanded endothelial progenitor cell recruitment for ischemic neovascularization. Circulation. 2003;107:1322-8.
18. Vasa M, Fichtlscherer S, Aicher A, Adler K, Urbich C, Martin H, et al. Number and migratory activity of circulating endothelial progenitor cells inversely correlate with risk factors for coronary artery disease. Circ Res. 2001;89:E1-7.
19. Tepper OM, Galiano RD, Capla JM, Kalka C, Gagne PJ, Jacobowitz GR, et al. Human endothelial progenitor cells from type II diabetics exhibit impaired proliferation, adhesion, and incorporation into vascular structures. Circulation. 2002;106:2781-6.
20. Zhou B, Ma FX, Liu PX, Fang ZH, Wang SL, Han ZB, et al. Impaired therapeutic vasculogenesis by transplantation of OxLDL-treated endothelial progenitor cells. J Lipid Res. 2007;48:518-27.
21. Kondo T, Hayashi M, Takeshita K, Numaguchi Y, Kobayashi K, Iino S, et al. Smoking cessation rapidly increase circulating progenitor cells in peripheral blood in chronic smokers. Arterioscler Thromb Vasc Biol. 2004;24:1442-7.
22. Vasa M, Fichtlscherer S, Adler K, Aicher A, Martin H, Zeiher AM, et al. Increase in circulating endothelial progenitor cells by statin therapy in patients with stable coronary artery disease. Circulation. 2001;103:r21-6.
23. Min TQ, Zhu CJ, Xiang WX, Hui ZJ, Peng SY. Improvement in endothelial progenitor cells from peripheral blood by ramipril therapy in patients with stable coronary artery disease. Cardiovasc Drugs Ther. 2004;18:203-9.
24. Bhaskar A, Gupta R, Kumar L, Sharma A, Sharma MC, Kalaivani M, et al. Circulating endothelial progenitor cells as potential prognostic biomarker in multiple myeloma. Leuk Lymphoma. 2012;53(4):635-40.
25. Naik RP, Jin D, Chuang E, Gold EG, Tousimis EA, Moore AL, et al. Circulating endothelial progenitor cells correlate to stage in patients with invasive breast cancer. Breast Cancer Res Treat. 2008;107(1):133-8.
26. Laufs U, Urhausen A, Werner N, Scharhag J, Heitz A, Kissner G, et al. Running exercise of different duration and intensity: effect on endothelial progenitor cells in healthy subjects. Eur J Cardiovasc Prev Rehabil. 2005;12:407-14.
27. Herbrig K, Haensel S, Oelschlaegel U, Pistrosch F, Foerster S, Passauer J. Endothelial dysfunction in patients with rheumatoid arthritis is associated with a reduced number and impaired function of endothelial progenitor cells. Ann Rheum Dis. 2006;65(2):157-63.
28. Egan CG, Caporali F, Garcia-Gonzalez E, Galeazzi M, Sorrentino V. Endothelial progenitor cells and colony-forming units in rheumatoid arthritis: association with clinical characteristics. Rheumatology (Oxford). 2008;47(10):1484-8.
29. Denny MF, Thacker S, Mehta H, Somers EC, Dodick T, Barrat FJ, et al. Interferon-alpha promotes abnormal vasculogenesis in lupus: a potential pathway for premature atherosclerosis. Blood. 2007;110(8):2907-15.
30. Moonen JR, de Leeuw K, van Seijen XJ. Reduced number and impaired function of circulating progenitor cells in patients with systemic lupus erythematosus. Arthritis Res Ther. 2007;9(4):R84.
31. Baker JF, Zhang L, Imadojemu S, Sharpe A, Patil S, Moore JS, et al. Circulating endothelial progenitor cells are reduced in SLE in the absence of coronary artery calcification. Rheumatol Int. 2012;32(4):997-1002.
32. Katsuki Y, Sasaki K, Toyama Y, Ohtsuka M, Koiwaya H, Nakayoshi T, et al. Early outgrowth EPCs generation is reduced in patients with Buerger's disease. Clin Res Cardiol. 2011;100(1):21-7.

33. Holmén C, Elsheikh E, Stenvinkel P, Qureshi AR, Pettersson E, Jalkanen S, et al. Circulating inflammatory endothelial cells contribute to endothelial progenitor cell dysfunction in patients with vasculitis and kidney involvement. J Am Soc Nephrol. 2005;16:3110–20.

34. Závada J, Kideryová L, Pytlík R, Vanková Z, Tesar V. Circulating endothelial progenitor cells in patients with ANCA-associated vasculitis. Kidney Blood Press Res. 2008;31(4):247–54.

35. Kuroi A, Imanishi T, Suzuki H, Ikejima H, Tsujioka H, Yoshikawa N, et al. Clinical characteristics of patients with Kawasaki disease and levels of peripheral endothelial progenitor cells and blood monocyte subpopulations. Circ J. 2010;74(12):2720–5.

36. Fadini GP, Tognon S, Rodriguez L, Boscaro E, Baesso I, Avogaro A, et al. Low levels of endothelial progenitor cells correlate with disease duration and activity in patients with Behçet's disease. Clin Exp Rheumatol. 2009;27(5):814–21.

37. Nevskaya T, Bykovskaia S, Lyssuk E, Shakhov I, Zaprjagaeva M, Mach E, et al. Circulating endothelial progenitor cells in systemic sclerosis: relation to impaired angiogenesis and cardiovascular manifestations. Clin Exp Rheumatol. 2008;26(3):421–9.

38. Avouac J, Juin F, Wipff J, Couraud PO, Chiocchia G, Kahan A, et al. Circulating endothelial progenitor cells in systemic sclerosis: association with disease severity. Ann Rheum Dis. 2008;67(10):1455–60.

39. Yamaguchi Y, Okazaki Y, Seta N, Satoh T, Takahashi K, Ikezawa Z, et al. Enhanced angiogenic potency of monocytic endothelial progenitor cells in patients with systemic sclerosis. Arthritis Res Ther. 2010;12(6):R205.

40. Del Papa N, Colombo G, Fracchiolla N, Moronetti LM, Ingegnoli F, Maglione W, et al. Circulating endothelial cells as a marker of ongoing vascular disease in systemic sclerosis. Arthritis Rheum. 2004;50(4):1296–304.

41. Del Papa N, Cortiana M, Comina DP, Maglione W, Silvestri I, Maronetti Mazzeo L, et al. Endothelial progenitor cells in systemic sclerosis: their possible role in angiogenesis. Reumatismo. 2005;57(3):174–9.

42. Tinazzi E, Dolcino M, Puccetti A, Rigo A, Beri R, Valenti MT, et al. Gene expression profiling in circulating endothelial cells from systemic sclerosis patients shows an altered control of apoptosis and angiogenesis that is modified by iloprost infusion. Arthritis Res Ther. 2010;12(4):R131.

43. Dogan S, Piskin O, Solmaz D, Akar S, Gulcu A, Yuksel F, et al. Markers of endothelial damage and repair in Takayasu arteritis: are they associated with disease activity? Rheumatol Int. 2014;34:1129–38.

44. Arend WP, Michel BA, Bloch DA, Hunder GG, Calabrese LH, Edworthy SM, et al. The American College of Rheumatology 1990 criteria for the classification of Takayasu arteritis. Arthritis Rheum. 1990;33:1129–34.

45. Kerr GS, Hallahan MS, Giordano J, Leavitt RY, Fauci AS, Rotten M, et al. Takayasu arteritis. Ann Intern Med. 1994;120:919–29.

46. Churdchomjan W, Kheolamai P, Manochantr S, Tapanadechopone P, Tantrawatpan C, U-pratya Y, et al. Comparison of endothelial progenitor cell function in type 2 diabetes with good and poor glycemic control. BMC Endocr Disord. 2010;10:5.

47. Malachias MVB, Barbosa ECD, Martim JF, et al. 7th Brazilian guideline of arterial hypertension. Arq Bras Cardiol. 2016;107(3 Suppl 3):79–83.

48. Xavier HT, Izar MC, Faria Neto JR, et al. V Brazilian guidelines on dyslipidemia and the prevention of atherosclerosis. Arq Bras Cardiol. 2013;101(4 Suppl 1):1–20.

49. Tripathy NK, Chauhan SK, Nityanand S. Cytokine mRNA repertoire of peripheral blood mononuclear cells in Takayasu's arteritis. Clin Exp Immunol. 2004;138:369–74.

50. Park MC, Lee SW, Park YB, Lee SK. Serum cytokine profiles and their correlations with disease activity in Takayasu's arteritis. Rheumatology (Oxford). 2006;45(5):545–8.

51. Arraes AED, Souza AWS, Mariz HA, et al. F-Fluorodeoxyglucose positron emission tomography and serum cytokines and matrix metalloproteinases in the assessment of disease activity in Takayasu's arteritis. Rev Bras Reumatol. 2016;56(4):299–308.

52. Grisar J, Aletaha D, Steiner CW, Kapral T, Steiner S, Säemann M, et al. Endothelial progenitor cells in active rheumatoid arthritis: effects of tumour necrosis factor and glucocorticoid therapy. Ann Rheum Dis. 2007;66:1284–8.

53. Ablin JN, Boguslavski V, Aloush V, Elkayam O, Paran D, Caspi D, et al. Effect of anti-TNF alpha treatment on circulating endothelial progenitor cells (EPCs) in rheumatoid arthritis. Life Sci. 2006; 17;79(25):2364–9

s

31

Prevalence and factors associated with diagnosis of early rheumatoid arthritis in the South of Brazil

Rafael Kmiliauskis Santos Gomes[1,2,4*], Ana Carolina de Linhares[3] and Lucas Selistre Lersch[3]

Abstract

Background: Rheumatoid arthritis (RA) is an autoimmune inflammatory disease characterized by peripheral and symmetrical polyarthritis. It can be divided into Very Early Rheumatoid Arthritis (VERA) diagnosed up to 3 months of symptoms and late onset (Late Early Rheumatoid Arthritis – LERA), diagnosed between 3 and 12 months. Currently, it is recommended to evaluate the patient with joint symptoms as early as possible, and the first 12 weeks of manifestations represent the ideal phase for the diagnosis, favoring a better evolution of the treatment. The present study aimed to determine the prevalence of early diagnosis of rheumatoid arthritis, mean time of diagnosis and to determine possible associated factors in the municipality of Blumenau, Santa Catarina, Brazil.

Methods: A cross-sectional study using the 1987 American College of Rheumatology diagnostic criteria to select patients attended at primary or secondary health care units in Blumenau, Santa Catarina, southern Brazil, in 2014. Diagnostic time was verified by self-report of the time elapsed between the onset of symptoms and the diagnosis made by a rheumatologist. To test the associations, the chi-square test, the Wald linear trend test and the Poisson regression analysis were used.

Results: The mean time of diagnosis was 28 months. The prevalence of diagnosis up to 3 and 12 months was 27. 7% and 64.8%, respectively. Obesity was associated with time diagnosis in both periods. The 0–4 years category of the variable education was associated only with the period up to 12 months.

Conclusion: The mean time of diagnosis was similar to the national context. Among socioeconomic factors, lower education was associated with the diagnosis of late onset RA. The anthropometric variable presented a progressive increase in the prevalence due to the longer time to diagnosis.

Keywords: Rheumatoid arthritis, Prevalence, Diagnosis, Epidemiology

Background

Rheumatoid arthritis (RA) is an inflammatory autoimmune disease characterized by peripheral and symmetric polyarthritis [1]. It can be divided into Very Early Rheumatoid Arthritis (VERA) diagnosed up to 3 months of symptoms and late onset (Late Early Rheumatoid Arthritis - LERA), diagnosed between 3 and 12 months [2]. It is estimated that the disease affects between 0.5 and 1% of the adult world population. Its complications can lead to deformity and destruction of joints, due to the erosion of bone and cartilage [3]. These complications can cause severe joint damage with loss of functional capacity, so the importance of early diagnosis and immediate treatment [4].

Currently, it is recommended to evaluate a patient with joint symptoms as early as possible, since the critical period of the first 12 weeks of manifestations represents the ideal phase for the diagnosis, favoring a better evolution of the treatment [5, 6],. Despite this, the world reality differs from that recommended. In Saudi Arabia, an average time of approximately 30 months was verified [7], whereas in England, the ERAN study found a period of approximately 4 months for the diagnosis [8]. In Brazil, a study from São Paulo verified that the average

* Correspondence: gomesmed2002@ibest.com.br
[1]Specialty Center of the City of Blumenau, Blumenau, Santa Catarina State (SC), Brazil
[2]Specialty Center of the City of Brusque, Brusque, SC, Brazil
Full list of author information is available at the end of the article

waiting time between the beginning of the symptoms and rheumatologic evaluation was on average 39 months[9] This situation could be modified with early referral to the specialist and immediate diagnosis of the disease [10].

A Canadian study showed that younger, higher socioeconomic level and female subjects consulted more quickly with specialists, so they were diagnosed earlier [11]. Another study, conducted in Venezuela, showed a significant difference in diagnosis time between private and public health centers. This demonstrates that several factors influence the establishment of the diagnostic interval and initiation of therapy in patients with RA [12].

The prognostic consequences of diagnostic delay may be irreversible, such as deformities and functional limitation by persistent inflammation and progressive joint damage [13]. One can also cite the presence of work incapacity [9] and for daily tasks [14]. Another consequence would be the greater refractoriness of conventional synthetic disease-modifying antirheumatic drugs (csDMARD), leading to an increased risk of immunobiological use, depending on the severity and progression of the disease [15]. This would increase the costs of drug treatment, mainly affecting the Unified Health System (SUS) [16].

The present study aimed to determine the prevalence of early diagnosis of rheumatoid arthritis, the mean time of diagnosis and to determine possible associated factors in the city of Blumenau, Santa Catarina, Brazil.

Methods

This cross-sectional, population-based study was conducted between July 2014 and January 2015 with individuals 20 years of age or older with rheumatoid arthritis according to the American College of Rheumatology criteria of 1987, of both sexes, resident in the municipality of Blumenau, southern region of Brazil.

The formula for calculating the sample size required to estimate the prevalence of an event in a simple random sample was used considering the following parameters: 0.5% RA prevalence (1110 patients), 50% prevalence of exposure and unknown outcome, 5% sample error and 95% confidence level. The participants were recruited from all primary care centers (Unidades Básicas de Saúde – UBS), the specialty outpatient clinic and the specialty pharmacy of the municipality. Sample loss occurred when households were visited twice, once on the weekend and again in the evening, and no resident was at home, the resident had moved or refused to participate in the study on both occasions. The data collection team consisted of a local supervisor docente and 8 medical academics of the Regional University of Blumenau (Universidade Regional de Blumenau – FURB) previously trained to conduct structured interviews at

home and, if necessary, by telephone. Quality control was performed in 20% of respondents, who were interviewed for the second time using a short questionnaire.

The dependent variable was the diagnostic time of rheumatoid arthritis analyzed in two periods: up to 3 months and 12 months. The independent variables were defined as: a) demographic factors: sex, age in completed years, ranging from 20 to 39, 40-49 for adults and ≥ 60 years for the erderly b) socioeconomic factors: education in years of completed study, divided into 0–4, 5–8 and ≥ 9 years, current monthly personal income in minimum wages before diagnosis of the disease categorized in the first tertile (lowest), second tertile and third tertile (highest); c) anthropometric factors: body mass index (BMI - kg / m^2) subdivided according to the World Health Organization (WHO) in ≤ 24.9 for ideal weight, between 25 and 29.9 for overweight and ≥ 30 for obesity; d) disease-related factors: total disease time in months diagnosed by the rheumatologist, categorized between 0 and 24 months and > 24 months of disease, type of medical care in the last 12 months, classified in three groups, the Unified Health System (Sistema Único de Saúde – SUS; free, public healthcare system), Public-Private Healthcare (supplementary healthcare system), and the private healthcare (fee-for-service care) defined according to the Ministry of Health (Ministério da Saúde – MS), number of consultations with rheumatologist in the last 12 months, categorized between 0 and 2 and ≥ 3 consultations, current use of cs DMARD, current use of biological disease-modifying antirheumatic drugs (bDMARD) - tumor necrosis factor inhibitors / TNFi (adalimumab, etanercept, infliximab), HAQ (Health Assessment Questionnaire), ranging from 0 to 1 (mild impairment), 1.1 to 2 (moderate) and 2.1 to 3 (severe), the presence of bone erosions in the radiography of hands; and e) labor factor: current professional situation (working, health insurance, disability retirement, retirement for time of service).

The data was entered in a system developed for this study with output in the format of the excel table and later the final file was exported to Stata 10.0 program (Stata Corp., College Station, USA). The variables of interest were analyzed for their distributions using average, standard deviation, median for continuous variables; and frequency and percentage for the categorical ones.

To test the association between symptom time and diagnosis of rheumatoid arthritis in months with independent variables, the chi-square test and, where appropriate, Wald's linear trend test were used. Then, the Poisson regression analysis was performed to verify the association of the factors studied with the dependent variable, estimating the crude and adjusted prevalence ratios (PR), the respective 95% confidence intervals and the value of p.

Table 1 Description of the sample and the prevalence of the diagnostic time of up to 3 and 12 months of symptons according to the independente variables in patients with rheumatoid arthritis of Blumenau, Santa Catarina, Brazil, 2014

Variables	Sample		Diagnostic up to 3 months			Diagnostic up to 12 months		
	N	%	Prevalence(%)	CI 95%	p	Prevalence(%)	CI 95%	p
Total	296	100,0	27,7%	(22,5–32,8)		64,8%	(59,3-70,3)	
Sex (n = 296)					0,098[a]			0,708[a]
Male	48	16,2	37,5	(23,2-51,7)		62,5	(48,2-76,7)	
Female	248	83,8	25,8	(20,3–31,2)		65,3	(59,3-71,2)	
Age in years (n = 287)					0,227[b]			0,893[b]
20–39	16	5,6	12,5	(5, 7–30,7)		62,5	(35,8-89,1)	
40–59	146	50,9	26,7	(19,4–33,9)		65,7	(57,9-73,5)	
≥ 60	125	43,5	29,6	(21,5–37,7)		64,1	(55,4-72,5)	
Education in completed years (n = 284)					0,447[b]			0,093[b]
0–4	106	37,3	27,4	(18,6–36,2)		70,5	(61,5-79,5)	
5–8	76	26,7	21,1	(11,6–30,4)		64,4	(53,4-75,4)	
> 9	102	35,9	32,1	(23,1- 41,1)		59,4	(49,9-68,9)	
Current monthly personal income in minimum wages (n = 248)					0,799[b]			0,493[b]
Third tertile (higher)	82	33,1	28,5	(18,7–38,4)		59,5	(48,8-70,2)	
Second tertile	82	33,1	25,6	(15,9–35,2)		65,8	(55,3-76,3)	
First tertile (lower)	84	33,8	26,8	(17,1–36,6)		64,6	(54,1-75,2)	
Body mass index (Kg/m^2) (n = 285)					0,012[b]			0,001[b]
≤ 24,9	110	38,6	36,3	(27,2–45,4)		75,4	(67,2-83,6)	
25–29,9	113	39,7	24,7	(16,7–32,8)		61,9	(52,8-71,1)	
≥ 30	62	21,7	19,3	(9,2–29,3)		51,6	(38,8-64,4)	
Type of service in the last 12 months (n = 269)					0,166[b]			0,515[b]
Public healthcare system	113	42,1	23,8	(15,9–31,8)		64,6	(55,7-73,4)	
Supplementary healthcare system	84	31,2	27,3	(17,7–37,1)		65,4	(55,2-75,7)	
Fee-for-service care	72	26,7	33,3	(22,3-44,3)		69,9	(58,6-80,2)	
Total number of consultations with a rheumatologist in the last 12 months (n = 281)					0,165[b]			0,069[b]
0–1	42	15,0	33,3	(18,4-48,2)		69,1	(54,4-83,6)	
2–3	126	44,9	23,0	(15,5 –30,4)		58,7	(50,0-67,4)	
≥ 4	113	40,1	30,9	(22,3–39,6)		69,9	(61,3-78,4)	
Disease time in months (n = 235)					0,193[a]			0,102[a]
0–24	37	15,7	37,8	(21,4-54,2)		75,6	(61,1-90,1)	
> 24	198	84,3	27,2	(21,1-33,5)		61,6	(54,7-68,4)	
Use of cs DMARD (n = 296)					0,396[a]			0,994[a]
Yes	202	68,2	29,2	(22,8-35,5)		64,8	(58,2-71,4)	
No	94	31,7	24,4	(15,6-33,3)		64,8	(55,1-74,7)	
Use of TNFi (ADA + ETA+IFX) (n = 288)					0,960[a]			0,592[a]
Yes	75	26,1	28,0	(17,5-38,4)		61,3	(50,1-72,6)	
No	213	73,9	27,6	(21,6-33,7)		64,7	(58,3-71,2)	
HAQ (n = 165)					0,904[b]			0,211[b]
0–1 (mild)	65	39,4	24,6	(13,8-35,3)		55,3	(42,9-67,7)	
1,1–2 (moderate)	59	35,7	32,2	(19,9-44,4)		69,4	(57,3-81,5)	
2,1–3 (severe)	41	24,9	24,3	(10,6-38,1)		65,8	(50,7-81,0)	

Table 1 Description of the sample and the prevalence of the diagnostic time of up to 3 and 12 months of symptons according to the independente variables in patients with rheumatoid arthritis of Blumenau, Santa Catarina, Brazil, 2014 *(Continued)*

Variables	Sample		Diagnostic up to 3 months			Diagnostic up to 12 months		
	N	%	Prevalence(%)	CI 95%	p	Prevalence(%)	CI 95%	p
Presence of radiological changes (erosions) in hands (n = 237)					0,814[a]			0,665[a]
No	89	37,5	26,9	(17,5–36,3)		66,2	(56,2-76,3)	
Yes	148	62,5	28,3	(21,1–35,7)		63,5	(55,6-71,3)	
Current professional situation (237)					0,325[b]			0,132[b]
Working	77	32,5	23,3	(13,7 – 33,1)		59,7	(48,5 – 70,9)	
Health insurance	29	12,2	24,1	(7,5 – 40,7)		55,1	(35,9 – 74,4)	
Disability retirement	65	27,5	27,6	(16,5 – 38,8)		60,1	(47,7 – 77,2)	
Retirement for time of service	66	27,8	30,3	(18,9 – 41,6)		72,2	(61,9 – 83,7)	

csDMARD conventional synthetic disease-modifying antirheumatic drugs, *TNFi* tumor necrosis factor inhibitors *ADA* adalimumab, *ETA* etanercept, *IFX* infliximab, *HAQ* health assessment questionnaire; CI 95%: confidence interval of 95%
[a]Chi-square test [b]Wald's linear trend test

For the input in the final model, all the variables that presented a value of $p < 0.20$ in the crude analysis were taken into account. The regression model adjusted for those variables that maintained the value of $p \leq 0.05$ or adjusted the final model. For the inclusion of the variables in the regression model, the researchers chose sequentially to include the variables: demographic, socioeconomic, anthropometric, related to the disease and professional situation.

This research was submitted to the research ethics committee of the University of São Paulo (USP) and FURB (protocol n°.339 / 13 and 133/12, respectively) and approved; all participants signed the informed consent form.

Results

A total of 336 patients were identified. After excluding deceased patients and those who refused to participate in the study or patients without data for any variable, 296 patients were included in the study.

The majority of the sample consisted of females (83.8%) and adults (50.9%) with mean age and standard deviation (SD) of 58.1 years (SD: 11.5), ranging from 27 to 89 years. Regarding education, the majority of patients had 0 to 4 years of completed study (37.3%), with a mean of 7.7 years (SD: 4.4). Regarding the disease-related characteristics, the mean disease duration was 126 months (SD: 100), ranging from 0 to 420, mean HAQ of 1.3 (SD: 0.8) and that the majority of the population was using cs DMARD (68.2%). The majority of individuals presented overweight BMI, mean of 26.6 kg / m² (SD: 4.9).

Regarding the factors related to the diagnosis time, it was observed that the sex variable, for diagnosis up to 3 months, prevailed among males; for diagnosis up to 12 months in the female sex. In relation to age, for diagnosis up to 3 months, preponderated in the population of 60 years or more; and for 12 months, from 40 to 59 years. Regarding education, individuals with more than 9 years of study predominated, for diagnosis up to 3 months; for diagnosis up to 12 months, the population with 0 to 4 years of study. Patients with a diagnosis established up to 3 months had income in the third tertile (highest), and for 12 months in the second tertile (intermediate). Regarding the variables related to the disease, it was observed that individuals who had a disease time of less than 24 months had a higher prevalence of early diagnosis for both periods. In addition, there was a progressive increase in the prevalence of obese individuals over time. Regarding the total number of consultations with rheumatologists in the last 12 months, the majority of patients diagnosed up to 3 months had 0 to 1 consultation, and those diagnosed up to 12 months, consumed a greater number of consultations, 4 or more (Table 1).

It was verified in the crude regression analysis that the dependent variable up to 3 months showed a tendency of association with sex and age, whereas education only for up to 12 months. Regarding the anthropometric variable, it was observed that in the two time intervals analyzed, the BMI was associated with the category of values ≥ 30, since the longer the diagnosis, the greater the prevalence of obese individuals. The care performed by the SUS showed an associative tendency of lower prevalence with diagnosis in the very early period of the disease in relation to the private care. Patients diagnosed in both periods used fewer consultations than the reference category (2 to 3 visits in 12 months). Regarding the current professional situation, among the patients diagnosed up to 12 months, there was a trend of increasing form 11% to 34% in the health insurance in relation to the patients who remained working. Of the individuals diagnosed for up to 3 months, 16% had a prevalence of disease time greater than 24 months, whereas for the interval of up to 12 months, the prevalence increased to 57%.

Table 2 Crude and adjusted regression analysis of diagnostic time up to 3 months and independent variables in patients with rheumatoid arthritis in Blumenau, Santa Catarina, Brazil, 2014

Variables	Crude analysis			Adjusted analysis		
	(PRc)	CI 95%	p	(PRa)	CI 95%	p
Sex (n = 296)			0,146			0,154**
Male	0,84	(0,6-1,0)		0,85	(0,6-1,0)	
Female	1			1		
Age in years (n = 287)			0,200			0,267**
20–39	1			1		
40–59	0,83	(0,6-1,0)		0,84	(0,6-1,0)	
≥ 60	0,80	(0,6-1,0)		0,81	(0,6-1,0)	
Education in completed years (n = 284)			0,459*			0,314**
0–4	0,93	(0,7-1,1)		0,90	(0,7-1,0)	
5–8	1,08	(0,9-1,2)		1,07	(0,9-1,2)	
> 9	1			1		
Current monthly personal income in minimum wages (n = 248)			0,801*			0,622**
Third tertile (higher)	1			1		
Second tertile	1,01	(0,8-1,2)		1,01	(0,8-1,2)	
First tertile (lower)	0,97	(0,8-1,1)		0,95	(0,7-1,1)	
Body mass index (Kg/m^2) (n = 285)			0,010			0,031
≤ 24,9	1			1		
25–29,9	1,18	(0,9-1,4)		1,16	(0,9-1,4)	
≥ 30	1,26	(1,0-1,5)		1,23	(1,0-1,5)	
Type of servicee in the last 12 months (n = 269)			0,177			0,623**
Public healthcare system	0,87	(0,7-1,0)		0,95	(0,7-1,1)	
Supplementary healthcare system	0,95	(0,8-1,1)		0,96	(0,8-1,1)	
Fee-for-service care	1			1		
Total number of consultations with a rheumatologist in the last 12 months (n = 281)			0,165			0,163**
0–1	0,86	(0,6-1,1)		0,85	(0,6-1,0)	
2–3	1			1		
≥ 4	0,89	(0,7-1,0)		0,89	(0,7-1,0)	
Disease time in months (n = 235)			0,247*			0,605**
0–24	1			1		
> 24	1,16	(0,8-1,5)		1,07	(0,8-1,3)	
Use of csDMARD (n = 296)			0,383*			0,283**
Yes	1			1		
No	1,06	(0,9-1,2)		1,12	(0,9-1,3)	
Use of TNFi (ADA + ETA+IFX) (n = 288)			0,960*			0,277**
Yes	0,99	(0,8-1,1)		0,88	(0,7-1,0)	
No	1			1		
HAQ (n = 165)			0,901*			0,587**
0–1 (mild)	1			1		
1,1–2 (moderate)	0,89	(0,7-1,1)		0,86	(0,6-1,1)	
2,1–3 (severe)	1,01	(0,8-1,2)		0,92	(0,6-1,3)	

Table 2 Crude and adjusted regression analysis of diagnostic time up to 3 months and independent variables in patients with rheumatoid arthritis in Blumenau, Santa Catarina, Brazil, 2014 *(Continued)*

Variables	Crude analysis			Adjusted analysis		
	(PRc)	CI 95%	p	(PRa)	CI 95%	p
Presence of radiological changes (erosions) in hands (n = 237)			0,814*			0,306**
No	1			1		
Yes	0,98	(0,8-1,1)		1,13	(0,8-1,4)	
Current professional situation (237)			0,324*			0,637**
Working	1			1		
Health insurance	0,99	(0,7-1,2)		0,99	(0,7 – 1,4)	
Disability retirement	0,94	(0,7-1,1)		0,89	(0,6 – 1,1)	
Retirement for time of service	0,91	(0,7-1,1)		0,95	(0,7 – 1,2)	

csDMARD conventional synthetic disease-modifying antirheumatic drugs, *TNFi* tumor necrosis factor inhibitors, *ADA* adalimumab, *ETA* etanercept, *IFX* infliximab, *HAQ* health assessment questionnaire, *PRc* crude prevalence ratio, *PRa* adjusted prevalence ratio; CI 95%: confidence interval of 95%
* Value of $p > 0,20$ excluded from the adjusted analysis. ** Value of $p > 0,05$ excluded of final model

In the adjusted analysis, the variables sex, age, total number of consultations, time of disease and current professional situation lost power of association with both diagnostic periods, excluded from the final model. The BMI remained in the final model in the two periods represented by the obesity category, respectively, with a prevalence of 23% and 107% higher in relation to the ideal weight patient. The variable education remained in the model for the diagnosis period up to 12 months, with 59% higher prevalence in the category of 0–4 years of study. (Tables 2 and 3).

Discussion

The present study observed that the mean time from onset of symptoms to diagnosis was 28 months. The prevalence of the diagnosis of very early rheumatoid arthritis was 27.7%, whereas in the late initial period it was 64.8%. Although the majority of the patients received the diagnosis up to 12 months, the others presented a great diagnostic delay, which increased the mean time of diagnosis of the disease.

The research identified that the lower educational level of the patient was directly related to the diagnosis later than 12 months. Also, there was a progressive increase in the prevalence of obesity between the diagnostic periods.

Previous studies conducted in other Brazilian cities showed a diagnostic time of approximately 8 [17], 12 [18] and 39 months [9], showing that the present study is within the national intervals, and presented similarity to a study in Brasília, whose time was 27 months [19]. The international literature offers a variety of data, such as a mean time of 6 months in European countries [20], 30 months in Saudi Arabia [7] and up to 33 months in Colombia [21]. These data show that there are contributing factors for the diagnostic time that differ according to locality. The prevalence of patients diagnosed in the

first 3 months of the symptoms is in line with both national (35.3%) [17] and international data, which show values of 1–50% [22] and 32–38% [23]. The prevalence found in the period was found to be better than that found in Sri Lanka (0.7%) [24], but worse than that found in Uruguay (45%) [25] and Norway (50%) [26].

Possible association factors with RA diagnosis time, including social and demographic profile, were analyzed. It was observed that the sex and age of the patients were not related to the dependent variables, as was found in studies carried out in Belgium [27], Norway [26] and England [28] and contrary to a Canadian study that states that women and younger individuals have less diagnostic time [29]. In the present study, patients with less years of study had a later diagnosis, this data contradicts Venezuelan and Canadian literature, where there was no association with this variable [12, 30]. This may occur due to the possible relationship of lower education and income; and consequent greater use of the public health system, which generates more waiting for consultation with a specialist. In Blumenau, this waiting time for consultation is up to 2 months (unpublished data).

It is known that obesity is a frequent condition in patients with RA [31, 32]. According to the present study, when we compared patients with a later diagnosis in relation to the very early, they were more strongly associated with BMI. For the authors' knowledge, this is the first article to demonstrate this association and should be confirmed in the future research. As justification, it is suggested that patients with greater time to diagnosis have more difficulty controlling the disease and therefore use more drugs, such as glucocorticoid, which may influence the weight gain [33]. The result could also occur due to a more advanced disease, which leads to greater disability, favoring the sedentary lifestyle and increased BMI of the patient.

Table 3 Crude and adjusted regression analysis of diagnostic time up to 12 months and independent variables in patients with rheumatoid arthritis in Blumenau, Santa Catarina, Brazil, 2014

Variables	Crude analysis			Adjusted analysis		
	(RPc)	CI 95%	p	(PRa)	CI 95%	p
Sex ($n = 296$)			0,704*			0,720**
Male	1,08	(0,7-1,6)		1,07	(0,7-1,6)	
Female	1			1		
Age in years ($n = 287$)			0,894*			0,920**
20–39	1			1		
40–59	0,91	(0,4-1,7)		0,91	(0,6-1,7)	
≥ 60	0,96	(0,4-1,8)		0,95	(0,4-1,8)	
Education in completed years ($n = 284$)			0,094			0,041
0–4	1,37	(0,9-2,1)		1,59	(1,1 - 2, 5)	
5–8	1,20	(0,7-1,8)		1,29	(0,7-2,1)	
> 9	1			1		
Current monthly personal income in minimum wages ($n = 248$)			0,496*			0,741**
Third tertile (higher)	1			1		
Second tertile	0,96	(0,6-1,4)		0,91	(0,5-1,4)	
First tertile (lower)	1,11	(0,7-1,6)		1,07	(0,7-1,6)	
Body mass index (Kg/m^2) ($n = 285$)			0,001			0,001
$\leq 24,9$	1			1		
25–29,9	1,55	(1,0-2,3)		1,62	(1,0-2,4)	
≥ 30	1,97	(1,2-2,9)		2,07	(1, 3 - 3,1)	
Type of servicee in the last 12 months ($n = 269$)			0,515*			0,997**
Public healthcare system	0,86	(0,5-1,3)		1,01	(0,6-1,6)	
Supplementary healthcare system	0,97	(0,6-1,4)		0,90	(0,5-1,4)	
Fee-for-service care	1			1		
Total number of consultations with a rheumatologist in the last 12 months ($n = 281$)			0,074			0,223**
0–1	0,75	(0,4-1,2)		0,79	(0,4-1,3)	
2–3	1			1		
≥ 4	0,72	(0,5-1,0)		0,79	(0,5-1,1)	
Disease time in months ($n = 235$)			0,134			0,115**
0–24	1			1		
> 24	1,57	(0,8-2,8)		1,76	(0,8-3,5)	
Use of csDMARD ($n = 296$)			0,994*			0,744**
Yes	1			1		
No	0,99	(0,7-1,3)		1,08	(0,6-1,7)	
Use of TNFi (ADA + ETA+IFX) ($n = 288$)			0,588*			0,217**
Yes	0,91	(0,6-1,2)		0,75	(0,4-1,1)	
No	1			1		
HAQ ($n = 165$)			0,227*			0,867**
0–1 (mild)	1			1		
1,1–2 (moderate)	0,68	(0,4-1,1)		0,78	(0,6-1,1)	
2,1–3 (severe)	0,76	(0,4-1,2)		0,82	(0,6-1,3)	

Table 3 Crude and adjusted regression analysis of diagnostic time up to 12 months and independent variables in patients with rheumatoid arthritis in Blumenau, Santa Catarina, Brazil, 2014 (Continued)

Variables	Crude analysis			Adjusted analysis		
	(RPc)	CI 95%	p	(PRa)	CI 95%	p
Presence of radiological changes (erosions) in hands (n = 237)			0,668*			0,877**
No	1			1		
Yes	1,08	(0,7-1,5)		1,03	(0,6-1,6)	
Current professional situation (237)			0,125			0,088**
Working	1			1		
Health insurance	1,11	(0,6-1,8)		1,34	(0,8 – 2,1)	
Disability retirement	0,99	(0,6-1,4)		0,85	(0,5 – 1,3)	
Retirement for time of service	0,67	(0,4-1,1)		0,68	(0,4 – 1,1)	

csDMARD conventional synthetic disease-modifying antirheumatic drugs, TNFi tumor necrosis factor inhibitors, ADA adalimumab, ETA etanercept, IFX infliximab, HAQ health assessment questionnaire, PRc crude prevalence ratio; PRa: adjusted prevalence ratio; CI 95%: confidence interval of 95%
* Value of p > 0,20 excluded from the adjusted analysis. ** Value of p > 0,05 excluded of final model

As for the time of disease, an average of 126 months was found, higher than that found in another Brazilian study that was 92 months [34]. There was no statistical association between diagnosis time and disease time, but patients with a recent disease had an earlier diagnosis, whereas patients with a longer disease period (> 2 years) had a later diagnosis, as observed in international studies [22, 35].

The symptoms of RA can be initially attenuated with symptomatic drugs, however, the specific treatment for the disease is done with cs DMARD and, when they do not achieve adequate control of disease activity, TNFi drugs, which are bDMARD medications [36, 37]. In this study, there was no significant association in the use of cs DMARD and / or TNFi and time to diagnosis. Despite this, it was possible to observe that patients diagnosed up to 3 months would have less need to use cs DMARD when compared to those diagnosed up to 12 months. This finding was also found in the Leiden cohort (Netherlands), stating that there was a higher remission rate without the use of cs DMARD in patients evaluated within 3 months [5]. Regarding the use of TNFi, in earlier diagnosis, there would be less need to use, as found in an Italian study [22].

In the present study, patients had an average of 3.4 consultations in the last year with a rheumatologist, similar to the national data [16, 38]. No statistical association was found regarding the number of consultations with rheumatologists in the last year and the diagnostic interval. However, it was observed that when the diagnosis was made within 3 months, patients consumed fewer visits in the last year compared to those diagnosed within 12 months. This is probably due to better control of the disease when diagnosed earlier, requiring fewer consultations during the year.

It was seen that as the time to diagnosis increased, the prevalence of patients with an intermediate or worse HAQ also increased, although there was no association with the dependent variable. A study conducted between 2007 and 2009 with 1795 patients also showed that individuals diagnosed earlier were able to maintain lower values of HAQ in their follow-up [22]. Non-association could be attributed to a smaller sample of patients when compared to the other variables.

The presence of radiological alterations in hands was observed in the majority of the patients, a result that may have occurred because most of the patients in the sample had more disease time and therefore the availability of resources was more precarious than the ones we have currently, and could favor greater joint damage. In addition, it was initially observed that the later the diagnosis, the greater the prevalence of erosions in the patients hands, as evidenced in a work performed with patients in the state of São Paulo [39].

The results showed a trend that the later the diagnosis, the lower the prevalence of patients being able to retire due to length of service. Brazilian literature confirms this information when it cites that the delay in diagnosis increases the individual's incapacity to work [9]. Regarding the type of care, most of the patients in the sample used the SUS in the last year. In spite of this, there was a tendency of a higher prevalence of the diagnosis of very early RA in the private service when compared to SUS of the order of 13%. As justification, it is assumed that individuals diagnosed earlier would have a higher economic level to obtain faster service.

Some limitations should be considered in this research. The transversal design of the study makes it impossible to determine cause and effect between the exploratory variables and the outcome. Based on the obtained results, the possibility of characteristic reverse causality in cross-sectional studies is highlighted. Other factors to take into account concern the possibility of memory bias in collecting some information attenuated by the common feature of RA being a chronic injury. The agreement between the answers of the first and the second questionnaire including the dependent variable was 82% (unpublished data).

Conclusion

Therefore, this research reinforces the need to know the factors that may delay the earlier diagnosis of RA; and thus decrease the chances of the best results for the patient. It was evidenced that the socioeconomic factor, lower education, was associated with a later initial diagnosis. As a result of the longer diagnosis time there was a progressive increase in the prevalence of obesity among patients. We suggest that more studies be carried out regarding this theme in order to know the local realities, in order to speed up the access of care of the individuals affected by the disease, reinforcing the importance of the early diagnosis.

Abbreviatons

bDMARD: Biological disease-modifying antirheumatic drugs; BMI: body mass index; csDMARD: Conventional synthetic disease-modifying antirheumatic drugs; FURB: Blumenau Regional University Foundation; HAQ: Health Assessment Questionnaire; LERA: Late Early Rheumatoid Arthritis; MS: Ministry of Health; PR: Prevalence ratios; RA: Rheumatoid arthritis (RA); SD: Standard deviation; SUS: Unified Health System; TNFi: Tumor necrosis factor inhibitors; USP: University of São Paulo; VERA: Very Early Rheumatoid Arthritis; WHO: World Health Organization

Authors' contributions

RKSG contributed to elaboration, literature review, statistical analysis and article writing. ACL e LSL contributed to writing and literature review. All approved final version for submission in journal.

Competing interests

The authors declare that they have no competing interests.

Author details

[1]Specialty Center of the City of Blumenau, Blumenau, Santa Catarina State (SC), Brazil. [2]Specialty Center of the City of Brusque, Brusque, SC, Brazil. [3]School of Medicine, Regional University of Blumenau (Universidade Regional de Blumenau – FURB), Blumenau, Brazil. [4]Centro de Referência Policlínica Lindolf Bell, Rua: Dois de Setembro, 1234 - Itoupava Norte, 3° andar, sala 1. CEP, Blumenau, SC 89052-003, Brazil.

References

1. American College of Rheumatology Subcommitte on Rheumatoid Arthritis Guidelines. Guidelines for the management of rheumatoid arthritis. Arthritis Rheumatology. 2002;46:328–46.
2. Da Mota Licia Maria Henrique, Laurindo Ieda Maria Magalhães e Dos Santos Neto Leopoldo Luiz. Artrite reumatoide inicial: conceitos. Rev Assoc Med Bras 2010; 56(2):227–229.
3. Da Henrique MLM, Alfonso CB, Viegas BC, Alves PI, Stange R-FL, Barros BM, et al. Guidelines for the diagnosis of rheumatoid arthritis. Rev Bras Reumatol. 2013;53(2):141–57.
4. Cheung PP, Dougados M, Andre V, Balandraud N, Chales G, Chary-Valckenaere I, et al. Improving agreement in assessment of synovitis in rheumatoid arthritis. Joint Bone Spine. 2013;80(2):155–9.
5. der Linden Michael V, Saskia le C, Karim R, der Woude Diane V, Rachel K, Tom H, der Helm-van Mil Annette V. Long-term impact of delay in assessment of patients with early arthritis. Arthritis Rheumatology. 2010; 62(12):3537–46.
6. Nell VP, Machold KP, Eberl G, Stamm TA, Uffmann M, Smolen JS. Benefit of very early referral and very early therapy with disease-modifying antirheumatic drugs in patients with early rheumatoid arthritis. Oxford J. 2004;43:906–14.
7. Hussain W, Noorwali A, Janoudi N, Baamer M, Kebbi L, Mansafi H, et al. From symptoms to diagnosis: an observational study of the journey of rheumatoid arthritis patients in Saudi Arabia. Oman Med J. 2016;31(1):29–34.
8. Kiely P, Williams R, Walsh D, Young A. Contemporary patterns of care and disease activity outcome in early rheumatoid arthritis: the ERAN cohort. Rheumatology. 2009;48:57–60.
9. Melo V, Aguiar F, Baleroni T, Novaes G. Análise temporal entre início dos sintomas, avaliação reumatológica e tratamento com drogas modificadoras de doença em pacientes com artrite reumatoide. Ver Fac Ciênc Méd Sorocaba. 2008;10(2):12–5.
10. Combe B, Landewe R, Lukas C, Bolosiu HD, Breedveld F, Dougados M, et al. EULAR recommendations for the management of early arthritis: report of a task force of the European Standing Committee for International Clinical Studies Including Therapeutics (ESCISIT). Ann Rheum Dis. 2007;66(1):34–5.
11. Feldman DE, Bernatsky S, Haggerty J, Leffondré K, Tousignant P, Leffondré K, et al. Delay in consultation with specialists for persons with suspected new-onset rheumatoid arthritis: a population based study. Arthritis Rheum. 2007;57:1419–25.
12. Rodríguez-Polanco E, Al Snih S, Kuo YF, Millán A, Rodríguez MA Lag time between onset of symptoms and diagnosis in Venezuelan patients with rheumatoid arthritis. Rheumatol Int 2011; 31(5):657–65.
13. Da Mota LM, Cruz BA, Brenol CV, Pereira IA, Fronza LS, Bertolo MB, et al. Consensus of the Brazilian Society of Rheumatology for diagnosis and early assessment of rheumatoid arthritis. Rev Bras Reumatol. 2011;51(3):199–219.
14. James F, Patricia S, Halsted KGH. Measurement of patient outcome in arthritis. Arthritis Rheum. 1980;23:137–45.
15. Ministério da Saúde. Portaria SCTIE no 66, de 6 de novembro de 2006. Protocolo Clínico e Diretrizes Terapêuticas – artrite reumatoide. Diário Oficial da União 2006.
16. Bagatini BF, Raquel BC, Estima MAC, Nair LS, Rocha FM. Estudo de custo-análise do tratamento da artrite reumatoide grave em um município do Sul do Brasil. Cad Saúde Pública. 2013;29(1):81–91.
17. Da Mota Licia M, Ieda L, Leopoldo N. Características demográficas e clínicas de uma coorte de pacientes de artrite reumatoide inicial. Rev Bras Reumatol. 2010;50(3):235–48.
18. David Juliano M, Mattei Rodrigo A, Mauad Juliana L, Almeida Lauren G, Nogueira Marcio A, Poliana M, et al. Estudo clínico e laboratorial de pacientes com artrite reumatoide diagnosticados em serviço de reumatologia em Cascavel, PR, Brasil. Rev Bras Reumatol. 2013;53(1):57–65.
19. Cunha BM, de Oliveira SB, dos Santos-Neto LL. Coorte Sarar: atividade de doença, capacidade funcional e dano radiológico em pacientes com artrite reumatoide submetidos à artroplastia total de quadril e joelho. Rev Bras Reumatol. 2015;55(5):420–6.
20. Karin R, Rebecca S, Kanta K, Andrew F, Jacqueline D, Hans B, et al. Delays in assessment of patients with rheumatoid arthritis: variations across Europe. Ann Rheum Dis. 2011;70:1822–5.
21. Ruiz O, Salazar JC, Londoño PJ, Saiibi DL, Molina JF, Santos P, et al. Cambio en la capacidad funcional, calidad de vida y actividad de la enfermedad, en un grupo de pacientes colombianos con artritis reumatoide refractaria al tratamiento convencional, que recibieron terapia con infliximab como medicamento de rescate. Revista Med. 2009;17(1):40–9.
22. Elisa G, Fausto S, Laura BS, Alessandro C, Francesca B-P, Roberto C, et al. Very early rheumatoid arthtitis as a predictor of remission: a multicentre real life prospective stydy. Ann Rheum Dis. 2013;72:858–62.
23. Jessica N, Elisabeth B, Floris G, Cornelia A, Tom H, Marcel P, et al. Improved early identification of arthritis: evaluating the efficacy of early Arrthritis recognition clinics. Ann Rheum Dis. 2013;72:1295–301.
24. Atukoorala I, Wljewickrama P, Gunawardena MPH, Atukorala K, Weerathunga D, Dharmasena D. The community prevalence of early rheumatoid arthritis and health seeking behavior of affected individuals. Int J Epidemiol. 2015;44(1): 2016–207.
25. Palleiro D. Diagnostic delay in rheumatoid arthritis. J Clin Rheumatol. 2006;12:41.
26. Palm O, Purinszky E. Women with early rheumatoid arthritis are referred later than men. Ann Rheum Dis. 2005;64:1227–8.

27. De Cock D, Meyfroidt S, Joly J, Van Der Elst K, Westhovens R, Verschueren P. A detailed analysis of treatment delay from the onset of symptons in early rheumatoid arthritis patients. Scand J Rheumatol 2014;43:1–8.

28. Kumar K, Daley DM, Carruthers D, Situnayake C, Gordon K, Grindulis CD, et al. Delay in presentation to primary care physicians is the main reason why patients with rheumatoid arthritis are seen later by rheumatologists. Rheumatology. 2007;46:1438–40.

29. Feldman Debbie E, Sasha B, Jeannie H, Karen L, Pierre T, Yves R, et al. Delay in consultation with specialists for persons with suspected new-onset rheumatoid arthritis: a population-based study. Arthritis Care & Research. 2007;57(8):1419–25.

30. Cheryl B, Juan X, Pope Janet E, Gilles B, Carol H, Boulos H, et al. Factors associated with time to diagnosis in early rheumatoid arthritis. Rheumatol Int. 2014;34:85–92.

31. Junior RSD, Ferraz AL, Oesterreich AS, Schmitz WO, Shinzato MM. Caracterização de pacientes com artrite reumatoide quanto a fatores de risco para doenças vasculares cardíacas no Mato Grosso do Sul. Rev Bras Reumatol. 2015;55(6):493–500.

32. Rachel Z, Marcia D, Thelma S. Perfil nutricional na artrite reumatoide. Rev Bras Reumatol. 2013;54(1):68–72.

33. Michael G, Joshua B. The obesity epidemic and consequences for rheumatoid arthritis. Curr Rheumatol Rep. 2016;18(1):6.

34. Almeida Maria do Socorro TM, Almeida João Vicente M, Bertolo Manuel B. Características demográficas e clínicas de pacientes com artrite reumatoide no Piauí, Brasil – avaliação de 98 pacientes. Rev Bras Reumatol. 2014;54(5):360–5.

35. Jennifer A, George W, Verhoeven Arco C, Felson David T. Factors predicting response to treatment in rheumatoid arthritis: the importance of disease duration. Arthritis & Rheumatism. 2000;43:22–9.

36. Jasvinder S, Kenneth S, Louis B Jr, Elie A, Raveendhara B, Matthew S, et al. 2015 American College of Rheumatology Guideline for the treatment of rheumatoid arthritis. Arthritis Care Res. 2015;67(10):1335–486.

37. Monika S, John W, David S, Angela Z, Pamela R, Robert L, et al. Economic aspects of treatment options in rheumatoid arthritis: a systematic literature review informing the EULAR recommendations for the management of rheumatoid arthritis. Ann Rheum Dis. 2010;69:996-–1004.

38. Vaz Andrey E, Faria Wilmar A Jr, Lazarski Cristina FS, Do Carmo Humberto Franco, Da Rocha Hermínio Maurício. Perfil epidemiológico e clínico de pacientes portadores de artrite reumatóide em um hospital escola de medicina em Goiânia, Goiás, Brasil. Medicina (Ribeirão Preto) 2013;46(2):141–153.

39. Louzada-Junior P, Souza BDB, Toledo RA, Ciconelli RM. Análise descritiva das características demográficas e clínicas de pacientes com artrite reumatoide no estado de São Paulo, Brasil. Rev Bras Reumatol. 2007;47(2):84–90.

Permissions

The contributors of this book come from diverse backgrounds, making this book a truly international effort. This book will bring forth new frontiers with its revolutionizing research information and detailed analysis of the nascent developments around the world.

We would like to thank all the contributing authors for lending their expertise to make the book truly unique. They have played a crucial role in the development of this book. Without their invaluable contributions this book wouldn't have been possible. They have made vital efforts to compile up to date information on the varied aspects of this subject to make this book a valuable addition to the collection of many professionals and students.

This book was conceptualized with the vision of imparting up-to-date information and advanced data in this field. To ensure the same, a matchless editorial board was set up. Every individual on the board went through rigorous rounds of assessment to prove their worth. After which they invested a large part of their time researching and compiling the most relevant data for our readers.

The editorial board has been involved in producing this book since its inception. They have spent rigorous hours researching and exploring the diverse topics which have resulted in the successful publishing of this book. They have passed on their knowledge of decades through this book. To expedite this challenging task, the publisher supported the team at every step. A small team of assistant editors was also appointed to further simplify the editing procedure and attain best results for the readers.

Apart from the editorial board, the designing team has also invested a significant amount of their time in understanding the subject and creating the most relevant covers. They scrutinized every image to scout for the most suitable representation of the subject and create an appropriate cover for the book.

The publishing team has been an ardent support to the editorial, designing and production team. Their endless efforts to recruit the best for this project, has resulted in the accomplishment of this book. They are a veteran in the field of academics and their pool of knowledge is as vast as their experience in printing. Their expertise and guidance has proved useful at every step. Their uncompromising quality standards have made this book an exceptional effort. Their encouragement from time to time has been an inspiration for everyone.

The publisher and the editorial board hope that this book will prove to be a valuable piece of knowledge for researchers, students, practitioners and scholars across the globe.

List of Contributors

Penélope Esther Palominos, Ricardo Machado Xavier and Rafael Mendonça da Silva Chakr
Universidade Federal do Rio Grande do Sul (UFRGS), Programa de Pós Graduação em Ciências Médicas (PPGCM), Rua Ramiro Barcelos 2400, segundo andar, Porto Alegre 90035-903, Brazil
Department of Rheumatology, Hospital de Clinicas de Porto Alegre, Rua Ramiro Barcelos 2350, sexto andar, Porto Alegre 90035-903, Brazil

Andrese Aline Gasparin, Nicole Pamplona Bueno de Andrade and Fernanda Igansi
Universidade Federal do Rio Grande do Sul (UFRGS), Programa de Pós Graduação em Ciências Médicas (PPGCM), Rua Ramiro Barcelos 2400, segundo andar, Porto Alegre 90035-903, Brazil

Laure Gossec
Sorbonne Universités, UPMC Univ Paris 06, Institut Pierre Louis d'Epidémiologie et de Santé Publique, GRC-UPMC 08 (EEMOIS); Department of Rheumatology, Pitié Salpêtrière Hospital, AP-HP, 47-83 Boulevard de l'Hôpital, 75013 Paris, France

Ana Paula Monteiro Gomides, Licia Maria Henrique da Mota and Leopoldo Luiz Santos-Neto
Programa de Pós-Graduação em Ciências Médicas, Faculdade de Medicina, Universidade de Brasília, UnB, CEP, Brasília, DF 70910-900, Brazil

Josierton Cruz Bezerra
National Social Security Institute, Brasília, Brazil

Eduardo José do Rosário e Souza
Santa Casa de Misericórdia Hospital of Belo Horizonte, Belo Horizonte, Minas Gerais, Brazil

Rafaela Maria de Paula Costa and Letícia Nunes Carreras Del Castillo Mathias
Medical Sciences, State University of Rio de Janeiro, Rio de Janeiro, Brazil
Orthopedics Service, Pedro Ernesto University Hospital, State University of Rio de Janeiro, Rio de Janeiro, RJ, Brazil

Themis Moura Cardinot
Medical Sciences, Rural Federal University of Rio de Janeiro, Seropédica, RJ, Brazil

Gustavo Leporace
Biomedical Engineering, Federal University of Rio de Janeiro, Rio de Janeiro, RJ, Brazil

Liszt Palmeira de Oliveira
State University of Rio de Janeiro, Rio de Janeiro, RJ, Brazil
Orthopedics Service, Pedro Ernesto University Hospital, State University of Rio de Janeiro, Rio de Janeiro, RJ, Brazil

Francisco Vileimar Andrade de Azevedo, Fabrício Oliveira Lima and Carlos Ewerton Maia Rodrigues
Post-Graduate Program in Medical Sciences, University of Fortaleza (UNIFOR), Fonseca Lobo 560 apto. 1202, Aldeota, Fortaleza, Ceará CEP 60175020, Brazil

Jozélio Freire de Carvalho
Division of Rheumatology, Federal University of Bahia, Salvador, Bahia, Brazil

Andrea Rocha de Saboia Mont'Alverne
Division of Rheumatology, University of Fortaleza (UNIFOR), Fortaleza, Brazil

Juleimar Soares Coelho de Amorim
Ciências da Reabilitação, Instituto Federal de Educação, Ciência e Tecnologia do Rio de Janeiro – IFRJ, Rio de Janeiro, RJ, Brasil
Colina, Manhuaçu, Brazil

Renata Cristine Leite and Renata Brizola
Centro Universitário Filadélfia – UNIFIL, Londrina, PR, Brasil

Cristhiane Yumi Yonamine
Saúde Coletiva, Centro Universitário Filadélfia – UNIFIL, Londrina, PR, Brasil

Vanessa Hax, Ana Laura Didonet Moro, Ricardo Machado Xavier and Odirlei Andre Monticielo
Division of Rheumatology, Hospital de Clínicas de Porto Alegre, Universidade Federal do Rio Grande do Sul, 2350 Ramiro Barcelos St, Room 645, Porto Alegre, RS 90035-903, Brazil

Rafaella Romeiro Piovesan
Medical School Student, Universidade Federal do Rio Grande do Sul, Porto Alegre, Brazil

Luciano Zubaran Goldani
Division of Infectious Diseases, Hospital de Clínicas de Porto Alegre, Universidade Federal do Rio Grande do Sul, Porto Alegre, Brazil

Thiago Costa Pamplona da Silva, Marilda Guimarães Silva and Samuel Katsuyuki Shinjo
Division of Rheumatology, Faculdade de Medicina FMUSP, Universidade de Sao Paulo, Av. Dr. Arnaldo, 455, 3° andar, sala 3150 - Cerqueira César, Sao Paulo CEP: 01246-903, Brazil

Josielli Comachio, Mauricio Oliveira Magalhães, Ana Paula de Moura Campos Carvalho e Silva and Amélia Pasqual Marques
Department of Speech, Physical and Occupational Therapy, School of Medicine, University of Sao Paulo, Cipotânea, n 51, Cidade Universitária, Sao Paulo, Brazil

Graziela Sferra da Silva, Mariana de Almeida Lourenço and Marcos Renato de Assis
Faculty of Medicine of Marilia (Famema), Marília, SP, Brazil

Darcisio Hortelan Antonio and Claudia Saad Magalhaes
Pediatrics Department, Botucatu Medical School, Graduate Program in Public Health of UNESP, Sao Paulo State University UNESP, Avenida Prof. Mario Rubens Guimarães Montenegro SN, Campus da Unesp, Rubião Junior, CEP, Botucatu, SP 18618-687, Brazil

Norma Celia González-Huerta, Verónica Marusa Borgonio-Cuadra and Antonio Miranda-Duarte
Departments of Genetics, Instituto Nacional de Rehabilitación "Luis Guillermo Ibarra Ibarra", Calzada México-Xochimilco No. 289, Arenal Guadalupe, Tlalpan, CP 14389 México City, Mexico

Eugenio Morales-Hernández
Departments of Radiology, Instituto Nacional de Rehabilitación "Luis Guillermo Ibarra Ibarra", Calzada México-Xochimilco No. 289, Arenal Guadalupe, Tlalpan, CP 14389 México City, Mexico

Carolina Duarte-Salazar
Departments of Rheumatology, Instituto Nacional de Rehabilitación "Luis Guillermo Ibarra Ibarra", Calzada México-Xochimilco No. 289, Arenal Guadalupe, Tlalpan, CP 14389 México City, Mexico

Mariana de Almeida Lourenço, Flávia Vilas Boas Ortiz Carli and Marcos Renato de Assis
Marília School of Medicine, R. Pedro Martins, 209. Marília/SP – Brazil, Marília, São Paulo CEP 17519-430, Brazil

Rafael Kmiliauskis Santos Gomes
Specialty Center of the City of Blumenau, Blumenau, Santa Catarina State (SC), Brazil
Specialty Center of the City of Brusque, Brusque, SC, Brazil.
Centro de Referência Policlínica Lindolf Bell, Rua: Dois de Setembro, 1234 – Itoupava Norte, 3° andar, sala 1, Blumenau, SC CEP: 89052-003, Brazil

Luana Cristina Schreiner, Mateus Oliveira Vieira and Patrícia Helena Machado
School of Medicine, Regional University of Blumenau (Universidade Regional de Blumenau – FURB), Blumenau, Brazil

Moacyr Roberto Cuce Nobre
Clinical Epidemiology Unit, Heart Institute, University Hospital, School of Medicine, University of São Paulo (Universidade de São Paulo – USP), São Paulo, SP, Brazil

Diego Sales de Oliveira, Rafael Giovani Misse and Samuel Katsuyuki Shinjo
Division of Rheumatology, Faculdade de Medicina FMUSP, Universidade de Sao Paulo, Av. Dr. Arnaldo, 455, 3° andar, sala 3150 - Cerqueira César, Sao Paulo 01246-903, Brazil

Fernanda Rodrigues Lima
Division of Rheumatology, Hospital das Clinicas HCFMUSP, Faculdade de Medicina, Universidade de Sao Paulo, Sao Paulo, Brazil

Pedro S. Franco, Renato R. Azevedo, Fernando G. Ceccon and Felipe P. Carpes
Applied Neuromechanics Research Group, Federal University of Pampa,Uruguaiana, BR 472 km 592, Po box 118, Uruguaiana, RS ZIP 97500-970, Brazil
Graduated Program in Physical Education, Federal University of Santa Maria, Santa Maria, Brazil

Cristiane F. Moro and Mariane M. Figueiredo
Applied Neuromechanics Research Group, Federal University of Pampa,Uruguaiana, BR 472 km 592, Po box 118, Uruguaiana, RS ZIP 97500-970, Brazil

Liete Zwir, Melissa Fraga, Monique Sanches, Carmen Hoyuela, Claudio Len and Maria Teresa Terreri
Universidade Federal de São Paulo (UNIFESP), Rua Guilherme Moura, São Paulo 95, Brazil

Andrei Pereira Pernambuco
Departamento de Morfologia, Instituto de Ciências Biológicas da Universidade Federal de Minas Gerais (UFMG), Avenida Presidente Antônio Carlos, 6627 - Pampulha, Belo Horizonte, MG CEP 31270-901, Brazil
Centro Universitário de Formiga, MG. Avenida Doutor Arnaldo de Senna, 328. Água, Vermelha, Formiga, MG CEP 35570-000, Brazil
Universidade de Itaúna, MG. Rodovia MG, 431 Km 45, s/n - Campus Verde, Itaúna, MG CEP 35680-142, Brazil

Lucina de Souza Cota Carvalho
Departamento de Morfologia, Instituto de Ciências Biológicas da Universidade Federal de Minas Gerais (UFMG), Avenida Presidente Antônio Carlos, 6627 - Pampulha, Belo Horizonte, MG CEP 31270-901, Brazil.
Hospital Mater Dei, Avenida do Contorno, 9000 - Barro Preto, Belo Horizonte, MG CEP 30110-064, Brazil

Luana Pereira Leite Schetino
Departamento de Morfologia, Instituto de Ciências Biológicas da Universidade Federal de Minas Gerais (UFMG), Avenida Presidente Antônio Carlos, 6627 - Pampulha, Belo Horizonte, MG CEP 31270-901, Brazil.
Universidade Federal do Vale do Jequitinhonha e Mucuri - Campus I. Rua da Glória, n° 187 – Centro, Diamantina, MG CEP 39100-000, Brazil

Débora d' Ávila Reis
Departamento de Morfologia, Instituto de Ciências Biológicas da Universidade Federal de Minas Gerais (UFMG), Avenida Presidente Antônio Carlos, 6627 - Pampulha, Belo Horizonte, MG CEP 31270-901, Brazil

Janaíne Cunha Polese
Pós-Graduação em Ciências da Reabilitação da Universidade Federal de Minas Gerais, Avenida Presidente Antônio Carlos, 6627 - Pampulha, Belo Horizonte, MG CEP 31270-901, Brazil

Renato de Souza Viana
Santa Casa de Caridade de Formiga, MG. Rua Doutor Teixeira Soares, 335 - Centro, Formiga, MG CEP 35570-000, Brazil

Pablo Arturo Olivo Pallo, Fernando Henrique Carlos de Souza, Renata Miossi and Samuel Katsuyuki Shinjo
Division of Rheumatology, Faculdade de Medicina FMUSP, Universidade de Sao Paulo, Av. Dr. Arnaldo, 455, 3 andar, sala 3150 - Cerqueira César, CEP 01246-903 Sao Paulo, Brazil

Elis Carolina de Souza Fatel
Postgraduate Program, Health Sciences Center, State University of Londrina, Londrina, Paraná, Brazil
Department of Nutrition, University of Fronteira Sul, Rodovia PR 182 Km 466, CEP 85770-000, Realeza, Paraná Postal Code 253, Brazil

Flávia Troncon Rosa
Postgraduate Program, Experimental Pathology, State University of Londrina, Londrina, Paraná, Brazil

Andréa Name Colado Simão
Department of Pathology, Clinical Analysis and Toxicology, University Londrina, Londrina, Paraná, Brazil

Isaias Dichi
Department of Internal Medicine, University of Londrina, Londrina, Paraná, Brazil

Fernando Henrique Carlos de Souza, Renata Miossi and Júlio Cesar Bertacini de Moraes
Division of Rheumatology, Hospital das Clinicas IICFMUSP, Faculdade de Medicina, Universidade de Sao Paulo, Sao Paulo, Brazil

Eloisa Bonfá and Samuel Katsuyuki Shinjo
Division of Rheumatology, Faculdade de Medicina FMUSP, Universidade de Sao Paulo, Sao Paulo, Brazil

Alexandro Andrade, Sofia Mendes Sieczkowska and Guilherme Torres Vilarino
Health and Sports Science Center, CEFID / Santa Catarina State University – UDESC, Florianópolis, SC, Brazil
Laboratory of Sports and Exercise Psychology - LAPE, Florianópolis, SC, Brazil. 3Regional University of Blumenau - FURB, Blumenau, SC, Brazil

Ricardo de Azevedo Klumb Steffens
Health and Sports Science Center, CEFID / Santa Catarina State University – UDESC, Florianópolis, SC, Brazil

Laboratory of Sports and Exercise Psychology - LAPE, Florianópolis, SC, Brazil
Regional University of Blumenau - FURB, Blumenau, SC, Brazil

Leonardo Alexandre Peyré Tartaruga
Human Movement Sciences and Pneumological Sciences, UFRGS- Federal University of Rio Grande do Sul, Porto Alegre, RS, Brazil
Research Laboratory of Exercise – LAPEX, Porto Alegre, RS, Brazil

Clovis A. Silva
Pediatric Rheumatology Unit, Hospital das Clinicas HCFMUSP, Faculdade de Medicina, Universidade de Sao Paulo, Rua Joel Jorge de Melo, 600 apto 121, Vila Mariana, São Paulo, SP 04128-081, Brazil
Division of Rheumatology, Hospital das Clinicas HCFMUSP, Faculdade de Medicina, Universidade de Sao Paulo, São Paulo, SP, Brazil

Kátia T. Kozu, Adriana M. Sallum and Lucia M. Campos
Pediatric Rheumatology Unit, Hospital das Clinicas HCFMUSP, Faculdade de Medicina, Universidade de Sao Paulo, Rua Joel Jorge de Melo, 600 apto 121, Vila Mariana, São Paulo, SP 04128-081, Brazil

Nadia E. Aikawa, Rosa M. R. Pereira and Eduardo Borba
Division of Rheumatology, Hospital das Clinicas HCFMUSP, Faculdade de Medicina, Universidade de Sao Paulo, São Paulo, SP, Brazil

Cynthia Savioli
Division of Dentistry, Hospital das Clinicas HCF-MUSP, Faculdade de Medicina, Universidade de Sao Paulo, São Paulo, SP, Brazil

Rafael Mendonça da Silva Chakr and Ricardo Machado Xavier
Serviço de Reumatologia, Hospital de Clínicas de Porto Alegre, Ramiro Barcelos Street 2350, Porto Alegre Zip code 90035903, Brazil
Programa de Pós Graduação em Ciências Médicas, Universidade Federal do Rio Grande do Sul (UFRGS), Ramiro Barcelos 2400, Porto Alegre Zip code 90035903, Brazil
Faculdade de Medicina, Departamento de Medicina Interna, Universidade Federal do Rio Grande do Sul (UFRGS), Ramiro Barcelos 2400, Porto Alegre Zip code 90035903, Brazil

Penélope Esther Palominos
Serviço de Reumatologia, Hospital de Clínicas de Porto Alegre, Ramiro Barcelos Street 2350, Porto Alegre Zip code 90035903, Brazil
Programa de Pós Graduação em Ciências Médicas, Universidade Federal do Rio Grande do Sul (UFRGS), Ramiro Barcelos 2400, Porto Alegre Zip code 90035903, Brazil

Laure Gossec, Sarah Kreis
Institut Pierre Louis d'Epidémiologie et de Santé Publique. Pitié-Salpetrière Hospital, AP-HP, Rheumatology Department, Sorbonne Universités, UPMC Univ Paris 6, GRC-08, 83 Boulevard de l'Hôpital, 75013 Paris, France

Charles Lubianca Kohem
Serviço de Reumatologia, Hospital de Clínicas de Porto Alegre, Ramiro Barcelos Street 2350, Porto Alegre Zip code 90035903, Brazil
Faculdade de Medicina, Departamento de Medicina Interna, Universidade Federal do Rio Grande do Sul (UFRGS), Ramiro Barcelos 2400, Porto Alegre Zip code 90035903, Brazil

Ana Laura Didonet Moro
Serviço de Reumatologia, Hospital de Clínicas de Porto Alegre, Ramiro Barcelos Street 2350, Porto Alegre Zip code 90035903, Brazil

César Luis Hinckel
Faculdade de Medicina, Departamento de Medicina Interna, Universidade Federal do Rio Grande do Sul (UFRGS), Ramiro Barcelos 2400, Porto Alegre Zip code 90035903, Brazil

Willemina Campbell
Patient Research Partner, Group for Research and Assessment of Psoriasis and Psoriatic Arthritis (GRAPPA), University Health Network, Toronto Western Hospital, 399 Street Toronto, Bathurst, ON M5T 2S8, Canada

Maarten de Wit
Department of Medical Humanities, Patient Research Partner, VU University Medical Centre, de Boelenlaan 1089a, 1081 HV Amsterdam, Netherlands

Niti Goel
Patient Research Partner; Advisory Services, Quintiles; Division of Rheumatology, Duke University School of Medicine, Durham, North Carolina 27705, USA

Melek Kechida, Rim Klii, Sonia Hammami and Ines Khochtali
Internal Medicine and Endocrinology Department, Fattouma Bourguiba University Hospital, 1st June Avenue, 5000 Monastir, Tunisia

Sana Salah
Physical Medicine and Rehabilitaion Department, Fattouma Bourguiba University Hospital, Monastir, Tunisia

Rim Kahloun
Ophtalmology Department, Fattouma Bourguiba University Hospital, Monastir, Tunisia

Samuel Katsuyuki Shinjo and Marilda Guimarães Silva
Disciplina de Reumatologia, Faculdade de Medicina FMUSP, Universidade de Sao Paulo, Sao Paulo, Brazil

Adriana Maluf Elias Sallum and Clovis Artur Silva
Instituto da Criança, Hospital das Clinicas HCMFUSP, Faculdade de Medicina, Universidade de Sao Paulo, Sao Paulo, Brazil

Suely Kazue Nagahashi Marie and Sueli Mieko Oba-Shinjo
Laboratório de Biologia Molecular e Celular, Faculdade de Medicina, Universidade de Sao Paulo, Sao Paulo, Brazil

Deborah Hebling Spinoso
Department of Physical Education, São Paulo State University, UNESP, Rio Claro, SP, Brazil
Departamento de Fisioterapia e Terapia Ocupacional, Universidade Estadual Paulista, Avenida Hygino Muzzi Filho, 737, CEP, Marília, SP 17525-000, Brazil

Natane Ceccatto Bellei
Department of Physiotherapy and Occupational Therapy, São Paulo State University, UNESP, Marília, SP, Brazil

Nise Ribeiro Marques
Department of Health Sciences, University of the Sacred Heart, USC, Bauru, SP, Brazil

Marcelo Tavella Navega
Lecturer in Musculoskeletal Physiotherapy Department of Physiotherapy and Occupational Therapy, São Paulo State University, UNESP, Marília, SP, Brazil

Aline Defaveri do Prado
Rheumatology Unit, Nossa Senhora da Conceição Hospital, Porto Alegre, RS, Brazil
Rheumatology Department, Sao Lucas Hospital, Faculty of Medicine of Pontifical Catholic University of Rio Grande do Sul (PUCRS), Av. Ipiranga, 6690/220, Porto Alegre 90610-000, Brazil

Henrique Luiz Staub, Melissa Cláudia Bisi and Inês Guimarães da Silveira
Rheumatology Department, Sao Lucas Hospital, Faculty of Medicine of Pontifical Catholic University of Rio Grande do Sul (PUCRS), Av. Ipiranga, 6690/220, Porto Alegre 90610-000, Brazil

José Alexandre Mendonça
Rheumatology Unit, Pontifical Catholic University of Campinas (PUCCAMP), Campinas, SP, Brazil

Joaquim Polido-Pereira and João Eurico Fonseca
Rheumatology Research Unit, Instituto de Medicina Molecular, Faculdade de Medicina, Universidade de Lisboa, Lisbon, Portugal
Rheumatology Department, Hospital de Santa Maria, Lisbon Academic Medical Centre, Lisbon, Portugal

Izabel M. Buscatti, Katia Kozu, Victor L. S. Marques, Roberta C. Gomes and Adriana M. E. Sallum
Pediatric Rheumatology Unit, Children's Institute, Hospital das Clinicas HCFMUSP, Faculdade de Medicina, Universidade de Sao Paulo, São Paulo, Brazil

Henrique M. Abrão
Universidade de Santo Amaro – UNISA, São Paulo, Brazil

Clovis A. Silva
Pediatric Rheumatology Unit, Children's Institute, Hospital das Clinicas HCFMUSP, Faculdade de Medicina, Universidade de Sao Paulo, SP, Av. Dr. Eneas Carvalho Aguiar, 647 - Cerqueira César, São Paulo, SP 05403-000, Brazil

Hisa Costa Morimoto and Anamaria Jones
Rheumatology Division, Universidade Federal de São Paulo, São Paulo, Brazil

Jamil Natour
Disciplina de Reumatologia, Rua Botucatu, 740, Sao Paulo, SP 04023-090, Brazil

Luiz Samuel Gomes Machado, Ana Cecilia Diniz Oliveira, Patricia Semedo-Kuriki, Alexandre Wagner Silva de Souza and Emilia Inoue Sato
Rheumatology Division, Escola Paulista de Medicina UNIFESP (Universidade Federal de São Paulo), Rua Doutor Diogo de Faria, 561, apt 12, Vila, Clementin São Paulo-SP CEP: 04037-000, Brazil

Rafael Kmiliauskis Santos Gomes
Specialty Center of the City of Blumenau, Blumenau, Santa Catarina State (SC), Brazil

Specialty Center of the City of Brusque, Brusque, SC, Brazil
Centro de Referência Policlínica Lindolf Bell, Rua: Dois de Setembro, 1234 - Itoupava Norte, 3° andar, sala 1. CEP, Blumenau, SC 89052-003, Brazil

Ana Carolina de Linhares and Lucas Selistre Lersch
School of Medicine, Regional University of Blumenau (Universidade Regional de Blumenau – FURB), Blumenau, Brazil

Index

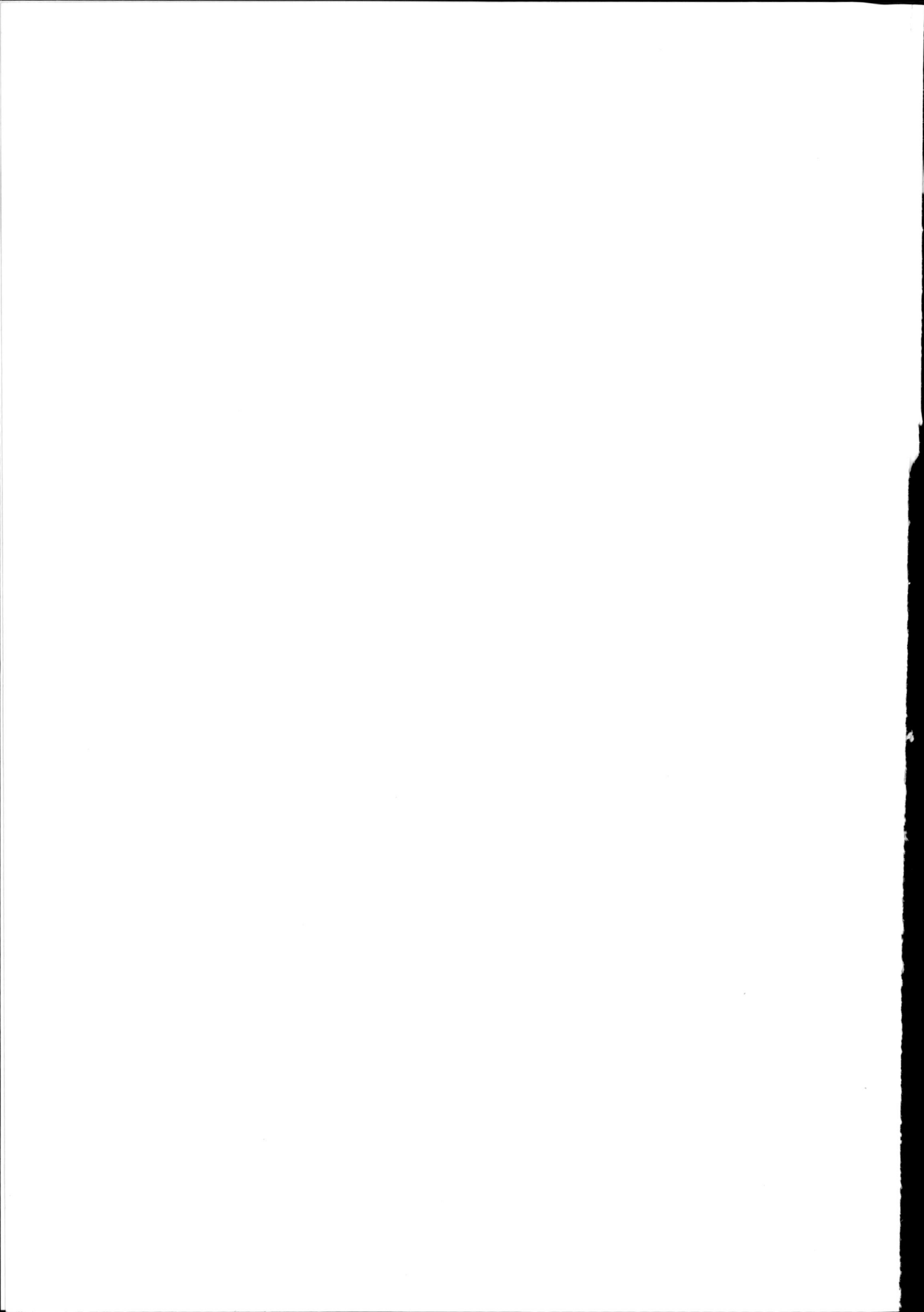